The Physics of Diagnostic Imaging

The Physics of Diagnostic Imaging

David J. Dowsett
Patrick A. Kenny
Mater Hospital Dublin, Ireland
University College Dublin, Ireland

R. Eugene Johnston
University of North Carolina,
Chapel Hill, North Carolina,
United States of America

CHAPMAN & HALL MEDICAL
London · Weinheim · New York · Tokyo · Melbourne · Madras

Published by

Chapman & Hall, an imprint of Thomson Science, 2—6 Boundary Row, London SE1 8HN, UK

Thomson Science, 2—6 Boundary Row, London SE1 8HN, UK

Thomson Science, 115 Fifth Avenue, New York, NY 10003, USA

Thomson Science, Suite 750, 400 Market Street, Philadelphia, PA 19106, USA

Thomson Science, Pappelallee 3, 69469 Weinheim, Germany

First edition 1998

© 1998 Dowsett, Kenny & Johnston

Thomson Science is an imprint of International Thomson Publishing   I(T)P

Printed in Great Britain by T.J. International, Padstow

ISBN   0 412 40170 3

∞

Printed on acid-free text paper, manufactured in accordance with ANSI/NISO Z39.48-1992 (Permanence of Paper).

We wish to dedicate this book to an individual who has had considerable influence on the authors, both personally and professionally.

Dr Bernard (Randy) Brill has been a colleague who has given encouragement, provided stimulating ideas and opened avenues for our professional development. Randy Brill has served as a mentor and friend and in this small way hope we can show our gratitude.

Units of measurement were pondered by the cartful, barrowful and bucketful. Time was a backward rote of names and mishaps...

(Seamus Heaney *"The First Kingdom"*)

Thus the Seer, with vision clear, sees forms appear and disappear in the perpetual round of strange mysterious change...

(Henry Wadsworth Longfellow *"Rain in Summer"*)

Contents

Foreword

1   Basic mathematics for radiology

    1.1   Expressions   1
    1.2   Notation   1
    1.3   Fractions and ratios   4
    1.4   Reciprocal value   5
    1.5   Logarithms   5
    1.6   Proportional quantities   8
    1.7   Graphs   9
    1.8   Calculus   11
    1.9   Volumes and Surfaces   14
    1.10   Trigonometry   16
    1.11   Oscillations and waves   17
    1.12   Basis statistics in radiology   18

2   Basic physics for radiology

    2.1   International system of Units   29
    2.2   Force, mass, momentum   29
    2.3   Work, energy, power   30
    2.4   Density, pressure   32
    2.5   Heat   34
    2.6   Sound   38
    2.7   Waves and oscillations   40
    2.8   Electromagnetic radiation   42
    2.9   Atomic and nuclear structure   46
    2.10   Magnetism   49
    2.11   Electricity   51
    2.12   Electronics   60

3   X-ray production and properties: Fundamentals

    3.1   Introduction   64
    3.2   X-ray tube design   67
    3.3   The x-ray spectrum   75
    3.4   Electrical characteristics   81
    3.5   X-ray tube rating   83

4   X-ray production and properties: Specific machine design

    4.1   The supply generator   90
    4.2   Control circuits   96
    4.3   Exposure control   99

| | 4.4 | X-ray tube design | 101 |
| | 4.5 | Equipment | 103 |

5   Interaction of X and γ-radiation with matter

	5.1	General interactions with matter	107
	5.2	Interactions with the atom	112
	5.3	Subject contrast	122
	5.4	Radiation dose	124

6   Interaction of radiation with matter : Detectors

	6.1	Radiation detection	128
	6.2	Film as a detector	129
	6.3	Gas detectors	129
	6.4	Luminescent detectors	134
	6.5	Practical detector	138
	6.6	Semiconductor detectors	142
	6.7	Efficiency and sensitivity	142

7   Photography and the film image.

	7.1	The photographic principle	149
	7.2	Film sensitometry	154
	7.3	Intensifying screens	161
	7.4	Film processors	168
	7.5	Phosphor imaging plate	169

8   The analog image : Film and video

	8.1	Vision	175
	8.2	Image detector surface	177
	8.3	Image quality factors	182
	8.4	Scatter and grids	190
	8.5	Image quality measurement	197
	8.6	Hardcopy devices	206

9   Special procedures: Low kilovoltage, high kilovoltage imaging

| | 9.1 | Low kilovoltage imaging | 200 |
| | 9.2 | High kilovoltage imaging | 222 |

10   Fluoroscopy

	10.1	Fluoroscopic image	368
	10.2	Performance parameters	232
	10.3	The fluoroscopy system	237
	10.4	Feedback controls	244
	10.5	Specific system designs	247

11 Computers

11.1	Computer architecture	254
11.2	Central processing unit (CPU)	256
11.3	Bulk storage	260
11.4	Data input/output	264
11.5	Software	265
11.6	Networking	267

12 The digital image

12.1	Signal input	274
12.2	The image matrix	276
12.3	Digital image quality	279
12.4	Digital image processing	281
12.5	Picture Archiving and Communications - (PACs)	287

13 Digital fluoroscopy (df) and digital subtraction angiography (dsa)

13.1	Basic components	297
13.2	Digital fluorography	299
13.3	Digital subtraction angiography	304
13.4	Digital subtraction programs	308
13.5	Machine performance	311

14 Linear and computed tomography

14.1	Introduction	314
14.2	Linear tomography	314
14.3	Computed axial tomography (CAT or CT)	317
14.4	Image signals and data handling	327
14.5	CT image reconstruction	329
14.6	Equipment and image quality	334
14.7	Image artifacts	338
14.8	Radiation exposure	340

15 Nuclear medicine : Basic principles

15.1	Nuclear parameters	344
15.2	Decay schemes	347
15.3	Specific activity	354
15.4	Radionuclide production	356
15.5	Laboratory instrumentation	364
15.6	The gamma camera	368
15.7	Camera performance	371
15.8	Collimator properties	377

16   Nuclear medicine : Radiopharmaceuticals and imaging equipment

16.1	Radiopharmaceuticals	383
16.2	Dosimetry	387
16.3	Planar imaging	397
16.4	Tomography: SPECT	399
16.5	Tomography: PET	407
16.6	Comparative studies	411

17   Ultrasound principles

17.1	Ultrasound properties	415
17.2	Interaction with matter	421
17.3	The ultrasound transducer	425
17.4	The ultrasonic field	431

18   Ultrasound imaging

18.1	Ultrasound imaging	436
18.2	Image processing	431
18.3	Transducers	446
18.4	Image artifacts	453
18.5	Blood velocity measurement	454
18.6	Safety	459

19   Magnetic resonance: Principles

19.1	Introduction	466
19.2	The proton in a magnetic field	467
19.3	Relaxation time constants	473
19.4	Pulse sequences	478
19.5	Signal measurement	480

20   Magnetic resonance imaging

20.1	The main magnet	486
20.2	The MRI system	491
20.3	Imaging pulse sequences	500
20.4	Fast imaging techniques	508
20.5	Image quality	515
20.6	Choice of MRI system	519
20.7	Image artifacts	521
20.8	Magnetic spectroscopy MRS	522

21 Radiation protection : Radiobiology and risk estimation

21.1	Radiation interaction with tissue	527
21.2	Biological damage	531
21.3	Natural and man-made radiation	537
21.4	Risk estimates	538

22 Radiation protection: Clinical practice

22.1	Dosimetric quantities	543
22.2	Staff radiation exposure	547
22.3	Patient radiation exposure	554
22.4	Hospital radiation protection	560
22.5	The X-ray room	560

23 Equipment quality control

23.1	Quality assurance program	569
23.2	Quality control equipment	571
23.3	Conventional radiology	576
23.4	Film image	579
23.5	Mammography	586
23.6	Fluoroscopy	591
23.7	Computed tomography	596
23.8	Nuclear medicine	598
23.9	Ultrasound	602
23.10	Magnetic Resonance Imaging	607

24 Appendices

611

Index

623

Foreword

The major problem associated with teaching the physics of diagnostic imaging is its changeability. Over the last twenty years radiology has seen the most dramatic improvements in non-invasive imaging using x-rays, gamma rays, high frequency sound and high frequency radio-waves. Over the last ten years the quality of these images has enabled visualization of early pathological changes both in anatomy and function. The last five years has seen the emphasis change to low radiation dose techniques which demand more efficient imaging methods and during the last two years most of these images have been appearing routinely in digital format. With digital systems a truly filmless environment can exist promising easy and rapid transmission of images, patient information and quality control data across countries, continents and oceans. This complex scenario provides difficulties when trying to understand modern developments, teach students or set examinations.

This book is primarily an introduction to current methods, fundamental principles and applications. The reader is encouraged to explore specialist publications armed with this basic information.

Steve Pizer was an important pivotal figure in the early stages of this book. The authors also wish to thank and acknowledge the help given by the following scientists in reading the various chapters, supplying information and offering advice on content: David Washburn, Brendan Coburn, Guy Lamartine, John Broderick, John Winder, Jørgen Thanning, Peter Wells.

In spite of their expertise, errors may have crept through. For these the authors are entirely responsible.

DJD
PAK
REJ

1997

Basic mathematics for radiology

1.1 Expressions   1.7   Graphs
1.2 Notation   1.8   Calculus
1.3 Fractions and ratios   1.9   Volumes and surfaces
1.4 Reciprocal values   1.10 Trigonometry
1.5 Logarithms   1.11 Oscillations and waves
1.6 Proportional quantities   1.12 Basic statistics in radiology

1.1 EXPRESSIONS

Mathematics plays a very important role in radiology and some knowledge of basic math and formulas is necessary in order to fully appreciate certain applications. As radiology becomes more complex (radionuclide activity, digital imaging, magnetic resonance, axial tomography etc.) quite simple mathematical procedures often explain complex details more effectively than words or diagrams.

Simple formulas can often be employed which reveal hidden difficulties such as accuracy of counting radioactive samples, or radiation dose measurements or x-ray exposure levels which can suggest corrective measures.

This chapter serves only for reference and identifies those areas of radiology where a knowledge of mathematics can reveal greater understanding.

SI Units Basic physical constants have standard SI abbreviations which are used throughout this book; these are given in Table 1.1. The year and gram sometimes have non-standard abbreviations and these are also included. The complete set of basic SI units along with their derived units, which are formed by combining base units for measuring physical quantities (e.g. pressure, radiation dose etc.) are given in Chapter 2.

Other systems of units are still in common use. The centimeter-gram-second system (cgs units) was used prior to the SI units and other units such as the micron (10^{-6}m), angstrom (10^{-10}m) and curie (3.7×10^{10} disintegrations per second) are frequently encountered in radiology. None of them is a recognized SI unit.

Table 1.1 Basic physical constants (SI and cgs)

Quantity	SI unit	cgs unit
Mass	kilogram (kg)	gram (g) (gm)*
Length	meter (m)	centimeter (cm)
Time	second (s)	second (s)
(derived)	minute (min)	
	hour (h)	
	day (d)	
	year (a) (yr)*	

* non-standard abbreviation

1.2 NOTATION

The common symbols most frequently used in radiology are listed in Table 1.2. The order of priority when calculating a mixed equation is:

1. Bracketed functions ($x+y$) etc.

Table 1.2   Common arithmetic symbols

Symbol	Function	Symbol	Function
+	addition	$\neq$	does not equal
−	subtraction	$\approx$	approximately equals
× or *	multiplication	$\equiv$	exactly equal to
÷ or /	division	$\propto$	proportional to
$\sqrt{x}$ or Sqrt (x)	square root	>	greater than
x^2	square	<	less than
$\log_{10}x$ or $\ln x$	logarithm base$_{10}$ or e	$\pm$	range of + and − values
$\tan(x)$ $\sin(x)$ $\cos(x)$	trigonometry functions	Δx	small change in x
=	equals	Σ	sum of samples

2. Squares and square roots x^2 $\sqrt{x}$
3. Multiply and divide × * ÷ /
4. Addition and subtraction +, −

Common prefixes which are used to express multiples or fractions of standard quantities are given in Table 1.3. Examples of prefix use would be kilogram kg, microsecond µs, millimeter mm. Less common would be nanometer nm, used for measuring wavelength, and mega-becquerel MBq used for nuclide activity levels

Table 1.3   Prefixes used for constants

Factor	Prefix	Symbol	Example
10^9	giga-	G	GBq
10^6	mega-	M	MJ, MBq
10^3	kilo-	k	kg, kW
10^{-2}	centi-	c	cm, cGy
10^{-3}	milli-	m	mm, mGy
10^{-6}	micro-	µ	µs, µCi
10^{-9}	nano-	n	nm, ns

1.2.1 Conventional notation

Integers   A single whole digit, for example: 1, 2, 3, 24, 135, 1 000 000 are all integers. Integers are used when only whole numbers make sense, such as sample numbers, radioactive counts or object numbers (patients, films etc.).

Fractions   Figures that are not whole numbers i.e. 3.1416 are fractions. If the value has a fixed number of decimal places i.e. 2.5, it is a **rational number**. If the fraction represents values such as π, e, $\sqrt{2}$ or ⅓ then the decimal places are infinite and it is an **irrational number**, for example: π is 3.14159.... e is 2.71828....

Precision   The precision or accuracy of a fraction is dependent on the number of **significant figures**. A value 1.23456 of six significant figures is accurate to five **decimal places**. Alternatively a value, such as π, can be rounded off to four decimal places, so 3.14159 becomes 3.1416. The **least significant** figure is 9.

Rounding off is applied to calculations when extreme accuracy is not important. The value for π at 3.14159 is correct to 6 significant figures but in certain circumstances 4 significant figures are sufficient. Greater precision is required when measuring values with small differences in order to show a distinction i.e. linear attenuation coefficients at high kilovoltages.

1.2.2 Scientific notation

This is used for describing very large and very small numbers in mathematical operations without introducing large quantities of zeros. The format is $a \times 10^n$ where the **mantissa** is a having a value 1 to 9 and the index is n which can be a positive or negative integer. Typical examples would be:

123.4	$\equiv$	1.234×10^2
0.0001234	$\equiv$	1.234×10^{-4}
12 340 000.0	$\equiv$	1.234×10^7

Practical examples of scientific notation used in radiology would be the old (non-SI) units of activity, the curie (Ci) where 1 μCi is 0.000001 Ci or 1.0×10^{-6} Ci and its equivalent SI unit, expressed in disintegrations per second, as the becquerel (Bq) where $1\mu Ci \equiv 37\times10^3$ Bq or 37kBq.

The index of 10^{-6} is shorthand for 'move the decimal point 6 places to the left' and 10^3 'move the decimal point 3 places to the right'. Similarly a mega-becquerel MBq is1×10^6 dps. The speed of light which traveled through a vacuum at 30,000,000,000cm s^{-1} is more conveniently written as 3.0×10^{10}cm s^{-1} or 3.0×10^8 m s^{-1}.

Rules for addition and subtraction require that the units (e.g. gram, kilogram or meter, cm) and the exponents agree. An example manipulating mixed indices and quantities is shown in Box 1.1. Only the integer numbers are added or subtracted. The exponents remain unchanged.

Box 1.1

Addition of mixed indices

Example A (activities measured in curies)
Adding 1.575mCi to 43 μCi
1.575mCi is 1.5750×10^{-3} Ci or 1575.0×10^{-6} Ci
43.0 μCi is 43.0×10^{-6} Ci
Add mantissas to give 1618×10^{-6} Ci
(or 1.618mCi)

Example B (different units m and cm)
Combine 1.75×10^{-6} m + 5.43×10^{-6} cm

1.75×10^{-6} :	1.75×10^{-6} m
5.43×10^{-6} cm:	0.0543×10^{-6} m

Add mantissas 1.7643×10^{-6} m (1.7643μm)

NB The integers could be subtracted using the same principle

Multiplication and division In this case the integers are multiplied or divided; the exponents are added or subtracted. The units can be multiples of the same base. (seconds, microseconds etc.) Box 1.2 gives examples of multiplying and dividing dissimilar quantities.

Box 1.2

Multiplication and division of values

Example A (indices added)
The speed of light is 3.0×10^8 m s^{-1}
How far will it travel in 2 ns (2×10^{-9} s)
$= (3.0\times10^8) \times (2\times10^{-9})$
$= 6.0\times10^{-1}$m
$= 0.6$m

Example B (addition and subtraction)
A light year is the distance traveled by light in one year. There are 365 × 24 × 60 × 60s in one year = 3.15×10^7s. Distance traveled in meters:
$= 3\times10^8$m × 3.15×10^7s
$= 9.45\times10^{15}$m
Distance in miles (1.6×10^3m = 1mile):
$= (9.45\times10^{15}) \div (1.6\times10^3)$
$= 5.81\times10^{12}$ miles

Floating point This notation is used to represent a very wide range of numerical values in a similar fashion to scientific notation but is found commonly associated with computer format. The notation as before is $a\times10^n$ but the mantissa is restricted to be greater than 0.1 but less than 1.0 so:

123.4	is	0.1234×10^3
567.8	is	0.5678×10^3
0.0000789	is	0.789×10^{-4}

The index or **exponent** governs movement of the decimal point as before, to the right for positive values and to the left (adding zeros) for negative values.

The exponent is further simplified so the above numbers are represented with their relevant exponents as 0.1234E3, 0.5678E3 and 0.789E–4. This format is commonly accepted by calculators and computer programs (i.e. spreadsheets).

1.2.3 Negative numbers

Negative numbers simplify the handling of decreasing quantities. The answer to several subtraction calculations can give negative quantities i.e. $7-9 = -2$. An **absolute** value to this sum, where the sign is removed, is 2 and can be obtained by squaring and then taking roots :

$$\sqrt{(7-9)^2} = 2$$

This procedure is frequently used to remove negative quantities in statistics. An absolute number in an equation is bounded by vertical lines: $|7-9| = 2$

Binary numbers   These use $Base_2$ instead of the decimal $Base_{10}$. Since only one of two conditions can exist (1 or 0 representing 'on' or 'off') this format is used by computers, each figure is called a **bit**. This format is more fully discussed in Chapter 12.

1.2.4 Complex numbers

If the equation $x^2+2x+2=0$ is solved then it yields $(x+1)^2+1=0$ which then simplifies to $x+1 = \pm\sqrt{-1}$ where $x = -1 \pm\sqrt{-1}$.

The quantity $\sqrt{-1}$ does not exist as an entity and is not a real number, however the equations are not impossible so $\sqrt{-1}$ exists as an imaginary number and is denoted by i or j in an equation. A complex number has the form $a+ib$ where a and b are the real numbers.

Although complex numbers are rather artificial they are extremely useful for solving practical problems and play a very important role in waveform analysis involving frequency and phase that will be met when dealing with Fourier Analysis and frequency phase relationships in magnetic resonance imaging MRI.

1.3 FRACTIONS AND RATIOS

Quantities are commonly compared with reference values either as fractions (half, third etc.) or as percentages (50%, 33% etc.)

1.3.1 Percentages

Percentage change   The term percentage literally means 'for each hundred values'; abbreviated to %. Although this strict definition is commonly misused and expressions using '150%' and 'over 400%' are seen in some literature, this is not correct and should not be used in scientific work; ×1.5 and ×4 should be substituted. The symbol '%' (parts per hundred or percent) has been modified as '‰' for parts per thousand.

Fractional error   When measurements are carried out there is always inaccuracy associated with the measurement i.e. length, weight, activity, radiation exposure. If the original value is known V_o along with the nominal value V_n then the fractional error f is:

$$f = \frac{V_n - V_o}{V_o} \qquad (1.1)$$

Common examples of percentage calculations are given in Box 1.3

Box 1.3

Application of percentages

The original value V_o of 80 undergoes a reduction to a new value of 72 V_n. The new value as a percentage of the original is:

$$\frac{V_n}{V_o} \times 100\% = 90\%$$

The percentage change is :

$$\frac{V_n - V_o}{V_o} \times 100\% = 10\%$$

The ratio of signal to noise (SNR)

When a particular signal is measured in the presence of noise the pure signal is 12 units and the noise is 2 units.

The SNR is $1: \dfrac{12}{2}$ or $1:6$

If the noise content increases to 6 units.

The SNR is $1: \dfrac{12}{6}$ or $1:2$

NB A decrease in the ratio signifies degradation of the perceived signal.

Ratios Comparisons can also be made by comparing a reference with an unknown; the reference value is **normalized** to 1 so if the calculation yields 2.5 to 10 the **ratio** is 1:4. Box 1.3 also gives a worked example where ratios are commonly employed in radiology to give a 'signal to noise' ratio where a recorded signal is measured in the presence of noise.

So an object moving a distance in a certain time has a velocity measured as **meters per second** or m s^{-1}. Similarly thermal conductivity, measured as joules per second, is J s^{-1} and acceleration, measured as meters per second per second, is m s^{-1} s^{-1} or m s^{-2}. Volume measurements use the cube power so density is represented as kg m^{-3}.

1.4 RECIPROCAL VALUES

A reciprocal value describes quantities that are **inversely** related, as x increases then y decreases:

$$y = \frac{1}{x} \qquad (1.2)$$

Alternatively eqn. 1.2 can be expressed as:

$$y = x^{-1} \qquad (1.3)$$

An inverse relationship plays an important role in radiology between distance d and radiation intensity I so that:

$$I = \frac{1}{d^2} \qquad (1.4)$$

This forms the basis of the inverse square law which plays an important role in radiology.

Reciprocal values are frequently used for describing measurements. For instance kilometers per second or grams per cm^3 can be given as kg/s or g/cm^3 however these should be expressed as kg s^{-1} and g cm^{-3}. An example demonstrating the derivation of this format is: If an object moves a fixed distance (meters) in a given time (seconds) then:

$$\frac{distance\ (m)}{time\ (s)} = meters\ per\ second$$

This can be rearranged as:

$$distance \times \frac{1}{time}$$

Since the reciprocal of time can be expressed as time^{-1} then from eqn.1.3:

$$\frac{1}{time} = \frac{1}{second} = s^{-1} \qquad (1.5)$$

1.5 LOGARITHMS

The logarithm of a decimal number is the exponent or power to which the base must be raised to produce the number. There are two common logarithmic bases:

- Base$_{10}$ (10^x) used for log$_{10}$: these are common logarithms.
- Base$_e$ (e^x) used for log$_e$ (or ln) as natural logs where $e = 2.71828$ to 6 significant figures. It describes many common phenomena found in radiology, particularly the absorption of radiation (x-radiation, sound or radiofrequencies) and decay of radioactive material.

For both base$_{10}$ and base$_e$ their exponents have indices that are not whole numbers i.e. $10^{2.6078}$ and $e^{0.693}$ the log values are 2.6078 and 0.693 respectively.

Logarithmic quantities using base$_{10}$ and base$_e$ have the following inverse relationships:

$$\log_e 2 = 0.693 \qquad e^{0.693} = 2$$
$$\log_{10} 2 = 0.301 \qquad 10^{0.301} = 2$$

1.5.1 Logarithm to base$_{10}$ (log$_{10}$)

There is a difference between tables of logarithms and calculator/computer logarithms. Tables are designed to give convenient similar log values for numbers having the same digits i.e. 2.0 and 0.2 which are both given a value 3010 so a different set of tables for integers and fractions are not needed. Logarithms given by calculators and computers use the true log values where 2.0 is 0.3010 as before but 0.2 is −0.6989. Logarithms to Base$_{10}$ were originally used for simplifying complex calculations but the introduction of scientific calculators has superseded their use for this purpose.

The manipulation of decimal numbers is simplified when using logarithms since complex calculations can be reduced to addition, subtraction, multiplication and division as shown in Tab. 1.5

Table 1.4 Logarithms simplify calculations

Decimals	Logarithms
Multiply ($a{\times}b$)	Add (log a + log b)
Divide (a/b)	Subtract (log a − log b)
Square (a^2)	Multiply by index (log a ×2)
Roots ($\sqrt[3]{a}$)	Divide by root (log a/3)

Examples of log$_{10}$ in radiology   Logarithms to Base$_{10}$ are commonly used in radiology to calculate optical density and decibel ratings.

Photographic optical density *OD* is measured as a log$_{10}$ value of incident I_i and transmitted I_t light where:

$$OD = \log_{10} \frac{I_i}{I_t} \qquad (1.6)$$

A worked example of eqn.1.6 for film density, represented as light intensity transmitted by a light box through the film, is given in Box 1.4. The logarithmic log$_{10}$ scale is again found in ultrasound imaging, when it is used for measuring sound intensity (watts cm^{-2}) as the **decibel** (dB) which is represented as a rounded log value.

Table 1.4 gives approximate dB levels showing that a change in 3dB (a change from log 1.0 to log 2.0) doubles sound intensity.

Table 1.5   Log values give decibel intensities

Intensity (watts cm^{-2})	log$_{10}$ value	dB
1	1.0000	0
2	0.3010	3
3	0.4771	5
4	0.6020	6
5	0.6989	7

Box 1.4

Film density as log$_{10}$ values

The optical density of film (OD) is defined in eqn. 1.6 as:

$$\log_{10} \frac{\text{Intensity of Incident light}}{\text{Intensity of Transmitted light}}$$

$$= \log_{10} \frac{I_i}{I_t}$$

If I_i = 2000 and I_t = 200 then: $\log_{10} \frac{2000}{200}$

$$= 3.3010 \text{ minus } 2.3010 \text{ so OD} = 1$$
(10% transmission)

Similarly if I_i = 2000 and I_t = 20 then   OD = 2
(1% transmission)

If I_i = 2000 and I_t = 1000 then   OD = 0.3
(50% transmission)

NB

An OD value change of 0.3 doubles or halves the transmission (compare this with the dB change of 3.0 in sound intensity).

1.5.2 Natural logarithms to base$_e$ (log$_e$ x or ln$x$)

In biological and physical processes the exponential function e is common to many growth and decay processes and can be used to describe, for instance, absorption of radiation and decay of radioactivity.

Growth and the origin of e   The process of growth can be expressed as:

$$G = G_o (1+1/t)^t \qquad (1.7)$$

Where G is the final value and G_o the original value. The factor $1/t$ is the increment added at time t; for $t=2$ the equation $e=(1+1/t)^t$ becomes $(1+\frac{1}{2})^2 = 2.25$. For large values of t in eqn.1.7 the value e becomes 2.71828... This irrational figure is adopted as the base of **napierian** or **natural logarithms**.

The exponential law The common formula used in radiology which uses the exponential function e is:

$$N = N_o \times e^{-y} \qquad (1.8)$$

Where N_o is the original activity and N is the value representing new activity influenced by y. The parameter y is a mixed value whose components depend on the particular application. The general formula for **exponential decay** is eqn.1.8 above.

It can also be applied to the absorption of radiation; the two components for the product y are:

- μ which describes the absorption efficiency of the material.
- x the thickness of the material.

So eqn. 1.8 becomes:

$$N = N_o\, e^{-\mu x} \qquad (1.9)$$

As two values N and N_o now represent **radiation intensities** they now become I_o (incident intensity) and I_x (intensity after adding absorber with thickness x). Equation 1.9 becomes perhaps the most familiar equation in radiology:

$$I_x = I_o \times e^{-\mu x} \qquad (1.10)$$

This formula was originally used by J. Lambert (1728-77; German physicist) to describe light absorption and is called Lambert's Law. It is an important basic formula used in radiology where exponential change is seen such as the absorption of electromagnetic radiation (x- or γ–radiation) by various materials (tissue, aluminum, lead etc.). It can also describe the decay of radioactive isotopes e.g. ^{131}iodine or ^{99m}technetium when I_x and I_o become activity levels.

If the radiation intensities are measured using eqn.1.10, then the separate indices can be found:

$$\frac{I}{I_o} = e^{-\mu x} \qquad (1.11)$$

Inverting eqn.1.11 removes the negative value so:

$$\ln \frac{I_o}{I} = \mu x \qquad (1.12)$$

An example of eqn.1.12 use for calculating absorber thickness necessary to reduce x-ray beam intensity is given as an example in Box 1.5.

The thickness of absorber that reduces the beam intensity by ½ is the half-value-layer and with this measurement the basic formula can be used to derive the attenuation coefficient of materials. This is shown in Box 1.6 and will receive added importance in Chapter 3.

Box 1.5

Attenuation of radiation

What thickness x of lead is required to reduce radiation by 90% if the attenuation coefficient (μ) of lead is 27.72cm^{-1} at the given keV

Let $I_o = 100$ and $I_x = 10$ then using eqn. 1.5
$$\ln \frac{100}{10} = 2.3025 \text{ so } x = 0.08\text{cm } (0.8\text{mm})$$

Applications Applying the formula shown in eqn.1.10 to problems concerning radioactive decay two values exponent values (μ and x) now change to:

- Time t when activity is measured
- The **half-life** of the nuclide $t\frac{1}{2}$

8 *Physics of Diagnostic Imaging*

Box 1.6

Reducing intensity by half: the half-value-layer (HVL)

Derivation of the attenuation coefficient. By definition adding a half-value-layer (HVL) will reduce I_0 to $\dfrac{I_0}{2}$

so from eqn.1.10: $\dfrac{I_0}{2} = I_0 \times e^{-\mu \times HVL}$

and $e^{-\mu \times HVL} = 0.5$ or $e^{\mu \times HVL} = 2$

Simplifying $\ln 2 = \mu \times HVL$ ($\ln 2 = 0.693$)

so $\mu = \dfrac{0.693}{HVL}$

Example: Find the attenuation coefficient μ if a 0.45cm of aluminum reduces the beam intensity by half.

$$\mu = \frac{0.693}{0.45} \approx 1.5 \text{ cm}^{-1}$$

Box 1.7

Isotope decay

Example A T½ for ^{99m}Tc is 6h. Original activity was 800MBq. How much remains after 1 day? From eqn 1.13: $A_t = A_o \times e^{-\lambda \times t}$

Where A_o is original activity (800MBq). Activity after time t (24hrs) is A_t and λ, the decay constant for ^{99m}Tc is 0.1155 h:
$$A_t = A_o \times e^{-0.1155 \times 24}$$
$$= 800 \times 0.06253$$
$$= 50\text{MBq}$$
This formula is also valid for mCi.

Example B The original activity of ^{131}iodine (t½ 8 days) on Day 0 was 400MBq in 2cm^3 saline. On Day 5 130MBq is required. What volume must be drawn up?
Total activity Day 5 is
$$A_t = 400 \times e^{-(0.693\times5)/8}$$
$$= 400 \times 0.65$$
$$= 260\text{MBq in 2cm}^3$$
so 1cm^3 will give the required 130MBq

---

so the formula now becomes:

$$A_t = A_o \times e^{-\lambda t} \qquad (1.13)$$

Where A_o is the original activity and A_t is the activity at time t. The arguments derived in Box 1.6 where μ can be obtained from the half-value-layer apply to radioactive decay. Instead of HVL a half-life is introduced so when the measurement time t equals $t½$ a similar expression can be derived for λ:

$$\lambda = \frac{0.693}{t½} \qquad (1.14)$$

similarly $e^{-\lambda \times t½} = 0.5$ and $\ln 2 = \lambda \times t½$. Since the fraction λ does not vary this is the **decay constant** for the isotope. Box 1.7 calculates the activity for a short half-life isotope ^{99m}technetium using this constant.

Exponential growth The exponential law also describes growth processes. An example from nuclear medicine would describe an increased growth of radioactivity in an isotope generator (^{99}Mo/^{99m}Tc), or in MRI for describing the rate at which the proton axis regains equilibrium during T1 time in MRI

1.6 PROPORTIONAL QUANTITIES

Although two quantities x and y may be directly **proportional** to each other they are not necessarily equal so: $y \propto x$ could signify $y = kx$ where k is a constant. In radiology x-ray intensity is proportional to tube current (mA). Parameters are **inversely proportional** when $y \propto 1/x$ which restates eqn.1.2 and describes a function where if x is doubled y is halved. The radiation dose from a point source measured at a surface varies as the **inverse square** of the distance d already seen in eqn.1.4 restated now as $y\ (dose) \propto 1/d^2$; the quantities dose and distance are not defined so an equals sign cannot be used.

This important relationship will be discussed further in a later section.

1.7 GRAPHS

A graph illustrates the relationship between sets of numbers or quantities (usually two) plotted as a series of points or lines with reference the set of axes. The most common type of graph is the Cartesian graph with uniform scales, shown in Fig.1.1. This shows:

- The horizontal axis (the *x*-axis) or **abscissa** which usually contains the **independent variable** (time, distance, kilovoltage)
- The vertical axis (the *y*-axis) or **ordinate** contains the measured or **dependent variable** (size, exposure, attenuation)

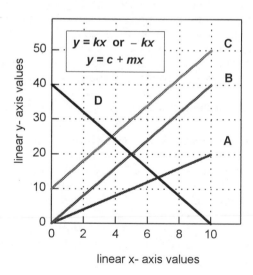

linear x- axis values

Figure 1.1 Examples of three linear graphs described in the text. A and B have different slopes but the same origin (zero). C is offset by 10 and D shows a negative relationship with *y*.

1.7.1 Linear graphs

The straight-line relationships shown in Fig.1.1 are given when:

$$y \propto x \text{ or } y = c + mx \text{ or } y = c - mx$$

Where *c* is the intersect with the *y*-axis (the off-set) where the line does not intersect zero and *m* is the slope or angle of the line.

The examples in Fig.1.1 show A and B having different slopes but no offset. Graph C shows an offset from zero and graph D shows a negative relationship where $y = -mx$.

If data are missing on a graph then it is valid to **interpolate** the missing values and fill in the unknowns by reference to neighboring points. **Extrapolation** infers the extreme values of a given range, either the highest or the lowest, however, this can produce questionable results and must be used with care.

A common radiology example where extrapolation is used is the relationship between radiation dose and the incidence of leukemia. Here the lower values are extrapolated since there are insufficient real measurements from observed results; this is investigated in Chapter 22. In certain cases a series of experimental results are plotted and then a formula derived describing the relationship between *x* and *y*; this is an **empirical** approach. A series of measurements can also conform to a set formula for instance a straight-line or exponential and the measured values then fit a set formula (i.e. inverse or exponential function).

1.7.2 Non-linear graphs

Non-linear relationships are found when value *x* does not have a uniform relationship with value *y*. Common functions found in radiology are squared values $y = x^2$ and inverse relationships $y = 1/x$. Squared values x^2 are plotted in Fig.1.2(a). Practical examples would be the intensity of x-ray output increasing as the square of the kilovoltage ($I \propto V^2$). **Inverse** values where $y = 1/x$ are

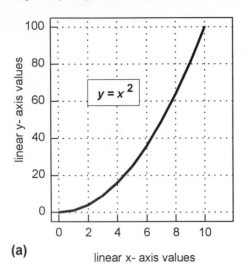

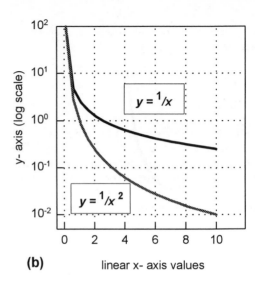

Figure 1.2 (a) A non-linear relationship plotted where $y = x^2$. (b) The inverse function showing $y = 1/x$ and $y = 1/x^2$

plotted in Fig.1.2(b). Common examples in radiology would be $1/d^2$ (inverse square law) and the probability of a photo-electric reaction with energy varying as $1/E^2$.

1.7.3 Logarithmic functions.

The common **exponential functions** of the type e^x and e^{-x} are plotted in Fig.1.3(a). where the curve for e^x shows a rapidly increasing curve typically seen in x-ray tube rating charts plotting tube current versus filament current at high kV settings.

The negative curve for e^{-x} is a very common function in radiology since it describes both radioactive decay and photon (electro-magnetic) attenuation. When dealing with a simple exponential function a **semi-log** plot, where the x-axis is linear but the y-axis is logarithmic, will yield a straight-line. This is shown in Fig.1.3(b) where the same functions e^x and e^{-x} are straight lines. This is most useful since it only requires the two or three points of a known exponential function in order to plot the entire relationship. Figure 1.3(c) shows an example where radiation absorption is being measured; only 2-3 points are needed to give the complete function. A linear plot would require many points in order

to give the same accuracy to a curve shown in Fig.1.3(a).

A multiple exponential function (2 or more exponential functions combined) can also be separated on a semi-log plot. Fig.1.4(a) shows the fast and slow phases of a tissue clearance curve. These can be approximately separated by drawing a line along the flat section of the graph, representing the slow phase meeting the y-axis.   These extrapolated values are then subtracted from the original graph revealing the fast slope.

Other logarithmic functions   The exponential function $1 - e^{-x}$ plotted in Fig.1.4(b) is commonly seen in radiology since it describes conditions which are reaching saturation e.g. growth of activity in isotope production (^{99m}Tc growth in a ^{99}Mo/^{99m}Tc generator) or returning to an equilibrium state such as a proton magnetic moment in nuclear magnetic resonance.

The Power law   The function $y = A + x^n$ where A and n are constants may be rewritten as $\log y = \log A + \log x \times n$. As A is a constant then $\log A$ is also a constant so $\log y = \log x \times n$. This plots a straight line on log/log axes and obeys the **power law**.

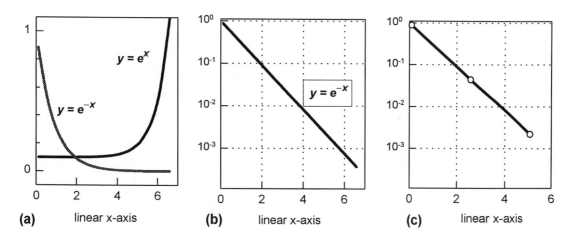

Figure 1.3 **(a)** The two exponential functions $y = e^x$ and $y = e^{-x}$ plotted on linear x and y axes. **(b)** The same functions e^{-x} plotted on a linear x-axis and a log y-axis (semi-log scale) yield straight lines. **(c)** An exponential curve only needs 2 to 3 readings for its completion (e.g. plot for HVL).

Examples of functions obeying the power law commonly found in radiology are:

$$y = x^2$$
$$y = x^{-2} \quad (\text{or } 1/x^2)$$
$$y = x^{\frac{1}{2}} \quad (\text{or } \sqrt{x})$$
$$y = x^{-\frac{1}{2}} \quad (\text{or } 1/\sqrt{x})$$

In radiology they are seen for functions describing kV^2, Z^3, $1/d^2$ and $1/E^2$; each of these gives a straight line obeying the power law.   An example for $1/d^2$ is shown in Fig. 1.5(a).

1.8 CALCULUS

Problems often occur with graphed quantities where a rate of change of one measurement with another is required, such as the change of heat loss from an x-ray tube with time or the change of intensity with distance. The rate of change can be calculated by using **differential calculus**. The complete or part area under a curve is also a common requirement (the intensity of radiation given by a particular x-ray spectrum for instance) and

this is calculated using **integral calculus**. The differential and integral calculus forms the foundation for many techniques used in radiology and a revision of its basic properties is relevant. This section is a springboard to further reading; a detailed description is not necessary at this point. The hypothetical function $f(x)$ where $y=f(x)$, describing the y value being some operation on x and is plotted in Fig. 1.5(b), illustrates the fundamental points.

1.8.1 Differential calculus

This describes the **derivative** of a function or the gradient of a curve marked as the slope in Fig. 1.5(b). It is concerned essentially with the rate of change of one quantity with respect to another. If $f(x)$ denotes any function of x and $y = f(x)$ then the derived function is:

$$\frac{dy}{dx}$$

Simple examples where differential calculus is used in radiology would be the rate of heat loss from an x-ray tube and the decay rate of

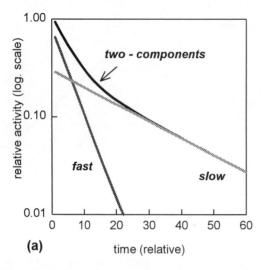
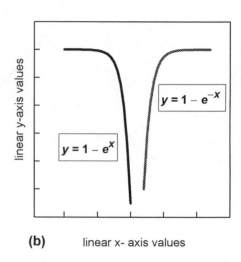

(a) time (relative)   **(b)** linear x- axis values

Figure 1.4   **(a)** A fast and slow phase tissue clearance which can be separated from the two-part composite exponential curve. The slow phase is first extrapolated back to time zero and these extrapolated figures subtracted from the composite curve to give the fast phase. **(b)** Exponential growth using the function $y = 1 - e^{-x}$. The function $1 - e^x$ is rarely met in radiology but is included here for completion.

a radioactive isotope together with the attenuation of radiation by an absorber. Film contrast is often expressed as a derivative curve superimposed on the characteristic curve.

Exponential decay   Equations 1.8 and 1.9 describing radioactive decay can be derived from first principles. Let the amount of undecayed nuclei at time t be $N = f(t)$, then $-dN/dt$ represents rate of decrease at that time so:

$$\frac{dN}{dt} = -kN \qquad (1.15)$$

where k is a positive constant. Eqn 1.15 is really the same as the basic equation in Box 1.8 expressed as a negative quantity so:

$$\frac{dt}{dN} = -\frac{1}{kN} \qquad (1.16)$$

and in a similar fashion to the second equa-

tion in Box 1.8:

$$t = -\frac{1}{k}\ln N + C$$

this is usually expressed as $N = A\,e^{-kt}$ where A is a constant. If at $t = 0$, N equals N_o, then A is replaced by N_o and the formula becomes:

$$N = N_o\,e^{-kt} \qquad (1.17)$$

This is the fundamental equation describing exponential decay or absorption. For radioactive decay the constant k is replaced by the decay constant λ.

Higher order differentials   If $f'(x)$ is the first derivative then $f''(x)$ is the second derivative taking the form:

$$\frac{d^2 y}{dx^2}$$

Second derivatives describe how the rate of change is itself changing, examples would be accelerations. This is sometimes applied to cardiology when studying the rate of change

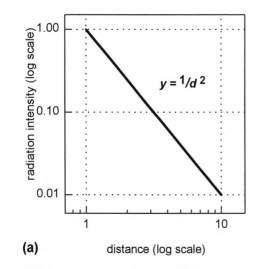

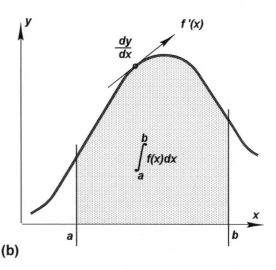

Figure 1.5 **(a)** A log-log plot obeying the power law. The general formula would be $y = x^n$ where n is a fixed index: i.e. ½ –½ , 2, 3. The example shows the inverse square law relationship ($y = 1/d^2$) **(b)** The use of differential and integral calculus for analyzing a curve.

of wall motion. So the first derivative would be rate s^{-1} and the second derivative would be acceleration describing second per second or s^{-2}.

1.8.2 Integral calculus

Integration is the inverse of differentiation. The integral of a function $f'(x)$ with respect to x is written as $\int f'(x).dx$. The symbol $\int$ is the old English for S which is used here to represent 'sum'. The **definite integral** $f(x)$ as defined by an interval a to b in Fig.1.5(b) takes the form

$$\int_a^b f(x) \cdot dx \qquad (1.18)$$

where a and b are the lower and upper limits of an area for the variable x.

Numerous approximations are available for calculating integrals. The Trapezoidal Rule places strips under the curve having trapezium shapes whose individual areas are summed to give the required curve area. Simpson's rule improves accuracy by using strips bounded by a parabolic shape which more closely approximates the shape of the curve.

Improper or infinite integral This is the case if one or both of the limits tends to infinity (a or $b = \infty$) such as the area under a continuous x-ray spectrum. Equation 1.18 now takes the form:

$$\iint f(x,y) \cdot dx \cdot dy \qquad (1.19)$$

This is an example of double integration for a two-dimensional array (x, y matrix) is often seen in image analysis and manipulation.

Box 1.8

The exponential decay of an isotope.

Using the basic form:

$$\frac{dy}{dx} = ky \; (k = \text{constant}) \text{ and } x = \int \frac{dy}{ky} = \frac{1}{k}\ln y + C$$

which simplifies to $y = A\,e^{-kx}$ where A is a constant

NB This basic formula for radioactive decay, attenuation of radiation through matter and heat loss

1.9 VOLUMES AND SURFACES

The emission of radiation from a point source occurs equally in all directions creating a sphere of radiation. This is **isotropic** emission and applies commonly to a radioactive source. The x-ray tube focal spot does not emit isotropically due to forward absorption by the anode.

When measuring isotropic radiation sources with a flat detector it is important to realize that the detector surface, being flat, can only capture a very small proportion of the total activity emanating from the source. A basic knowledge of planar and volume geometry is therefore useful in radiology for understanding detector efficiency.

1.9.1 Volumes

Solid geometry The geometry of a three dimensional (3D) body is applicable to irradiation of volumes and surfaces from a point source (x-ray or gamma ray). The relevant formulas are:

- Surface area $4\pi r^2$
- Spherical volume $4\pi r^3/3$

The inverse square law This can be derived by reference to spherical geometry shown in Fig.1.6(a). It is a very important concept in radiation exposure. The intensity of radiation from an isotropic source is measured at r_1 and r_2. This is the photon density per unit area. The energy emitted is E so the intensity at the surface of the small sphere I_{r_1} is:

$$I_{r_1} = \frac{E}{4\pi r_1^2} \qquad (1.20)$$

and for the intensity I_{r_2} is:

$$I_{r_2} = \frac{E}{4\pi r_2^2} \qquad (1.21)$$

The intensity of radiation varies as $1/r^2$, the inverse square of the distance - if the intensity at 2m is 100 then at 4m it will be 25.

Steradian This is the solid angle used in spherical geometry so $4\pi = 12.56$ steradians, to 4 significant figures, which is the complete central angle of a sphere; the 100% collection efficiency is known as **4π geometry** and can only be achieved by a detector which completely surrounds the source.

Detector efficiency e This is given by the equation

$$e = \frac{\Omega}{4\pi} \times 100\% \qquad (1.22)$$

Where Ω is the solid angle subtended by the detector surface. The efficiency of a spherical detector having 4π geometry is approached by a nuclear medicine 'Dose Calibrator' where a radioactive source is placed inside a gas detector. There is a slight loss of efficiency due to the sample aperture which is the detector entrance. This is described in Chapter 15.

1.9.2 Surface detectors

Flat or surface detectors are manufactured in a variety of sizes, rectangular as well as round. If a circular detector shown in Fig.1.6(b) is taken (radius r or diameter d) and the hypotenuse is L then the geometry of a cone can be employed:

- Detector area πr^2
- Detector circumference $2\pi r$ or πd
- Conic angle $\Omega = \pi r^2/L^2$

Using these formulas the efficiency of a planar detector can be calculated as shown in Fig 1.6(b) (examples would be a gamma camera or an image intensifier face). For surface detectors with a detector area $A = \pi r^2$ then the conic angle subtended by the detector is:

$$\Omega = \frac{A}{r^2} \qquad (1.23)$$

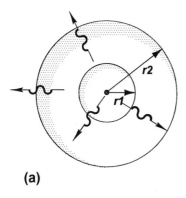
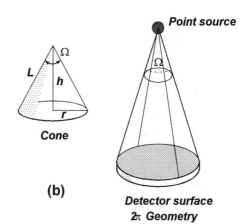

(a)

(b)

Detector surface
2π Geometry

Figure 1.6 **(a)** Isotropic emission from a source. Intensity measured at the surface of two spheres having radius r_1 and r_2 (in text). **(b)** Planar Detector efficiency showing the detector surface subtending the solid angle Ω with the point source.

The value of 6.28 steradians is the central angle of a hemisphere representing a surface detector; this is called **2π geometry**. Geometrical detector efficiency for 2π geometry (surfaces) is determined by two factors:

- Area of detector
- Source to detector distance.

These factors define the solid angle 'subtended' by the detector relative to the source and eqn.1.22 is used for calculating the efficiency. Calculated examples are given in Box 1.9.

Radian This is the basic unit for a plane angle Ω shown in Fig.1.6(b), which is $360/2\pi$ or $57.2958°$, to six significant figures. The radian is based on the constant proportionality between the radius and the circumference of a circle. The definition of a radian is the angle subtended (at the center) by an arc equal in length to the radius of the circle. The circumference equals $2\pi r$ so a circle contains 2π radians. A complete $360°$ rotation is 2π radians or 6.283... so 1 radian ≈ $57.3°$. The radian and steradian are supplementary SI units.

Box 1.9

Detector efficiency

Using the eqn.1.23 for the angle $\Omega = \dfrac{A}{r^2}$
the efficiency for a 10mm² detector at:
(a) 25mm (b) 50mm is:

(a) $\dfrac{10}{25^2} = 1.6\times10^{-2}\ \Omega$

$e = 1.6\times10^{-2}/4\pi \times 100\%$

At 25mm = 0.127% which would be 1.27% for a 100mm² detector surface.

(b) $\dfrac{10}{50^2} = 4.0 \times 10^{-3}\ \Omega$

$e = 4.0\times10^{-3}/4\pi \times 100\%$

At 50mm = 0.032%

NB The geometrical efficiency of a 2π detector is extremely small

---

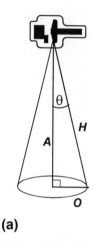

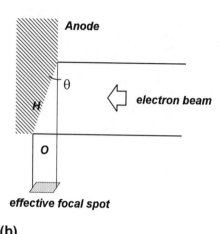

(a)   **(b)**

Figure 1.7 **(a)** The useful field of view given by an x-ray tube can be calculated using tan θ as shown in the text. 'A' is adjacent side, 'O' opposite side and 'H' hypotenuse. **(b)** The effective focal spot size of an x-ray tube target can be calculated from the anode angle and length of the target area.

1.10 TRIGONOMETRY

Tangent The geometric definition is a straight line which touches the circumference of a circle at only one point. However it is also a trigonometric value relating angle of a triangle to side dimensions. If a right angled triangle represented in Fig.1.7(a) has sides adjacent A, opposite O and the hypotenuse H, relative to angle θ then:

$$\tan \theta = \frac{A}{O} \qquad (1.24)$$

The useful field of view is calculated in Box 1.10.

Sine A sine of an angle in a right angled triangle is given by the ratio of opposite over hypotenuse.

$$\sin \theta = \frac{O}{A} \qquad (1.25)$$

The effective focal-spot size of an x-ray tube can be calculated from knowledge of the anode angle and its sine value: Fig.1.7(b) shows the dimensions involved and a worked example is given in Box 1.10. The important geometry of **sine-waves** will be covered in later chapters

Cosine This is the third member of the family of trigonometric functions having the relationship:

$$\cos \theta = \frac{A}{H} \qquad (1.26)$$

It is included for completeness. Its value in radiology is discussed in Chapter 2 where sine/cosine values play an important role in waveform analysis and alternating current power supplies.

Box 1.10

Tangent example from Fig.1.7(a):
Angle θ = 20°
Adjacent side A = 100cm (1m)
Field of view = 2× (0.364 × 100) = 36×2 = 72cm

Sine example from Fig.1.7(b)
If the hypotenuse A is 3mm and the anode angle θ = 20° then the effective focal spot:
$A \times \sin \theta = 3 \times 0.342 = 1$mm

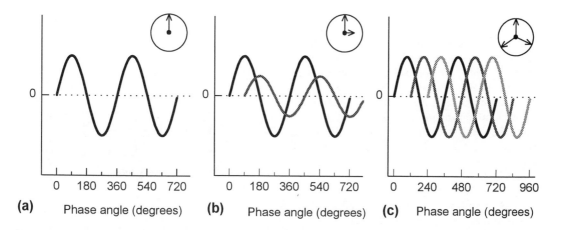

Figure 1.8 **(a)** The geometry of a sine-wave showing wavelength and amplitude. The two waveforms in **(b)** have a different amplitude and phase which is identified by the arrow position and size in the phase diagram (90° phase difference). The 3-phase waveform in **(c)** (AC power supply) shows a 120° phase difference.

1.11 OSCILLATIONS AND WAVES

Signals used in radiology for image formation are commonly either continuous (video) or undergo a decay process after a finite length of time (radio-waves). Continuous signals are **periodic** and decaying signals are **transient**. A continuous sound wave, an electromagnetic emission or the AC mains supply would demonstrate a periodic signal whilst a magnetic resonance signal or an ultrasound pulse would be transient.

1.11.1 The sine-wave

The simplest type of periodic signal is the sine-wave, shown in Fig. 1.8(a) where the signal varies as:

$$y = A \times \sin(\omega + \theta) \qquad (1.27)$$

where A is a constant representing amplitude, ω the angular frequency $2\pi f_0$ where f_0 is the number of repetitions per unit time or the wave **frequency** measured in hertz (Hz). The variable θ is the initial **phase** angle with respect to the time origin in radians. The distance between zero crossing points is the wavelength λ so that if n oscillations pass a given point in unit time the velocity of the wave is $V = \lambda \times n$.

Angular velocity The waveform repeats itself every 360° so the phase relationships between waveforms, where one leads or lags the other, can be simply described by using a circular **phase diagram** shown in the top left of Figs. 1.8(a), (b) and (c). For two waveforms having different phase relationships in Fig. 1.8(b), the angular velocity is $\theta_2 - \theta_1 = \Delta\theta$ expressed in **radians**. Figure 1.8(b) shows two sine-waves with the same frequency but different amplitude, *A1* and *A2*, and phase. The phase diagram indicates the amplitude difference and 90° phase shift.

A 3-phase sine-wave with equal amplitude and 120° phase shift is shown in Fig. 1.8(c). Its phase diagram shows the same 120° phase shift between each waveform. This is the common waveform in 3-phase AC power supplies.

1.11.2 Waveform analysis

The signals most commonly encountered in radiology (ultrasound, MRI, image data, etc.) consist of mixed waveforms having different frequency, amplitude and phase. These signals can be separated and their individual characteristics measured by using Fourier analysis (J.B. Fourier, 1768-1830, French mathematician). Fourier's theorem states that a composite waveform (or function $x(t)$) comprising different frequencies, phase and amplitude can be treated as a series of the form:

$x(t) =$
$A_O + A_1 \times \sin(\omega_t + \theta_1) + A_2 \times \sin(2\omega_t + \theta_2)$
$+ \quad A_3 \times \sin(3\omega_t + \theta_3) + A_4 \times \sin(4\omega_t + \theta_4) +$
$\ldots\ldots\ldots A_n \times \sin(n\omega_t + \theta_n)$ \hfill (1.28)

$A_1 \ldots A_n$ represent the peak amplitude of the fundamental and harmonic component of the series; $\theta_1 \ldots \theta_n$ represent the phase relationships between the fundamental and harmonics at time t. So a complex waveform seen in image data (CT) or ultrasound, for instance, can be decomposed into the sum of its individual sine-waves where the fundamental frequency is:

$$f_O = \frac{\omega}{2\pi}$$ \hfill (1.29)

In order to simplify the principle of Fourier analysis without introducing complex variables a demonstration of its analytical ability is given in Fig.1.9 for a rectangular waveform combining eqns. 1.28 and 1.29 to give:

$$x(t) = \frac{A}{2} + \frac{2A}{\pi} \times \sin(\omega_t) + \frac{2A}{3\pi} \times \sin(3\omega_t) +$$
$$\frac{2A}{5\pi} \times \sin(5\omega_t) + \ldots + \frac{2A}{n\pi} \times \sin(n..\omega_t) \quad (1.30)$$

The first two terms then the next 3 in eqn.1.30 are plotted in Fig.1.9 showing that increasing the number of terms more closely approaches the original rectangular waveform.

When a waveform analysis is attempted the more terms that are included the greater the accuracy, however a large number of terms is obviously impractical so a truncated Fourier series is employed.

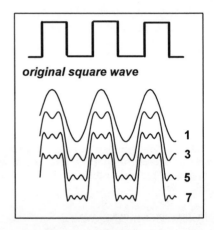

Figure 1.9 An example of Fourier analysis of a rectangular waveform (square wave) showing the results of using increasing numbers of terms in eqn. 1.30

1.12 BASIC STATISTICS IN RADIOLOGY

Statistical analysis allows accurate predictions and sensible decisions to be made, sometimes on incomplete measurements or data sets. Each **data set** or sample may come from the same **population** (i.e. population heights or weights) or may come from two different populations (i.e. population heights in country A versus country B).

In radiology the data sets are commonly count or density measurements taken from different organs or tissues in an image or sample activity counts (GFR counts) or a group of physiological measurements (heart rate, body temperature) from a group of patients undergoing a particular investigation (new contrast agent or drug). These quantities taken from a population are **variables**. It is rarely possible to measure an entire population so a population sample must be taken. The size of the sample depends on the variation within the population.

1.12.1 Sample distribution

The degree of variability of a series of measurements, such as photon flux on a detector surface, are subject to random variations. For comparative measurements it is not necessary to count the total number of events (usually impossible anyway) providing the equipment is stable. A sample series of count rates or densities is only required. However even under the most careful experimental conditions a series of repeat observations with a constant level of activity will give variable results. The distribution of this variability can be analyzed to give useful information about counting characteristics etc.

Three basic distributions are used for describing different data characteristics. These are, in order of complexity: Binomial, Poisson and Gaussian (Normal) distributions.

Binomial distribution This describes the probability of an event occurring p or not occurring q. If a certain population has a disease content of 10% then the probability of a certain selected person having the disease is $p= 0.1$ or not having the disease is $q = 0.9$, then $p+q=1$. The probability that two people selected from this population will have the disease or be normal is obtained by expanding $(p+q)^2$ which is p^2 for both having the disease $2pq$ for one being normal and one having the disease and q^2 for both being normal. The simple algebraic relationship leads to the expansion:

$$p^2+2pq+q^2 = (p+q)^2 \qquad (1.31)$$

Similarly the probabilities from a population of n individuals can be derived by expanding $(p+q)^n$. This forms the binomial distribution which plays an important role in population sampling and having confidence that a sample from this population accurately represents the population distribution.

During sampling we do not know the value of p but are trying to infer its value. In application a sample of a definite size is taken and a note is made of the number of times a certain event is observed. The binomial distribution can be a useful tool for quality control procedures in radiology where equipment performance is being documented. An example of this application for estimating the film rejection rate in a department and judging whether the rejection rate has gone up or down is calculated in Box 1.11

From the above distribution we may calculate the mean μ and standard deviation σ values of the number of reject films per sample. These are $\mu = np$ and $\sigma = \sqrt{npq}$. Substituting the values from this exercise gives $\mu=1.0$ and $\sigma = 0.894$.

Box 1.11

Example of binomial distribution

A certain radiology department has a 20% rejection rate for its film radiographs (processor spoilage, technical error etc.). This is particularly high so a study was designed where a group of five films ($n=5$) was selected at the end of each clinical session. There were 12 sessions per day so at the end of the year 4380 groups of 5 films had be analyzed.

For a 20% rejection rate $p=0.2$ and $q=0.8$. Since $(p+q)^n = (0.2+0.8)^5$ this expands to give:

$$p^5+5p^4q+10p^3q^2+10p^2q^3+5pq^4+q^5$$

Inserting the figures gives the individual values:
$(0.2)^5 + 5(0.2)^4(0.8) + 10(0.2)^3(0.8)^2 \ldots\ldots$ etc.

This expansion is the binomial distribution for the different outcomes as the relative expected frequencies.

Poisson distribution (SD Poisson 1781-1840, French mathematician). In most practical applications the binomial distribution is not appropriate since we do not know the value of n in the expression $(p+q)^n$. This is true for example when studying the number of counts registered by a detector or intercepted by an imaging surface.

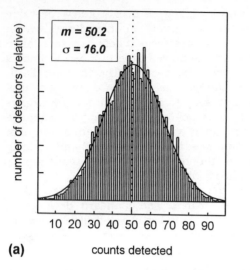

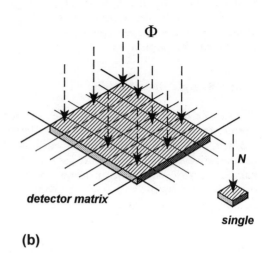

(a)   counts detected   **(b)**

Figure 1.10   **(a)** A Poisson and normal distribution superimposed **(b)** A detector surface and a single detector exposed to a uniform x-ray fluence.

A Poisson distribution is shown as a histogram portion in Fig.1.10(a) representing the random distribution of counts collected over a uniformly exposed detector surface, represented in Fig.1.10(b) constructed from 10×10 detectors having individual areas of 1cm^2.

The Poisson distribution can be used to answer the question 'how many x-rays m are intercepted by a detector in an array of detectors?' (or a certain fixed area of an imaging surface). If the number N of individual detectors (or areas shown in Fig.1.10(b)) is large and the probability P of an x-ray photon falling on a single detector is small then the variable x is the number of x-rays detected. The Poisson probability $P(x)$ which would describe this is:

$$P(x) = \frac{m^x}{x!} \cdot e^{-m} \qquad (1.32)$$

Where e is the exponential constant.

The probability of recording a certain count value is calculated in Box 1.12. Since factorials are used this example uses low count values. Since the variance of this distribution is:

$$\sigma^2 = (x - m)^2 = m \qquad (1.33)$$

The standard deviation of a Poisson distribution is $\sqrt{m}$. This is very useful in radiology when the distribution or noise of a particular measurement is required. If a particular count is 100 the expected noise or signal variation would be 10 or 10% whereas if the count is increased to 10,000 the expected noise is 100 reducing its effect to 1%.

The Poisson distribution may only be applied in cases where the expectation of m is constant from reading to reading as would be the case when collecting counts for a fixed period of time.

Box 1.12

Probability of registering a certain count.

From a detector counting background activity, what is the probability of registering a count of 7 when the average count is 5 using eqn.1.32:

$$P(x) \quad = \frac{(5)^7}{7!} \times e^{-5}$$
$$= 0.10$$

Normal or Gaussian curve The frequency of occurrence of a certain random event can be assigned to the mathematical families described by the binomial or Poisson distributions. While these distributions enable the study of discrete events (i.e. probability of occurrence or counts seen per unit time) it does not allow the study of continuous random variable distributions where the investigation does not involve individual counts or events but estimations or measurements of the entire population are made.

Continuous variables seen in radiology would be:

- weight of individuals in a population
- attenuation coefficient of separate tissue samples (i.e. bone) in a population.
- uptake of radioactive tracer in normal tissue of a population group.
- bone mineral concentration in a population
- T1 and T2 times of various discrete tissue types.

If a large number of events described by these examples are recorded then the Poisson distribution approaches a continuous distribution shown by the curve envelope in Fig.1.10(a). This is a bell-shaped curve commonly referred to in statistics which describes a continuous, normal or Gaussian distribution (KF Gauss 1777-1855, German mathematician). The bell shape is described by the general formula:

$$y = \frac{1}{\sigma\sqrt{2\pi}} \cdot e^{-(t^2/2)} \qquad (1.34)$$

where $t = \frac{x - \bar{x}}{\sigma}$. The normal curve extends to infinity in either direction (asymptotic) and the area under the curve represents probability and the constant $1/\sqrt{2}$ ensures that the total area is unity. The parameter σ in eqn. 1.34 is the standard deviation of the mean value x.

Probability tables can be used for estimating the number of items in a certain population which would fall into a specified standard deviation band and Box 1.13 gives an example of their use in a calculation concerning numbers of individuals in a population having a certain bone density. The standard deviation will be described later.

Box 1.13

Expected probability.

For a middle aged population of 2000 the bone mineral concentration was measured as 1.0g cm^{-2} with a standard deviation of 0.01g cm^{-2}. What would be the expected number of people having a BMC of 0.98g cm^{-2} from this population.

$$t = \frac{0.98 - 1.0}{0.01} = -2.0$$

Consulting a table of t values gives a probability value of 0.023 for t=2.0 and 2000×0.023 = 46, which would be the expected number of normals having this low value in our population of 2000.

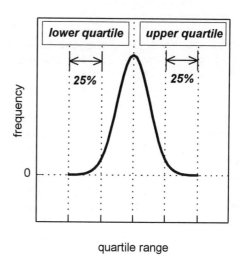

Figure 1.11 Quartile divisions of the normal curve

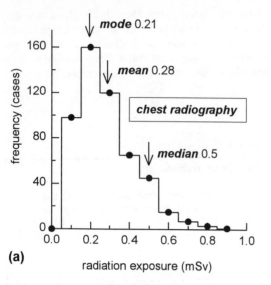

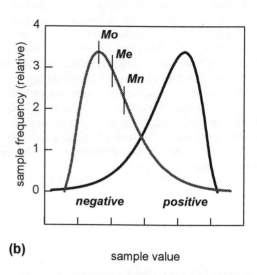

(a)

(b)

Figure 1.12 **(a)** Data example of chest exposure during plain film radiography representing the spread of entrance dose from a selection of hospitals. This data is used to calculate the mode, mean and median of this negative skewed distribution. **(b)** Continuous distributions showing negative and positive skewdness the mean *Mn*, mode *Mo* and median *Me* points are marked.

1.12.2 Measures for data spread

The crudest measure of overall spread is the distance between highest and lowest data values; this is the **range** but this is strongly influenced by **outlier** presence or abnormally high or low values.

The population can be simply divided into four groups (Fig.1.11) giving **quartiles**. The lower quartile being the lowest 25% and the upper quartile being the highest 25%, the inter-quartile range occupies the middle 50% and is a good measure of dispersion being immune from outlier interference. The median and quartiles are special cases of a general scheme for dividing a distribution by **quantiles**. As an example the data table in Table 1.6 shows a frequency range stretching from an exposure dose of 0.1 to 0.9mSv but from 0.6 onwards only small numbers are involved and this range figure gives a false impression. Other measures of dispersion are therefore required. The data given in this table is plotted in Fig.1.12(a).

These measurements represent the surface doses reported by various hospitals for chest radiography. The itemized dose values *x*, their frequency of occurrence *f* and the product of *fx* listed in the table are used in calculations. These data show a skewed distribution and separate mean, median and mode values of the distribution can be identified in the figure.

The mean The arithmetic mean $\bar{x}$ is the most common average value quoted for a set of data and is commonly found by adding together the individual values and dividing by the number of items. The data set featured as a grouped frequency distribution in Table 1.5 does not lend itself to this method of calculation so the mean is calculated from the frequency distribution in the table as:

$$\bar{x} = \frac{\Sigma fx}{\Sigma f} \qquad (1.35)$$

where Σf and Σfx values are the sum values. The arithmetic mean value for this data set is 0.28 and is marked on Fig.1.12(a).

The median This is the value of the item *x* which lies in the center of the distribution with half the data on one side and half on the other. It is calculated as $(n+1)/2$ where n is the number of items in the distribution. The median of the data plotted in Fig.1.12(a) is 0.5. If the position of the central point in the distribution is important then the median can be a useful average. This is the case where the data set contains extreme values which distort the overall picture. The median is immune to these and gives a more correct picture of frequency distribution. The disadvantage however is that the median value is unsuitable for calculation.

Table 1.6 Data for exposure dose during chest radiography plotted in Fig.1.12(a)

Dose (mSv) x	Frequency f	fx
0.1	98	9.8
0.2	160	32.0
0.3	120	36.0
0.4	65	26.0
0.5	45	22.5
0.6	15	9.0
0.7	7	4.9
0.8	3	2.4
0.9	1	0.9
Totals:	$\Sigma f = 514$	$\Sigma fx = 143.5$

The mode In some instances neither the mean nor median give the best description of a data set (this is the case for the skewed distribution in Fig.1.12(a)). The mean value is influenced by all the values and does not draw attention to extreme values which may be of significance. The median is the central value, dividing the data set in half, but this value may be unrepresentative, as it is in this case. The mode however is that value in a data set which occurs most frequently. The mode can be obtained by inspection (roughly) or by calculation (exactly) using the formula:

$$mode = L + \frac{f_M - f_L}{(f_M - f_L)+(f_M - f_H)} \times C \quad (1.36)$$

where L is the lower limit of the modal group (0.15) as the class intervals are 0.5-1.5, 1.5-2.5 etc., f_M is the frequency of the modal group (160), f_L the frequency of the neighboring lower group (98) and f_H the frequency of the higher neighboring group (120). The class or item interval distance C is 0.1. Using this equation the exact modal value is found to be 0.21.

The mean, mode and median values are identical in a normal distribution but if the distribution is not normal, containing extreme values (larger or smaller), then the distribution is skewed and the mean, mode and median do not coincide; negative and positive skewed distributions are demonstrated in Fig.1.12(b). These are commonly found in image dis-tribution maps where localized high count regions (organ uptake) will skew the data.

1.12.3 Standard deviation σ

A more stable value of data spread in a distribution comes from calculating how each variable differs from the mean value. This is the derivation of **variance** and the square root of the variance is the standard deviation. Standard deviations have been calculated already for binomial and Poisson distributions. A continuous distribution of n items requires a more complex calculation however:

$$\sigma = \sqrt{\frac{\Sigma(x-\bar{x})^2}{n-1}} \quad (1.37)$$

The normal distribution shown in Fig.1.13(a) plots the standard deviation as the x-axis the various areas of the normal curve and shows that the area covered from $\sigma = -1$ to $+1$ is 66% and from σ -2 to +2 covers 96% and σ -3 to +3 covers 99.8%.

The two sample populations shown in Fig.1.13(b) are of different size and give different standard deviations. They could be superimposed so giving the same mean value but their standard deviation value would distinguish them.

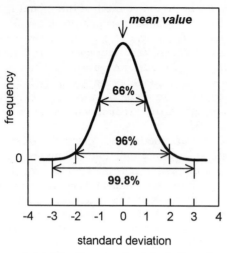 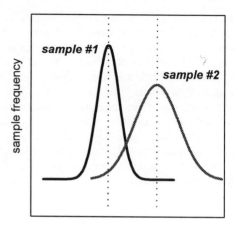

population distribution

Figure 1.13 (a) The standard deviation plotted on the *x*-axis and the areas under the normal curve that they cover. **(b)** Sample spread showing sample #1. with a narrow standard deviation and Sample #2 with a larger standard deviation. These samples could be from different populations (e.g. diseased and normal).

Standard error When samples are taken from a large population there is always an uncertainty between the sample mean and the parent population mean (the mean value for the entire count distribution). This is simply measured as:

$$standard\ error = \frac{\sigma}{\sqrt{n}} \qquad (1.38)$$

The standard error becomes smaller as the number of items increases. The standard error is most useful when calculating confidence limits which a selected quality control measurement should keep within.

Coefficient of variation A measure of spread within the sample uses the standard deviation expressed as a percentage of the mean:

$$CV = \frac{\sigma}{\bar{x}} \times 100\% \qquad (1.39)$$

From Table 1.7 it can be seen that larger sample sizes give smaller variations.

Table 1.7 Coefficient of variation

Observed count	σ	CV(%)
10	±3.2	31.6
100	±10.0	10.0
1000	±31.6	3.16
10000	±100.0	1.0

1.12.4 Statistics of counting

There will always some degree of error when collecting count data for imaging or sample quantitation. The sample accuracy or image quality depends on the number of counts taken or stored, as seen in Table 1.7. If the total counts collected are 100, 1000, 10,000 then the standard deviations are roughly 10, 32 and 100 showing that it requires about 1000 counts to achieve a coefficient of variation of 3%. To express the deviation in terms of counting rate the total time taken is used as a divisor. For 1000 counts in 10 seconds the deviation is:

$$\sqrt{\frac{1000}{10}} = 10 \text{ counts s}^{-1}$$

The counting rate would be expressed as 100 ± 10 counts s^{-1} which indicates that there is a 68.3% probability (1σ) that the counting error is <10 counts s^{-1} or 10%. If 10,000 counts are collected over 100 seconds the uncertainty remains the same (10 counts s^{-1}) but the accuracy is now 1%. The greater the number of counts collected (which could be met either as a count rate sample or in an image pixel) the smaller the error due to statistical fluctuations.

Background counts There is always a background count due to either natural radiation or interfering radiation sources. These can be caused by:

- Other radioactive sources in the vicinity i.e. patients, natural radiation or other active samples, in the case of sample counting.
- Scattered radiation from other parts of the body in the case of radiography.

When the sample count is large compared with the background the standard error can be estimated with little error. When the background and sample counts are not greatly different then the background must be considered. It should be noted that percentages and ratios are comparative measurements and so should not be used as data in any form of statistical analysis.

Sampling interval This plays an important role when measuring dynamic events. Fig.1.14 illustrates two sampling intervals *A* and *B*. The under-sampling in *A* misses detail of the fast changes in the initial stages of a tissue or organ uptake which is shown in *B* having many more samples. Over-sampling does not add to the information but requires more storage space and takes longer to analyze.

1.12.5 Sample data analysis

Only a brief introduction will be given to statistical analysis routines. A list of suitable statistics books for the medical scientist is given at the end of the chapter. Problems which require the use of statistics can usually be reduced to one of three basic tests:

- A significant **difference** between two data sets from different populations. Finding a trend in a sample: the **regression**
- Testing for the similarity between samples: the **correlation**.

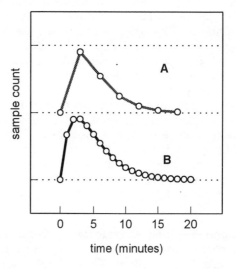

Figure 1.14   Activity-time curves obtained from a kidney GFR study. Under-sampling (A) misses the fast vascular changes revealed in (B) which has more samples.

Difference between samples   This is broadly divided into:

- **parametric** tests where population quantities are used i.e. means, variances, or standard deviations
- **non-parametric** tests that do not use population parameters and present the data often in the form of scores or ranks.

If we wish to test the hypothesis that two data

sets plotted in Fig.1.13(b) are significantly different and do not form part of the same larger population, then a simple Student's 't' test will indicate if the sample mean value could have come from a population with a known mean and estimated standard deviation value. Most books on statistics will give the basic Student's 't' formula for this computation giving also the corrections that must be made for small sample numbers. More rigorous methods of analysis are available, as for example the analysis of variance (Anova) tests for the variance within each sample.

Non-parametric tests that have a lower overall power than their parametric equivalent utilize scores or ranking marks in their dataset. These, of course, would be distribution free, not having means, variances or standard deviations. Examples would be a ranking of (say) 1 to 5 to describe the confidence of visualizing a lesion in a particular radiograph, which has been processed in two different ways (gray scale or color for instance).

The Tukey quick-test decides whether two independent ranked samples could have been drawn from the same population. A Mann-Whitney test is equivalent to the 't' test which scores the difference between the medians of two distributions. The Kruskal-Wallis test is the non-parametric version of an Anova.

Regression and Correlation These tests determine how variables x and y are related linearly. The graph in Fig.1.15 is a scatter diagram which gives a rough idea how the variables x and y are related (if at all). A number is needed however that is a measure of how linear the relationship is between x and y: this is the **sample correlation coefficient** r; ranging from -1 to $+1$. A value of $+1$ indicates perfect linear relationship where y increases with x; a value of -1 indicates a perfect negative relationship, a decreasing value of y with x. Zero indicates total random distribution between x and y.

The correlation coefficient is a measure of the linear relationship between x and y but it does not indicate what the relationship is. It is often necessary to know the trend of the relationship for certain values of x, so that a

prediction can be made: if a value for x is given then the probable value of y can be calculated. The slope of the **regression line** will give this.

Both x and y for the correlation coefficient are random variables; it is not known *a priori* the distribution or relationship. The regression analysis, however, can select certain values of x (fixed population characteristics) so they are not random. The y values retain their random nature since these are not controlled.

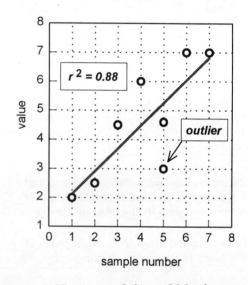

Figure 1.15 A set of data which shows some positive correlation characteristics ($r = 0.88$). A regression analysis shows a rough linear relationship using a least squares calculation.

KEYWORDS

2π surface: relating to a flat radiation detector

4π surface: relating to a volume radiation detector

abscissa: the horizontal x-axis of a graph usually holding the independent variable

coefficient of variation: a measure of dispersion as the standard deviation expressed as a percentage of the mean.

correlation coefficient: a measure of association between two random variables. If one variable changes with the other then they are said to be correlated.

data set (or set): a collection of numbers that usually have one common property.

decimal place: the figures to the right of the decimal point giving a specified degree of accuracy.

deterministic: a model where all events are inevitable consequences of antecedent causes. An effect seen at a predefined point (count rate, dose etc.)

dispersion: the spread of a distribution (see standard deviation and quartile)

e: symbol for the transcendental number 2.718 282... used as the base for the natural logarithm (also see exponential)

extrapolation: estimation of a value of a variable beyond known values

exponent: indicator for decimal point shift (left or right) in scientific notation, or in an exponential function x^n then n is the exponent.

exponential: most commonly used when the exponent is the power of e. The exponential of x is e^x

floating point: a method of writing real numbers as $a \times 10^n$ or aEn where $a<1$ but ≥ 0.1 and n is the integer exponent directing decimal point position '−' left, '+' right. For example 0.564E−1 = 0.0564. A format also used in computing.

Fourier analysis: a method of waveform analysis

histogram: a chart which displays grouped data.

integer: a whole number

interpolation: estimation of a value of a variable between two known values.

isotropic: emitting in all directions (spherical emission)

least squares: a way of estimating the best fit straight line for a plotted set of values

logarithm: the power to which a fixed number, the base, must be raised to obtain a given number. Abbreviated to log for base$_{10}$ and ln for base$_e$.

normal distribution: a continuous distribution of a random variable with its mean, median and mode equal.

null hypothesis: usually based upon the assumption that nothing special is different between two samples. a statistical test challenges this assumption. if the significance of the difference (probability) is sufficiently large then the null hypothesis is rejected

ordinate: the y-axis of a graph

outlier: observation which is far removed from the others in a set.

parametric (non-parametric): pertaining to exact measurement (count density, weights, temperature etc.). Non-parametric measurements are scores or ranks.

power law: a function giving a straight line when plotted on log-log axes.

quantile: general name for the values of a variable which divide its distribution into equal groups.

quartile: the value of a variable below which three-quarters (first or upper quartile) or one-quarter (3rd or lower quartile) of a distribution lie.

radian (rad): the SI unit of plane angle where one rad is 57.2958°

rational (irrational) number: having a fixed number of decimal places. An irrational number would be π or e

regression: a test which calculates the best fit for a straight line through a set of points on a graph when y is the dependent variable and x the independent (see least squares).

scientific notation: a numerical form similar to floating point: $a \times 10^n$ or aEn where a is a number 1 to 10 and n is a whole number as before, i.e. $5.64E{-}2 = 0.0564$

significance: a probability of rejecting the null hypothesis. $p = 0.05$ borderline significance, $p = 0.01$ significant, $p = 0.001$ highly significant

sine wave: a wave-function where $y = \sin(x)$

skew: a distribution where mean, mode and median do not coincide.

standard deviation: a measure of sample dispersion. square root of the variance.

standard error: standard error of the sample mean. A comparison of the sample mean with the parent mean $\sigma/\sqrt{n}$

steradian: the solid angle in spherical geometry

stochastic: an entirely random process.

variable, continuous: a variable that may take any value.

variable, dependent: a variable dependent on another. usually placed on the y-axis.

variable, discrete: the opposite to continuous. a variable that may only take certain values.

variable, independent: a variable not dependent on another, usually placed on the x-axis.

variance: a measure of dispersion.

Recommended reading

Colton, T. *Statistics in Medicine*, Little Brown

Porkess, R. *Dictionary of Statistics*, Collins Reference

2
Basic physics for radiology

2.1 International system of units
2.2 Force, mass, momentum
2.3 Work, energy, power
2.4 Density, pressure
2.5 Heat
2.6 Sound

2.7 Waves and oscillations
2.8 Electromagnetic radiation
2.9 Atomic and nuclear structure
2.10 Magnetism
2.11 Electricity
2.12 Electronics

2.1 INTERNATIONAL SYSTEM OF UNITS

The Système International (SI) has been chosen as the standard measurement system in physics. A few units have already been given in Sec.1.1, a complete set of basic units is given in Tab.2.1. If all the quantities in a calculation are expressed in SI units then the answer will hold the SI unit format.

Table 2.1   SI Base Units

Quantity	Name	Symbol
Length	meter	m
Mass	kilogram	kg
Time	second	s
Temperature	kelvin	K
Electric current	ampere	A
Luminous intensity	candela	cd
Amount of substance	mole	mol

A table of derived SI units is given in the Appendix, along with two supplementary units: the radian and the steradian, which are units for plane and solid angles respectively.

Non-metric measurements: mile, pound, inch and gallon are not used, however certain metric non-SI units are still retained and equivalent SI units are given in Tab.2.2 for these.

Table 2.2 Frequently encountered non-SI units and their equivalents.

Non-SI	SI-unit	Application
angstrom 10^{-10}m	10^{-9}m (nm)	wavelength
micron 10^{-6}m	10^{-9}m (nm)	wavelength
erg	joule (J) (10^{7}erg)	energy
curie	becquerel (Bq)	activity
g cm^{-3}	kg m^{-3}	density
mm Hg	pascal (Pa)	pressure

2.2   FORCE, MASS, MOMENTUM

Force is that which alters or tends to alter the motion of a body. The force with which the earth attracts a body is the **weight** of a body; its **mass** is the amount of substance in the body. Weight differs according to the object's position on earth. Outside the earth's gravitational pull, in space, an object will be in a weightless condition but its mass would not have changed.

Momentum is the product of the mass and the velocity of the body. These are fundamental concepts and play an important role in x-ray tube design since a heavy rotating metal anode gives considerable problems concerning force, mass and momentum.

2.2.1   Force

The Newton N is the force F which gives a mass of 1kg an acceleration of 1m s^{-2} so:

$$F = ma \qquad (2.1)$$

All objects fall with the same acceleration due to the earth's gravity which is about 9.8m s^{-2} (neglecting air resistance).   The force on a mass of 1kg due to gravity, from eqn. 2.1, is 1×9.8 = 9.8N
If the mass is 100kg then the force due to gravity is 980N, so mass and weight are proportional (mass∝ weight). A common balance compares masses but a spring balance will indicate weights since it will be influenced by gravity.

2.2.2 Mass

Newton's first law recognizes that objects have a reluctance to move when they are at rest. They also have a reluctance to stop when they are moving; this is the object's **inertia**.
  The mass of the object is a measure of the amount of matter and its inertia and is expressed in kilograms. The force of attraction on an object's mass, due to gravity, is its **weight** as already stated above.

2.2.3 Momentum

  The momentum of a moving object is mass times velocity. Force F is momentum change per second (mass × velocity change). As velocity change per second is acceleration a then momentum is also described by eqn.2.1.

The conservation of momentum   This is a fundamental law of physics which is central when considering elastic and inelastic collisions between objects (radiation and orbital electrons). In both cases although there may be a change in energy the total momentum is conserved. An example of conservation of momentum and momentum change during braking is given in Box 2.1.

Box 2.1

Conservation of momentum and momentum change

A mass A colliding with a stationary mass B using the basic formula $F = ma$.

Example A
Mass A of 0.5kg has a velocity of 1.5m s^{-1}. Its momentum is 0.5×1.5 = 0.75 m s^{-1}.
This collides with a stationary object B of mass 1kg. The total mass is now 1.5kg.

Velocity on collision is $\dfrac{0.75}{1.5}$ kg = 0.5m s^{-1}
So original momentum 0.5×1.5 is the same as the resultant momentum 1.5×0.5

Example B
A mass of 50kg moving at 1m s^{-1} has a momentum of 50×1 = 50 kg m s^{-1}. A mass with a momentum of 150 kg m s^{-1} comes to rest in 6s. The momentum change per second is
$$\frac{150}{6} = 25N$$
Shortening the time to 0.5 second increases the momentum change is 300N

The braking force required to bring an object to rest depends on time to rest. Rotating parts in radiology (x-ray tube anode, CT fan beam assembly) produce problems during acceleration and braking; in practice their momentum change is reduced by decreasing the object mass.

2.3   WORK, ENERGY, POWER

Work   This is done when a force F moves a body a certain distance d.   The work done is $F \times d$ and is measured in **joules** (J).

Energy   This is the ability to do work and is also measured in joules. The total energy of a closed system remains constant, however it may be transformed. It may take the form of mechanical energy which can be either potential or kinetic energy. Other forms of energy are electrical, chemical and heat.

Power The rate of doing work or the time taken to do an amount of work. The SI unit is the watt (W) and 1J = 1W s.

Friction This causes energy losses which are commonly seen as an increase in system heat. Since friction always opposes motion a moving body experiences a frictional force. This is not confined to solids, it is also experienced by fluids and gases caused by viscous drag between layers of molecules.

2.3.1 Work

Work W is the force F multiplied by the distance d moved by the force:

$$W = F \times d \qquad \text{joules} \qquad (2.2)$$

One joule of work is a force of 1N moving through a distance of 1m. The capacity to do work involves either kinetic or potential energy.

$$1J = 1\ N\ m$$

2.3.2 Energy

Potential energy is the energy of a body due to its condition or state. Examples would be given by batteries (power supplies) or gravitation. The amount of potential energy is measured by the work the system performs until the energy source reaches its ground state.

Kinetic energy This increases with mass m and velocity v. If an object is brought to rest in time t the final velocity is zero so from eqn 2.1:

$$F = ma = \text{momentum change s}^{-1} = \frac{mv}{t}$$

If over the distance d, moved by the object in a time t, the velocity diminishes uniformly from v to zero, then:

$$d = \text{average velocity} \times \text{time} = \frac{v}{2} \times t$$

Work done (kinetic energy) is E_k and

$$E_k = F \times s = \frac{mv}{t} \times \frac{vt}{2}$$

The time t cancels to give:

$$E_k = \tfrac{1}{2} mv^2 \qquad (2.3)$$

Equation 2.3 defines **kinetic energy** and a calculated example is given in Box 2.2.

Forms of kinetic energy

- Translational where the entire object moves.
- Rotational given by object spin.
- Vibrational where small masses move back and forth.

Simple gas molecules, having one atom (hydrogen, helium, oxygen etc.) only have translational kinetic energy. More complex gas molecules (H_2O, NH_4) may have rotational and vibrational kinetic energy.

Box 2.2

Kinetic energy

An object of mass 2kg moves with a velocity of 1m s^{-1}. From eqn 2.3 it has a kinetic energy of:

$$= \tfrac{1}{2} mv^2 = \tfrac{1}{2} \times 2 \times 1^2 \text{ Joules}$$
$$= 1\ J$$

If the velocity is doubled the kinetic energy will increase ×4 so a 2kg object at 2m s^{-1}:
$$= \tfrac{1}{2} \times 2 \times 2^2 \text{ J}$$
$$= 4\ J$$

Conservation of energy This is a basic physical law that states: in a given system, the total amount of energy is always constant although the energy may change from one form to another (i.e. electrical energy into light and heat energy). The total amount of energy is obtained by adding the kinetic and potential energies.

2.3.3 Power

This is defined as the rate of doing work (spending energy) per second:

$$Power = \frac{work\ done}{time\ taken}$$

it is measured in joules per second the SI unit being watts W.

$$1\ W = 1\ J\ s^{-1}$$

Electrical energy is measured in joules and electrical power in watts as shown in Box 2.3

Heat units HU when electrons bombard the anode of an x-ray tube their energy in converted into x-rays and heat. The heat capacity of an anode is commonly expressed in Heat Units HU which depend on the applied kilovoltage V and the electron density or current I per unit time s so:

$$HU = V \times I \times s \qquad (2.4)$$

The conversion to and from joules is:

$$HU \times 0.74 = joules \qquad (2.5)$$
$$joules \times 1.35 = HU$$

The energy rating for x-ray anodes range from 250kJ to 3.5MJ and eqns. 2.4 and 2.5 will be used in later chapters when describing x-ray tube heat rating.

Box 2.3

Work / Power relationships.

Electrical energy
The total amount of energy required to generate 1kW of electrical work for 1 hour is:
$$1000 \times (60\times60) = 3.6\times10^6 = 3.6MJ$$

Electrical power
1800 Joules of work are completed over a period of 5 minutes. The power generated is:

$$1800/(5\times60) = 5\ W$$

Summary

- Mass is a measure of inertia (units: kilogram). Force is mass × acceleration (newton)
- Momentum is mass × velocity
- Work is force × distance (joules)
- Energy is the capacity for doing work (joules)
- Power is the rate of doing work (joules s^{-1} or watt)
- The efficiency of a system is power obtained divided by power supplied. This is never 100% due to heat production and loss.

2.4   DENSITY, PRESSURE

2.4.1   Density

The physical density of a body ρ is its mass (kg) divided by its volume (m^3). The density will be the same for any object made of the identical material; it will vary if the material's composition is changed. Density is also a term used in radiology to describe the opacity of a photographic image; the two terms are obviously not related.

Density of a substance ρ is its weight relative to volume, so:

$$\rho = \frac{mass}{volume} \qquad (2.6)$$

The SI unit is kg m^{-3} although non-SI g cm^{-3} is often used. A conversion factor of 10^{-3} converts g cm^{-3} to kg m^{-3}. So if 50g of aluminum displaces 18.5cm^3 of water its density is:

$$\rho = \frac{50}{18.5} = 2.70g\ cm^{-3}\ or\ 2700\ kg\ m^{-3}$$

The density of elements (aluminum, tungsten, uranium) usually follow their atomic number

(Z) however there are exceptions as shown in Tab.2.3. Water has a density of 1000kg m^{-3} (1g cm^{-3}) and this liquid is used as a reference for density measurements. The relative density for aluminum is therefore just 2700. The density of a substance divided by the density of water is the specific gravity or relative density; for a gas the relative substance is usually air.

Table 2.3   Density of some materials

Atomic No. Z	Material	Density kg m^{-3}
	Air	1.225
	Water	1000
13	Aluminum	2700
26	Iron	7870
29	Copper	8900
42	Molybdenum	10200
73	Tantalum	16600
74	Tungsten	19320
76	Osmium	22480
79	Gold	19300
82	Lead	11340

The Mole   is the amount of substance which contains as many elementary entities as there are atoms in 0.012kg of carbon (^{12}C). the elementary entities may be atoms, molecules, ions, electrons or other particles or groups of particles as shown in Box.2.4. The number of elementary particles is a constant known as **Avogadro's constant** and is 6.022 ×10^{23} mol^{-1}

2.4.2 Pressure

Pressure may be caused by the weight of material pressing on its surface or by collisions of atoms or molecules of gas within a container (i.e. gas radiation detectors); it acts in all directions. The SI unit is the pascal (B. Pascal 1623-62: French mathematician). This is related to the newton as one pascal (Pa) equals 1Nm^{-2}. Atmospheric pressure is about 1.01×10^5 Pa or approximately 10^5 Nm^{-2}.

The non-SI unit mm Hg extensively used in

medicine is retained by agreement and is related:

$$1mm\ Hg = 1.33\times10^2\ Pa$$

Standard atmospheric pressure previously given as 760mm Hg is now taken as 10^{5}Pa.

Box 2.4

Molar quantities

Example 1. (Molar solution)
Sodium chloride (saline) has a molecular weight of 23 + 35 = 58 and so one liter contains 58g for a 1.0M solution and 5.8g for a decimolar solution 0.1M

Example 2. (Electron density *e*)
Atoms per mole = 6.022×10^{23} = *N*
Atomic mass = *A*   Atoms per unit mass = *N/A*
Since Z (atomic number) = electron number

Electron density $e = N \times Z/A$

	Z	A	e (×10^{23})
H	1	1	6.02
O	8	16	3.01
N	7	14	3.01
C	6	12	3.01
I	53	127	2.50
Ba	56	138	2.44
Pb	82	207	2.38

NB
Lighter elements have greater electron density. This plays an important part in x-ray interactions.

Pressure *p* is defined as the force per unit area:

$$p = \frac{total\ force\ on\ surface\ F}{area\ of\ surface\ A} \qquad (2.7)$$

Hence pressure is not the same as force and the result of eqn.2.7 is measured in newtons per square meter (Nm^{-2}). This is true for incompressible substances solids and liquids.

Gas laws   The variation of pressure, volume and temperature on a gas, Boyle's Law (Robert Boyle 1627-91; Irish physicist) together with Charles' Law (JA Charles,1746-

1823; French physicist) form basic relation-ships in physics and also feature in the pro-pagation of sound through air.

Boyle's Law states that pressure is inversely proportional to volume at constant temp-erature and Charles' Law states that volume and temperature are proportional at constant pressure. Summarizing these two statements gives:

$$PV/T = \text{a constant} \tag{2.8}$$

The gas laws play an important academic role in the derivation of the SI scale for temperature. The increase in volume per unit volume of gas at 0°C per °C rise in temperature keeping pressure constant forms a volume coefficient *a*:

$$\frac{\text{increase in volume from } 0^\circ C}{\text{original volume at } 0^\circ C \times \text{temperature rise}}$$

This is a constant whose accurate measure-ments indicate a value of 3.6609×10^{-3} or $1/273.15$ °C^{-1} for all gases.

Charles' Law states that a given mass of gas increases by $1/273.15$ of its volume at 0°C for every degree rise in temperature at constant pressure.

Lord Kelvin (1824-1907; British physicist) originated his Kelvin temperature scale where 0°C is 273.15K and 0K (zero K or absolute zero) is –273.15°C, the magnitude of each division is identical: 1°C is the same size as 1K. The degree kelvin K is the SI unit of temperature.

Standard temperature and pressure (stp) In order to make comparisons (i.e. relative density) many measurements are made at standard temperature and pressure (stp). The standard temperature is 298.15K (25°C) and the pressure is 10^5Pa (about 760mm Hg).

2.5   HEAT

Heat is a form of energy that gives atoms and molecules increased movement or kinetic energy. Thermodynamics is the study of heat transfer. Since heat is a form of energy it can be measured in joules and watts.

Heat is transmitted from one place to an-other by **conduction**, **convection** and **radiation**. All of these play a very important part in radiology equipment (x-ray tubes, generators).

2.5.1 Temperature

Two temperature scales are used for measuring change in heat output:

- Celsius or centigrade: 0°C is melting ice and 100°C is boiling water both at normal pressure 10^5 N m^{-2}
- Kelvin: Zero degrees Kelvin (0K) is absolute zero, equivalent to –273.15°C The melting point of ice is therefore 273.15K.
- Celsius and Kelvin scales have the same magnitude so a one degree change in either scale is the same.

The kelvin is the SI Unit and its derivation has been given from the gas laws stated above.

2.5.2   Thermal capacity

Specific heat or specific heat capacity
(J kg^{-1} K^{-1}) The specific heat of a substance is the heat required to increase the temp-erature of 1kg by 1K (or 1°C). As an example 42 joules of heat would increase the temperature of:

2g water	by 5 °C
2g Aluminum	by 20 °C
2g Copper	by 50 °C

Table 2.4 lists values of specific heat for common substances and the reason for choosing water and oil for heating and cooling liquids is obvious from their capacity to both store and transport heat. Water is a good reservoir for excess heat or a good cooling

medium whereas aluminum and copper take up heat rapidly and since they are also good heat conductors, are able to conduct it away rapidly. The specific heat of gases varies according to pressure.

Table 2.4 Specific heats of common materials

Substance	Specific heat (J kg^{-1} K^{-1})
Water	4180
Oil	2130
Aluminum	910
Copper	386
Tungsten	136

Thermal capacity (J K^{-1} or °C^{-1}) This is the characteristic of the material independent of its size or shape and is the heat required to raise its temperature by 1K or 1°C. The thermal capacity of 1000 liters of water is larger than that of 1cm^3 of water.

Latent heat (J kg^{-1}) The amount of heat per unit mass that is added to or removed from a substance undergoing a change of state i.e. from solid to liquid or liquid to gas. If heat is applied to ice the temperature of the ice remains at 0°C until all the ice has changed to water. The heat required to change the ice to water is the hidden or latent heat.

Latent heat of fusion A change of state from solid to liquid. The definition is the quantity of heat required to change 1g of the solid, at the melting point, to a liquid at the same temperature. Ice has a latent heat of fusion of 336 joules.

Latent heat of vaporization A change of state from liquid to vapor. The definition is the quantity of heat required to change 1g of substance from its liquid to its vapor state at the boiling point. This is 2260 joules for steam, so a great deal of energy is removed from the system when water changes from liquid to steam.

Table 2.5 Latent heats (MJ kg^{-1})

Substance	LH (vaporization)
Water	2.260
Alcohol	0.850

Evaporation This is the change of liquid to vapor. Liquids vary in the ease with which they change. Liquids which evaporate easily have a low boiling point e.g. volatile liquids. Latent heat is needed to change from liquid to vapor and this heat is absorbed (taken) from the surface. Liquids with large latent heats (water) remove heat more effectively. Table 2.5 lists the latent heats for two liquids, water and alcohol, in MJ kg^{-1} showing the much larger latent heat for water.

2.5.3 Thermal transfer

Conduction Heat is conducted by molecular vibration along the material and sets up vibrations which is communicated to other molecules. Heat is transferred along the substance without any alteration in the position of the molecule.

Thermal conductivity The speed of heat transfer, measured in watts per meter per degree kelvin (or Celsius) W m^{-1} K^{-1} (°C^{-1}). It is the characteristic of the material independent of size or shape. Table 2.6 lists conductivities and melting points of some important substances to radiology.

The heat current can be large for materials with high values of thermal conductivity; these are good heat conductors such as silver and copper. Copper is used for conducting heat in the x-ray tube. Tungsten is a fair conductor of heat but has a high melting point so is ideal for the x-ray tube target. Molybdenum is a poor heat conductor so is used as the anode stem protecting the bearings from conducted heat. Substances with small values would be poor heat conductors but good insulators (air and oil); they transfer heat by convection.

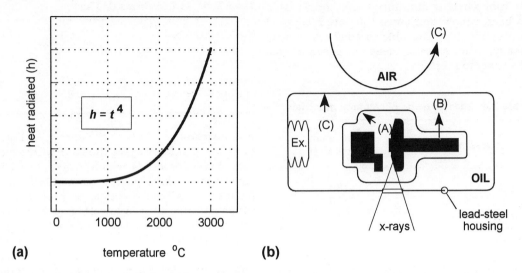

Figure 2.1   **(a)** Heat radiated from a surface is proportional to the fourth power of its temperature. **(b)** Heat loss from an x-ray tube housing. Heat is radiated from the anode (A) conducted away from the glass/ceramic tube case by conduction through the bearing (B) and convection currents through the oil (C) then by the surrounding atmospheric air. Expansion of the oil is taken up by the bellows (Ex)

Table 2.6 Materials useful to radiology

Substance	Therm. cond. $(W\,m^{-1}\,K^{-1})$	Melting point °C
Silver	427	961
Copper	401	1083
Aluminum	237	660
Tungsten	178	3377
Molybdenum	140	2607
Nickel	89	1453
Glass	0.9-1.3	1127
Oil	0.15	
Water	0.59	0
Air	0.02	

Convection In liquids heat causes a fluid to expand making it less dense so it rises. The cold denser fluid takes its place. The heat in this case is carried by moving molecules. This can be achieved by natural convection or by pumping (forced convection).

In gases the convection of heat occurs more readily since gases expand considerably more when heated. Convection currents in air remove heat from a x-ray tube housing to the atmosphere. Oil and then water circulation (forced convection) remove heat from large x-ray installations (CT).

Radiation   The transfer of heat by conduction and convection requires a material medium either solid, liquid or gas, for its transport but heat can be transmitted through a vacuum by radiation (infra-red). The radiation from a body depends on the nature of its surface and on its temperature t; it also depends on its area. The intensity I of radiation emitted by a body is proportional to t^4. Thus a doubling of the surface temperature increases the heat intensity by 2^4 or ×16. The relationship $I \propto t^4$ is plotted in Fig.2.1(a) showing the rate of heat loss increases with the temperature of the surface. This is a most important factor when operating an x-ray tube near its maximum rating since heat loss radiated from the anode is highest at this point.

Emission and absorption For a given temperature a body radiates most heat when its surface is matt black and least when it is highly polished; graphite is an ideal radiator so it is most useful in x-ray tube anode construction. A blackened surface is both a good emitter and absorber. A polished surface is a poor absorber and emitter but is a good reflector of heat.

Relevance to radiology From the simplified sketch of an x-ray tube housing in Fig.2.1(b) it is evident that conduction, radiation and convection play a vital role in removing excess heat from an x-ray tube during operation. Choice of material and the dimensions influence heat transfer. The tungsten target reaches extremely high temperatures (about 3000 °C) and although it has a high melting point it also has a low specific heat so excess heat must be removed quickly. This is achieved by radiation from the anode surface ($\propto t^4$). Surface area is best increased by adding graphite which increases the surface area without adding undue weight. Molybdenum is chosen as a support stem since its low thermal conductivity protects the bearings of the rotating anode (see Table 2.6). Radiated heat is absorbed by the x-ray tube envelope (glass or ceramic/metal) which is then conducted to an oil bath which loses heat by convection to the atmosphere. Oil is chosen as a heat conducting medium mainly for its insulating properties and high boiling point. Its thermal conductivity is poor but since it has a relatively high specific heat (Table 2.4) it acts as a good heat reservoir.

2.5.4 Expansion

Most materials expand when their temperature increases. Gases show the greatest expansion of all on heating. Expansion in metals is measured as a coefficient of linear expansion which is defined as the increase in length, per unit length, for a temperature changes of 1K, an example is given in Box 2.5.

The coefficient of expansion for materials used in radiology are listed in Tab. 2.7.

Expansion causes problems in x-ray tube construction where conducting metal contacts are brought out through the insulating glass envelope. The excessive heat produced during x-ray production would cause failure at these joints unless glass and metal are closely matched for their expansion properties. Low expansion glass and metal alloys are used to achieve this.

Table 2.7 Expansion of some common materials

Solid	Expansion $(10^{-5} K^{-1})$
Glass	0.8
Lead	2.9
Aluminum	2.3
Copper	1.7
Molybdenum	0.5
Tungsten	0.45

The relatively small expansion shown by molybdenum and tungsten make these ideal metals for x-ray tube construction where considerable heat is experienced, however heavy duty anodes are protected from non-uniform expansion by placing stress-cuts along their circumference.

Heating effect by compression This is the converse of expansion by heating and can only be observed in gases, since solids and liquids are incompressible. Compression increases the gas density so more molecules collide with the surface and therefore more kinetic energy is turned into heat.

Box 2.5

Expansion of metal

1 meter of steel increases its length to 1.10m when the temperature rises by 90°C.
The Linear Coefficient of Expansion is:

$$\frac{1.10}{1000 \times 90} = 1.22 \times 10^{-5} K^{-1}$$

NB As the coefficient is a percentage value no units of measurement are included.

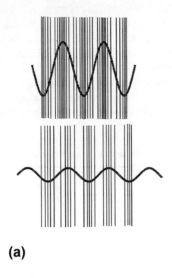

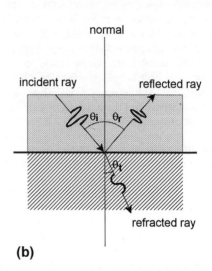

(a)   **(b)**

Figure 2.2   (a) Sound energy transmitted by compression and rarefaction giving a pressure equivalent sine waveform. **(b)** Reflection and refraction of the incident sound wave. The incident angle θ_i and angles of reflection θ_r and refraction θ_t are marked.

2.6   SOUND

Sound is a longitudinal wave made up of areas in a material (air, tissue, water etc.) where the density and pressure are higher (compression) or lower (rarefaction) than normal. Figure 2.2(a) illustrates the compression and rarefaction events. The amplitude of the wave corresponds to denser compression events. High frequency is represented by denser packing of the compression and rarefaction events.

Velocity of sound in medium depends on density ρ and elasticity K: the velocity of sound v in a gas obeys:

$$v = \sqrt{\frac{K}{\rho}} \qquad (2.9)$$

Boyle's Law states that gas volume is inversely proportional to pressure:

$$V \propto \frac{1}{P}$$

and as gas density is proportional to pressure then sound velocity is independent of pressure changes. From Charles' Law at constant pressure $V \propto T$; since $V \propto 1/\rho$ then $1/\rho \propto T$. Therefore at constant pressure:

$$\text{velocity} \propto \sqrt{T} \qquad (2.10)$$

A list of sound velocities is given in Tab.2.8. where the velocity of sound in air is approximately 330m s^{-1} being independent of pressure but proportional to $\sqrt{T}$ as stated above.

Table 2.8   Sound velocity in m s^{-1}

Material	Velocity
Air	330
Helium	1000
Water	1540
Soft Tissue	1540
Bone	4080
Aluminum	6400

2.6.1 Reflection and refraction

Reflection Sound is reflected from a smooth surface. Smooth is defined as any unevenness in the surface is much less than the wavelength; this gives **specular** reflection. A rough surface will give **non-specular** reflection.

For specular reflection, shown in Fig.2.2(b), the angle of incidence is equal to the angle of reflection. The angle of incidence θ_i between the direction of motion of the incident wave and the normal (perpendicular from the surface) is equal to the angle of reflection θ_r.

Refraction The sound wave may be partially reflected and the remaining wave front traveling through the new medium. The **transmitted** wave will change direction depending on material composition. The beam is refracted owing to the fact that the speed of sound is different in the two materials. The frequency of the sound will not change but the wavelength will. This will be less in the material in which the wave travels more slowly. The angle between the refracted wave and the normal is the angle of refraction.

Snell's Law (W. Snell 1591-1626; Dutch physicist) The sine of the incident angle divided by the sine of the angle of refraction is a constant. This constant is the refractive index.

$$refractive\ index = \frac{sin\,\theta_i}{sin\,\theta_t} \qquad (2.11)$$

2.6.2 Intensity

Intensity is the sound power per unit area and proportional to pressure squared: $I \propto P^2$. Sound intensity is measured $J\ s^{-1}\ m^{-2}$ or $W\ m^{-2}$. As an example normal conversation has an intensity of 10^{-7} to $10^{-4}W\ m^{-2}$ and the threshold of hearing is $10^{-12}\ W\ m^{-2}$. Ultrasound is measured in $10^{-3}\ W\ m^{-2}$ ($mW\ cm^{-2}$)

The decibel (Alexander Graham Bell 1847-1922; British inventor) is a ratio measure of relative powers or intensities. It uses a logarithmic scale. Relative **intensities** are measured as:

$$dB = 10\ log_{10}\frac{I}{I_o} \qquad (2.12)$$

where I_o is the reference sound level commonly 10^{-12} W m^{-2} at 1kHz at audible levels. A sound level of 20dB is ×10 more intense than a 10dB sound level. A 3dB change halves or doubles the sound intensity. When comparing the pressure or **amplitude** differences a factor of 20 is used:

$$dB = 20\ log_{10}\frac{A}{A_o} \qquad (2.13)$$

Whereas the half power value is 3dB in eqn.2.12, the half amplitude is 6dB in eqn.2.13. The attenuation given by a material is quoted as dB mm^{-1}; this is the attenuation coefficient α. Decibel scales are compared in Appendix I.

The speed of sound is frequency independent but α is influenced strongly by frequency. For soft tissue $\alpha=0.1$dB mm^{-1} so 3cm of tissue will reduce the intensity by 50%; bone will give $\alpha=1.3$dB mm^{-1} attenuation. The attenuation coefficient is the sum of the individual coefficients for scatter and absorption.

Intensity and amplitude By reference to Chapter 1 Fig.1.6(a) a sound pressure wave P passing through two spheres of radius r_1 and r_2 gives an intensity:

$$I = \frac{P}{4\pi r^2} \qquad (2.14)$$

The total energy passing through *sphere$_1$* must equal *sphere$_2$*. Since $4\pi r^2$ is the surface area of a sphere then the average intensity falls off as the **inverse square** from the point source. So the in intensity of a spherical wave decreases as $1/r^2$. The **amplitude** A decreases with distance as $1/r$ since:

$$A_2 = A_1\left[\frac{r_1}{r_2}\right] \qquad (2.15)$$

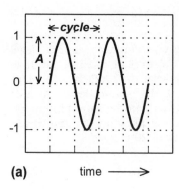 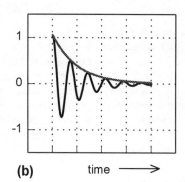 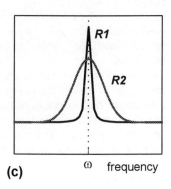

Figure 2.3   (a) A sine waveform showing amplitude, wavelength, measured as a complete cycle. (b) a damped sine-wave showing exponential loss of amplitude. (c) a frequency ω at resonance giving a strong peak intensity.

Further properties of sound, as related to medical imaging, are discussed in Chapter 17.

2.7   WAVES AND OSCILLATIONS

Oscillations in the form of sound or radio-frequency waveforms play a most important part in radiology. The interactions of sound waves and radio-waves show the same general behavior:

* harmonic motion
* signal decay
* signal resonance.
* interference between signals having different frequency and phase.

The waveform characteristics of oscillating signals can be analyzed using a Fourier transform as previously described in Chapter 1.

2.7.1 Simple harmonic motion

Simple harmonic motion occurs when the force acting on a system is directly pro-portional to its displacement x from a fixed

point. The variation of x with time follows a sine relationship:

$$x = a \sin \omega t \qquad (2.16)$$

where a is the amplitude of the waveform or the greatest displacement from the equi-librium position. The constant ω equals $2\pi f$ where f is the frequency of oscillation mea-sured in cycles per second or hertz (Hz). The period T of the waveform which is a measure of the time to undergo one complete cycle is $1/f$ so $\omega = 2\pi/T$. Each time the waveform completes a cycle it moves forward a distance λ, the wavelength. Equation 2.16 is used to plot the sine-wave in Fig.2.3(a). In one second when f vibrations occur the wave moves forward a distance $f\lambda$. Hence the velocity c of the waves, which is the distance a peak moves in one second, is:

$$c = f\lambda \qquad (2.17)$$

2.7.2 Damping and resonance

The amplitude of vibration of a simple harm-onic motion shown in Fig.2.3(a) does not remain constant but becomes progressively

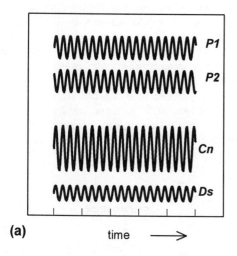

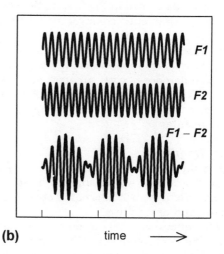

Figure 2.4 **(a)** Constructive (Cn) and destructive (Ds) interference of two waveforms with the same frequency but different phases P1 and P2. **(b)** A beat frequency caused by slightly different frequency waveforms F1 and F2.

smaller (the exception here is an electro-magnetic wave). A vibration undergoing loss of energy shows damping Fig.2.3(b).

The amplitude of a mechanical vibration (pendulum swing) undergoes damping due to the air's viscosity, an electrical waveform undergoes damping due to energy loss within the circuit. As damping is increased the oscillations die away more quickly. So a waveform is influenced by energy input. If this oscillating energy is influenced by a retarding force, electronic or mechanical (friction), then the oscillation amplitude decreases exponentially which is shown by the decay envelope of Fig.2.3(b).

Resonance   In order to keep a damped system, which is losing energy, in continuous oscillatory motion some outside periodic force must be introduced. The frequency of this force is called the forcing or driving frequency. The frequency of the undamped waveform is the system's natural frequency.

When the forcing frequency is equal to the natural frequency of the system then **resonance** occurs producing the greatest power output; the peak frequency ω in Fig.2.3(c) is the resonant frequency. This is of practical use in radiology where an oscillating system (e.g. ultrasound transducer crystal or tuned MRI inductive circuit) is the same as the frequency of the driving force (electrical pulse). Considerable energy is absorbed at resonant frequency from the system supplying the external force.

The two resonant signals shown in Fig.2.3(c) are a strong resonant signal and a slightly damped signal. The amplitude of the oscillations at resonance will be less if the system is strongly damped the curve will also be broader. The resonance coupling is enhanced when the frequencies are equal; resonance causes a dramatic increase in signal amplitude at the resonant frequency. This is the principle behind radio frequency (RF) reception: an RF receiver is tuned to be in resonant with the RF transmitter.

2.7.3 Interference

Constructive / destructive   When waveforms having the same frequency but slightly different phase combine they interfere with each other as shown in Fig.2.4(a) . Waveforms **in-phase** (coherent) constructively interfere and produce a resultant of greater amplitude (*Cn*). Waveforms **out of phase** (incoherent) show destructive interference (*Ds*). Increasing phase differences give greater degrees of destructive interference until a 180° phase difference cause the signal to disappear giving a zero resultant.

Beat frequency If two waveforms have slightly different frequencies (Fig. 2.4(b)) then phase differences will change with time and wave interference will alternate between constructive and destructive.

These alterations of intensity cause an overlaying beat-frequency. The beat frequency is the difference between the two original wave frequencies. The frequency variation modulates the amplitude of the resultant wave which will have a frequency equal to the average frequency of the two waves.

Transverse waves These are propagated by vibrations perpendicular to the direction of the wave travel. Examples of these waves are shown by waves seen on water and electromagnetic waves (light waves).

Longitudinal waves The vibrations occur in the same direction as the direction of travel. The most common example is a sound wave where compressions and rarefactions move along with the speed of the waveform, each particle vibrating about a mean position transferring energy to the next particle.

2.8 ELECTROMAGNETIC RADIATION

Electromagnetic energy is transmitted by both an electric and magnetic field oscillating together opposed 90° to each other; this is diagrammatically shown in Fig.2.5. This is self sustaining, the changing electric field producing a magnetic field and vice versa. All electromagnetic waves travel through a vacuum with the same speed c which is

3.0×10^8 m s^{-1}; this is a constant. There is no known limit on wavelength which can range from several kilometers to 10^{-14}m. The energy content of an electromagnetic wave is a multiple of the basic quantum: the **photon**.

The electromagnetic spectrum encompasses extremely low frequencies and wavelengths from radio-waves and visible light to ultra-violet, x-rays and gamma radiation. Each frequency band has unique properties but the wave character is identical having an electrical and magnetic component.

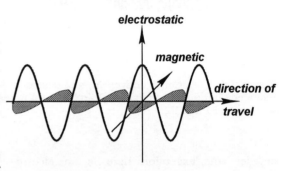

Figure 2.5 Electromagnetic energy is transmitted with a 90° opposed dual electrical and magnetic component.

2.8.1 Dual characteristic of electromagnetic radiation

The dual characteristics of electromagnetic radiation which behaves both as particles (photons) and waves seem to conflict. Discrete packets of energy called **quanta** or **photons** have energy which is related as:

$$E = hf \qquad (2.18)$$

where f is frequency in hertz (Hz $\equiv$ cycles s^{-1}) and h is Planck's Constant, (Max Planck; 1858-1947; German physicist). This is a conversion factor used in eqn.2.18 to enable the answer to be expressed as Joules per second where

$$h = 6.62 \times 10^{-34} \text{ J s}$$

Wave energy increases with frequency. The frequencies f of some electromagnetic radiations are:

Red Light	3.7×10^{14}Hz
Blue light	7.5×10^{14}Hz
Ultra-violet	4×10^{15}Hz
X-rays	5×10^{17}Hz
Gamma radiation	5×10^{19}Hz

In comparison radio and television waves (FM and UHF) are much lower down the scale having frequencies between 80MHz and 1GHz (80×10^6 to 1×10^9Hz). The complete EM spectrum is listed in Appendix II.

Radiation energy This is a function of wavelength λ and frequency f since $c = \lambda f$ and consequently $f = c/\lambda$ where c is the speed of light (3.0×10^8 m s^{-1}). Albert Einstein (German/US physicist:1879-1955) introduced the idea of photon energy E being a function of frequency and Planck's Constant broadening Planck's equation (eqn.2.18):

$$E = hf = mc^2 \qquad (2.19)$$

The mass-energy relationship demonstrated by this equation enables electron mass to be expressed as either:

$$9.1 \times 10^{-31} \text{ kg} \qquad \text{or}$$

$$0.511 \text{ MeV (mega-electron volts)}$$

The electron volt is a measure of radiation energy since the joule is too large a quantity being 6.24×10^{18} eV or conversely 1eV equal to 1.6×10^{-19}J. Wavelength and energy can be converted by utilizing eqn.2.17: $c = \lambda f$, since it then follows that $f = c/\lambda$ this function can be substituted for f in eqn.2.18 to give:

$$E = \frac{hc}{\lambda} \qquad (2.20)$$

Using the constants stated above:

$$
\begin{aligned}
hc \quad &= (6.62 \times 10^{-34}) \times (3.0 \times 10^8) \\
&= 1.98 \times 10^{-25} \text{ J}
\end{aligned}
$$

Since 1keV = 1.6×10^{-16} J the answer can be expressed in kilo-electron volts (keV) providing the wavelength is given in nanometers (nm) so:

$$E = \frac{1.24}{\lambda \text{ (nm)}} \text{ keV} \qquad (2.21)$$

Alternatively the answer can be given in electron volts if the wavelength is in meters:

$$E = \frac{1.24 \times 10^{-6}}{\lambda} \qquad (2.22)$$

The interrelationship between frequency, wavelength and energy is explored in Box 2.6 for visible light, ultra-violet and x-rays.

Box 2.6

Radiation energy as electron volt

Red light Wavelength 700nm (7×10^{-7} m)

$$f \quad = \quad c/\lambda \quad = \quad 4.28 \times 10^{14} \text{ Hz}$$

$$E \quad = \quad 1.24 \times 10^{-6}/7 \times 10^{-7} \quad = \quad 1.77 \text{eV}$$

Blue light Frequency f is 7.5×10^{14}Hz

$$\lambda = c/f = 3.0 \times 10^8 / 7.5 \times 10^{14} = 4 \times 10^{-7} \text{ m}$$

$$E \quad = 1.24 \times 10^{-6}/4 \times 10^{-7} \quad = \quad 3.1 \text{ eV}$$

Alternatively $E = hf$ (where $h \equiv 4.13 \times 10^{-15}$ eV) then (4.13×10^{-15}) $\times$ (7.5×10^{14}) = 3.1 eV

Ultra-violet frequency = 4×10^{15}Hz

$$\lambda \quad = 3.0 \times 10^8/4 \times 10^{15} = 75 \text{nm}$$
$$E \quad = 16 \text{ eV.}$$

X-ray A continuous spectrum from 60 to 120keV has a wavelength range from 0.02 to 0.0099nm and a frequency range from 1.5 to 3.0×10^{19} Hz.

Electromagnetic spectrum properties A summary of the formulas and values that are commonly used in radiology is given in Tab.2.9. Electromagnetic radiation exhibits the following:

- Electric and magnetic vectors are 90° opposed
- Wave/particle-photon duality
- Very broad range of frequency and wavelength.
- Polarization of the wave (orientation in a single plane commonly seen in radio and visible wavelengths)
- Speed in vacuum 3.0×10^8m s^{-1} (is a constant)
- Unaffected by external electrical or magnetic fields
- Absorption by material follows an exponential law.

Table 2.9 Summary: Electromagnetic units

Measure	Eqns.	Values
Velocity c	$c = f\lambda$	$c = 3.0 \times 10^8$ m s^{-1}
Wavelength λ	$\lambda = c/f$	λ in m or nm
Frequency f	$f = c/\lambda$	f in Hz
Planck's constant h		6.62×10^{-34} J s^{-1} 4.13×10^{-15} eV
Electron mass e		$e = 9.1 \times 10^{-31}$kg $= 0.511$MeV $= 1.6 \times 10^{-19}$C
Energy E	$E = hc/\lambda$	$hc = 1.24 \times 10^{-6}$ eV

2.8.2   Light optics

The production of light from an intensifying screen, video screen or laser is an essential process in radiology for producing images. The behavior and distortion of light when passing through different materials determines the quality of the final image whether on film or video screen.

Light undergoes reflection, refraction and interference. Constructive interference occurs when two waves, in phase, combine to give a wave of larger amplitude. Destructive interference occurs when the waves are out of phase. Coherent sources have the same frequency and are in phase. This short description of light behavior will be covered in more detail in the relevant chapters.

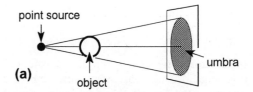

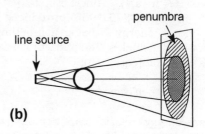

Figure 2.6 (a) A point source projecting an object as a pure shadow (umbra). A broader light beam from a line source **(b)** causes a secondary shadow (penumbra) whose dimensions are determined by parameters f, i and o identified in the text.

Umbra and penumbra A point source of light projects a sharp shadow onto a screen. Figure 2.6(a) demonstrates that when this ceases to be a point source then image unsharpness causes shadowing. The degree of shadowing depends on the of the focal spot f and its position relative to the object and image plane.

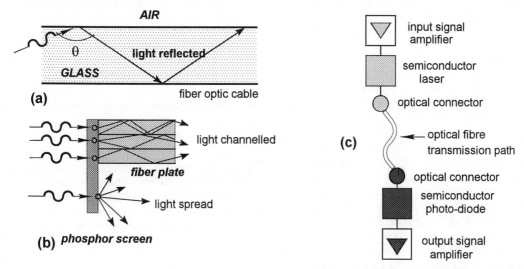

Figure 2.7 (a) Fiber optic principle: only when the critical angle is reached does total internal reflection occur. (b) A fiber optic plate on a phosphor screen (image intensifier) prevents light diffusion. (c) Fiber optic fiber used for digital signal transmission between two computer workstations.

The parameters *i* and *o* in Fig.2.6(b) determine the penumbra dimension *p* (unsharpness) so that:

$$p = \frac{i \times f}{o} \qquad (2.23)$$

Umbra and penumbra effects are shown by x-rays since they are produced by fine and broad focal spots and mimic the light effects described here. The geometry of an x-ray beam also obeys eqn.2.23.

Color RGB Video color displays use the primary colors of red, green and blue to form their images. These can be mixed to give any particular color scale. The thermal scale has become popular as a logical continuous scale using a 'temperature gradient' of red, orange, white to represent increasing count densities or activities.

The Laser (light amplification by stimulated emission of radiation) A strong mono-chromatic coherent light source can be produced by causing many atoms to make transitions from one excited state to another so that all the light waves are in phase (coherent). Many materials can be made to lase: ruby, carbon dioxide, helium/neon. These are high power devices commonly found in laser film formatters

Semiconductor lasers are low power devices producing red/infra-red light used for optical transmission and reading laser-disks and CD-ROMs.

Fiber optic effects Light travels at a constant 3×10^5 km s^{-1} in a vacuum. However when it enters a transparent medium (glass) the speed of light is less by a factor of about 1.5 (2×10^5 km s^{-1}). This factor is the refractive index of the material. When light passes from one medium to another this change in speed causes the light to bend. Under certain conditions the light ray will be reflected back into the more dense medium: this is **total internal reflection**. Light rays in glass are totally internally reflected if their angle of incidence is increased beyond a critical angle (42°). Figure 2.7(a) shows light rays within glass being refracted at the interface with a less dense medium (air).

Images can be transferred along a bundle of **coherent** fibers where the position of the fibers is identical at the start and the end of the bundle length. Figure 2.7(b) shows an optical fiber plate (short length of coherent fibers) applied to a phosphor screen; this light pipe prevents light scatter so reducing image data loss that would occur by viewing the phosphor screen directly. Tapering the fiber bundle can either minify or magnify the image.

The light beam can be piped along a glass rod or fiber. An optical fiber for this purpose is typically 0.125 and 0.5mm in diameter and signal losses are about 0.5 dB km^{-1} resulting in a small signal loss of about 10% per km. Signals can be transmitted over about 50km without amplification. A simplified transmission scheme is shown in Fig. 2.7(c).

Radiology applications Fiber optics play an important part in image intensifier signal collection in fluoroscopy explained in Chapter 10. It is also playing an increasing role in computer data transmission over local area networks (LAN's in Chapter 11).

2.8.3 Radio waves and transmission

Radio waves are a form of electromagnetic radiation produced by oscillating electrons in an inductor (coil). The waves are transferred to an aerial which at low frequencies can be a short length of wire but at higher frequencies a system of conductors is necessary to shape the transmitted beam or increase the ability to detect radio waves of a certain frequency band.

Very high frequency (VHF) radio waves (20 to 80MHz) are the signal in magnetic resonance imaging. At these frequencies it is essential to maintain impedance matching otherwise the signal strength will be reduced.

Interference from other radio transmissions is reduced by using efficient narrow-band transmission and receiving circuits (high Q). These resonate at narrow precise frequencies (see resonance in Fig.2.3(c)).

2.9   ATOMIC AND NUCLEAR STRUCTURE

The atom is the fundamental unit from which all matter is made. The essential features are shown in Fig.2.8.   All atoms consist of:

- Electron shells forming orbits
- A nucleus which is the central mass consisting of protons and neutrons.

The atom is neutral having an electron charge equal to the nuclear charge. Atoms of the separate elements have different numbers of protons forming the nuclear charge (+) balanced by different numbers of electrons (–).

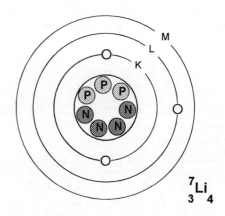

Figure 2.8   A representation of the atom showing a nucleus with 3 protons and 4 neutrons together with the K, L and M electron orbits; the 3 proton charges are balanced by 3 electrons. This would represent a lithium atom.

The **nucleus** of an atom is a small positively charged mass at the center of the atom; its size is approximately ×10^4 to 10^5 smaller than the atom itself but contains almost all the mass of the atom since an electron is about ×2000 less massive than a proton.

The important components of an atom are listed in Tab.2.10 giving their electrical charge and mass. The neutrino, which takes part in beta decay, and the photon which forms the electromagnetic radiation (gamma radiation), have neither charge nor mass. The positron can be treated as a positively charges electron and will be further discussed in Chapter 15 on nuclear medicine. The neutron is a neutral particle that only increases the nuclear mass without altering the nuclear charge.

Table 2.10 Fundamental atomic particles

Particle	Charge	Mass
Electron	−1	∼ 0
Positron	+1	∼ 0
Proton	+1	1
Neutron	0	1
Neutrino	0	0
Photon	0	0

If an atom gains or loses an electron it acquires an electrical charge and becomes an **ion**. Metals commonly lose electrons and become positive ions, non-metals gain electrons becoming negative ions. This is commonly seen in ionizing salt solutions which dissociate so:

$$NaCl \text{ in solution} \rightarrow Na^+ + Cl^-$$

also sodium and chlorine in their elemental state:

$$Na - e^- \rightarrow Na^+$$
$$Cl + e^- \rightarrow Cl^-$$

In both cases Na^+ and Cl^- are ions. If energy (hf from eqn. 2.18) is delivered to a system (e.g. a gas) in the form of x- or gamma radiation then it will ionize giving a positive ion and a free electron:

$$Xe + hf \rightarrow Xe^+ + e^-$$

The xenon is then ionized and the ionized events ($Xe^+ + e^-$) can form an electrical signal, which is the basis of a gas detector for ionizing radiation. Ionization events can occur with any element and are most important reactions in radiology.

2.9.1   Electron orbits

Electrons orbit around the nucleus in shells. The nucleus and its surrounding concentric shells of orbiting electrons makes up the complete atom.

The electron (discovered by J J Thomson 1856-1940; British physicist) is a negatively charged particle. Electron orbits form shells around the nucleus; the closest orbit to the nucleus is designated K followed by L, M, N etc., drawn in Fig.2.8. There are maximum numbers of electrons that can occupy each orbit (quantum number).

K:	2 electrons
L:	8 electrons
M:	18 electrons
N:	32 electrons
O:	50 electrons

Electrons and some other fundamental particles (protons) have **spin** or **angular momentum**. This is always the same for a certain particle type and is a whole number. Angular momentum for protons is important in radiology when describing nuclear magnetic resonance.

The electrons are held in their orbits by electrostatic forces called **binding energies.** These are greater for the K-shell electrons and get successively weaker for the outer orbits. Binding energies for any particular K-shell will be greater for nuclei with large positive charges (large atomic number: Z). Examples of some of the binding energies are given in Tab.2.11.

The removal of an electron from an orbit can only be achieved if the binding force is overcome. Most energy is needed for the K-shell electrons; these are more closely bound. The outer shell electrons are more easily removed and take part in chemical reactions; these are the **valency** electrons.

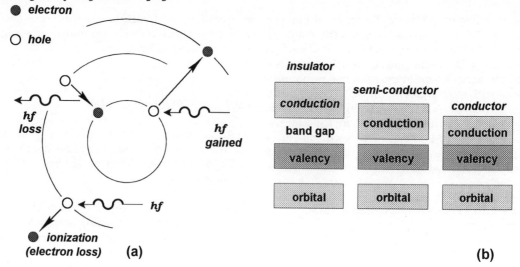

Figure 2.9   **(a)** Electron orbits showing transition from one energy level to another. A transition is accompanied by energy equal to the energy difference between the two levels taken in (photon absorbed) or given out (photon emitted). **(b)** Bands of conduction and valency separated by a varying width band gap in solid insulators, semi-conductors and conductors.

Table 2.11   K-shell binding energies

Element	Z	K-shell energy (eV)
Carbon	6	0.28
Nitrogen	7	0.4
Oxygen	8	0.5
Phosphorus	15	2.1
Sulfur	16	2.5
Calcium	20	4.0
Molybdenum	42	20.0
Barium	56	37.4
Iodine	53	33.2
Tungsten	74	69.5
Lead	82	88.0
Uranium	92	115.6

Ionization   Since the positive charge on the nucleus is balanced by the negative charges of the electrons removal of any electrons give the remaining structure a positive charge. This is an *ion* and the process is ***ionization***. The positive ion is unstable until the vacant orbit is filled by a free electron. If the K-electron is removed then the vacancy can be filled by an electron from the L-shell leaving a vacancy which then attracts its neighboring electron and so on, producing a cascade.

Figure 2.9(a) illustrates electron movement between orbits. The L-electron jumping into the K-orbit loses energy in the form of electromagnetic radiation. Other electron jumps involve less energy for their transition and give lower energy radiation (ultraviolet). A transition from a higher orbit to a lower one (the ground state) emits electromagnetic radiation. The K and L shell transitions emit x-ray photons which are **characteristic** for the atom.

Excitation   Electrons in the outer shells can receive enough energy to be moved into an upper orbit, placing the atom into a state of **excitation** (Fig.2.9(a)). They stay there for a short time before returning to their original orbit emitting electromagnetic radiation: visible or ultraviolet. These events play an important role in luminescence, which is found in some radiation detectors and screen materials (Chapter 6). Excited atoms are also more active chemically and are considered in tissue radiation dosimetry (Chapter 21).

2.9.2 Elements and compounds

The periodic table places the elements in order of their atomic number. Each row of the periodic table signifies the start of a new electron shell so elements which have similar chemical properties appear in the same part of the table. Metals tend to be on the left (Na, Ca etc.) and non-metals (I, Xe etc.) tend to be on the right of the table.

When atoms form solid compounds or crystals the energies of the orbitals change slightly so single energy levels become ranges of energy called energy bands shown in Fig.2.9(b), these are:

- the **valence band** where the valence electrons are found
- the **conduction band** where there are both electrons and spaces for more electrons. The electrons are mobile and materials which have a conduction band are the only ones which can conduct electricity at room temperature.
- the **forbidden band** is the range of energies between two energy bands which is not occupied by electrons. The electron must cross this band gap to occupy a higher electron band. The band gap is large in insulator materials, very narrow in semiconductors and does not exist at all in conductors.

These bands are most important in radiology since they play a significant role in semiconductor electronics and radiation detector operation.

The energy levels of the electron orbitals in an atom and the energies necessary to eject the electron from its orbital during the ionization process play an important role in the interaction of radiation with matter. The electron undergoes a transition when moving from one orbital to another either absorbing energy when going to a higher orbital from its ground state or emitting energy (usually in the form of a photon) when descending into a lower orbital.

2.9.3 The nucleus

The nucleus of an atom is characterized by its charge:

- the atomic number Z and
- atomic mass or mass number A.

The atomic number Z is the number of protons; the atomic mass A is the sum total of protons and neutrons N. The full description of the element X is given as:

$$_{Z}^{A}X_{N}$$

Examples for hydrogen, carbon and lead would be:

$$_{1}^{1}H_{0} \qquad _{6}^{12}C_{6} \qquad _{82}^{208}Pb_{126}$$

More simply they can be represented as:

$$^{1}H \qquad ^{12}C \qquad ^{208}Pb$$

The proton adds mass and charge to the nucleus the neutron, being neutral, adds mass without charge.

Isotopes are defined as a change in atomic mass without change in atomic number (loss or gain of neutrons). An unstable nucleus produces alpha α, beta β or gamma γ radiation in order to achieve stability; this is fully discussed in Chapter 15.

2.10 MAGNETISM

A magnetic field B is the force equivalent in magnetism to an electrostatic charge producing an electrostatic field which sets up lines of charge around an object. The SI unit for the magnetic field is the tesla T. (N. Tesla 1856 -1943; Croatian physicist).

A **magnetic flux** is set up by the magnetic field. The unit for the magnetic flux per unit area at right angles to the direction of the magnetic field B (magnetic line density) is the **weber** Wb where $1Wb = 1T\ m^{-2}$. The motion of an electric charge (a flowing current) is always accompanied by a magnetic flux. The insertion of ferromagnetic material (iron, cobalt, nickel) within a magnetic flux causes the atoms within the material to align themselves and a permanent magnet is formed. Permanent magnets have a north and south pole (compared to positive and negative charges in electrostatics). Lines of force connect these poles which form the magnetic flux lines shown in Fig.2.10(a).

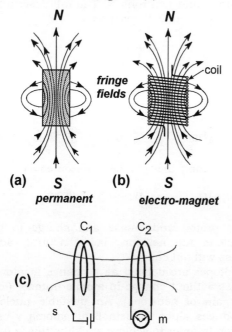

Figure 2.10 **(a)** Magnetic flux field lines surrounding a permanent magnet and **(b)** magnetic induction seen in a coil carrying an electric current. **(c)** current induction in a second solenoid.

2.10.1 Magnetic Induction

Magnetic effect of current A current carrying wire shows the following points:

- A magnetic field surrounds it.
- The magnetic field is perpendicular to the current.

The magnetic effect shown by a current

carrying wire can be increased by winding the wire into a coil (a solenoid), so concentrating the lines of magnetic force. A solenoid is constructed from a multi-turn coil, shown in Fig.2.10(b); an iron core will concentrate the magnetic flux still more, this is the basis of an electromagnet which loses its magnetization when the current is switched off.

Electromagnetic induction If a magnet is moved within a coil a current is induced in the coil. The coil can be moved producing the same effect. This is the principle behind the dynamo and alternator, producing electric energy from mechanical energy.

Induction by current If two coils (C_1 and C_2 in Fig.2.10(c)) are placed closely together and C_1 energized by switching a battery in circuit, causing a growth of a magnetic field, then this induces a current in C_2. The current in C_1 must be changing to induce a current in C_2. This is the principle behind the transformer to be discussed later.

Magnetic strength This is dependent on the pole strength m_1 and m_2 at a distance d. These attract or repel each other with a force F so that:

$$F = K \times \frac{m_1 \times m_2}{d^2} \qquad (2.24)$$

where K is a constant. The force obeys the inverse square law. Intensity of the magnetic field is measured as:

$$F = \frac{m_1 \times m_2}{p \times d^2} \qquad (2.25)$$

Where p is the permeability of the medium which is large for ferromagnetic materials (p for air=1). In coils C_1 and C_2 (described above) the magnetic flux would be p times as great if the coils are wound over a magnetic core material (soft-iron); this is exploited in transformer design.

Domain theory of magnetism Ferromagnetic materials are crystalline and small regions within these crystals have strong resultant magnetism but this is randomly distributed so the bulk material shows no magnetism. These tiny regions are called **domains**. It is the realignment of these domains which achieves the magnetic property. Total realignment gives saturation and magnetization of the material is at a maximum when all domains point in the same direction.

The domains can be disturbed by heat and vibration so the magnetic property is gradually lost. Audio or video magnetic recordings gradually become noisier as the magnetic signal on the tape is lost over time. MRI permanent magnets very slowly lose magnetic strength for the same reason.

Field change A small field produces strong magnetization in soft iron so this is an ideal ferromagnetic material but steel requires a stronger electric field so is not an ideal magnetic material.

Ferrite (a ceramic iron material) gives a large field change for a large electric field; it quickly saturates and retains this saturated condition when the electric field is removed. This property makes ferrite a valuable magnetic material for recording analog and digital information on tape or disk.

Eddy current losses A changing magnetic flux in the coil produces a flux change in the core material (soft-iron) which causes eddy current losses seen as heat. Eddy currents can be reduced if the core is laminated. At higher frequencies (radio frequencies) soft iron is not suitable and sintered iron particles are used (ferrite). Eddy current losses cause serious problems in MRI.

Shielding It has already been seen that ferromagnetic materials serve to concentrate the magnetic flux. Soft iron (mu-metal) is a common material used for shielding against magnetic interference and can be placed around sensitive equipment (image intensifiers, photomultiplier tubes etc.), since it can concentrate quite weak magnetic fields reducing the external magnetic flux and so protecting devices which are surrounded by the material.

2.11 ELECTRICITY

Electricity and the properties of electricity are obviously of prime importance to radiology. The high voltages associated with **static electricity** and their electrostatic effects are essential for electron beam control in x-ray tubes, image intensifiers and video display tubes. As the name electrostatics implies the properties do not depend on organized electron flow but rather distribution of positive and negative charges on a body. **Current electricity** is concerned with the flow of electrical energy by charge carriers (electrons) between two points having a potential difference between them. This difference is the electromotive force (emf) measured in volts and can be treated as a form of potential energy in both static and current electricity.

2.11.1 Electrostatics

This is the branch of physics that deals with static or very high voltages (relevant to x-ray generators and x-ray tubes).

Electric charge Static electric charges arise when electrons are transferred from one object to another. An object with excess electrons has a negative charge and conversely an object having lost electrons has a positive charge. The basic measurement of charge is the **coulomb** C (Charles Coulomb 1736-1806; French physicist):

$$1 \text{ coulomb} = 6.24 \times 10^{18} \text{ electrons}$$

Each electron has a charge Q of 1.6×10^{-19} C per electron. This is a fundamental constant usually called the elementary charge. The rest mass of the electron is also a fundamental constant being 9.1×10^{-31} kg. The charge and energy of an electron beam is calculated in Box 2.7.

Box 2.7

The charge of an electron beam

If Q coulombs flows during t seconds then:

$$I = \frac{Q}{t} \text{ amps}$$

$$Q = I \times t$$

Example 1

If $I = 4$ C s^{-1} $t = 10$ seconds then

$\qquad\qquad$ $Q = 40$ coulombs.

Example 2

X-ray exposure for 100mA at $t = 0.5$s (50mAs) then $I = 0.1$ coulombs s^{-1} and $Q = 0.05$ coulombs or 50 milliCoulombs (mC)

So x-ray exposure in mAs is equivalent to mC.

The **energy gained by electron** beam in a x-ray tube. If 3×10^{17} electrons representing 50mA (1.6×10^{-19}C each electron) move along an x-ray tube at 120keV. Then energy gained is:

$$
\begin{aligned}
E \; &= QV \text{ joules} \\
&= (3 \times 10^{17}) \times (1.6 \times 10^{-19}) \times (120 \times 10^3) \\
&= 5760 \text{ joules}
\end{aligned}
$$

Laws of Electrostatics   These laws state that similar charges (−, − or +, +) on separate bodies repel; unlike charges (+ and −) attract. The force of two charged bodies is proportional to their charge $F \propto q$. The attractive or repulsive force F of a charge q over a distance d has the relationship :

$$F \propto \frac{1}{d^2}$$

this has already been expressed as the inverse square law in Chapter 1.

also $\qquad$ $F = \dfrac{q_1 \cdot q_2}{d^2}$ $\qquad\qquad$ (2.26)

which is analogous to the magnetic force in eqn.2.24. Here F is the force exerted on two objects with charge q_1 and q_2 at a distance d.

The inverse square law also applies to charged bodies. This equation describes Coulomb's law which plays an important part in x-ray tube design for defining electron beam dimensions.

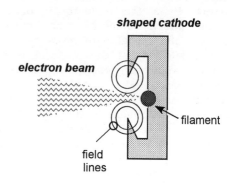

Figure 2.11 Static field set up around shaped points in an x-ray tube filament cup assembly

Electric field   The force is proportional to the charge ($F \propto q$) and every charge produces an electric field in the space around it:

$$\text{Electric field} = \frac{F}{q} \qquad\qquad (2.27)$$

The charges will be closer giving a stronger electric field where the conductor is most curved. A sharp edge will have a very high electric field; this property has valuable applications to the design of focusing cups in x-ray tubes. Figure 2.11 shows how sharp edges can be used for controlling the dimensions of an electron beam produced by an electrically heated filament.

The Volt   (AG Volta 1745-1827; Italian physicist) Before an electric current can flow there must be a pressure difference or driving force between the electrodes. This is called a potential difference (PD) which is measured in volts V and applies to both static and current electricity. It is the work done in moving 1 Coulomb so 1V = 1 J C^{-1}. The volt as a unit exists as multiples listed in Tab.2.12.

Table 2.12 Multiples of the volt

Megavolts (MV:10^6)	Static electricity (millions of volts)
kilovolts (kV:10^3)	X-ray high voltage (20-150kV) Domestic supply and batteries (1.5 - 240V)
milliVolts (mV:10^{-3})	Physiological signal level (ECG) (10-100mV)
microVolts (µV:10^{-6})	Radio signal strength e.g. MRI (1-10µV)

Box 2.8

The energy equivalence of an electron volt

The electron velocity v at 1 volt is 6×10^5 m s^{-1}
The rest mass m is 9.1×10^{-31} kg
so

$\frac{1}{2}mv^2 = 0.5 \times (9.1\times10^{-31})\times (6\times10^5)^2$
or 1.6×10^{-19}J
This is the **energy equivalent** of 1eV

Similarly the electron velocity at 100kV is
$1.6\times10^{-19}\times(1\times10^5) = 1.6\times10^{-14}$J
so

$\frac{1}{2}mv^2 = 1.6\times10^{-14}$
Velocity v is 1.88×10^8 m s^{-1} at 100kV which is about $^2/_3$ the speed of light .

NB
Relativistic effects (mass-velocity) play a small part in electron velocity.

The electron volt eV This has been previously mentioned in Sec.2.8.1 and is a measure of energy necessary since traditional units of energy (Joule) are much too large to describe electrostatic attractive forces. The electron volt is the energy acquired by an electron when it moves between a potential difference of 1 volt. The electron volt has multiples keV, MeV. Equivalent values of the electron volt are:

$$1eV = 1.6\times10^{-19}J$$
$$h = 4.13\times10^{-15} eV$$

There is a clear distinction between electrical potential difference (voltage: 50kV, 100kV etc.) and energy (electron volt: 50keV, 100keV etc.). Energy equivalence and velocity of an electron beam is calculated in Box 2.8.

Application to radiology Electrostatic forces are responsible for accelerating electrons in an x-ray tube. Electrostatics are also employed to control the dimensions of an electron beam. Figure 2.11 shows a filament cup whose sharp edges carry a strong electric field and this negative potential can repel the electron beam, controlling its dimensions and also switching off the beam, if the charge is high enough.

2.11.2 Current electricity

Direct Current (DC) is given by batteries, dynamos and rectified power supplies. It is used as the final power supply for radiology equipment whether driving high voltage x-ray tubes or low voltage semiconductor circuits.

The Ampere (AM Ampère 1775-1836; French physicist). Electrical current is caused by the transport of electrons and is measured in amperes A:

$$1 A = 1 \text{ coulomb per second (C s}^{-1})$$

As one coulomb represents the charge on 6×10^{18} electrons one ampere would be this number of electrons per second passing in a conductor. Smaller currents are measured in milliAmps (mA; 10^{-3}A) and microAmps (mA; 10^{-6} A). The volt can be described in terms of current flow since it is the difference of electrical potential between two points on a wire carrying a constant current of 1A when the power dissipation is 1W, so:

$$1V = 1W A^{-1}$$

X-ray tube current is measured in mA and x-ray exposure is measured in mA per unit time i.e. mA seconds mAs and from the above definition of a coulomb:

$$1\text{mAs} = 1\times10^{-3} \text{ coulomb (1mC)}$$

Energy gain   The energy gained by an electron when it is accelerated from one electrode to another (video/television tube, x-ray tube) can be calculated as shown in Box.2.9. A summary of electrical measurements is given in Tab.2.13 along with constants useful for radiation calculations.

Table 2.13   Summary: Electrical units

Measure	Parameter	Relationships
Electric charge Q	Coulomb C	$1C = 6.24\times10^{18}e$
	charge/electron	$1.6\times10^{-19}C$
Potential difference PD	volt V	$1V = 1J\ C^{-1}$
Energy E	joule J	$J = QV$
	electron volt eV	$1J = 6.24\times10^{18}$ eV
		$1eV = 1.6\times10^{-19}J$
Current I	ampere A	$Q = I\times t$
		$1A = 1C\ s^{-1}$
		$(6.24\times10^{18}\ e\ s^{-1})$

Power and resistance   (George Simon Ohm 1787-1854; German physicist) Ohm's Law states that current I and voltage V are proportional providing temperature and resistance R of the conductor are constant. So $I \propto V$ and V/I is a constant.

The unit of resistance is the **ohm** Ω. One ohm maintains a current of one amp at one volt so that:

$$R = \frac{V}{I} \tag{2.28}$$

Variations of this basic formula of eqn 2.28 are: $I = V/R$ and $V = IR$

Box 2.9

Electrical energy

Energy gain
Energy W (1 volt = 1 JC^{-1})
    Since $Q = I\times t$ then
              $W = IVt$ Joules

50,000 volts (50kV) at 50mAs (50mA for 1s)
Energy consumed $= 0.1 \times 50\text{kV} \times 0.5$ J
                        $= 2500$ J

Electric power
A 100W electric light bulb at 220 volts consumes $W/V = 0.45$ amp and at 110 volts consumes 0.9 amp
Commercial Electric Power is measured in kilowatts kW. Electrical Energy consumed is expressed as kW × time which is the kW hour.
So 4 × 100W lamps burning for 8 hours consume: 100 × 4 × 8 = 3.2 kW hour (regardless of supply voltage)

$$1\text{kWh} = 3.6\times10^6 \text{ J}$$

Heating effect of electric current   This depends on

- The electric current being passed I
- The resistance of the circuit R
- The time spent t

The following laws can be established:

- For a constant current I and fixed resistance: Heat produced $\propto$ time spent
- For a constant resistance and fixed time: Heat produced $\propto I^2$

Joule's Laws of electrical heating summarize these findings. The heat developed in a wire is proportional to:

- The time spent
- The current squared I^2
- Resistance of the conductor (wire)
    $P = I^2 Rt$ joules

Electrical power P relationships are derived

as:

$$\frac{energy\ delivered}{time\ taken}\ joules\ s^{-1}$$

$$P = \frac{IVt}{t} = IV\ J\ s^{-1}$$

Since 1 watt = 1 J s^{-1} and $P = IV$ then:

$$W = IV\ watts \qquad (2.29)$$

Examples of electrical power calculation are give in Box 2.9 and a summary of units in Tab.2.14.

Table 2.14 Summary: Resistance and power

Measure	Parameter	Relationships
Resistance (R)	ohm (Ω)	$I = V/R$ $R = V/I$ $V = IR$
Power (P)	watt (W)	$P = IV$ $P = I^2R$ $P = V^2/R$ $E = W/Q$ $1W = 1J\ s^{-1}$ $1J = 1\ W\ s$ $1kWh = 3.6 \times 10^6\ J$ $W = EQ$ $W = I^2R\ t$ $= V^2 t/R$ $= V I t$

Power loss Deriving electrical power P as:

$$P = IV \qquad (2.30)$$

and restating Ohm's Law as $V = IR$.

Then $\qquad P = I \times (IR)$

or $\qquad\quad P = I^2R \qquad (2.31)$

Similarly since $I = V/R$

then $\qquad P = V \times (V/R)$

or $\qquad\quad P = V^2/R \qquad (2.32)$

Which gives 3 standard formulas (eqn.2.30,

2.31, 2.32) relating power with voltage, current and resistance. Since all conductors have some electrical resistance, no matter how small, power is always lost when transporting electricity. Box 2.10 illustrates this for 500V, 10kV and 100kV power lines.

Box 2.10

Power loss

For a cable of resistance 2Ω supplying a 100W lamp: At 110 volts ~1 amp is flowing so the power lost in the cable is $I^2R = 1 \times 2 = 2$ watts Or 2% of the lamp power is lost in the cable.

At 220 volts ~0.5 amp is flowing and the power lost in the cable is $0.25 \times 2 = 0.5$watts Or 0.5% of the available power is lost.

Power transmission

Supplying 1MW to a small town over a cable with a resistance of 10Ω can use:
500V at 2000amps or
10,000V at 100amps or
500,000V at 2amps
(all delivering the required 1MW).

Power loss is I^2R
500V there is total power lost in the cable.
10,000V   10% of the power is lost
100,000V   0.1% of the power is lost

NB Power transmission uses highest practical voltage to minimize power loss.

Conductor dimensions If a is the cross-sectional area of a conductor then providing the length L is constant its resistance is proportional to cross-sectional area. So that:

$$R \propto \frac{L}{a^2} \qquad (2.33)$$

If the diameter of the wire is doubled (increasing the area a) then resistance decreases by ¼.

2.11.3 Alternating current and voltage

Alternating Current (AC) is produced by generators/alternators and electrically oscillating circuits. It is used for transmitting electrical power over long distances, eventually appearing as the domestic mains supply; it is more easily controlled than DC.

Alternating current is produced at the power station by a generator capable of delivering many thousands of volts at a very high current. This is stepped up prior to transmission along the high voltage power lines; the voltages sometimes exceed 500 000 volts. High voltage transmission reduces power lost in the cables as demonstrated in Box 2.10. Power loss can be reduced by either:

- Increasing the supply voltage
- Reducing cable resistance

The transmitted high voltage is successively stepped down in order to supply cities, towns, streets and eventually individual consumers. A single and 3-phase AC waveform is shown in Fig.2.12. Each phase of the 3-phase supply is separated by 120°, which transmits electrical energy with much greater efficiency than a single phase supply.

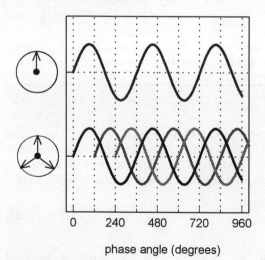

0   240   480   720   960

phase angle (degrees)

Figure 2.12   A single and a 3-phase supply. The polar diagram indicates that the 3 phases are 120° out of phase with each other.

The transformer   The valuable property of alternating current is that it can be easily changed from high to low values and vice-versa with very little loss; this is achieved with a transformer. A transformer, Fig.2.13(a), consists of two coils primary n_p and secondary n_s wound on a soft iron core in the case of low frequency power supplies (50 or 60Hz. Sintered ferrite cores are used for high frequency transformers (>1000 Hz).

The following relationship applies to transformers where E_p and E_s are the voltages at the primary (n_p) and secondary (n_s) windings:

$$\frac{E_s}{E_p} = \frac{n_s}{n_p} \qquad (2.34)$$

The parameters n_p and n_s are the number of turns so the ratio n_s/n_p is the turns ratio in eqn.2.34. A step-up transformer has a turns ratio >1 and a step-down transformer <1.

The current in a transformer changes inversely with the voltage; the energy in the transformer obeys the conservation of energy, thus the energy in the secondary at any instant equals the power supplied to the primary. If I_s and I_p and the secondary and primary currents then:

$$I_s \times E_s = I_p \times E_p$$

and
$$\frac{I_s}{I_p} = \frac{E_p}{E_s} = \frac{n_p}{n_s} \qquad (2.35)$$

Thus in a step-up transformer (shown schematically in Fig.2.13(b)) with a turns ratio 60:1 (voltage increases) the currents are stepped down in the ratio 1:60. A step-down transformer will increase current in the secondary winding but at a reduced voltage. In practice there is a loss of energy in the transformer due to eddy currents which are induced in the iron core by the changing magnetic flux in the windings; these losses can be reduced if the core is laminated.

The current needed for an x-ray machine is calculated in Box 2.11 and shows that very high main supply currents are necessary for the high voltages required.

The voltages induced in the secondary winding of a transformer depend on the size of the primary and secondary windings. For 50/60Hz supplies the average x-ray generator transformer is particularly large and occupies a great deal of space in the x-ray room (approximately a 0.5m cube).

Box 2.11

X-ray generator supply

What is the mains current I_p required to supply an x-ray generator capable of giving 125kVp at 100mA. The mains voltage is 220V.

$$I_p = \frac{E_s \times I_s}{E_p} = \frac{(125 \times 10^3) \times (100 \times 10^{-3})}{220}$$

$$= 56 \text{ amps}$$

A 110V supply would require 112 amps.

NB X-ray equipment requiring high currents commonly employ high voltage 3-phase supplies.

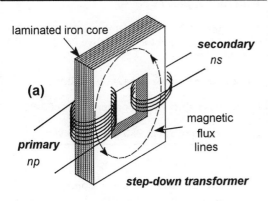

(a)

laminated iron core

secondary ns

magnetic flux lines

primary np

step-down transformer

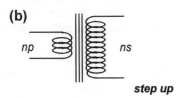

(b)

np   ns

step up

Figure 2.13 (a) A step-down transformer showing the primary and secondary windings on an iron core and **(b)** an electrical schematic for a step-up transformer.

High frequency transformers Extremely compact high voltage transformers can be designed by increasing the AC supply frequency since the induced secondary voltage E_s is influenced by the cross-sectional area of the transformer core A and the number of turns n and the frequency:

$$E_s = (A \times n) \times f \qquad (2.36)$$

The transformer size can be reduced substantially by increasing the supply frequency and maintaining E_s constant in eqn.2.36. This is accomplished by first converting the 50/60Hz supply to DC and then electronically converting this to a much higher frequency using a high frequency converter. High voltage transformers can be small enough to fit with the x-ray tube itself in CT machines. Box 2.12 illustrates the reduction in transformer size with increasing frequency of supply.

The x-ray system contains various transformer designs. A step-up transformer supplies the very high voltage necessary to generate the x-rays. A step-down transformer supplies the low voltage for the filament of the x-ray tube. These are commonly combined in the same transformer tank complete with oil coolant. An isolation transformer with equal turns ratio is used in order to separate the mains supply from the machine power supply; this reduces electrical shock hazards to personnel using the equipment.

A single winding auto-transformer is sometimes employed in order to compensate for power loss in the high voltage cables.

Impedance Z this is the AC parameter analogous to resistance in a DC circuit. For AC supplies it is a complex function of resistance, inductance and capacitance of the circuit as well as the frequency of supply. The unit of impedance is the same as the DC unit (the ohm Ω; see Ohm's Law) and similarly we can write $V = IZ$ or $I = V/Z$. In certain AC circuits it is important to match the impedances when the supply is connected in order to prevent undue power loss. This is most important when dealing with radio-frequency (high frequency AC) circuits that are used in magnetic resonance imaging.

Box 2.12

High frequency transformer

Transformer size decreases with increased frequency. The basic formula is $E_s = (A \times n) \times f$.
For an x-ray tube supply of 100keV and a relative overall size $(A \times n)$ for 50Hz transformer of 2000:

2000×50Hz	= 100keV
1666×60Hz	= 100keV
1000×100Hz	= 100keV
20×5kHz	= 100keV
10×10kHz	= 100keV

So operating a generator frequency of 10kHz, instead of 50Hz, reduces the transformer size by ×200

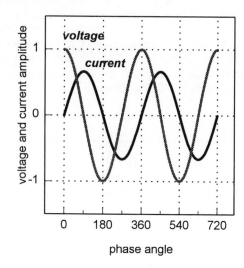

Figure 2.14   AC power voltage and current waveform for an inductive load where voltage and current show a 90° phase difference.

Box 2.13

Real and apparent power

The applied AC voltage and current to a system including an inductor (inductive load) is 440 volts at 50amps

The **apparent power** is 440×50 = 22kVA

A 12° phase shift gives a power factor of 0.84

so the **true power** is 22×0.84 = 18.5kW

2.11.4 AC power

The electrical power in a DC circuit is the product of current and voltage. The power in alternating current (AC) circuits is measured similarly but this is only valid when the current and voltage waveforms are in phase, which is the case with purely resistive circuits, e.g. heaters and light bulbs.

With electrical loads that include inductors e.g. motors, transformers, the voltage and current are not in phase as shown by Fig.2.14. The degree of phase-shift is expressed by the power factor (cos φ) or phase angle, so that the relationship between true power *P* measured in kW and apparent power *S* measured in kVA is $P = S \times \cos \varphi$. Box 2.13 gives an example of real and apparent power measurements when the voltage and current waveforms are out of phase.

Root-Mean-Square RMS. Comparing the electrical energy *W* produced by a direct current *I* flowing through a resistance *R* for a time *t* and an alternating current flowing through the same resistance both producing the same power as heat requires a measure of root mean square for the alternating current which is defined as that value of steady current which would dissipate heat at the same rate in a given resistance which for direct current is given by:

$$W = I^2 \times R \times t \qquad (2.37)$$

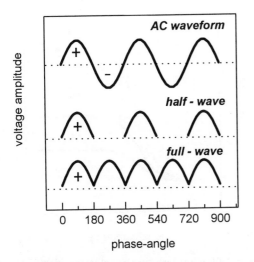
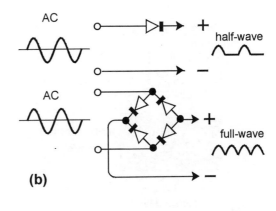

(b)

Figure 2.15 **(a)** The rectified AC waveform undergoing half-wave rectification (only positive cycles used) and full-wave rectification where both positive and negative cycles are used for the rectified DC supply. **(b)** The half-wave and full-wave circuits using diode rectifiers.

If a current is continuously varying (AC) the electrical energy is not converted into heat energy at a constant rate. The sine wave for a mains supply shows maximum energy when the current is maximum and zero when the current is zero. For this reason a mean value is derived called the root mean square (RMS) value. The RMS value of an AC power source, restating the above definition, is simply that value of DC which produces the same heating effect. For any sinusoidal waveform the RMS value is:

$$\frac{peak\ value}{\sqrt{2}} \qquad (2.38)$$

The quoted mains supply is always given as its RMS value, the peak voltages are obtained by multiplying by √2 (or 1.414) which gives the results listed in Tab.2.15. It is planned to 'harmonize' European and UK voltages to a common 230V by the year 2000.

Table 2.15 Mains supply voltages

RMS value	Peak value
115	162 (USA)
220	311 (Europe)
240	339 (UK)

2.11.5 Rectification

The convenience of an AC supply for transmitting electric current and its ease of voltage change by transformers is offset by the problems associated with rectifying the alternating waveform and converting it to a DC supply since the AC supply cannot be used for driving x-ray generator units or electronic equipment. Rectification is achieved by using one-way current devices (diodes), which in early machines used thermionic emission but in present day equipment use semiconductors.

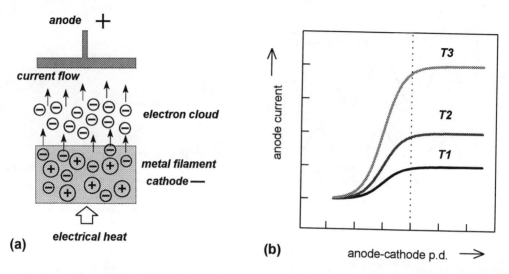

Figure 2.16 (a) Thermionic emission from a heated metal filament creating an electron cloud. There is a high potential difference between anode and cathode causing a current flow. **(b)** The thermionic emission efficiency depends on the temperature of the filament . The current flow (anode current) increases with increased filament temperature (T1 to T3)

These rectifiers only allow passage of current in one direction so their output has a single polarity. A half-wave rectifier uses a single diode and is 50% efficient since it does not utilize the negative half of the AC waveform. A full-wave rectifier uses 4 diodes and is 100% effective in utilizing all the AC power.

2.12   ELECTRONICS

The control of electrical circuits by thermionic or semiconductor devices is central to the equipment used in diagnostic imaging. The control of high voltages associated with x-ray production was, in the past, performed by mechanical switching but is now almost universally performed by electronic devices. Electronics is divided into analog and digital circuits. Analog devices are amplifiers which deal with varying signal voltages representing the x-ray spectrum, sound or radio waves. Digital devices act as very fast switches and feature mostly in logic circuits of control systems and computers.

2.12.1   High Voltage electronics

Thermionic emission   When heat is applied to a wire filament electrons close to the surface gain energy and leave the metal forming a cloud. The concentration of electrons causes a negative space charge which repels further electron emission. Placing a positive charged electrode (anode) above the filament will draw electrons so a current will flow. Electrons only flow from the negative cathode (filament) to the positive anode. As the filament temperature is increased from T1 to T3 in the simple device shown in Fig.2.16(b) the curves show that the current increases non-linearly reaching a saturation point or plateau. The saturation current level depends on the applied voltage between cathode (*x*-axis) and anode.

As well as being non-linear this device is also unidirectional (a diode), allowing current to pass from cathode to anode (not vice-versa) which removes the negative half of the alternating current; this is the rectification action.

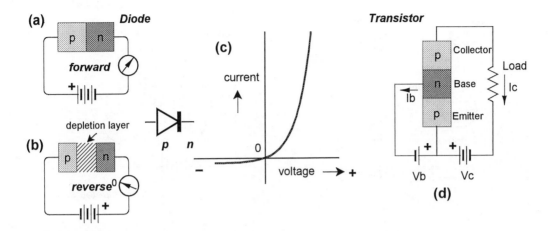

Figure 2.17 (a) Forward biased diode conducting current (b) Reverse biased diode where a depletion layer has formed preventing current flow. (c) The response of a diode to a negative and positive voltage showing its non-linear response in the forward direction. (d) A 3-layer device, a transistor, which amplifies a small base signal.

2.12.2 Low Voltage Electronics

Semiconductors These have all but replaced vacuum tube devices (valves). The x-ray tube is perhaps the remnant vacuum tube device that has not been replaced. Semiconducting materials are silicon, germanium and gallium arsenide; the first predominates. These materials are doped with impurities to produce n-type and p-type semiconductors. Electrons are main conductors or majority carriers in n-type semiconductors. The p-type semiconductors have 'holes' or orbital gaps as majority carriers.

The n-type and p-type semiconductors are combined to form the p-n junction diode. The junction diode exhibits different properties when connected to different polarity (+,–).

Semiconductor diode Before current supply is connected a small **depletion layer** exists between the p- and n-boundary. Electrons migrate from the n-type a small way into the p-type layer. Holes from the p-type also migrate into the n-type material.If the positive pole of a battery is connected to the p-type and the negative pole to the n-type then a current flows Fig.2.17(a); the diode is then **forward biased**. Reversing the polarity causes a wide depletion layer to be formed Fig.2.17(b) and no current is able to flow; the diode is **reverse biased**. When a p-n junction is part of a circuit and the voltage varied from negative to positive as plotted in Fig.2.17(c) current only flows when the diode is forward biased. Current flow does not obey Ohm's Law since current flow shows an exponential relationship. The junction diode acts as a rectifier for AC waveforms. They have replaced all thermionic diodes in x-ray equipment giving a large reduction in size and cooler operation.

Amplification Three layer semiconductor devices are used for signal amplification. These are transistors which includes two p-n junctions in a sandwich. (Fig.2.17(d)). A transistor can be either p-n-p or n-p-n. The three regions are **collector**, **base** and **emitter** with the load commonly in the collector

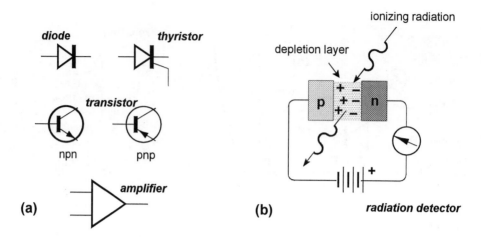

Figure 2.18   **(a)** Semiconductor circuit symbols commonly used in radiology equipment **(b)** a semiconductor radiation detector

circuit (common emitter circuit).   In the absence of a current (*Ib*) in the circuit (base-emitter) there is only a very small current through the load resistor (*Ic*). When a voltage *Vb* is applied charge carriers called 'holes' (electron vacancies) are introduced which cause a current to flow in the base-collector circuit. The current *Ic* through the load is much higher than the current *Ib* and so amplification has taken place; a small base current controls a much larger collector current. Basic semiconductor devices are shown as schematics in Fig.2.18(a): a diode, p-n-p and n-p-n transisitors, a thyristor which is used as a fast switching device in high power circuits (x-ray generators) and a general symbol which represents an amplifier circuit.

Switching Devices   The basic transistor circuit can be modified to form a switching circuit where a small signal can switch large collector loads on and off. Millions of micro-transistors can form fast switching devices which are incorporated into integrated logic devices for computers.

Radiation Effects   A reversed bias junction diode is sensitive to penetrating radiation (x-rays, γ-rays). Ionization causes carriers to be formed and a current flows proportional to radiation intensity. This is represented in Fig.2.18(b). Efficiency is low for x and gamma radiation since the depletion zone is small. The depletion layer width is determined by the applied voltage and is typically 10-30μm. Since Z for germanium (32) is higher than silicon (14) then germanium makes a more efficient detector. Small p-n diodes are used for small scale x-ray detectors, useful for surface dose measurements and automatic exposure controls.

KEYWORDS

ampere A: is a measure of electrical current; $1C \ s^{-1}$ represents 6.24×10^{18} electrons s^{-1}

Avogadro's constant: number of particles in 1 mole 6.022×10^{23}

coulomb C: the SI unit of charge $1A = 1C \ s^{-1}$

density ρ: mass per unit volume kg m^{-3} or non-SI unit of g cm^{-3}

elastic collision: in which the kinetic energy of the colliding bodies is the same after collision as before. No energy change.

electron charge   e: the charge on the electron 1.602×10^{-19} C and 1C = 6.24×10^{18} electrons

electron volt eV: a measure of electro-magnetic radiation energy particularly photons 1eV = 1.59×10^{-19} J

energy: ability to do work (potential and kinetic energy)

gravity g: gravitational constant 9.78 m s^{-2} at the equator; 9.832 m s^{-2} at the north pole.

intensity: the power carried by a wave or oscillation dived by the area over which it arrives (W m^{-2})

internal reflection: this occurs when the reflection angle is >90°

joule J: the SI unit of work 1J = 1 N m

kelvin K: the SI unit of temperature 0K = −273.15°C

kinetic energy: the energy due to motion so that $E = \frac{1}{2}mv^2$

momentum: mass × velocity measured as kg m s^{-1}

newton N: the SI unit of force $F = ma$ measured as kg m s^{-1}

ohm Ω: the measure of electrical resistance when 1A flows at a potential difference of 1V

pascal Pa: the SI unit for pressure measured in N m^{-2} and 1mm Hg = 1.33×10^{2}Pa

potential energy: chemical, gravitational, electrical and elastic are all examples.

power: the rate of work done per unit time measured as J s^{-1}

refraction: the change in the direction of a wave front when passing from one medium to another.

refractive index: the ratio of the sine of angle of incidence to the sine of the angle of refraction.

specular reflection: reflection at a smooth border where the surface unevenness is much less than the wavelength.

tesla T: the SI measure of magnetic field strength where 1T = 1N m^{-1} at 90° to the field

volt V: a measure of electrical potential difference where 1V = 1 J C^{-1}

watt W: the SI unit of mechanical or electrical power where 1W = 1 J s^{-1}

wavefront: a line that joins all points on a wave that have the same phase.

weber Wb: the unit of magnetic flux

3

X-ray production and properties: Fundamentals

3.1 Introduction
3.2 X-ray tube design
3.3 The x-ray spectrum

3.4 Electrical characteristics
3.5 X-ray tube rating

3.1 INTRODUCTION

On Friday 8th November 1895 Wilhelm Conrad Röntgen (1845-1923: German physicist), while experimenting with high voltages using a Crooke's Tube (an evacuated tube with electrodes inserted), noticed that invisible radiation was being produced that penetrated the soft tissue of his hand revealing skeletal structure. He called the radiation 'x-rays': x-denoting their unknown origin. Within a year of their discovery x-rays were being used for medical imaging. In 1901 Röntgen received the first Nobel Prize for physics. In 1913 W.D. Coolidge (USA engineer: 1873-1975) produced the electrically heated cathode tube: the forerunner of all modern x-ray tubes.

3.1.1 X- and γ-radiation

The principle of x-ray generation is relatively simple. A beam of high energy electrons from a heated **filament** (situated in a cathode assembly) bombards a positively charged heavy metal target, the **anode**.

The electrons mostly react with the target's orbital electrons producing heat (99%). The remaining electrons interact with the target nuclei giving a **continuous** x-ray spectrum made up from many photon energies; a **poly-energetic** spectrum. X-ray photon energy from the tube can be controlled by varying the electrical supply high voltage. The diagnostic range has a **peak energy** (kVp) from 40 to 140kVp; mammography utilizes a lower energy from 20-30 kVp.

Figure 3.1(a) shows that an x-ray tube can be treated as a electronic diode since the electrons only travel one direction, having a heated filament at one end which acts as the source of electrons and an anode at the other. Electrons emitted by the filament are accelerated across a vacuum by applying a high voltage, colliding with the anode to produce x-radiation. X-rays are formed by electrons changing direction within the vicinity of a heavy nucleus (tungsten). Since there is a direction change the electrons lose energy in the form of electromagnetic radiation.

Gamma radiation In contrast to x-rays gamma radiation, although similar to x-radiation in many respects, is produced during nuclear decay and has discrete energies forming a line spectrum. It is mostly mono-energetic although some nuclides emit more than one gamma energy. Gamma radiation, having discrete energies, is measured in keV and MeV; the useful diagnostic imaging range is 100keV to 0.511MeV.

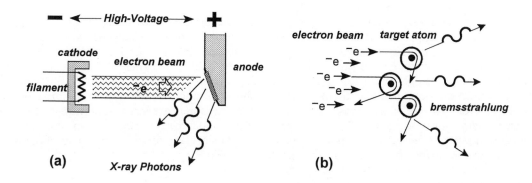

Figure 3.1 **(a)** The basic components of an x-ray tube. A hot filament is the electron source embedded in a metal cathode (negative charge) The electron beam is attracted toward the target anode (positive charge) causing bremsstrahlung events. **(b)** Bremsstrahlung production caused by electron deflection by heavy metal nuclei.

A non-nuclear source of gamma radiation is positron annihilation. X-rays are also produced from some types of nuclear decay: these processes are covered more fully in Chapter 15 (Nuclear Medicine).

3.1.2 Bremsstrahlung

The potential energy of the electron is the product of the electrostatic charge between the cathode and anode seen in Fig.3.1(a). Potential energy is transformed into kinetic energy as the electrons accelerate between cathode and anode.

The electrons penetrate the anode material passing close to its atomic nuclei. They are deflected from their initial path by the nuclear coulomb field of the heavy atoms (e.g. tungsten) causing changes in velocity (both acceleration and deceleration) simply illustrated in Fig.3.1(b). During their changes in velocity (deflection) they lose energy in the form of electromagnetic radiation which is called braking radiation or **bremsstrahlung**.

The deflection is dependent on the nuclear charge (atomic number Z) of the anode. Loss of kinetic energy through interactions with target electrons causes a great deal of heat energy which must be removed effectively in order to prevent anode melting.

Heat and light production (99%) together with x-rays (1%) obey the basic equation from Chapter 2:

$$E = hf \qquad (3.1)$$

where h is Planck's constant and f the frequency of the electromagnetic radiation.

The x-ray tube has a high vacuum so that gas molecules do not impede the electron beam and since very high voltages are used (from 20 to 150kV) the tube must be manufactured from robust insulating materials e.g. glass or ceramic.

Continuous x-ray spectrum Only a small proportion of the x-rays are created at the surface of the target, those formed deeper within the target material are absorbed. Energy transformations that yield x-radiation vary since the bombarding electrons approach the nuclei differently, there is consequently a spread of bremsstrahlung energies from maximum (where the entire electron energy is transformed into x-radiation) to the lowest energy x-ray emission when the electron is only slightly deflected by the nuclear field. Electron velocity increases with the applied high voltage but very few electrons lose all their energy in a single event giving a photon of maximum energy; most of them undergo multiple events where energy loss results in a mixed energy x-ray photons. The peak high tension applied to the tube does not represent the maximum x-ray photon energy (kV peak or kVp) owing to relativistic effects which reduce electron velocities. The resulting x-radiation takes the form of a continuous x-ray spectrum which is shown in Fig.3.2.

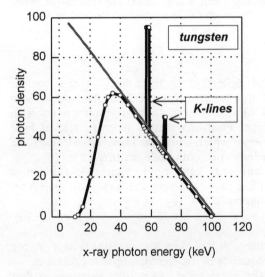

Figure 3.2   Continuous spectrum (gray line) shows that the lowest photon energies (below about 20keV) are removed by the x-ray tube glass wall giving an exit spectrum which is peaked. Characteristic line spectra are superimposed on this spectrum.

The lowest energy photons are removed since the beam of x-rays leaving the tube is filtered by the glass envelope. If low energy x-rays are required (e.g. mammography) then a thin

metal beryllium window must be used with its much lower density (1800 kg m^{-3}) than glass (4200 kg m^{-3}) giving a greater transparency to lower energy x-radiation.

Characteristic radiation   The collisions between the beam electrons and the inner orbital electrons (K and L shells) of the target create orbital vacancies. These are quickly filled accompanied by the emission of characteristic radiation in the form of line spectra which are seen superimposed on the continuous x-ray spectrum in Fig.3.2. The line spectra for tungsten occur at roughly 59 and 69keV.

3.1.3   X-ray beam intensity

X-ray production is a very inefficient process, most of the electrical energy is lost as heat. The approximate balance is:

Electron beam intensity	100%
Heat and light production	99%
X-radiation from anode surface	1%
Remaining after fixed filtration	0.5%
Remaining after added filtration (available x-rays for imaging)	0.1%

The **probability** p for bremsstrahlung events is low, about 1-5%, but increases with both atomic number Z of the anode material and the electron beam energy E, so that $p \propto Z{\cdot}E^2$. Substituting kV for E yields:

$$p \propto Z{\cdot}kV^2 \qquad (3.2)$$

This function follows a power law relationship. The **efficiency** η of bremsstrahlung production depends on:

$$\eta = k{\cdot}E{\cdot}Z \qquad (3.3)$$

k is a constant being $1.1{\times}10^{-9}$ for tungsten. The efficiency of bremsstrahlung production for tungsten and molybdenum, over a range of energies, is listed in Tab.3.1.   X-ray intensity increases with applied kV and density of anode material since both probability and efficiency are influenced by these two factors.

Table 3.1 Efficiency of x-ray Production

Tungsten (Z =74)	
20kV	0.162%
60kV	0.48%
100kV	0.814%
140kV	1.14%
Molybdenum (Z = 42)	
20kV	0.092%

Knowing the electron charge and the tube current, together with the exposure time (mAs), the available photons which form a chest radiograph can be estimated (Box 3.1). If allowances are made for x-ray pro-duction efficiency an approximate quantity can be derived that is useful for future calculations.

Box 3.1

Chest radiograph photon number

The number of x-ray photons produced during a standard radiograph of 60kV at 5mAs can be calculated approximately:

Number of electrons for 5mAs
Electron charge is 1.6×10^{-19} coulombs (C)
Since 1amp = 1C s^{-1} then C $s^{-1} \times$ seconds represent coulombs

$$5\text{mAs} = \frac{5 \times 10^{-3}}{1.6 \times 10^{-19}} = 3.13 \times 10^{16} \text{ electrons}$$

But owing to low production efficiency at 60kV only 0.5% produce useful x-rays. (Tab.3.1) So 60kV at 5mAs would give:

$3.13 \times 10^{16} \times 0.005 = 1.5 \times 10^{14}$ available x-ray photons.

In summary

- x-rays are produced by bombarding heavy metal targets with electrons: probability of production increases as kV^2.
- efficiency increases with applied kilovoltage and with target Z.
- bremsstrahlung radiation gives a continuous x-ray spectrum. The peak energy (kVp) equals the applied kV.
- Lowest photon energies are absorbed by tube wall. Lower energies can be retrieved by using beryllium window.
- characteristic x-rays are produced by dislodging K and L shell electrons from target.

3.2   X-RAY TUBE DESIGN

Diagnostic x-ray tubes are high precision units which are engineered to very close tolerances and are largely hand finished; they are therefore costly items.
The major problems of x-ray tube design are:

- Efficient production of x-radiation and efficient heat removal.
- Constant x-ray beam quality with desired geometry (beam profile)
- Reliable performance under a wide variety of loading conditions such as short duration/high loading (pulsed CT and DSA) and long duration low loading (fluoroscopy).

The majority of x-ray tubes employ **rotating anodes** since stationary anode x-ray tubes are only suitable for low output applications experienced in dentistry and small mobile x-ray units. Consequently rotating anodes are the most common x-ray tube design.
The important components can be identified from the detailed diagram of Fig. 3.3.

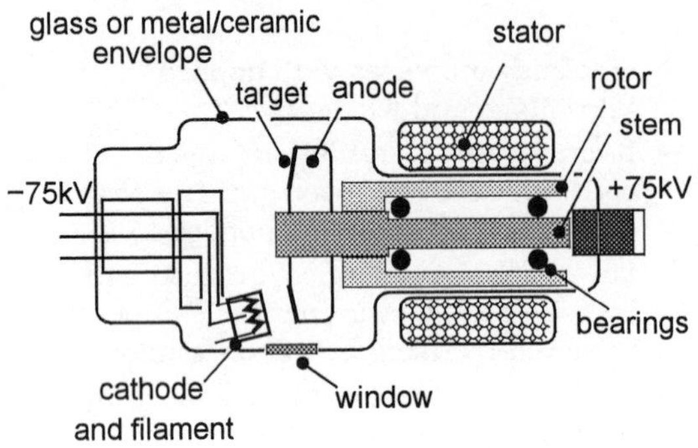

Figure 3.3   The details of a typical x-ray tube showing the position of the filament-cathode assembly with respect to the anode. A molybdenum axle supported by bearings (rotor) is driven by the external stator. High voltage negative and positive connections are shown.

Table 3.2   Melting point, specific heat and thermal conductivity of some important materials.

Material	M.Pt °C	Sp.Ht $J\,kg^{-1}K^{-1}$	Therm. Con. $W\,cm^{-1}K^{-1}$
W	3410	137	1.76
Mo	2617	253	1.38
Ni	1726	455	59
C	3800	730	0.07
Glass	1400	670	0.015

Metals used in construction   The various materials used in x-ray tube construction are listed in Tab.3.2 along with their properties. Specific heat capacity, heat conduction and melting point are very important parameters owing to the excessive heat produced by x-ray tubes.

Molybdenum has a larger heat capacity than tungsten and is used as a backing for the target and in the manufacture of the supporting stem for the anode disk.

Carbon, in the form of graphite, is used for increasing the radiating surface of the anode. It is ideal since it is a good heat radiator (black), has a low mass and a high melting point.

Copper has a large heat capacity together with superior heat conduction but a lower melting point which restricts its use and it is mainly found as electrical wires and as part of the anode rotor.

3.2.1   The cathode assembly

The basic design for the x-ray tube shown in Fig.3.1(a) shows the cathode and filament assembly consisting of a **filament**, made from tungsten wire, which is heated electrically to a high temperature so that electrons are 'boiled-off' from its surface. These electrons form the **tube current**. The filament is located within a negatively charged nickel **cathode** which is shaped so that a precise beam geometry is obtained.

The filament   This is manufactured from tungsten wire and is part of the cathode assembly. Together they provide a carefully shaped electron beam which bombards a precise target area on the anode. The cathode assembly is connected to the negative high voltage supply.

Filament supply   The power supply, which heats the filament, is low voltage AC from a filament transformer supplying 8-12volts. Since this is AC there is a superimposed low frequency ripple on filament emission and the x-ray tube current. High frequency transformers do not have this problem.

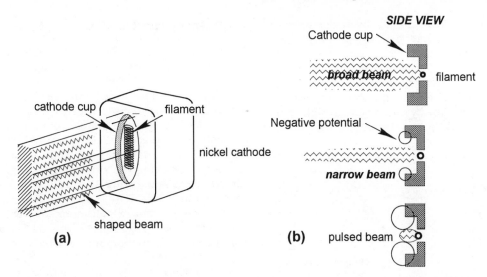

Figure 3.4 **(a)** The filament encased in a nickel cathode. The sharp edges of the cup shapes the electron beam . **(b)** The geometry of the electron beam is controlled by the applied negative voltage to the cathode. The bottom diagram shows how the beam can be switched off by applying a much higher negative voltage.

The cathode This houses the filament and is manufactured from nickel. The filament is located within a depression or **cup** having sharp contoured edges which electrostatically focus the electron beam. Figure 3.4(a) shows the complete cathode assembly. Exact focusing is achieved by altering the depth of the filament in the cathode during manufacture. The cathode cup can also be independently supplied with a high negative voltage which can dynamically alter the focal size or, if the negative charge is big enough, switch off the electron beam entirely. This is the **grid controlled** x-ray tube and is used in cinefluorography, digital subtraction angiography (DSA) units and computed tomography (CT) where rapid pulses of x-rays are required.

Figure 3.4(b) shows three examples of beam control obtained by using an increasing negative voltage on the cathode cup. A broad focus beam (top diagram) is about 1 to 2mm wide and a fine focus beam (middle) would typically be about 0.4 to 0.1mm wide. A high negative charge on the cathode edges (bottom diagram) switches off the electron beam entirely, and this control mechanism is used for giving precise x-ray pulses.

Tube lifetime The available electron density from the heated filament (emission current density) depends on the filament temperature. The relationship between filament temperature and emission current density is plotted in Fig. 3.5(a) and shows that for small changes in filament temperature there are large changes in emission current and hence x-ray tube current. Stable filament power supplies are therefore essential for consistent x-ray exposure.

The level of filament current significantly determines the lifetime of the x-ray tube. This is indicated by a typical lifetime graph in Fig. 3.5(b). For short exposures the filament temperature is 2500°C but would be lower for continuous use as in, say, fluoroscopy.

Space charge effect As electrons leave or are 'boiled-off' from the filament it becomes increasingly more positive owing to the loss of negative charge. The electrons tend to be attracted back towards the filament surface. At higher filament temperatures a cloud of electrons develops containing a constant stream of electrons both leaving and returning from the filament surface shown in

Fig.3.6(a). It has already been demonstrated in Chapter 2 that a positive charged body (anode) placed near the filament will attract some electrons from the cloud and therefore a current will pass between the filament and the anode. Electrons are injected into this dynamic system by the negative high voltage supply (–75kV) connected to the filament circuit.

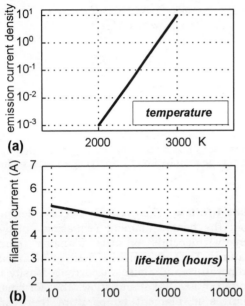

(a)

(b)

Figure 3.5 **(a)** The available electrons measured as an emission current increases rapidly with relatively small increases in filament temperature. **(b)** Increasing the filament current shortens tube life.

The tube current (current flow in diagram) depends on the applied anode voltage. At lower voltages (between 20 and 40kV) not all the available electrons are attracted from the filament. This limits the tube current and is the **space charge** effect. This effect is demonstrated by the shoulder region of the graph in Fig.3.6(b) between a tube voltage of about 10 and 50kV. Increasing the tube voltage overcomes this problem allowing higher tube currents shown by a large increase in tube current with applied tube kilovoltage in the graph.

3.2.2 Anode construction

Dental units and some small mobile x-ray units use stationary or fixed anode designs. The most efficient design however uses a rotating disc anode which enables higher x-ray output owing to more effective cooling.

The basic design of a simple rotating anode consists of a tungsten disk, typically between 90 and 200mm diameter, with an accurately beveled edge giving the **anode angle**; this has already been seen in Fig.3.1(a) but is given in more detail in Fig.3.7(a). It is attached to a molybdenum stem which connects with a rotor forming, together with the stator windings, an induction motor which rotates the anode at speed.

Since useful x-rays are produced at the surface of the anode the target area itself is made from thin metal alloy (tungsten-rhenium), about 1mm thick. This has the added advantage of easier heat removal and the rhenium content reduces surface pitting.

Graphite, being a very low mass material with a high melting point, is brazed onto the back of the anode which increases heat radiating efficiency in tubes that will experience high loading (DSA and CT).

Anode size Rotating anode disks are manufactured in many designs. The anode diameter determines the heat rating of the x-ray tube and therefore its thermal loading. The disk mass and surface area also play an important part.

From Fig.3.7(b) a larger anode diameter at the same rotational speed offers a longer track length of target and so the heat generated is spread over a greater area of metal. Larger discs therefore take higher loading (higher output). The 150mm anode gives a target length ×1.5 more than the 100mm anode and its target area is also larger. Anode disc diameters vary from 75 to 200mm depending on loading required. Larger anode diameters are used for high power applications such as fluoroscopy and CT. A larger disc diameter increases the heat capacity and also the area radiating heat but there is potential mechanical damage in the larger anode due to localized expansion.

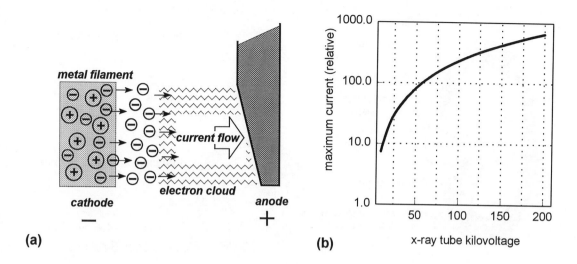

(a)

(b)

Figure 3.6 **(a)** A cloud of electrons surrounding the hot filament causing a space-charge effect. **(b)** The space charge effect decreases as the applied kilovoltage increases. Below 30kV it is a significant factor reducing tube current. The *y*-axis is plotted on a log scale.

This is prevented by cutting radial slots into the anode (the 150mm anode in Fig. 3.7(b)); these are **stress relieved** anodes. This technique is not usually applied to CT tubes since the slit surface would interfere with the high speed grid control producing the pulsed x-ray beam.

Exposure overload monitoring devices (Loadix) placed behind the anode to monitor heat output prevent x-ray tube ratings from being exceeded. Anode speed affects rating and Box 3.2 gives some examples for anode size and speed.

Box 3.2 Anode disk size and power rating

Anode diameter and power rating
(refer to Fig.3.7(b))
100mm diameter anode; 7mm track width:
Mean radius: (100–7mm) = 93mm
Track length = $2\pi \times {}^{93}/2$ = 292mm
***Anode rotation speed* 3000 rpm:**
Complete target area exposed every ${}^{60}/3000$
= 0.02 second
for 9000 rpm this would be 0.0066 second so the electron energy deposited in the anode is spread over a greater target area for faster rotational speeds.

3.2.3 Rotor and stator

The rotating anode forms part of an induction motor shown as the rotor and stator in Fig.3.3. The rotor, made from copper, is attached to the anode by a molybdenum stem. This revolves about a central axle which forms the positive electrode (+75kV). The axle bearing can consist of either ball-races, lubricated by a silver paste, or sleeve bearings. The latter allow greater surface contact and therefore more rapid cooling by conduction. Excessive heat transfer along the anode stem is restricted since molybdenum has relatively poor heat conductivity and most of the heat loss is by radiation from the anode surface toward the x-ray tube envelope (glass or metal). In some tubes employing sleeve bearings an oil circulation path passes along the axle. The anode rotational speed is either 3000 or 3400rpm at 50/60Hz supply frequency or 850-10000 using high frequency waveforms. For these higher speeds either the overall tube loading can be increased or finer focal spot sizes can be selected. Larger disc diameters require better support and the anode stem in these tubes is carried forward

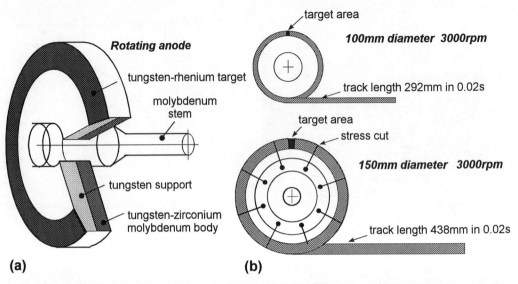

Figure 3.7   **(a)** The rotating anode construction showing a solid tungsten/ zirconium/ molybdenum base supporting a pure tungsten layer on which the thin (1mm thick) tungsten-rhenium alloy target is fused. **(b)** A 100mm diameter anode (top) showing the track length available during a 0.02s exposure time. Increased track length (150mm) allows greater heat dissipation for the same exposure time.

and supported by its own bearing, giving support both front and behind.

3.2.4 Focal spot

The x-rays do not originate from a single point on the anode surface, but from a rectangular area, the dimensions and angle of which are carefully calculated. This is shown as a target area in Fig.3.8(a) and forms the **real focal spot** of the electron beam. The anode angle determines the projected or **effective focal spot** size of the x-ray beam (sometimes called the apparent focal spot). The focal spot size influences the sharpness of the image and the tube rating.

Real and effective focal spots   The size of the effective focal spot is determined by the **line focus principle** and a calculation is given in Box 3.3 using the geometry shown in this figure. This calculation shows that the formation of a symmetrical effective focal spot from an angled real focal spot on the anode surface is achieved by choosing an angle that projects the same length as the real focal spot width.

Box 3.3

The line focus principle

From the diagram in Fig.3.8(a) The electron beam of width *A-A'* strikes the anode target area. The dimension *f* (which equals *CB*) is determined by: $sin\ \theta = {}^{opposite}/hypotenuse$ so the effective focal spot *BC* = $sin\ \theta \times AC$.

If *AC* is 2mm (real focal spot) the effective or apparent focal spot is then 0.2588×2 or 0.5mm. Doubling the real focal spot size (4mm) will give a 1mm effective focal spot.

Useful field of view   The smaller the angle θ the wider the track can be, as seen in Fig.3.8(b). In general the smaller the anode angle the wider the focal track which increases the power rating, however angle size also influences the field size of the x-ray beam at a given source to image distance (SID). Field size increases with anode angle, however so also does the effective focal spot size which will degrade image resolution, so a large area radiograph would be obtained at the expense of resolution.

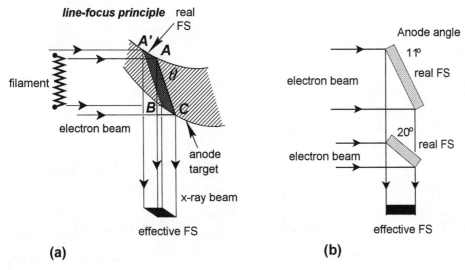

Figure 3.8   **(a)** The electron beam bombarding the target (shaded area). The anode angle θ of triangle A,B,C. is used for calculating the effective focal spot size. **(b)** Increasing the anode angle decreases the real focal spot area which reduces anode rating.

Conversely a smaller anode angle would give a smaller field size but a better resolution. The choice of anode angle depends on the application required and the SID. A smaller anode angle yields a larger focal spot and consequently higher heat rating or load. Stationary anode tubes have an energy dissipation of about 200W mm^{-2} s^{-1} of the actual focal spot size. A rotating anode has an energy dissipation of 1500W mm^{-2} s^{-1}

Dual focal spots   For many applications two focal spot sizes are necessary; a second smaller spot is used for higher resolution or magnified radiographs. Two methods are shown. In Fig.3.9(a) a single filament refocuses the electron beam electrostatically by varying the negative voltage on the cathode cup, so bombarding a smaller area on the anode track (see narrow beam in Fig.3.4(b)). Alternatively Fig.3.9(b) shows a double filament, each one directed to a different angled target, which requires a dual track anode to give two focal spot sizes.

Each method has its disadvantages. Figure 3.9(c) shows that the single track dual focus anode uses the central portion of the track for both fine and broad focus beams so greater wear will take place shortening tube life. Wear is reduced for a dual track dual focus design (lower picture in (c)) but the track length for the fine focal spot is shorter which will reduce its loading capability.

Heel effect   The photon intensity across the x-ray beam is not uniform. The uniformity changes with anode angle and gives a **heel effect** to the beam intensity. Collimating the useful field of view reduces the heel effect but does not eliminate it; Fig.3.10(a). The diagram of the field intensity patterns in Fig.3.10(b) shows that the heel-effect decreases with increase in anode angle (7°, 12° and 20°) but increasing the angle adversely affects image resolution and thermal rating (loadability). The heel effect only occurs in line with the cathode/anode axis and the plot of intensity across the beam in this axis, Fig.3.10(c), indicates the substantial drop (up to 25%) in beam intensity at the anode end of the tube. This is improved with increased SID as shown by the two plots for 70 and 110cm SID.

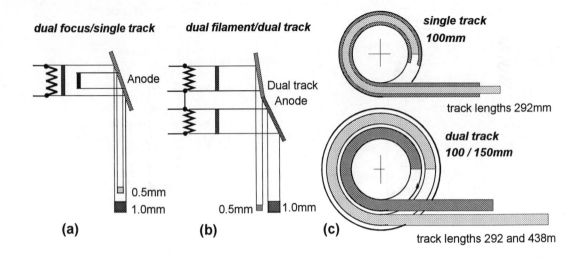

Figure 3.9 **(a)** Dual focal spot sizes can be obtained by altering the target size with different negative potentials on the filament cup or **(b)** by employing two filaments focused on different target angles. **(c)** Anodes showing single and dual target areas.

3.2.5 Tube enclosure

X-ray tube envelope Boro-silicate glass is the common material for tube construction since it conforms with manufacturing requirements. A high vacuum must be maintained in the x-ray tube for the electron beam so the surrounding envelope must be:

- strong enough to withstand atmospheric pressure.
- heat resistant to withstand considerable heat production by the anode.
- transparent to the heat radiated from the anode.

During the life of the tube metal atoms from the incandescent filament and those vaporized from the focal spot are deposited on the glass walls; this slowly reduces its insulator properties. The closer the electrodes are to the wall the more serious is this problem and gives design restrictions. Glass envelopes are particularly prone to breakdown but metal/ceramic enclosures repel ion deposits reducing the tungsten coating build up.

More compact tube design can be obtained by using a metal envelope which will be unaffected by vaporized metal and be a more efficient heat exchanger; it is also stronger. The insulating regions in metal tubes are made from ceramic material.

Housing The x-ray tube itself is enclosed in a sealed housing which is shown in Fig.3.11(a). Efficient removal of heat produced by x-ray production by the tube is essential. Circulating air is sufficient to cool mobile and mammography units (fan assisted cooling can halve tube cooling time), but circulating oil is necessary within the enclosure for cooling conventional and DSA equipment. The total heat capacity of the tube enclosure is largely dependent on the volume of oil it contains.

Radiation shielding X-rays are emitted from the tube in all directions and overall lead shielding must cover the complete housing assembly. Any leakage radiation is measured with the collimator diaphragms closed and should be less than $1mGy\ h^{-1}$ (100mR) at one meter and is usually less than 0.3mGy

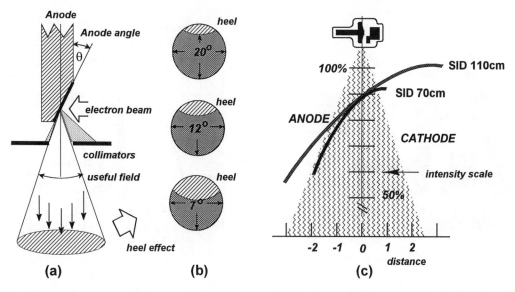

(a)   (b)   (c)

Figure 3.10   **(a)** The useful x-ray field is contained by the central beam and the outside margins of the beam are blocked by collimating the beam. **(b)** This useful field is still non-uniform due to the heel effect, influenced by anode angle. **(c)** The plot of beam intensity shows the variation along the anode to cathode axis for two source to image distances(SIDs): 70cm (shaded curve) and 110cm (black curve).

h^{-1} (30mR). An acceptable leakage figure for current x-ray equipment would be $\leq$0.5mSv h^{-1} at 150kVp. Since the beam intensity varies across the beam width in the anode-cathode axis (heel effect) a fixed lead diaphragm restricts beam dimensions yielding the useful beam width. Other adjustable diaphragms/collimators are used for varying the overall beam size for different field of views shown by the collimator diaphragm in Fig.3.11(a).

3.2.6 X-ray window

The glass window of the x-ray tube removes low energy x-ray photons (from 0 to ~20keV) and so provides **inherent beam filtration** (seen in Fig.3.2). Further filtration is still necessary however as photons from the low energy end of the spectrum play no part in image formation and are absorbed in the first few centimeters of soft tissue; this contributes to the patient radiation dose.

Fixed or **added filtration** (F in Fig.3.11(a)) is added to the beam to remove these lower energies. Inherent and fixed filtration to-

gether give the **total filtration**. The inherent filtration is equivalent to about 0.5mm aluminum but as the tube ages this increases due to vaporized tungsten and the fixed filtration (about 1.5 to 2.0mm aluminum) must be altered to compensate for this.

3.3   THE X-RAY SPECTRUM

The theoretical complete spectrum from an x-ray tube has already been shown as a straight gray line in Fig.3.2 but in practice several factors remove the lower energy photons:

- The depth of interactions within the target.
- X-ray tube wall thickness.
- Additional beam filtration.

The **maximum** beam energy (kVpeak or kVp) depends on the applied voltage which directly influences speed of the electron beam (kinetic energy). The x-ray **minimum** energy depends on the material through which the bremsstrahlung must pass.

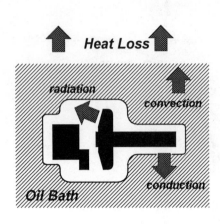

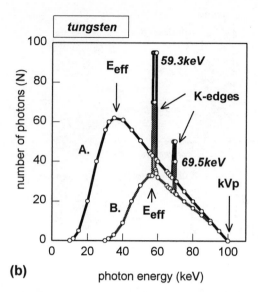

(b)

Figure 3.11   **(a)** Tube enclosure filled with oil which as the heat conduction system and radiation shield. **(b)** Continuous x-ray spectra from tungsten targets, before and after filtering, showing increase in effective energy (E_{eff}) and tungsten's characteristic K-lines.

3.3.1 Characteristic radiation

The common target materials tungsten, rhenium and molybdenum yield line spectra for their characteristic K-energies:

Tungsten:	69.5 and 59.3 keV
Rhenium:	71.6 and 61.1 keV
Molybdenum:	20.0 and 17.3 keV

Fig.3.11(b) shows an unfiltered (A) and filtered (B) continuous spectra from a tungsten anode showing the K shell radiation as superimposed line spectra which result from interactions with the electron beam and the K shell electrons. Smaller line spectra from the L shells would also be present.

3.3.2 Beam energy

Increasing the high voltage increases the overall intensity of the continuous spectrum. In Fig.3.12(a) the kilovoltage has been increased in three steps from 50, 80 and 120kV the peak energy values (kVp) follow

this. The choice of kilovoltage determines object (patient) penetration and image quality. Low kilovoltages give high contrast images (distinguishing soft tissue differences in mammography) since low energy x-ray photons are easily absorbed. Higher kilovoltages, due to their increased penetration, reduce con-trast differences and since beam intensity increases as kV^2 (eqn.3.2), the overall radiation reaching the film also increases (higher penetration). It will be seen in later chapters that film/screen sensitivity also improves with kV.

Effective energy This is the peak output identified on the curves in Fig.3.12(a) as E_{eff}. The beam's effective energy can be influenced by changing kVp and filtration. The intensity Q of the beam is seen to increase as $Q \propto kV^2$ so a 30% increase in kilovoltage approximately doubles x-ray beam intensity along with an increase in effective energy. The effective energy of a moderately filtered x-ray spectrum is very roughly $2/3$ kVp so 100kVp would translate as 70kV$_{eff}$.

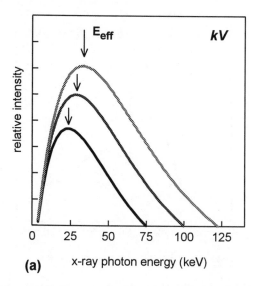

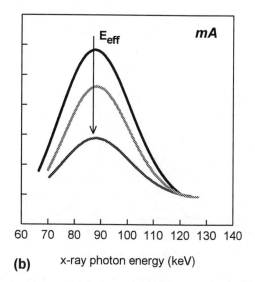

(a) x-ray photon energy (keV)

(b) x-ray photon energy (keV)

Figure 3.12 **(a)** The change of the x-ray spectrum with applied kilovoltage. Peak kilovoltages of 50, 80 and 120kVp show how the effective energy also changes. **(b)** Intensity of the x-ray beam increases with tube current (mA) but the effective energy remains the same.

Image density In order to achieve the same film density when increasing 50kV to 60kV then the exposure should be altered according to:

$$\left[\frac{kVp_{old}}{kVp_{new}}\right]^4 \text{ so } \left[\frac{50}{60}\right]^4 \approx 0.5 \qquad (3.3)$$

For each 10kV the exposure doubles or halves. Either the tube current (mA) or the exposure time (s) can be altered to maintain the same image (film) density. This effect lessens at higher kVs (85 to 120) for each 15kV increase doubles or halves exposure.
 The characteristic radiation energy does not change with voltage but its intensity increases contributing about 10% for a tungsten anode in the diagnostic range.

3.3.3 Current

Increasing the tube current mA does not influence beam quality. Its penetration is unaltered since only the intensity or **quantity** of x-ray photons increases as $Q \propto$ mA. Although the height of the curve changes overall shape remains the same so beam penetration is unaltered; beam quality remains the same (Fig.3.12(b)).
 In summary the overall quantity of x-ray photons produced by an x-ray tube depends on:

- anode material atomic number (Z)
- applied kilovoltage (kV)
- tube current (mA)

The beam intensity is the product of :

$$Z \times kV^2 \times mA \qquad (3.4)$$

This intensity value is influenced by the degree of beam filtration.

3.3.4 Beam filtration

The two spectra in Fig.3.13(a) (A and B) show the effect of adding filters which remove the lower x-ray energies. This changes the proportion of high to low energy photons in the spectrum so the effective energy increases. Aluminum is the common filter material for conventional radiography but higher kVp

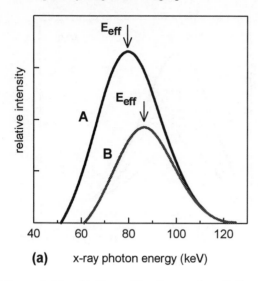

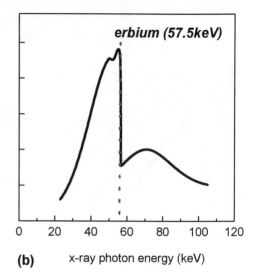

Figure 3.13 **(a)** Beam filtration preferentially removes lower energy photons and increases effective energy.   **(b)** Certain metals have K-edges that appear in the diagnostic range. There is maximum absorption at their K-edge. Erbium is shown here.

settings (CT at 125 or 140kVp) copper is used, together with aluminum.   Both aluminum and copper have low K-edges (Al at 1.6keV; Cu at 8.0keV) so these do not interfere at diagnostic energies. Removing low energy radiation from the beam significantly reduces patient entrance dose shown in Fig.3.14 where dose versus added beam filtration is plotted. Fixed filtration for a conventional x-ray tube is typically 1.2 to 1.5mm aluminum. The effect of filtration on the x-ray spectrum in Fig.3.13(a) shows the lower energies are preferentially removed and overall beam intensity is reduced but the effective energy E_{eff} is increased.

K-edge filtration   Metals with higher K-edge values (20 to 30keV) are useful filters in radiology since they preferentially remove higher energy photons. These filters are commonly found in mammography where they reduce patient radiation dose by removing energies above 28keV which only play a minor role in image formation for this examination. Common K-edge metals used for x-ray beam filtration are shown in Tab.3.3.

  Samarium is sometimes encountered as a K-edge filter in conventional radiography along with erbium whose effect on an x-ray spectrum in shown in Fig.3.13(b). The K-edge for tin is useful since this allows this metal to be used as lightweight shielding in light-weight protective aprons (see Chapter 5 Section 5.2.1).

Table 3.3 K-edge metals used as beam filters

Metal	*K-edge (keV)*
Molybdenum	20.0
Rhodium	23.2
Palladium	24.3
Tin	29.2
Samarium	46.8
Erbium	57.5

3.3.5   X-ray beam quality

Beam quality   This is defined as the penetrating power of the x-ray beam and subjectively describes the shape of the continuous spectrum. Changing the kilovoltage changes beam quality since the penetrating power alters and the increased cut-off point (kVp) changes the spectrum shape; the effective energy also changes. Other factors such as filtration and high voltage supply characteristics (single and 3-phase supply etc.) also change beam quality.

Tube current, although it changes the quantity of radiation, as seen in Fig.3.12(b), has no effect on the spectrum's effective energy so has no influence on the quality of the beam.

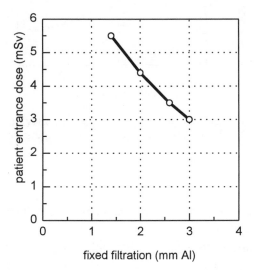

y-axis: patient entrance dose (mSv)
x-axis: fixed filtration (mm Al)

Figure 3.14 The reduction in patient surface dose with increased tube filtration. The thickness of fixed filtration depends on kVp.

The half-value-layer (HVL) This is a practical measure of x-ray beam **quality**. Thin aluminium foils of known thickness (from 0.1 to 2mm) are placed in a narrow beam of x-rays until the original intensity is reduced by half. The thickness of aluminium producing this is the half-value-layer (HVL) for the beam and is normally between 2.5-3.0mm for 80kVp x-rays. The half-value-layer will alter depending on spectrum shape. This is described further in Chapter 5.

Beam homogeneity A homogeneous photon beam (gamma source) would be attenuated in a simple exponential fashion by increasing the aluminium thicknesses (Fig. 3.15(a)).

For a single energy photon beam the HVL reduces beam intensity to half. A second HVL will bring the intensity to a ¼. For a homogeneous beam shown in Fig.3.15(a) the 1st and 2nd (primary and secondary) HVL are equal; slope M gives an HVL1 of 0.375mm and HVL2 of 0.75mm.

For a continuos (non-homogeneous beam) of x-rays (slope P) the primary and secondary HVL are not equal since lower energy photons are preferentially removed and the simple exponential law is not obeyed (HVL1 is 0.125mm but HVL2 is 0.375). A predominance of low energy photons in the x-ray beam will cause more inhomogeneity since the majority of these will be removed in the primary HVL leaving fewer to be removed in the secondary HVL. The difference between mono-energetic and poly-energetic radiation is shown when this second half-value-layer is measured. A low first HVL indicates the presence of low energy photons which play no part in image formation and only increase patient surface dose since the low energies are removed by the surface tissue. A high HVL indicates loss of useful medium energy x-ray photons which would have influenced image contrast. The HVL does not represent the fixed filtration of the beam but is influenced by it. The fixed filtration can be derived from the HVL value.

Equivalent energy This is defined as the energy of the mono-energetic beam which gives the same HVL as the x-ray spectrum. In other words, the single energy whose photons would be attenuated to the same extent as those of the mixed energies of the x-ray beam continuous spectrum. As an example a 100 kVp x-ray spectrum having an HVL of 5mm Al gives an attenuation coefficient of:

$$\mu = \frac{0.693}{\text{HVL}} = 1.38 \; \mu \; \text{cm}^{-1}$$

From the graph in Fig.3.15(b) this shows an equivalent energy of 40keV. This should not be confused with the effective energy which is the x-ray spectrum peak; a rough approximation for this would be $100 \times 2/3$ or $\sim 70 \text{kV}_{\text{eff}}$.

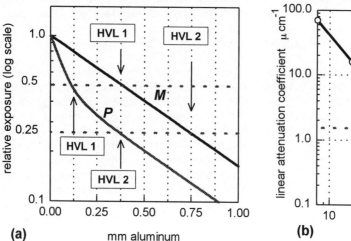

Figure 3.15 (a) The reduction of beam intensity to half its original value is a measure of its HVL **(b)** attenuation coefficient versus kilovoltage for aluminum. This curve can be used for finding the equivalent energy of a poly-energetic beam.

3.3.6 X-ray beam quantity

A subjective assessment of spectrum shape is given by beam quality. The **quantity** of x-radiation incident on a surface (e.g. patient) depends on area, time and energy. Measurements of radiation quantity are important for estimating the sensitivity of imaging devices and calculations in radiation dosimetry.
There are four important parameters that describe intensity:

Photon fluence	Φ	Photons cm^{-2}
Photon flux	ϕ	Photons cm^{-2} s^{-1}
Energy fluence	Ψ	MeV cm^{-2}
Energy flux	ψ	MeV cm^{-2} s^{-1}

For N photons of energy E incident on a surface area A for time t then:

Photon fluence (Φ) Is a measure of photon intensity per unit area expressed as:

$$\Phi = \frac{N}{A} \quad \text{photons cm}^{-2} \quad (3.5)$$

Photon Flux (ϕ) The photon fluence per unit time t is:

$$\phi = \frac{N}{A \cdot t} \quad \text{photons cm}^{-2} \text{ s}^{-1} \quad (3.6)$$

Energy Fluence (Ψ) Photon energy E deposited per unit area. For a mono-energetic beam this is simply ΦE MeV cm^{-2}

Energy Flux Density (ψ) For a mono-energetic beam this is simply ϕE but for a poly-energetic beam the proportion of each energy per unit time (E_i) gives the Energy Flux Density which is the sum of all the different energy components:

$$\psi = \Sigma \, (\Psi \times E_i) \quad \text{MeV cm}^{-2} \text{ s}^{-1} \quad (3.7)$$

The complete family describing the quantity of x-ray photons is used in Box 3.4 for calculating the quantity of x-rays used in a chest radiograph, using the basic quantity already calculated in Box 3.1

Box 3.4

X-ray beam quantitation

From the photon number 1.5×10^{14} calculated in Box.3.1 the x-ray fluence and flux for a chest radiograph of $60\mathrm{kV_{eff}}$ 5mAs over an area of $1500\ \mathrm{cm^2}$ would be:

The Photon Fluence

$$\Phi = \frac{N}{A} = \frac{1.5 \times 10^{14}\,\text{photons}}{1.5 \times 10^{3}\,\mathrm{cm^2}}$$

$$= 1.0 \times 10^{11}\ \text{photons cm}^{-2}$$

The Photon Flux

$$\phi = \frac{\Phi}{t} = \frac{1.0 \times 10^{11}}{0.05}$$

$$= 2.0 \times 10^{12}\ \text{photons cm}^{-2}\ \text{s}^{-1}$$

The Energy Fluence

$$\Psi = \frac{NE}{A}\ 1.0 \times 10^{11} \times 0.06$$

$$= 6.0 \times 10^{9}\ \text{MeV cm}^{-2}$$

The Energy Flux

$$\psi = \frac{\Psi}{t} = \frac{6.0 \times 10^{9}}{0.05}$$

$$= 1.2 \times 10^{11}\ \text{MeV cm}^{-2}\ \text{s}^{-1}$$

Energy flux density depends on the anode material, tube current and applied kilovoltage so that as already seen in eqn.3.4:

$$\psi \propto Z \times I \times E^2 \qquad (3.8)$$

Where Z is the atomic number, I the tube current and E the applied kilovoltage. A change in tube kilovoltage has a much greater effect on intensity than a change in tube current. From the above formula, increasing the kV by 10kV from 60 to 70 has the same effect on the energy flux density as increasing the tube current by roughly ×1.5.

3.4 ELECTRICAL CHARACTERISTICS

Factors influencing an x-ray tube electrical performance are:

- Filament current
- Maximum kilovoltage:
- Stationary anode: 70-90kVp.
- Rotating anode: 100-150kVp
- Tube current
- Exposure time

3.4.1 Filament current

The filament must be large enough to give a practical electron density but not too large, since this will cause focusing problems. The controlling factors are maximum operating filament temperature and filament size. Filament current is increased for low kVp work (mammography) to maintain tube current and compensate for the space charge limitation shown in Fig.3.6(b) for low kV values 20 and 40kV. Increasing filament emission with temperature has already been demonstrated in Chapter 2 , the space charge effect restricts tube current and its influence can be seen in Fig.3.16(a), (b).

In practice filament current is not switched on and off after each exposure but is kept in a standby mode (about 5mA) and increased to operating currents (4.5 to 5.5A) for exposures. When an exposure is made a preparation switch is first depressed which starts the anode rotating and increases the filament temperature from standby mode.

3.4.2 Tube voltage

The response of an x-ray tube to voltage is shown in Fig.3.16(a). When the filament is heated with electric current electrons are emitted from its surface as already described in Chapter 2 (space charge effect). When a high voltage is applied across the filament (part of the cathode) and the anode, some of the electrons from the space charge will travel across the tube providing the tube current; the higher the voltage the higher the current, as the graph shows.

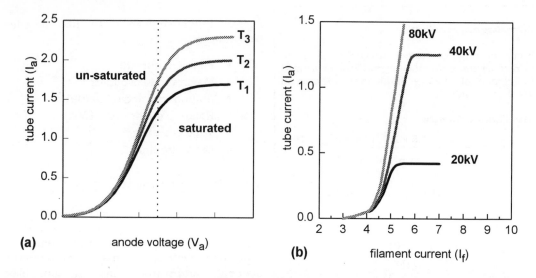

Figure 3.16   (a) The varaiation of anode current with anode voltage showing space charge limited region and saturated region for increasing filament temperatures (T1 to T3) (b) Tube kilovoltage and x-ray tube current for three kilovoltages showing saturation at 20 and 40kV.

The rising part of the curve is 'space charge limited' but as all the available elctrons are removed the curve shows a plateau region where increasing the voltage does not produce an increased tube current. At this point the tube is 'saturated'. The tube current, therefore, does not depend on the tube voltage but on the filament electron emission (i.e. filament temperature). The tube current is emission or temperature controlled; the height of the plateau region alters with filament temperature.

Fig.3.16(b) demonstrates this saturation effect by plotting tube current against filament current for separate high voltages. At low voltages (mammography) there is a tube current that cannot be exceeded in spite of filament current increase. Increasing the kilovoltage overcomes the space charge limitation and allows a higher tube current at 40kV. The operating tube voltage is determined by use. Mammographic tubes are designed for low voltage work (20-30kVp), modern CT up to 140kVp and some high

voltage chest x-ray tubes can approach 180kVp. Much lower filament currents are required for high kV work since the space charge effect is much less (see Fig.3.6(b)).

3.4.3 Tube current

Tube currents vary between 50 and 400mA for conventional radiography and up to 1000mA for fluorography, DSA and CT.

Mammography x-ray tubes operate at lower voltages (from 25 to 30kVp) placing their operating region below the saturation region seen in Fig.3.16(b). Increasing filament current, at fixed voltage, will not influence tube current under these conditions and so filament current is limited to prevent tube damage (see Fig.3.5(a)). Emitted electron density can be increased by increasing the temperature, Fig.3.16(a), or surface area of the filament. This is commonly achieved in mammography by operating dual (side-by-side) filaments focused on the same anode target area.

Grid control　If a sufficiently high negative voltage is applied to the sharp edges of the cathode cup (about 2kV) then the electron beam issuing from the filament can be cut off entirely (Fig.3.4(b)). A pulsed control voltage can be applied which can switch the beam on and off with very little inertia, so very sharp x-ray pulses, of the order of a few milliseconds duration, can be obtained. This is the method chosen for switching the x-ray beam in fluoroscopy (digital and cine) and computed tomography (CT).

3.5　X-RAY TUBE RATING

This is the total workload that can be placed on a tube combining the effects of kilovoltage (kVp), tube current (mA) and exposure time (s) for a certain focal spot size; this is the **electrical rating**. Anode **heat gain** and **heat loss** determines the **thermal rating** of the x-ray tube commonly referred to as loadability.

The workload (loading) or rating of an x-ray tube depends on factors which can be varied i.e.:

- Tube kVp
- Tube current
- Filament current and temperature
- Focal spot size
- Exposure time

Other factors, which are not variable but significantly influence tube rating are anode diameter and anode rotation speed.

3.5.1 Electrical Rating

Maximum kilovoltage　This is usually limited by the insulation of the tube and its oil filled housing. The maximum tube kilovoltage is limited in practice by electrical overload detection.

Maximum tube current　The curve in Fig.3.17(a) shows the maximum tube current for an x-ray tube operating at 80kV. Above the curve the x-ray tube will be overloaded and damaged by excess heat. In order to keep within the electrical rating the permissible maximum tube current decreases as the kV increases (Fig.3.17(b)). The tube current is varied by the filament current (filament heating) and the maximum allowable tube current depends on the tube kilovoltage. Increasing the size of the anode increases the maximum allowable tube current (Fig.3.17(c)).

Maximum power　The product of mA and maximum kV is the tube power: $P = kV \times mA$. This is the maximum power or rating that can be used without damaging the anode; however the rating at fast exposure times must be modified. At 3000 rpm the target lengths shown in Fig. 3.7(b) are completely exposed every 0.02 sec. so exposure times less than 20ms only use a part of this target length; for these the anode rating is independent of the exposure time so the rating curves flatten at shorter exposure times.

Kilowatt rating　This is usually measured from the rating curve for an exposure of 0.1s. In order to find the tube rating locate the intersection of the curve at the 100ms (0.1s) point on the *x*-axis (dotted line marked on graph in Fig.3.17(b)). This determines the tube current for the chosen kilovoltage on the rating curves. Since $P = IV$ watts then:

> 500mA for 60kV　= 30kW
> 375mA for 80kV　= 30kW
> 300mA for 100kV = 30kW

Box 3.5 demonstrates that increasing the real focal spot size can yield higher electrical rating. The anode angle is adjusted to give the same effective focal spot (line focus principle).

For very short exposure times (0.1s or less) **short term loadability** is determined by the size of the anode target. This depends on:

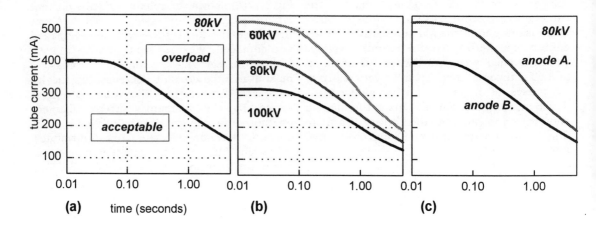

Figure 3.17   (a)   A simplified rating curve plotting time of exposure against maximum allowable tube current. Exposure rates below the curve are acceptable. The rating curve flattens for fast exposure times (<0.1s) **(b)** tube rating for three kilovoltage settings 60, 80 and 100kV; allowable tube current decreases with kV increase. **(c)**   Rating increases with size of anode; size A has a larger diameter than B.

- Speed of anode rotation
- Length of focal track
- Width of focal track

The smaller the anode angle the short term loadability can be increased however the anode angle size also determines the field size and heel effect. Anode cooling determines the **long term loadability** which is influenced by tube specification. If radiation is to be produced continuously, as in fluoroscopy, the tube loading is determined by the rate at which the heat can be dissipated. High mAs exposures permitted at low mA and long exposure times (e.g. 200mA at 1 second) may not be permitted at high mA and short exposure times (1000mA at 0.2 second). If the tube rating is exceeded then:

- Use a larger focal spot
- Use a higher speed rotation
- Reduce mA and increase exposure time

- Increase kVp and reduce mA or time
- Chose a sensitive film/screen combination which requires less exposure.

Box 3.5 Power rating for spot size and angle

Focal spot size and rating.

For a focal spot size and anode angle:
 11.6×3 for an angle 15°
10.26×3; angle 17°
8.7×3; angle 20°
Each gives an effective focal spot size of 3 × 3mm (see line focus principle).
 The power rating for a typical rotating anode is 1500W mm^{-2}, so for an anode angle of:

15°:	3 × 11.6 × 1500	=	52kW
17°:	3 × 10.26 × 1500	=	46kW
20°:	3 × 8.77 × 1500	=	39kW

NB: Smaller anode angles have higher ratings but give a larger heel effect

Radiographic techniques that use the maximum ratings of an x-ray tube produce target track roughening, so resolution slowly deteriorates and more tungsten becomes vaporized inside the tube enclosure, including the window area. This markedly reduces x-ray output since it acts as an effective filter. Operating at maximum ratings will considerably shorten the tube life so the tube should only be used at maximum rating if diagnostic quality demands it. Some specifications for three types of x-ray tube are given in Tab.3.4.

A large focal spot gives increased loading and reduced heel effect (Fig. 3.10(b)), however the effective focal spot will be large giving poor resolution images. A finer focal spot improves this but the tube's rating is reduced.

Improved resolution (smaller focal spot) leads to:

- Lower rating, a possible solution could be a larger anode diameter and/or faster rotation.
- Increased heel effect and less film coverage, a possible solution being to increase FFD but therefore less intensity $1/d^2$ requiring increased tube output (kV, mA, or time).

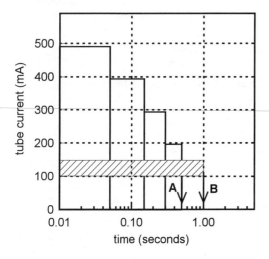

Figure 3.18 A rating curve demonstrating falling load showing the proportional exposures giving the required mAs calculated in Box 3.6 The shaded area shows the equivalent time for a constant current mAs.

Falling load If it can be arranged for the tube current to be high in the initial part of the exposure and then fall steadily during the exposure the same mAs can be achieved in a shorter time than would be the case for a constant current.

The falling load principle enables rapid multiple exposures to be made by driving the x-ray tube at near its maximum rating over the entire exposure time. Heat loss from the anode is most efficient at high working temperatures and the falling load principle keeps the high heating level constant.

The falling load principle is not suitable for very short exposure times when there would not be sufficient time for the multiple steps. The rating curve in Fig.3.18 shows the principle for the example in Box 3.6.

Box 3.6

Falling load calculation for Fig.3.18

From the example 60kV at 150mAs is required. The timing is proportioned as:

500mA at	0.05s	= 25mAs
400mA at	0.1s	= 40mAs
300mA at	0.15s	= 45mAs
200 mA at	0.2s	= 40mAs
Total time	0.5s giving	150mAs

The falling load provides 150mAs in 0.5s. (point A in Fig.3.18) . A constant load would require 1.0s (point B).

3.5.2 Thermal rating

The operating limits of an x-ray tube are influenced by three exposure factors:

1. Kilovoltage, chosen for particular investigation and penetration.
2. Exposure timing, chosen to reduce movement unsharpness.
3. Focal spot size, chosen for optimum resolution.

The heat generated at the anode by a combination of these factors determines the choice of tube design and its thermal rating. The overall heat loss from the x-ray tube and its housing is represented in Fig.3.19.

Heat generated   Factors 1 and 2 in the above list are a measure of the energy dissipated in the tube anode. This energy is proportional to kV and mA and exposure time. Since the majority of this energy appears as heat this product is the measure of power as described above. For a constant potential generator operating at 100kV and 300mA (see graph in Fig.3.17(b)) an electrical power of 30kW is dissipated in the anode. Since 1J = 1W s then for an exposure time of 0.02s the total heat energy is 30kW × 0.02 = 600 joules. This heat is deposited over a small area of the anode associated with the focal spot dimensions. Excessive heat can melt the target surface causing pitting and unequal expansion of the anode itself. A moderate form of this damage affects all x-ray tubes over their working life. A gradually pitted surface increases the size of the focal spot so resolution deteriorates and scatter from the uneven surface reduces tube output. Exposure factors are increased to compensate which accelerates the damage.

Target cooling   If there is no anode cooling then exposure (mAs) would depend only on focal spot size and the applied kilovoltage. Increased mAs or kilovoltage could only be used with large focal spots. This is not the case however since cooling by radiation, conduction and convection all remove heat from the anode during operation as Fig.3.19.

demonstrates. Forced air cooling accelerates heat loss, further increasing possible tube loading.

Exposure time   The optimum quality radiographs are achieved as a trade-off between tube current and time. The shortest time is usually chosen in order to minimize patient or organ movement (lung, heart). Since very short times would require damagingly large tube currents, exposure time is extended. This will, in turn, increase the total amount of heat generated and depend on its heat loss capabilities.

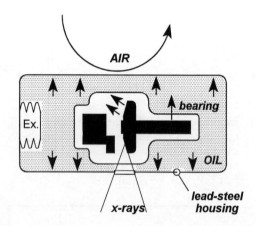

Figure 3.19   General heat loss from an x-ray tube enclosure relies on radiation from the anode, conduction from through the bearings and convection currents set up in the surrounding oil bath. All this heat is eventually lost from the tube housing to the surrounding air.

Table 3.4   Commercially available x-ray tube specifications

Tube type	Anode size mm	Angle	Focal spot mm	Heat storage	Long term loadability
Ceramic/Metal	200	9°	0.5/0.8	1.8MJ	3.2kW
CT Metal	100	10°	1.0	1.1MJ	1.5kW
Glass/Metal	90	9°	0.5/1.0	590kJ	300W

3.5.3   Anode heating and cooling

At the end of a short exposure the heat from the target is distributed by conduction throughout the anode mass. If this is not removed then the next exposure cannot take place without damaging the tube. Thus the heat capacity of the anode limits the number of exposures that can be made per unit time.

Loadability can be seen in three separate applications:

- Series loadability, where the tube is switched on and off for short periods over a long study time (angiography)
- Single exposure, maximum rating demanded for a short time (high kV chest radiography)
- Continuous loadability, where the tube is kept switched on at a lower level but for a long time.

Heat storage capacity The heat energy deposited in the target limits the workload and depends on:

- Exposure time
- Disk rotation
- Focal track length
- Focal spot size.

The heat stored in an anode mass depends on its heat capacity expressed in Heat Units (HU) or joules. Maximum heat storage capacity is related to: anode mass × specific heat × temperature rise. Since the first two are constant in any one tube, temperature rise is dependent on the anode heat capacity.

The early methods of measuring x-ray tube power used Heat Units which were the product of:

- tube kV × tube mA × exposure time (single phase)
- tube kV × tube mA × time×1.35 (3-phase)

A increase of 35% is added for a 3 phase or constant potential (or high frequency) supply due to improved efficiency. For an exposure of 70kVp at 10mAs the heat deposited would be 70k × 100 × 0.1 = 700HU for a single phase supply or 700×1.35 = 945HU for a 3-phase. Converting these values into joules uses the conversion figures: HU × 0.71 = joules or conversely: joules × 1.41 = HU. A conventional anode would have a typical heat storage capacity of 100kHU. This would increase to a few MHU for heavily loaded tubes (fluoroscopy and CT). Current metal/ceramic tubes can have a heat storage approaching 5MHU and a continuous load of 7kW.

Anode heating   A considerable quantity of heat is produced by bombarding the anode with an electron beam. During operation is glows red and sometimes white hot. This heat is removed by radiation from the anode to the enclosure wall (glass or metal) and also by conduction along the bearing. Sleeve bearings are replacing ball bearings in x-ray tube construction since they allow a greater heat loss by conduction which allows a higher tube rating.   Reflector plates behind the anode prevent excessive radiant heat from reaching the rotor-bearing mechanism.

Excessive heating of the anode will vaporize the target giving a rough surface which degrades the focal spot geometry, reducing x-ray output due to photon scatter from the rough target surface. It will also cause bearing damage. The vaporized anode material (tungsten) will increase the beam filtration (increased HVL), lowering image contrast.

Anode cooling   The   cooling   curve   in Fig.3.20 shows the number of heat units remaining per minute. The heat stored in an anode mass depends on its heat capacity. This is the heat storage capacity expressed in Heat Units or joules explained above.   The cooling curve in Fig. 3.20 shows the number of HU remaining per minute.

If the maximum heat capacity of the anode is 100,000 HU, then at a rate of 850HU s^{-1} this can be exceeded in 2½ minutes continuous exposure. For long exposure times, as in fluoroscopy, thermal equilibrium occurs when the heat generated by the electron beam is balanced by factors influencing heat loss (radiation, conduction, convection). The heating curves in Fig. 3.20 show that equilibrium would be achieved for this tube at about 500 HU s^{-1}, leveling out at the maximum heat rating of 100kHU The rate of radiant heat lost from the anode T_{loss} to the surrounding oil depends on the temperature difference between the anode T_a and the oil T_o so that:

$$T_{loss} = T_a{}^4 - T_o{}^4 \qquad (3.9)$$

The greatest heat loss occurs at high temperature differences. Doubling the values of T_a and T_o increases heat loss by ×16. Heat loss from the anode is most effective when the anode is operating near its maximum rating (falling load principle).

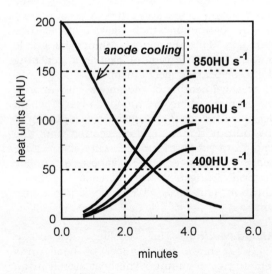

Figure 3.20 Example of a cooling curve and HU curves for a specific x-ray tube.

KEYWORDS

anode: The positive electrode of a thermion device. Commonly applied to the x-ray tube

beam filtration: The use of thin metal foil to remove low energy components from a poly-energetic beam.

beam homogeneity: A measure of how a poly-energetic beam compares to a mono-energetic beam of the same effective energy (E_{eff})

beam intensity: The number of photons per unit area (photon fluence).

beam quality: The penetrating power of the x-ray beam. Dependent on range of beam energies.

bearings: Rotational support for x-ray tube anode. Either ball or sleeve bearings are used.

bremsstrahlung: Generation of x-rays due to loss of electron energy (braking radiation).

cathode: A negative charged nickel support for the filament.

continuous spectrum: Poly-energetic x-ray spectrum.

energy (effective) E_{eff}: The modal energy of a poly-energetic beam.

energy (equivalent): Energy of a mono-energetic beam which would have the same HVL as the filtered x-ray beam.

energy (fluence): Ψ measured in MeV cm^{-2}

energy (flux): ψ measured in MeV cm^{-2} s^{-1}

falling load: using the maximum electrical rating to give a shorter exposure time.

filament cup: Part of the cathode assembly surrounding the filament which concentrates the negative charge, so shaping the beam.

filament: Coiled tungsten wire which is heated electrically to produce an electron cloud.

filter (K-edge): A high atomic number metal foil having a K-absorption edge in the diagnostic energy range.

filtration (fixed): Additional filter material added in order to remove low energy x-rays.

filtration (inherent): The filtration offered by the x-ray tube glass envelope.

filtration (total): Inherent + fixed filtration which should be at least 1.5mm aluminum for a 80kVp beam energy.

focal spot (effective): calculated from the line-focus principle.

focal spot (real): The dimensions of the anode target area.

half-value-layer (HVL): The thickness of aluminum which reduces the x-ray beam intensity by half. This should be at least 2.5mm aluminum at 80kVp.

heat units (HU): a measure of heat storage for an x-ray tube.

heel effect: the diminishing intensity across the x-ray beam toward the anode.

keV: Thousands of electron volts. Used as a precise measure of x-ray photon energy.

kV$_{eff}$: see effective energy

kVp: The peak photon energy of an x-ray beam

line focus principle: a formula for calculating a symmetrical focal spot using the electron beam angle and the real focus dimensions.

mAs: the product of tube current and exposure time

photon (fluence): Φ photons cm^{-2}

photon (flux): ϕ photons cm^{-2} s^{-1}

rotor: An integral part of the anode stem making up the induction motor.

space charge: accumulation of an electron cloud around a filament. More pronounced at low kV.

stator: the external winding surrounding the rotor section which completes the induction motor (see rotor).

useful field: the extent of the collimated x-ray beam.

window: the tube exit for the x-ray beam in the housing, which holds the fixed filtration.

4

X-ray production and properties: Specific machine design

4.1 The supply generator
4.2 Control circuits
4.3 Exposure control

4.4 X-ray tube design
4.5 Equipment

4.1 THE SUPPLY GENERATOR

A classic examination question in radiology physics: '*If an x-ray unit requires a highly stable DC supply for consistent x-ray output why is an AC supply used*' ? This question requires some thought before an accurate answer can be given.

The ideal generator is a **constant potential** generator which does supply the x-ray tube with a non-fluctuating constant DC using DC regulators for altering the high voltage. A DC battery supply for this unit would be absurd since a bank of batteries supplying 100kV for a reasonable length of time would occupy a very large space and would be excessively expensive.

The only practical solution is to use a **rectified** mains supply (single or 3-phase). All voltage fluctuations in the constant potential generator are equalized by regulating triode electronic tubes (valves) in the high voltage lines, giving a constant voltage with no ripple to the x-ray tube. The control circuits are in the high voltage side which provides very fast response times of <1ms. A constant potential generator is very expensive and occupies a large space; they are rarely found in diagnostic departments.

Basic generator design A typical x-ray generator derives its power from a single or 3-phase mains supply. The AC voltage levels

are increased or decreased by using power **transformers**. The AC is converted to a DC supply for the x-ray tube high voltage by using **rectifiers**. A general design for a **conventional** x-ray generator, that is a generator using mains frequency supplies, is shown in Fig.4.1 The specific features of a conventional generator are:

- Input transformer which allows adjustment of input mains voltage (primary) and output (secondary).
- A timer (older equipment only).
- A high voltage transformer increasing voltage levels up to 150,000 volts for the x-ray tube.
- A rectifier system converting high voltage AC to DC.
- A low voltage transformer reducing voltage levels to supply the tube filament 8 -12 volts.

The main supply can be either single-phase (110 or 220V) or three-phase (220 to 440V). An auto- or step-transformer (T1) allows adjustment to variations in the line supply (line compensation: M) manually or automatically. The reproducibility of the x-ray tube voltage is only ensured with stable line voltages. Response of automatic stabilizers is about 100ms so rapid changes in the mains supply may still be transferred to the x-ray tube voltage.

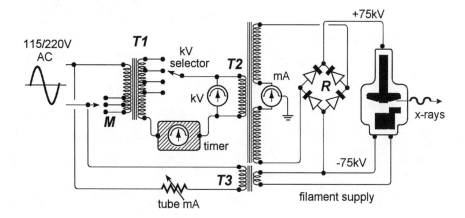

Figure 4.1 Simplified conventional generator showing basic components and controls described in the text.

The x-ray tube high voltage of about 150kV maximum is obtained from a step-up transformer (T2).

The exposure timing and switching takes place in the primary low voltage circuit (kV selector and timer). Timers in conventional generators are mainly electronic as mechanical timers are too slow and unreliable. Current equipment does not rely on a timer mechanism for halting the exposure. This is accomplished by feedback from an ionization chamber placed in the x-ray beam.

The high voltage generator itself consists of an oil filled tank which contains the high voltage transformer (T2) with its rectifiers (R). Also included in the bath is the filament transformer (T3) and high voltage switches. The high voltage is split as −75kV and +75kV with respect to earth so the insulation is only subjected to half the potential difference. The meter measuring the tube current (mA) is placed halfway in the secondary winding of T2 which is at earth potential.

4.1.1 Supply frequency

The AC mains supply has a cyclic frequency of 50Hz in Europe and 60Hz in the US. This variation can be responsible for small differences in generator performance.

Single phase supply The is the domestic mains supply at 115 volts in the US and 220, 240 volts in Europe. The waveform is shown in Fig.4.2(a) and (b). X-ray generators using this supply use two types of rectification.

Half-wave or **single-pulse** generators produce the pulsatile waveform shown in Fig.4.2(a) where only the shaded area is useful for x-ray production. Their efficiency is low giving power levels of about 2kW and these supplies are found in low power x-ray sets, such as dental and small mobile units. Single phase, **full-wave** rectified units produce the waveform in Fig.4.2(b); this is also known as a **two-pulse** generator for obvious reasons. This design makes better use of the supply power using both halves of the AC waveform and consequently higher x-ray outputs can be obtained; about 50kW maximum.

The half-wave system is the simplest requiring only a single rectifier. The full-wave system requires a four rectifier-bridge. A capacitor (C) can be added to smooth the pulsatile DC and reduce ripple. Supply frequency is superimposed on the rectified DC

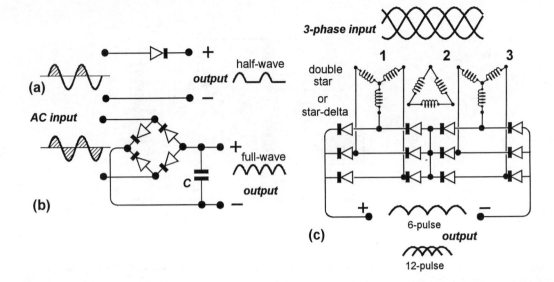

Figure 4.2   **(a)** Single phase waveform half-wave rectified using a single diode and **(b)** full-wave rectified using four diodes. **(c)** A three-phase supply showing star, delta, star transformer input and half-wave (6-pulse) or full-wave (12-pulse) rectified output.

as 'ripple'. This causes serious fluctuations in output and so broadens the x-ray spectrum. Typical ripple percentages are given in Tab.4.1 for single and 3-phase supplies.

Three phase supply   This waveform is shown in Fig.4.2(c) and has already been described in Chapter 2 as three sine-waves with a 120° phase difference. The supply is obtained from a special 3-phase mains supply (228 volts US, 440 volts Europe) using a star-delta transformer design. Half-wave rectification is produced from a **six-pulse** generator using twelve rectifiers in parallel as a double-star circuit shown in Fig.4.2(c). It gives a substantially higher output than two-pulse (single-phase) generators. They are found in medium power units of about 50kW or small generators used in older mammography equipment.

Full-wave rectification in 3-phase circuits uses a star-delta configuration as the input. This is a **twelve-pulse** generator and is used for high power supplies (≤150kW) such as old

model DSA or CT machines. The outputs for a 6 and 12-pulse generator are shown in Fig.4.2(c). The higher the pulse number the higher the efficiency of the power unit, producing an x-ray spectrum with a higher effective photon energy as shown in Fig.4.3(a) for the same kVp. This will allow faster exposures (less patient movement artifact) and less low energy photons, reducing patient dose. Anode heating during exposure can be kept constant (constant load) or can be reduced by feedback control under falling load conditions as described in Chapter 3.

The mains supply to the generator, whether it be single or 3-phase, can show variation particularly if it also supplies other equipment. This produces significant variation in supply voltage which is compensated manually or automatically by a separate transformer (an auto-transformer) which is shown in Fig.4.1 as 'M'. Single and 3-phase rectified power supplies now commonly feed high frequency generators since these offer superior control and stability.

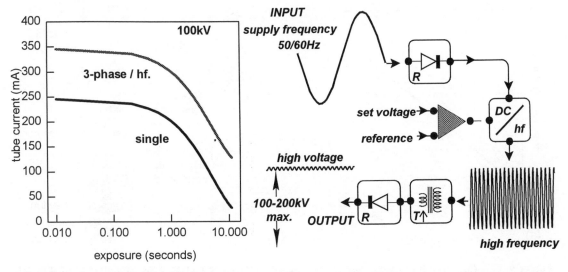

Figure 4.3 **(a)** Increased rating given by a 3-phase or a high frequency generator(gray curve) over the single phase (2-pulse) generator. The effective beam energy (E_{eff}) is also increased. **(b)** A high frequency waveform showing the mains frequency (50/60Hz) which is rectified supplying the high frequency generator. When rectified this high frequency gives a stable DC supply.

Table 4.1 Ripple values for generators

Generator	Ripple
Single Phase ½-wave	100%
Single Phase Full-wave	100%
	(15 - 20% smoothed)
3-Phase 6-pulse	13%
3-Phase 12-pulse	3%

4.1.2 High frequency generators

Medium and high frequency generators are now common for all x-ray equipment from mobiles, conventional, fluoroscopy, DSA and CT. They have many of the advantages of a constant potential generator giving very low ripple (<1%).

Figure 4.3(b) shows how the low frequency mains supply is first rectified to give a DC voltage which then supplies a high frequency generator (2 to 10kHz) which is rectified and supplies the x-ray tube circuits. The high frequency is rectified to give a very constant

DC high voltage. The generator design can utilize either single or 3-phase main supplies. These are full-wave rectified and smoothed to give a steady DC voltage which supplies a thyristor converter which switches the DC voltage producing a medium (up to 2000Hz) or high (up to 20kHz) square waveform. A high frequency transformer then converts this low voltage high frequency AC to kilovolt levels. Rectification and smoothing gives the high voltage DC for the x-ray tube. The thyristor converter can be controlled by low voltage signals to regulate its high-voltage output. There is a significant decrease in transformer size with increasing frequency for the same power output. Extremely compact transformer design is possible since cross-section A and number of turns n are related to output voltage V and AC frequency f as:

$$V = A \times n \times f \qquad (4.1)$$

This has obvious size advantages when designing compact generators for mobiles and CT units. There can be up to an 80%

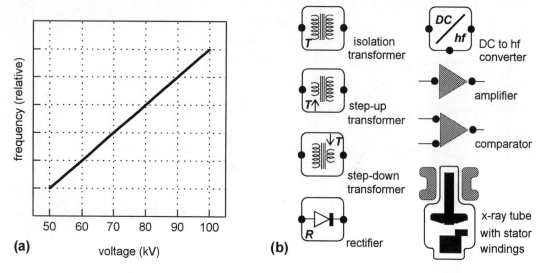

(a)

voltage (kV)

(b)

Figure 4.4   **(a)** Variation of high voltage output with small changes in generator frequency giving a control mechanism. **(b)** Building blocks used in high frequency generator schematics showing three types of transformer design, a full-wave semiconductor rectifier used for both medium and high voltage rectification. The DC to high frequency converter with its frequency control input. A single input/output amplifier and a two input comparator which detects signal differences.

reduction in transformer size over conventional 50/60Hz units for the same power output.

The tube kilovoltage can be electronically switched on and off at any point in time (no phase restrictions, unlike single and 3-phase units). Tube voltage is preset according to reference control value V_{ref} shown in Fig.4.3(b). Variation will influence output voltage and so can be regulated by slight frequency variation as plotted in Fig.4.4(a) and is independent of tube current. For power rating up to 50kW the generator is small enough to be built into a single housing with the x-ray tube. This is a 'single-tank' generator. For power ratings higher than 50kW the tube and generator housing are separate. Converter frequencies vary between 5 and 10kHz depending on manufacturer and after rectification yield a very low ripple DC voltage. Feedback regulation of the high voltage can give a response time of 200µs, so extremely stable output is possible giving <5% variation compared to between 10-20% for conventional single phase and 3-phase generators. The high frequency generator can

derive its power from either a single or 3-phase line supply which is rectified and then supplies the converter with power DC.

4.1.3 Generator performance

The general symbols used for describing high frequency generators are shown in Fig.4.4(b). Three types of transformer are commonly found: isolation, step-up and step-down. A common rectifier symbol serves for both medium voltage (115-240V) and high voltage (150kV); this is typically a full-wave semiconductor device. A DC to high frequency converter provides the 5 to 10kHz by switching the DC input; there is a third input for controlling the frequency level. A single input amplifier and a dual input comparator are common components. The comparator gives a signal output when input levels are different. An x-ray tube with stator windings completes the symbol family.

A general schematic for a high frequency generator unit is given in Fig.4.5 where high frequency converters, of different kinds, supply the x-ray tube high voltage, the filament

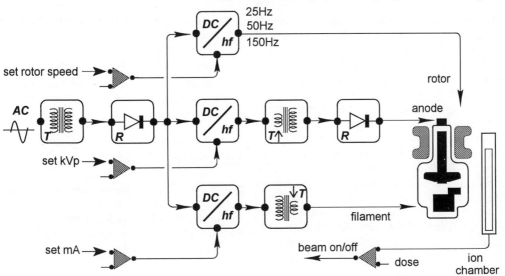

Fig. 4.5   Basic high frequency design showing the building blocks from Fig.4.4(b): the DC/high frequency converters, transformers, step-up T↑ and step-down T↓, and the various feedback controls for regulating kilovoltage, anode rotation speed and tube current. Film exposure is also controlled by feedback from an ion-chamber.

low voltage and also control the speed of the anode induction motor. Comparators are used as control devices accepting a reference input which can represent rotor speed, tube voltage or current and constantly comparing this with the measured value. A comparator circuit also monitors exposure from the x-ray beam, switching this off when a certain level has been reached.

Maximum rating   The insulation of the x-ray tube and housing have a maximum voltage rating usually less than the generator output. Maximum tube-current is controlled by both the filament current and tube kilovoltage as already seen in Chapter 3. The maximum tube current is determined by the filament rating and reduces with increasing tube kV.

The spectrum improvement shown in Fig.4.3(a) shows that since the 3-phase or high frequency generator is more efficient a higher effective energy can be obtained. In the electrical rating graphs of Chapter 3 the tube current plateau decreases as the kilovoltage is raised due to electrical power limitations which is the product of kV×mA. This rep-

resents the maximum power that can be focused on the anode for the shortest time without damage. It is not a filament current limitation but a thermal limitation and is relevant when very short exposures are taken (<0.1s).   Heat produced can be calculated from the electrical consumption. If the tube is being operated at 10kW for 0.05s then the total heat produced will be 10000×0.1 joules or 1000J. For shorter exposure times and a constant mAs this amount of heat will be produced in a shorter time over a smaller target area.

Overload   protection   The automatic overload monitors of the generator (excessive power) that prevent electrical overload cannot protect against thermal overload due to too short intervals between exposures. Thermal overload protection is provided by a small temperature detector (Loadix) placed in the x-ray tube housing behind the anode. This indicates   when   the   anode   radiant   heat exceeds a safe value and can feed information to a high frequency generator so that power input can be reduced from say 100% to 80%, which enables uninterrupted operation.

Cable resistance   High voltage generators are connected to the x-ray tube by means of two high voltage cables which deliver a split voltage i.e.–75kV and +75kV. This is for safety reasons since it gives symmetrical potential with regards to earth.

Supply cable resistance plays an important role in machine installation and these must be kept short if significant voltage drops at the generator are to be avoided during operation. A 10kW generator will draw up to 50 amps from the supply (depending on supply voltage) so even a small resistance of between 0.5 and 1Ω will cause a substantial voltage drop of the order of 50 volts. Any voltage drop is usually compensated by adjusting the auto-transformer setting.

Ripple   The cyclic variation, pulsation or ripple on the high voltage, described earlier, depends on the type of supply (single phase, 3-phase or high frequency). This is measured as the percentage of the peak value:

$$R = \frac{V_{max} - V_{min}}{V_{max}} \times 100\% \qquad (4.2)$$

The peak value of the x-ray tube supply is critical to image quality, since the proportion of ripple influences the x-ray spectrum. A large ripple content will reduce the available maximum voltage. Reproducibility of the generator output (stable kV) also influences the consistency of image quality. Variation in power output should be very low; 5-10% for conventional work and between 1-2% for mammography and DSA. It is less than 1% for CT.   Advantages of a high frequency supply are:

- Either a single or 3 phase supply can be used to provide the DC for the converter.
- Precise electronic control of the output with a response time of about200µs
- Fast switching of the tube voltage on and off during exposure.
- The tube voltage is independent of tube current
- Extremely compact high voltage

generator can be incorporated into tube assembly.
- Higher radiation output than conventional 3 phase supplies.
- Feedback controls vary or stabilize the x-ray tube voltage and current.

4.2   CONTROL CIRCUITS

Controlling high frequency generator kV output (eqn.4.1) is achieved by altering the frequency by a feedback control signal. In this way the kV can be finely adjusted within very close tolerances (<1%).

4.2.1 High voltage control

The high voltage control is shown in Fig.4.6. The sample signal is derived from a resistor divider circuit in the high voltage line and feeds one input of a comparator. When this a difference is found between sampled voltage and the set reference, a DC control voltage alters the frequency of the converter which alters high voltage level.   Tolerance levels better than 1% are essential for special applications such as subtraction angiography and CT. The x-ray beam is switched off rapidly after the required exposure by applying a low voltage logic signal to the converter; the speed of switching is compared in Tab. 4.2. Low inertia switching giving pulsed beams in CT and DSA uses grid-controlled x-ray tubes.

Table 4.2   Generator switching and rating.

Generator	Speed	Rating
Two pulse	20ms	2 - 50kW
Six-pulse	10ms	50kW at 100kV
Twelve-pulse	3ms	70kW at 100kV
Constant potential	20µs	150kW at100kV

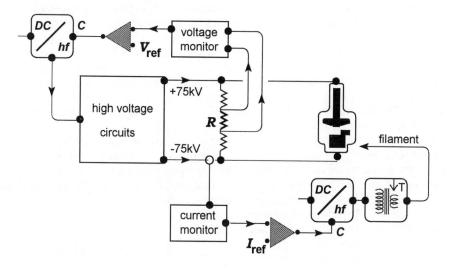

Figure 4.6   Stabilizing tube voltage and current by means of feedback controls from the high voltage output via a resistor chain (R). Tube current is monitored by a separate comparator circuit and is stabilized by adjustments to the filament supply.

4.2.2 Filament control and tube current

Slight variations in filament current produce large variations in the tube current which has already been seen in Chapter 3. The filament receives its power from an individual low voltage 'step-down' transformer shown both in the conventional circuit in Fig.4.1 and high frequency circuit in Fig.4.5. The transformer supplies between 8 to 12 volts at 6 amps. Since the filament current is 50/60Hz in the conventional AC supply, filament temperature alternates with the supply frequency giving a current ripple of about 10% which is super-imposed as ripple on the tube-current.

 The electron emission from the filament surface provides the tube current. Precise stabilization of the filament current by means of feedback controls is shown in Fig.4.6. Both kilovoltage and tube current are monitored so that when either are changed the filament current is adjusted to provide consistent output. If this feedback stabilization fails then there will be abrupt unregulated changes in the tube current when the kilovoltage settings are changed. Rapid response feedback control is most easily carried out with high frequency units. There are 3 levels of filament current

control during operation of the x-ray unit :

- A pre-heating current to maintain the filament winding in standby mode: about 2-3 amps. There is no electron emission so the x-ray tube current is zero.
- Filament operating at lowest rating gives a low tube current 0.1 to 4mA for fluoroscopy.
- High filament current for routine work. Exact pre-set values are used since a very small deviation in filament current gives significant tube-current variations.

4.2.3 Starter

An asynchronous motor consisting of a rotor (connected to the anode) and an external stator at ground (zero volts) potential drives the rotating anode. The asynchronous motor design allows a large gap between the stator and rotor. X-ray tubes with ball-bearings are accelerated before an exposure is made and then braked after exposure when the inertia of the anode plays an important part in braking. X-ray tubes with sleeve bearings are kept running throughout the working day since most wear occurs during braking, which is not necessary with this bearing.

The speed of starter rotation is the supply frequency×60. Conventional starters use either the line frequency direct which would give speeds of 3000rpm for 50Hz and 3600rpm for 60Hz, or use the third harmonic from a 3-phase supply which would give 9000 or 10800rpm respectively.

Figure 4.5 shows a starter circuit as part of the high frequency generator. Slow rotation of the anode (15 - 20Hz) is used for low output continuous screening (fluoroscopy) since there is reduced anode heating and slower speeds will reduce bearing wear. Medium frequency 50 - 180Hz is used for conventional work while 200 - 300Hz is reserved for special fast exposure times. Circuits monitor the anode rpm in order to indicate warning of worn bearings.

4.2.4 Exposure timing

Timing circuits   Control of x-ray exposure in conventional, mains driven, x-ray units was obtained by using mechanical timers, either clockwork or electrical. These have been discontinued since they are unable to offer fast switching rates necessary for effective x-ray exposure (0.01 to 0.05s) and have been replaced by either electronic, frequency controlled or exposure controlled timers.

Timer linearity   The radiation output should increase linearly with time for a given kV and tube current (mA). Tube current and exposure time both cause linear change in radiation output so their product mAs should also show a linear relationship. Fig.4.7(a) shows mAs plotted against exposure radiation dose (mGy) for 60, 80 and 100kVp showing the expected linear response which indicates that both exposure timing and the tube current regulation are working to specification. Exposure timing can be set manually or typically by feedback from an

exposure meter. Dose rate is measured by the built-in ion chamber situated either in front or behind the film cassette and switches the x-ray beam off when the integrated dose reaches a predetermined value set in the machine (dependent on film type and intensifying screen speed). Figure 4.7(b) shows such an arrangement fitted into a film cassette holder.

Several parameters control the exposure timing from a built-in ionization chamber. The output (radiation dose) from a generator is related to kilovoltage V tube current I and exposure time t as:

$$D = k \times V^n \times I \times t \qquad (4.3)$$

where k is a constant depending on anode material, filtration etc. and the power n depends on tube kilovoltage (for 50kV it is about 5, reducing to 3 at 150kV). The parameters in eqn. 4.3 are used by the exposure control to give consistent film density over a range of settings.

Electronic timing   devices use an R/C circuit (see Chapter 2) for producing switched variable time fractions. These are placed in the primary of the high voltage circuit of conventional machines controlling either a mechanical (relay) or electronic (thyristor or thyratron) switch: this is shown as the timer in Fig.4.1.   Frequency or pulse counting timers monitor the tube current for an appropriate number of cycles then switch off the high frequency generator.

Frequency or pulse counting timers   The product Q of tube current I and time t describes the exposure as the product of milliamps and seconds (mAs):

$$Q = I \times t \qquad (4.4)$$

When an exposure is made the selected tube kilovoltage is applied and the tube current, as measured by the feedback controls in Fig.4.6, is integrated over time t until the mAs product reaches its predefined value.

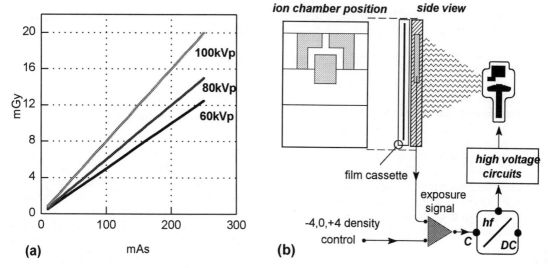

Figure 4.7 **(a)** There is a linear relationship between mAs and radiation output (mGy) for each kilovoltage setting. This is a good test for overall accuracy of generator regulation. **(b)** Automatic dose control from ion-chambers placed in front of the film cassette. Regions can be selected which cover the anatomy of interest (shaded areas). When the chamber output records an exposure value commensurate with the density setting the x-ray beam is switched off.

The tube voltage is then immediately switched off. Accurate reproducibility of the mAs value must be ensured since a small variation in mAs will cause a visible density change on the film image. The variation in mAs value ΔQ given by a high frequency generator depends on the tube current and switching frequency f so that:

$$\Delta Q = \frac{I}{2f} \qquad (4.5)$$

So for 1000mA and a 5kHz converter frequency the reproducibility would be ±0.1mAs.

4.3 EXPOSURE CONTROL

Ion chambers are commonly employed as automatic exposure control (AEC) devices for maintaining optimum film density for each kV and mA setting. Usually all that is required from the operator is a kVp setting; mAs is then chosen by the AEC for the particular film type and examination. The position of some commonly used exposure controls is shown in Fig.4.8

4.3.1 Automatic dose control devices

AEC units control exposure time for a pre-determined kV and mA. They are mostly flat ionization chambers made from radiolucent plastic which are placed in front of the film cassette in a common array pattern shown in Fig.4.7(b). This arrangement allows choice of AEC position for any patient study. Film density variation is selected by means of a feedback control to the generator converter as shown in the diagram. The dominant region of an image containing diagnostic information should maintain a specific optical density and these selected areas are placed within one of the separate automatic exposure controls (shaded areas on the diagram). These are either ion-chamber detectors or semiconductor device(s) which monitor the x-ray intensity in the chosen dominant area. AEC systems are used in fluoroscopy, conventional radiography and DSA.

Mammography uses a special balanced detector system behind the cassette. The reference signal which controls each exposure contains information about patient absorption and film/screen sensitivity. Three types of AEC are currently in use:

1. flat plate **ionization chamber** placed in front of the cassette. This is almost transparent to x-rays so does not interfere with the film image.
2. **semiconductor detector(s)** placed behind the cassette prevent image shadowing and are found in low exposure techniques such as mammography.
3. **photomultiplier** (Chapter 2) measures light intensity from an image intensifier acting as a brightness control and indirectly measuring radiation dose.

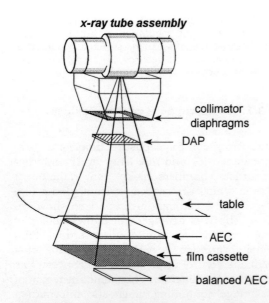

Figure 4.8 A variety of exposure controls and measuring devices fitted to the x-ray unit. The typical AEC is fitted in front of the film cassette but for mammography it occupies a central area behind the cassette. A dose-product meter (DAP) is fitted directly to the collimator housing.

All AEC systems have preset controls covering various radiographic procedures (extremities, chest, abdomen etc.). An over-ride film density correction control allows adjustment in detector sensitivity for variations in different film/screen sensitivities. This is shown as a −4, 0, +4 variable input in Fig.4.7(b). A mammography automatic exposure control is made behind the cassette and this is fully described in Chapter 9.

4.3.2 Dose-area product meters

A valuable requirement for any x-ray examination is to know the total dose received by the patient during a particular study. This information is provided by a dose-area product meter (DAP or diamentor).

The dose-area product is measured with a large area ion chamber placed directly below the tube collimator housing. Its position is shown in Figs.4.8 and 4.9(a).

The dose area product meter DAP is not an exposure control. It allows the radiation exposure to patients to be recorded and is the area integral of the air kerma over the surface area of the useful beam. It is measured in $Gy\ m^{-2}$ (replacing $R\ cm^{-2}$). Conversion factors are $1R\ cm^{-2} \equiv 0.87cGy\ cm^{-2} = 0.87\ mGy\ m^{-2}$. The DAP enables the total dose to be recorded for each patient examination, it can also display the total elapsed fluoroscopy time. With regular use the dose-area product meter can compare exposures for different patients and different techniques which is particularly useful for training. The detector consists of a large parallel-plate ionization chamber connected to a high input impedance amplifier. The charge collected by the chamber is proportional both to the chamber area and the x-ray dose. The chamber is fixed close to the x-ray tube housing (usually the diaphragm housing) where the x-ray dose is high and back-scattered radiation from the patient is minimal.

Figure 4.9(a) shows the independence of dose measurement with distance from the x-ray source. Since the chamber is transparent it does not interfere with any light beam positioning device. Table 4.3 lists the factors that do alter the dose area product. Under-couch x-ray fluoroscopy units are not ideal for dose-area product meters since the table acts as an additional filter in front of the patient.

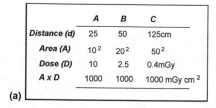

	A	B	C
Distance (d)	25	50	125cm
Area (A)	10^2	20^2	50^2
Dose (D)	10	2.5	0.4mGy
A x D	1000	1000	1000 mGy cm^2

(a)

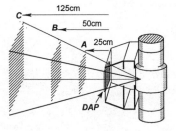

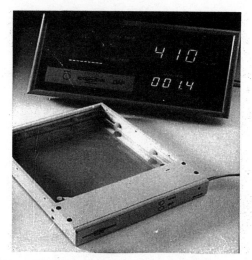

Figure 4.9 **(a)** Dose area product meter (DAP) showing distance independence as it registers dose (mGy or Gy) per unit area (cm^2). **(b)** A commercially available example (courtesy Gammex)

This is not the case (obviously) with over-couch designs. A commercial DAP is shown in Fig.4.9(b) with a large ion chamber and digital readout which can feed a paper printer for a permanent patient record.

Table 4.3 Factors influencing dose-area product

1	Tube Kilo-voltage	(kVp)
2	Tube Current	(mA)
3	Filtration	(mm Al)
4	Time	(minutes)
5	Area	(cm^2)

4.4 X-RAY TUBE DESIGN

4.4.1 Tube envelope

Glass has been the traditional material for x-ray tube construction but the modern metal ceramic x-ray tube has several advantages over glass :

- Scattered electrons from the anode are collected by the metal envelope.

- Improved heat conduction for size and increased rating possible due to more effective heat removal.
- Vaporised tungsten from the anode target condenses on a glass envelope more rapidly, destroying its insulating properties. A metal/ceramic envelope is protected from this.

The general features of a modern metal ceramic x-ray tube are shown in Fig.4.10(a) and the appearance of a modern metal cased x-ray tube is shown in the photograph of Fig.4.10(b). Additional improvements have increased tube performance by enlarging anode diameters and improving the bearings and their lubrication

4.4.2 Anode design

The design of the anode disk plays a crucial part in the performance of the x-ray tube. The body of the anode disk is a refractory alloy of molybdenum, titanium and zirconium (Fig.4.11(a)). The surface target is about 0.7mm thick consisting of a tungsten-rhenium alloy on a similar thickness of pure tungsten.

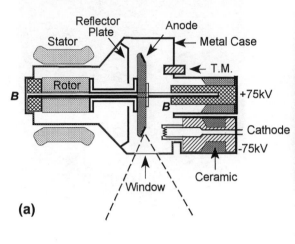

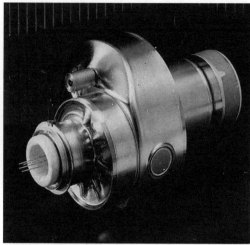

Figure 4.10 **(a)** Metal/Ceramic x-ray tube with a double bearing to carry the large anode. There is a thermal monitoring device (TM) for the anode. **(b)** Photograph of a modern metal ceramic x-ray tube (Philips Rotalix) showing the two large high tension connectors and the small thermal monitor attachment above them.

Tungsten-rhenium alloy permits higher thermal loading since it is not subjected to pitting. Increasing the diameter of the anode from the conventional 90/100mm to 200mm also gives higher loading and shorter exposure times. Special precautions are necessary to prevent distortion of larger anode disks due to local thermal expansion and Fig.4.11(b) shows stress slots cut around the disk circumference which prevent this. Disk volume is increased by backing the anode disk with graphite which gives minimum increase in weight but doubling the heat storage shown in anodes (b) and (c). A CT anode is sometimes flat in order to provide maximum metal thickness behind the focal spot; the angulation is achieved by a 9-11° cathode offset. Direct cooling of the anode is achieved in some tubes by circulating oil through a channel in the anode shaft.

Lubrication of anode bearing Air, water and oil are all obviously unsuitable for bearing lubrication at the high working temperatures of an x-ray tube. The lubricant commonly used is a metallic gallium alloy which is liquid at room temperatures. It has an extremely low vapor pressure, which is essential to maintain the vacuum conditions and provide good conduction of both heat and electric current. Some rotor bearings now use a sleeve design instead of a ball-bearing; the rotating shaft fits tightly into a hollow sleeve. Spiral grooves cut into the shaft improve metal lubricant circulation. The wear of these bearings is small and occurs during anode braking when there is direct mechanical contact between bearing surfaces. It is therefore recommended that the anode for these tubes is kept continuously rotating.

4.5 EQUIPMENT

Conventional radiography uses a short exposure having a small mAs and so x-ray tubes and generators can be of a moderate rating. Certain investigations however are more demanding and operate tube and generator near the maximum limits.

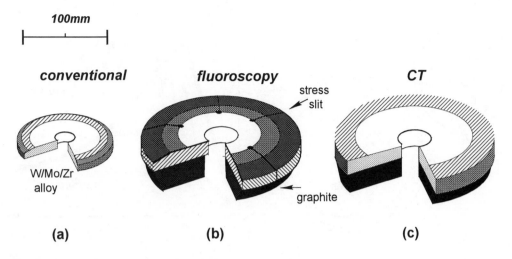

Figure 4.11   Anode designs for **(a)** conventional 100mm diameter anode made from a molybdenum/tungsten/zirconium composite with a rhenium/tungsten target, **(b)** an anode designed for a fluoroscopy system with stress slits and **(c)** a CT anode sometimes has a flat anode.

4.5.1 Tube thermal workload

The principal criteria involved for x-ray tube selection are the maximum tube voltage, the focal spot size and the thermal loadability for short, medium and long exposure times. The workload capacity of the x-ray tube is determined by the rapid rise in temperature of the focal spot.

A distinction is made between the rise in temperature for short load times (<0.1s: short term loadability) and the rise in temperature for longer load periods. Very short exposure times (0.01s) affect the rating of an x-ray tube since if the tube rotates at 3000 rpm equivalent to one revolution in 0.02 second then the focal spot area occupies only half the target circumference and the heat produced must be dissipated from this reduced area.

Figure 4.12(a) shows that only partial use is made of the available target area of 3000rpm anodes during fast exposure times; larger anodes rotating at increased speeds provide a solution to this problem. For short exposure times the current rating remains constant as shown by the electrical rating graphs of Chapter 3; the heat input rate remains constant even though the exposure time may

vary from 0.1 to 0.02s. The tube rating is therefore independent of exposure time at <0.1s so for very short time exposures the rating can clearly be improved by increasing the anode rotation speed. For very long load periods (e.g. fluoroscopy: long term loadability) a further limit is imposed by the thermal capacity of the anode and thermal dissipation to the surrounding cooling medium (oil). If an x-ray tube has experienced high load conditions then either the exposure power must be reduced or a pause must be made before the next set of exposures.

Load monitoring   The thermal state of the anode is monitored by a temperature sensor incorporated into the rear of the tube envelope behind the envelope (Loadix). The sensor is part of a feedback control circuit that considers the permitted load values for the tube, the intended number of exposures and the duration of each exposure so that tube ratings are not exceeded. Figure 4.12(b) illustrates the magnitude of the temperature rise that an anode may experience for different clinical applications: a single exposure from a high voltage chest-unit, a series of exposures during cardiac angio-

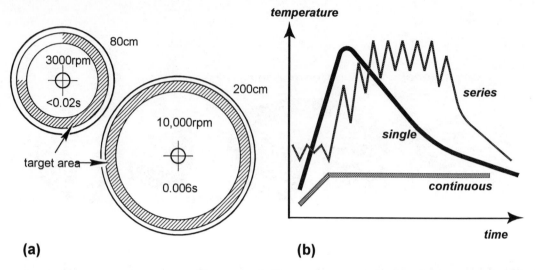

Figure 4.12   **(a)** The area of anode used when making a very fast exposure, showing the difference between a small diameter anode and a rapidly rotating large area anode used in high load applications such as chest radiography, fluoroscopy and CT. **(b)** the thermal load or loadability for various clinical examinations. The single exposure taken during a chest radiograph imposes a high thermal load which is then dissipated. A series of high exposures (angiography) places high demands on the tube whereas low tube current fluoroscopy imposes a continuous low thermal workload.

graphy and low power continuous use experienced in fluoroscopy screening.

Short-term loadability This applies to very short exposure times of 0.1s or less which applies to the flat region of the electrical rating graph shown in Chapter 3. This is determined by the size of the target region bombarded by the electron beam, which depends on the speed of anode rotation, length of the focal track and its width. The target angle is also critical since, in general, the smaller the angle the wider the focal track and therefore the greater the short-term loadability. Choice of anode angle is also determined by field size considerations.

Medium term loadability This is considered when the heat storage capacity for series of images is determined by the mass of the anode. The large thermal build up and dissipation during a single exposure (chest radiograph) and a series of exposures (cine-angiography) are compared with a low continuous exposure (screening during fluoroscopy) in Fig.4.12(b).

Long term loadability This requires rapid restoration of heat capacity by providing efficient cooling of the anode.

Series loadability This measure is defined as the load that the tube can withstand continuously for a period of say 20 seconds with a suggested cooling period of 120 seconds. It is proportional to the quantity of anode material or anode heat storage capacity. Series loadability is proportional to the diameter of the focal track. It is also determined by the length of the series of exposures but also by the cooling period between.

Batch loadability is the term used for describing a set of exposure series as would be experienced in CT examinations. An example of an acceptable load would be a batch of 2 minutes with a cooling period of 15 to 20 minutes before repeating the batch series. Doubling heat storage only usually gives an increase of about 40% in the batch loadability since heat dissipation plays an important role.

4.5.2 Applications

The specific requirements for clinical applications place different demands on the x-ray tube and generator. In **general radiography** for dentistry or small mobile applications only short term loadability is significant and simple stationary anode x-ray tubes can be used for these low power mobile x-ray sets. **Chest radiography** using high kilovoltage techniques also considers short term loadability but since the source to image distances (SID) are large the focal spot size can be quite large. Unsharpness is minimum for a 1.6mm focal spot at 2m SID and also a small anode angle can be used since field of view is not a critical factor at these distances. However since x-ray intensity obeys the inverse square law large tube currents are necessary in order to give adequate beam intensity for the very short exposure times (20ms) and tube loading is close to maximum. **Skeletal and abdominal** examinations demand critical tube loadability and focal sizes. Kilovoltages commonly employed are between 60 and 85kV to give sufficient contrast. The SID is usually small, between 40 and 100cm, requiring a larger focal spot size to give the field of view at these distances. However large focal spot sizes may be a limiting factor so dual focus tubes are employed giving a finer spot size for high definition work. A high tube load, upwards of 80 or 100kW, is sometimes required in order to give short exposure times.

The requirements for combined **radiography and fluoroscopy** are for high tube loadability particularly when long SID's are used, however where under-table work is carried out using short SID's the anode angle is critical to enable a practical field of view.

Continuous loadability is commonly found in fluoroscopic screening. During screening or fluoroscopy conditions continuous low tube currents are required. Directly controlled R/F systems (under-couch tube) require relatively small tube currents for fluoroscopy allowing simple heat loss from the tube. It is common practice to use a more slowly rotating anode (20Hz).

In order to cover a useful image field at an FFD of <100cm a large field of view is obtained if the anode angle is not too small (12°- 15°). Remote controlled R/F systems (over-couch tube) use larger SID's (~100cm) demanding greater output (doubling loadability up to 100kW) so a high output tube is necessary in order to freeze intestinal motion for spot filming by using fast exposure times of the order of 0.01 to 0.02s. Some basic specifications for high, medium and low rated x-ray tubes are given in Table 4.4.

Cardiology (Cine-angiography) Angiography and cine-cardiography both require series loadability which makes very high demands on the tube rating (Fig. 4.12(b)), particularly since high resolution pictures are required which demand small focal spot sizes. Cine-techniques are necessary to show rapidly moving vascular structures (cardiac walls and vessels): frame rates of up to 100-200 frames s^{-1}, exposure times of 8ms and run times of 5-10s. Small diameter catheters and stents also require high resolution pictures and focal spot sizes are typically 0.5mm. The upper limit of focal spot size is 0.8mm and loadability is very high for these continuous loads. The number of exposures is much higher than for GI studies and so requires a much higher tube loading.

Table 4.4 Specifications of three x-ray tubes of different rating.

	High load	*Medium load*	*Low load*
Anode diameter	200mm	100mm	60mm
Focal spots	0.5 and 0.8mm	0.2 - 1.0mm	0.4 - 0.6mm
Anode heat storage	1.8MJ	250 - 500MJ	70 - 100kJ
Application	CT, DSA	General	Mammography

Computed Tomography Since these x-ray tubes are heavily collimated in order to irradiate a thin slice of tissue only a small fraction of the x-rays generated are actually used for imaging. Fast image data processing means that the tube is quickly required to be ready for repeat exposures. Long term loadability is of prime importance and heat storage capacity and dissipation determines waiting time between slice acquisition. A large mass of graphite (Fig.4.11(c)), used to increase heat storage capacity, is not necessarily the best solution since stored heat must be lost quickly. This is most effectively achieved by using an oil cooled sleeve bearing to increase the conductive pathway and large diameter (200mm) all-metal anodes.

Mammography The x-ray tubes operate at between 25 and 30kVp so the anode heating is not a limiting factor and its mass can be kept low (Fig.4.11(a)). The filament rating however is critical owing to the space charge problems. Mammography is covered as a special topic in Chapter 9.

line frequency: either 50 or 60Hz

overload: a condition outside the safe operating either electrical or thermal which will damage the x-ray tube.

rating: limits imposed on kilovoltage, tube current and time for operating an x-ray tube.

rectification (full wave): both negative and positive AC waveform utilized in the DC output.

rectification (half wave): only utilizing the positive AC waveform for the DC output.

ripple: residual AC interference on the DC waveform.

starter: the electrical circuit driving the anode induction motor.

thyristor: a semiconductor switching device used for switching the DC waveform in a converter.

KEYWORDS

automatic exposure control: a radiation detector which monitors exposure and cuts off the x-ray beam

bearing: either ball or sleeve bearing support for the anode

converter: an electronic circuit which converts DC into high frequency alternating voltage.

feedback: the level of the output signal monitored in order to control accuracy.

generator (constant potential): a high power generator providing pure DC output.

generator (high frequency): a generator using a converter to produce a frequency between 5 and 10kHz.

5

Interactions of x- and γ-radiation with matter

5.1 General interaction with matter   5.3 Subject contrast
5.2 Interactions with the atom   5.4 Radiation dose

5.1 GENERAL INTERACTION WITH MATTER

The section of the electromagnetic spectrum of most concern to radiologists covers visible light, x-radiation and gamma radiation. The visible spectrum concerns the 'end product' which is the image or display. The higher energy x- and gamma radiation is concerned with image formation.

The difference between x- and gamma radiation concerns their origin. X-radiation is produced by the change in energy states of high energy or orbital bound electrons (K or L shells) or by the deceleration of an electron beam (x-ray tube). The energy change during these transformations is accompanied by electromagnetic radiation across a broad x-ray spectrum.

Gamma radiation originates almost exclusively from an atom's nucleus due to nuclear decay processes and appears as discrete energies and not a continuous spectrum. Nuclear decay and its associated radiation will be described in Chapter 15.

X-rays due the nature of their production have a mix of radiation wavelengths which produces a continuous spectrum. The x-ray spectrum for diagnostic purposes has an energy of 20 to 150keV; its wavelength can be calculated:

$$\lambda = \frac{1.24}{E} \qquad (5.1)$$

where E is in keV and λ in nm, so wavelengths would be 0.062nm to 0.0082nm respectively for these energies. These are very short wavelengths compared to visible light which ranges from 400 to 700nm.

Since gamma radiation occurs as discrete energies it is simpler to use for demonstrating general interactions with matter. The complexities that arise when considering the continuous spectrum of x-rays will be described later. A general diagram describing gamma photon behavior when penetrating an absorber is shown in Fig.5.1(a) where incident photons can be:

- Transmitted through the absorber unchanged
- Totally absorbed
- Scattered from the original direction retaining their original energy
- Scattered from the original direction but losing some of their energy.

The arrival of a 'useful' photon at the imaging receptor plane (i.e. film surface) depends therefore on two factors: photon **absorption** or photon **scatter** from the main beam.

5.1.1 Linear attenuation coefficient

The overall attenuation of radiation by matter can be readily explained by considering a

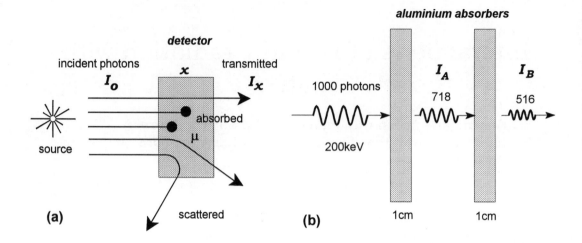

Figure 5.1 **(a)** General interactions of x-rays with matter showing transmission through the absorber unchanged; total absorption of the radiation or scatter of the radiation as different angles. **(b)** The fractional absorption of radiation through material for a photon energy of 200keV, this is explained in the text.

beam of monochromatic (single energy) photons incident on an absorbing material (e.g. aluminum). Figure 5.1(b) shows 1000 photons having an energy of 200keV incident on a 1cm thickness of aluminum. It is found that a certain number are removed from the beam leaving 718 photons transmitted as I_A. These are then incident on the second 1cm layer; the same fraction ($0.718 \times 718 = 516$) is transmitted as I_B.

This is the process of attenuation and is dependent on the absorber material and photon energy. The process of general radiation attenuation follows the exponential equation law described in Chap.2:

$$I_x = I_0 \cdot e^{-\mu x} \qquad (5.2)$$

Where I_0 is the original or incident intensity, I_x is the transmitted intensity through thickness x, e is the exponential function (2.7182...), μ is the attenuation coefficient for the absorber and x is its thickness. From eqn.5.2 the attenuation coefficient μ for a standard thickness (1cm) shown in our example of Fig.5.1(b) can be calculated since:

$$\frac{I_t}{I_0} = e^{-\mu x}$$

then

$$\frac{I_0}{I_t} = e^{\mu x} \quad \text{and} \quad \ln\frac{I_0}{I_t} = \mu x \qquad (5.3)$$

For the values 718 and 516 observed in Fig.5.1(b) the attenuation coefficient μ for 1cm aluminium and a photon energy of 200keV is:

$$\ln\left(\frac{718}{516}\right) = 0.33 \text{ cm}^{-1}$$

Box 5.1 investigates photon transmission through an absorber. The **logarithmic** difference between the transmitted photons is directly proportional to the difference in thickness x.

Exponential attenuation The graph in Fig 5.2(a) shows the attenuation of a mono-energetic beam as a simple exponential. The main factors to be remembered with transmission of radiation are:

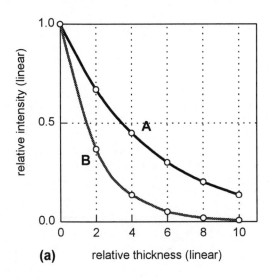

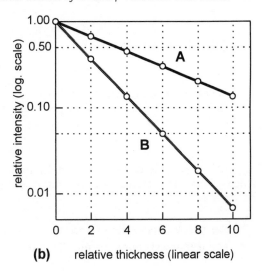

(a)   relative thickness (linear)   **(b)**   relative thickness (linear scale)

Figure 5.2   **(a)**   Exponential absorption of radiation in an absorber for two photon beam energies using a linear scale. **(b)** Using a log scale on the *y*-axis will give straight lines (semi-log. plot).

Box 5.1

Attenuation coefficient properties

Incident Photon Density: 1000
Thickness $B(x_B) = 2 \times$ thickness $A(x_A)$
Transmission for A is: $I_A = 718$
Transmission for B is: $I_B = 516$
The difference between the attenuated transmissions is constant but not directly proportional to the difference in thickness. Considering the logarithms of the transmissions:

$$I_A = I_o \cdot e^{-\mu x_A} \qquad I_B = I_o \cdot e^{-\mu x_B}$$

Taking log values both sides:

$$\ln I_A = -\mu x_A \qquad \text{and} \qquad \ln I_B = -\mu x_B$$

Then $\ln I_A - \ln I_B = \mu(x_B - x_A)$

so $6.57 - 6.24 = 0.33$

since in this example $A=1$ and $B=2$ the results gives the attenuation coefficient for aluminum at 200keV.

• the intensity is not halved as the thickness is doubled but decreases exponentially with thickness.
• the fraction absorbed depends on the photon energy.
• The linear attenuation coefficient is energy and material Z dependent

Both linear Fig.5.2(a) and semi-logarithmic plots Fig.5.2(b) are shown; the straight line semi-logarithmic plot has obvious advantages. The two curves (A) and (B) in Fig.5.2 show different rates of absorption that could be due to:

• different photon energies or
• different absorber properties.

For a given material a constant fraction is attenuated for equal added thicknesses of absorber.
 Box.5.1 uses the basic formula outlined above for overall photon attenuation and calculates the attenuation for two thicknesses of material A and B, where B doubles the absorber thickness. The worked example shows that:

- The fractional decrease in photon intensity is constant:
  1000 → 718 (~72%)
  718 → 516 (~72%)
- The difference in the $\log_n$ of the transmitted intensities is proportional to the difference in thickness of the material.

The critical parameters used in the equation which affect the attenuation of radiation in matter are:

- The **thickness** of the material x
- The **linear attenuation coefficient** μ

The linear attenuation coefficient itself is influenced by:

- atomic number Z
- material density ρ
- photon energy E

Thickness of the material x   Attenuation increases with the material (tissue) thickness, however the change in transmission of the photons (penetration) is not linearly dependent on the thickness i.e. doubling the thickness does not half the transmission but for a mono-energetic beam the fractional decrease is constant for equal thicknesses.

Half-value-layer   The linear attenuation coefficient μ for a particular tissue at a particular energy is a measure of the ability of the tissue to remove photons from a beam of x-rays. It is the fraction of photons (x- or γ-radiation) removed from a beam per unit thickness of absorber (m^{-1}). From the general exponential relationship of eqn.5.2:

$$I_x = I_0 \cdot e^{-\mu x}$$

the thickness x absorbing half the radiation is the half-value-layer or HVL where:

$$I_x/I_0 = 0.5 = e^{-\mu \cdot HVL}$$

Since $e^{-0.693} = 0.5$ then $\mu \times HVL = 0.693$

So
$$\mu = \frac{0.693}{HVL} \qquad (5.4)$$

This simple relationship is plotted in Fig.5.3 for intensity versus absorber HVL. The influence on the incident beam of a certain number of half-value-layers can be calculated from $1/2^n$ where n is the number of half-value-layers.

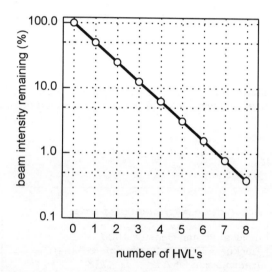

Figure 5.3   Half-value-layers n and intensity reduction using the function $1/2^n$. After four HVLs the intensity has been reduced to ~6% of the original.

The graph in Fig.5.4 shows the overall variation in μ over the diagnostic energy range for equal thicknesses of bone and water. As the photon energy increases the linear attenuation coefficient decreases. In practical terms the decrease in μ with increasing energy means that as the kV of an x-ray exposure increases the amount of **transmission** increases, but the change in transmission is greatest at low photon energies. Since **mammography** wishes to image differences between very similar soft tissues it uses low energy x-rays (between 26 and 28keV) to accentuate tissue detail. The differences in μ seen in Fig.5.4 between the three tissues - fat, soft tissue and bone - are greatest between energies of 10 and 30keV.

Transmission   Transmitted photons are responsible for exposing the film image and the image density obviously increases with photon number. The relative intensity of photons transmitted through 10cm of soft tissue is the inverse of the graph in Fig.5.4. A rapid increase is seen up to about 60keV then the transmitted photon intensity only increases slowly.

Beam hardening   Attenuation of a mono-energetic beam of photons (gamma radiation) follows simple rules but a poly-energetic x-ray beam loses lower energies more quickly than the higher ones. Although there is an overall reduction in the number of photons the average energy is higher than that of the incident beam. The beam is 'harder' and the attenuation coefficient will now be smaller.

5.1.2 Mass attenuation coefficient

This compares the attenuation characteristics of materials (μ) with reference to their density (ρ) in kg m^{-3}. It is calculated in Box 5.2, allowing comparison between μ and μ/ρ.

Photoelectric and scatter each have their own coefficients as mass absorption coefficient and mass scatter coefficient. The mass attenuation coefficient describes the probability of the total event. Lead has a μ value of 567m^{-1} for 100keV photons; its density is 11,350kg m^{-3}. Its mass attenuation coefficient is 567/11,350 = 0.05m^{-2} kg^{-1}. The mass attenuation does not depend on the physical state of the absorber (gas, liquid, solid), being independent of density.

As an example water exists in three states gas (water vapor), liquid and solid (ice), each having a different density, so the linear attenuation coefficient will be different for each state. Since the mass attenuation coefficient removes density differences the value for μ/ρ for each state will be the same. This is shown in Tab.5.1.

Table 5.1 Linear and mass attenuation for water

	μ	ρ	μ/ρ
Ice	0.196	0.917	0.214
Liquid	0.214	1	0.214
Vapor	1.28×10^{-4}	5.98×10^{-4}	0.214

Figure 5.5 plots the mass attenuation coefficient for bone, soft tissue and fat and when compared to the linear attenuation coefficient in Fig 5.4 it can be seen that when density differences are eliminated attenuation differences are reduced. The values of linear attenuation coefficient and mass attenuation coefficient for bone, soft tissue and fat at 20 and 150keV are listed in Tab.5.2. Differences between the tissue types are greatest for the linear attenuation coefficient and lowest for the mass attenuation coefficient and inversely proportional to the photon energy.

The mass attenuation coefficient provides a means of comparing the stopping power of

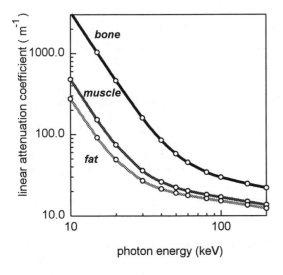

Figure 5.4   The linear attenuation coefficient μ for bone, soft tissue and fat.

different materials which is then independent of the state of the material. However the linear attenuation coefficient is more useful in radiology where organ thickness rather than masses are considered.

Table 5.2 Linear and mass attenuation for tissue

	Bone	Muscle	Fat
Linear Att. Coeff.			
μ 20	461	75	49
μ 150	24.6	15	13.5
Mass Att. Coeff.			
μ/ρ 20	0.28	0.074	0.054
μ/ρ 150	0.0149	0.0149	0.0150

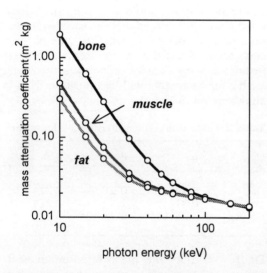

Figure 5.5 Mass attenuation coefficient matching bone, soft tissue and fat for attenuation coefficient in Fig.5.4

Summary Attenuation or reduction in transmission of ionizing radiation in matter depends on:

- Absorber thickness
- Material density
- Photon energy

The reduction of photon intensity is not linearly dependent on absorber thickness i.e. doubling of absorber thickness does not halve transmission.

- linear attenuation coefficient μ has units of m^{-1} or cm^{-1}
- mass attenuation coefficient μ/ρ has units of $m^2\ kg^{-1}$ or $cm^2\ g^{-1}$.

Box 5.2

Calculating μ for aluminum at 200keV

Density of aluminum 2700 kg m^{-3}
The HVL at 200keV is 2.1cm (0.021m)

The Linear Attenuation Coefficient μ is:
$$= \frac{0.693}{0.021} = 33.0m^{-1}$$
The Mass Attenuation Coefficient μ/ρ is:
$$= \frac{33.0}{2700} = 0.0122\ m^{-2}\ kg^{-1}$$
NB
Divide by 100 to convert to cm^{-1}
Multiply by 10 to convert to cm^{-2} g^{-1}

5.2 INTERACTIONS WITH THE ATOM

The interaction at the atomic level involves collisions with the electrons and nuclei of individual atoms which depend on material density and photon energy. Interactions with the atomic nucleus do not occur at photon energies used in diagnostic imaging so will only be mentioned briefly.

Electron interactions The terms 'free' and 'bound' electrons are used when describing photon interactions. Strictly speaking all electrons are held in orbits around a particular nucleus (ignoring conduction electrons in crystalline materials). When describing photon interactions an electron can be considered free when its binding energy is very small compared to the energy of the incident photon. For example while the M and N-shell electrons in lead with binding energies of 3.0 and 0.25eV may be treated as **free**, compared to x-ray diagnostic energies of 60-100keV, the K-shell electrons with a binding energy of 88keV are certainly **bound**.

Table 5.3 lists some important elements to radiology and their K and L-shell binding energies. For practical purposes the orbital electrons in low Z tissue elements (C, N and O) that have very small binding energies above the K-shell may be regarded as 'free' for the diagnostic x-ray energy range. In higher Z elements (calcium, barium, iodine) the K and L shells are treated as 'bound' and the orbitals above M are 'free' with respect to the x-ray photon energy.

Nuclear interactions If the photon energy exceeds 1.022MeV then nuclear interactions can take place with the formation of a positron and negatron (electron): this is pair formation. The positron forms a 'positronium' ion with a free electron which then rapidly undergoes mutual annihilation leaving two 0.511MeV gamma photons. X-ray photon energies do not reach this energy level in diagnostic imaging so pair formation will not be covered further. Positron decay does concern diagnostic imaging however and this will be covered in Chapter 15.

Table 5.3 The K and L shell binding energies

Z	Element	K-shell	L-shell
6	Carbon	283eV	low
7	Nitrogen	409eV	37 eV
8	Oxygen	542eV	41eV
13	Aluminum	1.56keV	117eV
15	Phosphorus	2keV	190eV
20	Calcium	4keV	438eV
29	Copper	8.9keV	1.1keV
42	Molybdenum	20.0keV	2.8keV
53	Iodine	33keV	5keV
56	Barium	37keV	6keV
74	Tungsten	69.5keV	12.0keV
82	Lead	88keV	16keV

5.2.1 Photoelectric effect

The photoelectric reaction plays a very important role in radiology and is encountered in the imaging process and radiation dosimetry.

The phenomenon was first studied by Albert Einstein (1879 to 1955; German/US physicist) who, in 1905, received the Nobel Prize for his work on the photoelectric interactions be-tween light of various wavelength and metal surfaces which illustrated the particulate (quantum or **photon**) nature of electro-magnetic radiation. Although this original work concerned visible light the photoelectric effect in radiology concerns higher energy electromagnetic radiation which are x- and gamma rays illustrated in Fig.5.6(a).

An incident photon (either x- or gamma) entering the electron sheath of an atom and having an energy greater than the binding energy of an inner orbital electron strikes or interacts with that electron. The incident photon is totally absorbed and the electron is ejected from its shell causing ionization. The orbital vacancy is filled by an electron from an outer orbit emitting characteristic radiation whose energy equals the difference in binding energy between the two shells.

Photoelectric absorption Figure 5.6(a) shows an interaction by the x-ray photon, of sufficient energy, with the K or L shell electron. The photon interacts by transferring all its energy to an inner K or L shell electron which is ejected from the atom as a photo-electron. The kinetic energy of the photo-electron E_k equals the photon energy hf minus the binding energy of the K or L electron E_b so:

$$E_k = hf - E_b \qquad (5.5)$$

The empty K or L shell is filled by an electron from one of the outer orbits. This electron transfer gives a characteristic x-ray and/or an Auger electron.

Excess photon energy is added to the kinetic energy of the electron.

$$hf = E_b + \tfrac{1}{2} mv^2 \qquad (5.6)$$

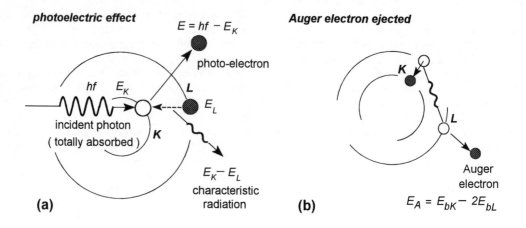

Figure 5.6   (**a**) The photoelectric reaction showing the incident photon ejecting a K-shell electron, which then becomes a photoelectron. The photon energy is entirely absorbed. (**b**) An Auger electron can be formed instead of characteristic radiation emission. The energy is transferred to and ejecting an L-electron.

where $\frac{1}{2}mv^2$ is the excess kinetic energy taken up by the electron.

The more tightly bound electrons of the atom are the major ones concerned with PE absorption and the most important electron orbit is the K-shell.   Maximum absorption occurs when the photon equals the K-electron binding energy. This gives rise to the steep K-edge in the absorption curves of Fig.5.7(a). A list of important K-edge energies is given in Tab.5.4.   For a photon energy of 100keV reacting with the K-electron of lead which has a binding energy of 88keV the photoelectron energy would be 100-88 or 12keV. Reacting with the L-electron (E_L=15keV) the photo-electron will have an energy of 85keV.

The probability of the photoelectric effect increases the closer the energy of the incident photon matches that of the electron. The probability of the photoelectric interaction is directly proportional to the cube of the atomic number Z^3 and inversely proportional to the cube of the energy $1/E^3$. The overall probability is described as: Z^3/E^3. The probability of an interaction between a 30keV photon and bone (calcium) is $12^3/40^3 = 0.027$ while that for soft tissue ($Z \equiv 7.4$) $7.4^3/100^3$ is 0.0004,

therefore photoelectric absorption is ×70 more likely for bone.

The photoelectron energy is absorbed by surrounding atoms. This is the major contribution to radiation dose in tissue. The vacancy or 'hole' left in the orbit is rapidly filled by an electron from a higher (less energy) orbit leading to an electron cascade as these higher orbit vacancies are filled. It is possible to lose energy from this reaction if the characteristic radiation is able to escape. However for soft tissues this photon energy is so low that it is absorbed.

It is not possible for a photon to give all its energy to a valency or 'free' electron since this process is not able to satisfy both conservation of energy and momentum together. This only happens with tightly bound electrons since the whole atom undergoes recoil enabling the reaction to comply with the conservation of momentum. Figure 5.6(a) shows the vacated orbit reoccupied by an electron from the adjacent orbit (i.e. L, M, N etc.) at the same time emitting excess energy as **characteristic radiation**.

Table 5.4 Some K-edge energies for important

elements in radiology.

Element	K-edge (keV)
Lead	88.0
Tungsten	69.5
Gadolinium	50.2
Lanthanum	39.0
Barium	37.4
Barium	37.4
Iodine	33.3
Tin	29.1
Silver	25.5
Molybdenum	20.0
Copper	9.0
Aluminum	1.6

In summary the characteristics of the photoelectric reaction are:

- The photoelectric event is greatest when the photon energy matches the electron binding energy.
- The probability decreases with increase in photon energy as $1/hf^3$ and increases with atomic number as Z^3
- The photoelectric effect (PE) contributes very strongly to attenuation at the lower diagnostic energies.

The PE effect depends on the atomic number Z of the attenuating material; photons whose energy is less than the binding energy will not be absorbed.

The probability of a PE reaction increases significantly as the energy of the incident photon approaches the binding energy of the electrons in a shell. Iodine, barium and rare earth intensifying screens (gadolinium and lanthanum) have K-shell binding energies that are in the diagnostic range to give optimum absorption.

Characteristic radiation The photoelectric event shown in Fig.5.6(a) results in an electron vacancy which is rapidly filled by a neighboring electron from (in this case) the L-shell emitting radiation in the process, the energy being:

$$hf = E_K - E_L \qquad (5.7)$$

The vacancy in the L-shell is similarly filled giving an electron cascade producing an emission spectrum of characteristic radiation. The number of characteristic photons is dependent on the number of electron shell vacancies. This is calculated for tungsten in Box 5.3. For high-Z materials (e.g. tungsten, lead and other shielding materials) the photoelectric reaction can be seen only as an attenuation process since the high energy characteristic radiation can escape taking part of the PE reaction with it (energy loss so only partial absorption) whereas for low Z materials (tissue) the very low energy characteristic radiation is completely absorbed within the tissue (no energy loss so PE effect shows complete absorption).

Auger electrons (P. Auger; French physicist 1899 to 1993). After a photoelectric reaction there is a vacancy in the K-shell which is normally filled by an L→K transition with the emission of a K-characteristic x-ray. Alternatively the energy involved in this transition may be transferred to one of the outer more loosely bound orbitals and these electrons will be ejected from their orbits as Auger electrons. This is a radiationless transition where the characteristic x-ray from the K-shell, produced during the photoelectric effect, is energetic enough to eject an electron from the L-shell. Fig.5.6(b) shows that two vacancies are created in the L-shell. The kinetic energy of an Auger electron is calculated as:

$$E_A = E_{bK} - 2E_{bL} \qquad (5.8)$$

Where: E_A is the energy of the Auger electron; E_{bK} the binding energy of the inner K shell; E_{bL} the binding energy of the outer L shell. The binding energy E_{bL} is represented twice in eqn.5.9 once for the transition energy and once to represent the ejected L shell electron. After an Auger event all the empty orbits will be filled to end the process. Auger events are an important consideration in radiology since they add to tissue dose.

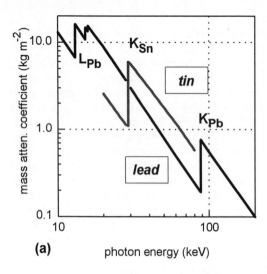

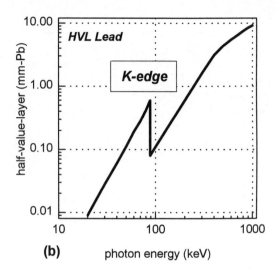

Figure 5.7   **(a)** Mass attenuation coefficient for lead and tin over the diagnostic energies. There is greater absorption for tin over the range 30-88keV due to its K-edge.   **(b)** The-half-value layer (HVL) for lead increasing with energy showing the K-edge effect. HVL for 80keV is 0.5mm but for 100keV it is 0.1mm.

The photoelectron is quickly brought to rest by the surrounding atoms of the absorber and its energy is given to them along with energy from any Auger electrons. The Auger electron has more energy than the photoelectron for diagnostic energies in heavy elements (tungsten, lead, etc.); however soft tissues have binding energies ranging from 0.28 to 0.53keV (carbon, nitrogen and oxygen) so the photoelectron would approximate to the incident photon energy.

Box 5.3

Characteristic radiation and Auger emission

Binding energy for **tungsten**
K-shell	69.5keV
L-shell	12.0keV
M-shell	1.8keV

Characteristic radiation (sum of transitions)
L to K, M to L etc. 69.5 – 12   = 57.5
                                    12 – 1.8   = 10.2
                                    1.8 – ~0   = 1.8
The total energy is therefore 69.5keV.

Auger electron energy. From eqn.5.9:
$$E_A = E_{bK} - 2E_{bL}$$
$$= 69.5 - 2 \times 12$$
$$= 45.5\text{keV}$$

Absorption edges   If the mass attenuation coefficient μ/ρ for photoelectric absorption is plotted as a function of energy in Fig.5.7(a) there is a rapid fall in μ/ρ with increasing energy. When the photon energy equals or exceeds the binding energy of the K-shell electrons there is a sharp increase in the photoelectric absorption coefficient.   If the energy of the photon just exceeds the electron binding energy then absorption increases substantially: the electron effective cross section for the photon is large.

Resonance between the photon energy and the K-shell electron binding energy removes a significant proportion of the photons seen as a sharp increase in absorption on the curve, which is the **K-edge**. For K electrons the absorption can increase by more than ×5. L-

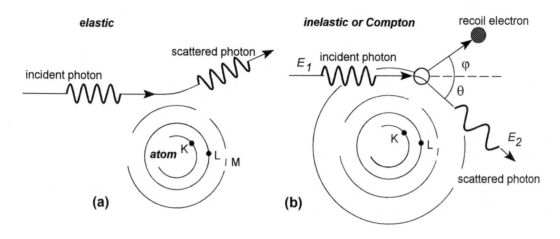

Figure 5.8 **(a)** Elastic or coherent scattering involving the atom as a whole **(b)** The Compton event showing the incident photon sharing its energy between the recoil electron and scattered photon.

shell electrons also show absorption edges as seen in the low energy region of the absorption curve for lead in Fig.5.7(a). Tin on a weight for weight basis is a better absorber between the energies 29 to 88keV despite having a lower atomic number (Sn $Z=34$, Pb $Z=88$). This would suggest that tin is a better shielding material than lead at diagnostic energies; however cost must be taken into consideration. Important elements whose K-edges appear within the diagnostic energy range are:

- X-ray Filters (molybdenum, rhodium, erbium etc.)
- Intensifying screen materials (tungsten, gadolinium etc.)
- Scintillation detectors (iodine, cesium)
- Contrast enhancing agents (barium, iodine)

Figure 5.7(b) shows the values of half-value thickness for lead over the diagnostic energy range. The K-edge at 88keV improves its shielding capabilities for nuclear medicine where gamma radiation from ^{99m}Tc (140keV) and ^{131}Iodine (364keV) fall after the K-edge and so less lead is required.

5.2.2 Radiation scattering

The general picture of attenuation in Fig.5.1(a) shows another process as well as absorption which can be responsible for preventing photons from reaching a target area (image receptor plane such as film). This is photon scattering and mostly involves electrons in the outer orbits. The scattered photon can assume any angle from >0° to 180°.

Coherent or elastic scattering (also known as Rayleigh/Thompson scattering). A photon can scatter elastically without electrons leaving their orbits (Fig.5.8(a)). Elastic or coherent scattering involves the atom as a whole. The photon passes in close proximity and the atom recoils, scattering the photon in the forward direction with no energy loss. About 10% of interactions involve elastic scattering in radiology.

Compton (inelastic) scattering This occurs if the incident photon interacts with an outer or unbound orbital electron shown in Fig 5.8(b). The electron has a binding energy which is negligibly small when compared with the photon energy. All electrons in soft tissue can be considered to be free electrons and in calcium (bone) all but the two K-shell electrons can be considered as free (18 out of 20 electrons per atom).

The probability of a Compton event depends on the probability of the photon encountering an electron. Absorber material characteristics such as atomic number do not enter into the Compton equation since the probability for a Compton interaction increases with the electron density and is independent of atomic number.

If the number of atoms in a mole is given by Avogadro's number N (6.203 × 10^{23}) then the number of atoms per unit mass is N/A where A is the atomic mass. The number of electrons per atom is given by its atomic number Z so the electron density can be calculated from:

$$N \times \frac{Z}{A} \quad \text{electrons g}^{-1} \quad (5.9)$$

The probability of a Compton event can be estimated from the number of electrons per cm^{-3} which is density (g cm^{-3}) × electrons g^{-1}. Compton interactions decrease slightly over the diagnostic energy range E following the relationship:

$$\frac{electron\ density}{E} \quad (5.10)$$

Table 5.5 lists the atomic number, atomic mass and electron densities of some important substances showing that scatter is dependent on the number of free electrons per unit volume. The number of electrons per gram shows a difference between dense materials (bone, lead etc.) and less dense materials (water, soft tissue etc.) Hydrogen has the highest electron density (6×10^{23} electrons per gram) so substances containing a lot of hydrogen will have more electrons and cause greater scatter (water, soft tissues).

Photon energy loss   The Compton process can be understood by considering the photon as a particle (quantum) with energy hf. The momentum (mass × velocity) of a photon is mc moving at the velocity of light, so:

$$mc = \frac{hf}{c} \quad (5.11)$$

The incident photon collides with an outer valency electron with energy E_1 and momentum hf/c. The electron recoils accepting a fraction of the photon energy. The geometry

Table 5.5   Important materials in radiology

Element	Z_{eff}	A	Electrons g^{-1}	Density	$Z:A$	Electrons cm^{-3}
Air	7.6	15.3	3.01×10^{23}	0.00129	0.49	3.80×10^{20}
Water	7.4	13.7	3.34×10^{23}	1	0.54	3.34×10^{23}
Muscle	7.5	14.5	3.36×10^{23}	1	0.51	3.36×10^{23}
Fat	5.9	10.2	3.48×10^{23}	0.91	0.57	3.16×10^{23}
Bone	13.8	27.7	3.00×10^{23}	1.85	0.49	5.55×10^{23}
Iodine	53.0	127.0	2.51×10^{23}	4.9	0.41	12.3×10^{23}
Barium	56.0	137.0	2.46×10^{23}	3.51	0.40	8.60×10^{23}
Lead	82.0	208.0	2.37×10^{23}	11.3	0.39	26.7×10^{23}

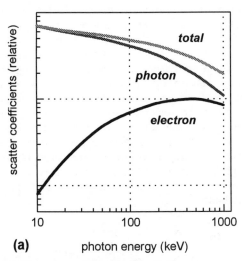

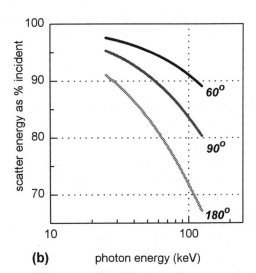

(a)   photon energy (keV)   **(b)**   photon energy (keV)

Figure 5.9   **(a)** The proportion of incident energy shared between scattered photon (mass scattering coefficient) and electron (mass absorption coefficient) making up the total attenuation.   **(b)** The energy of the scattered photon as a percentage of the incident energy for the diagnostic photon energy range for 60°, 90° and 120° scatter angles.

involved is shown in Fig.5.8(b) where the electron is scattered at an angle φ having gained kinetic energy from the incident photon. The scattered photon E_2 emerges at angle θ with a lower energy than the incident photon E_1. Conservation of energy and momentum yields the classic Compton equation that describes the **photon wavelength** shift:

$$\lambda_2 - \lambda_1 = \frac{h}{mc} \cdot (1 - \cos \theta) \qquad (5.12)$$

the constant h/mc in eqn.5.13 is the Compton wavelength and can be expressed in terms of **photon energy** instead of wavelength by substituting the rest mass of the electron m (0.511MeV). Equation 5.12 then becomes:

$$\frac{1}{E_2} - \frac{1}{E_1} = \frac{1}{511} \cdot (1 - \cos \theta) \qquad (5.13)$$

rearranging gives:

$$E_2 = \frac{E_1}{1 + (E_1 / 0.511) \cdot (1 - \cos \theta)} \qquad (5.14)$$

In contrast the difference in wavelength $\lambda_2 - \lambda_1$ described in eqn.5.12 depends upon h, m, c and the angle θ. Wavelength of the incident x-ray beam does not play a part, so, unlike energy, Compton scatter is independent of the incident wavelength, only the **wavelength difference** plays a role. It can be seen from eqn.5.15 that energy division between the Compton electron and the scattered photon depends on the incident photon energy E_1. At low energy the scattered photon retains a large fraction of the available energy; at higher energies there is a larger energy loss for the same scattering angle; the recoil electron receives an increased fraction. Fig.5.9(a) identifies the share in energy between the scattered photon and electron.

The mass absorption coefficient This determines the fraction of energy absorbed per unit mass and is defined as the fraction of beam energy absorbed per unit mass of absorber. It represents the average energy transferred to the electron. The higher the energy of the photon the greater the energy loss of the scattered photon and increasing energy of the recoil electron as shown in

Fig.5.9(a) From this graph the mass attenuation coefficient (total event) decreases with photon energy but the mass absorption coefficient increases with energy up to about 1MeV.

The mass scattering coefficient This is a measure of the average fraction of total beam energy remaining after a scatter event and from Fig.5.9(a) this photon component is seen to decrease with energy. Curves for the mass absorption coefficient and mass scattering coefficient cross at about 1.5MeV.

Scatter angle Figure 5.9(b) plots energy loss for scattering angles 60°, 90° and 180° over the diagnostic energy range showing greater energy loss for the scattered photon with increased photon energy and scatter angle. Calculations are given in Box 5.4.

Box 5.4

Compton scatter energy loss
(refer to Fig.5.8(b))

Calculating the percentage energy loss at a scatter angle of 60° for a 30keV and 100keV photon.

The basic equation (eqn.5.15):
$E' = E/(1 + (E/511) \times (1 - \cos \theta))$

For 30keV the scattered photon energy is:
$30/(1+(30/511) \times (1-0.5)) = 29$keV   (97%)

For 100keV the scattered photon energy is:
$100/(1+ (100/511) \times (1-0.5)) = 91$keV   (91%)

Conclusion:
Higher energy photons lose more energy to the recoil electron during Compton interactions (Fig.5.9(a) and (b)).

Scatter direction   The direction of the scattered radiation also depends on the energy of the incident beam. The proportions are exaggerated in Fig.5.10 but shows that as

the photon energy increases a forward angle of scatter is favored. The length of the radius indicates the probability of a photon being scattered in that direction and a forward angle is slightly favored in the diagnostic range as energy increases. The larger the angle of scatter the greater loss of photon energy to the electron so the scattered photon will have a low energy. At low scatter angles (forward scatter) a greater proportion of the photon energy is retained. Scattered photons degrade image quality since they do not represent attenuating values in the path of the beam.

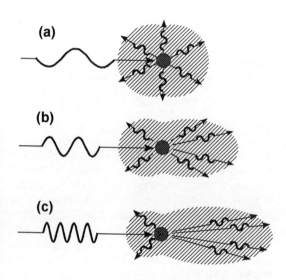

Figure 5.10 Scatter direction with energy: **(a)** low energy (20-30keV) **(b)** medium energy (50-80keV) **(c)** high energy (>100keV).

5.2.3. Pair formation

Interaction with the nucleus If the photon energy equals or exceeds 1.022MeV then it has sufficient energy to overcome nuclear electrostatic forces and the photon can be absorbed resulting in the formation of 2 particles of equal mass - a **positron** and an **electron**; this is **pair formation**. This pair formation event has only academic interest in diagnostic imaging since photon energies approaching 1MeV are rarely used.

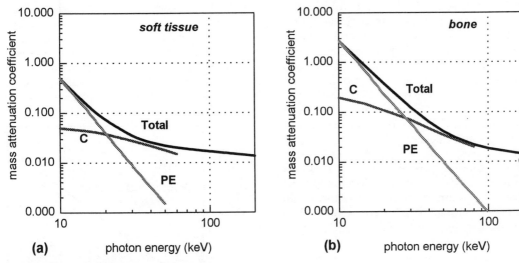

Figure 5.11   **(a)** The mass attenuation curves for soft tissue and **(b)** bone. The photoelectric and Compton components (PE and C respectively) make up the total attenuation process.

Positron Emission Tomography PET however is an example where a radionuclide decays by positron emission (β+) which then undergoes annihilation with a free electron. This can be treated as the complementary event to pair formation: energy converted to mass (x-ray photon producing positron and electron) or mass converted to energy (positron/electron undergoing annihilation to gamma radiation energy). These events are an excellent illustration of Einstein's famous formula $E = mc^2$ detailed in Box 5.5.

Box 5.5

Calculation for mass-energy relationship

Rest mass of electron/positron = 9.1×10^{-31}kg
Total mass m = 1.82×10^{-30}kg
Speed of light c = 3×10^8 m s^{-1}
        c^2 = 9×10^{16} m s^{-1}
$E = mc^2 = (1.82 \times 10^{-30}) \times (9 \times 10^{16})$ joules
    = 1.63×10^{-13} joules.
Since 1J = 6.24×10^{18} eV then energy can be expressed as $(1.63 \times 10^{-13}) \times (6.24 \times 10^{18})$ eV
        = 1.022MeV

This appears as two 180° opposed gamma photons having 0.511MeV each

---

5.2.4 Overall effects

The linear attenuation coefficient for a particular tissue at a particular energy is a measure of the ability of that tissue to remove photons from a beam of x-rays. The removal is due to the processes of:

• Photoelectric absorption; absorption coefficient

• Scattering (both coherent and Compton) and Compton attenuation coefficient

The linear attenuation coefficient μ is the sum of the photoelectric absorption coefficient (τ), the scatter coefficient (σ) and (where appropriate) the pair production coefficient (π). The latter is rarely experienced in diagnostic radiology.

The overall value μtot represented in the attenuation graph of Fig.5.4(a) and (b) is the combination of all three processes:

$$\mu_{tot} = \mu_\tau + \mu_\sigma + \mu_\pi \qquad (5.15)$$

Where μ_τ and μ_σ are the relevant attenuation coefficients: μ_σ is shared between coherent and Compton scatter. For completeness pair production is represented as μ_π.

The graphs in Fig. 5.11(a) and (b) show the percentage contributions to μ for soft tissue and bone for each process over the diagnostic energy range. As the photon energy increases the relative importance of the PE decreases and the curve flattens. The probability of a Compton interaction is small but its relative importance as an attenuating process increases as that of the photoelectric process decreases with energy.

The contribution of coherent scattering to the attenuation process is very small and relatively constant over the diagnostic range. Table 5.6 summarizes the important points associated with photon interactions with the atom in diagnostic imaging.

5.3   SUBJECT CONTRAST

Differential attenuation of photons in body tissue produces **subject contrast** which is directly responsible for the image information. The factors which affect the individual attenuation coefficients in eqn.5.15 will influence beam penetration. All the processes included in the equation lead to the attenuation of radiation as it passes through matter. Only some of the reactions lead to total or partial absorption of radiation. Low energy photons

are readily absorbed in soft tissue owing to the increase in PE so they do not contribute to image formation. Total absorption is given by the photoelectric effect and partial absorption by Compton scattering. A separate coefficient describes absorption which is the linear absorption coefficient or mass absorption coefficient.

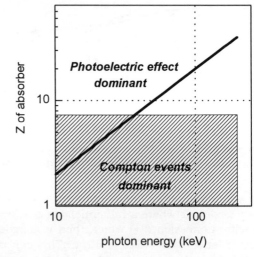

Figure 5.12   PE and Compton probability plotted on log-log scales for photon energy and effective atomic number Z_{eff} of the absorber. The shaded area represents a general soft tissue range.

Table 5.6   Summary of photon interactions with the atom in diagnostic radiology

Interaction	Factors	Process
Photon absorption		
Photoelectric	$\tau \propto \dfrac{Z^3}{E^3}$	Photon interacts with bound electron. Electron ejected. Orbital vacancy filled producing characteristic radiation or Auger electron
Photon Scattering		
Compton, inelastic incoherent	$\sigma \propto \dfrac{electron\ density}{E}$	Photon interacts with free electron. Energy shared between electron and scattered photon. Percentage energy loss increases with energy and scatter angle.
Rayleigh/Thomson elastic, coherent	$\mu_e \propto \dfrac{Z^2}{E}$	No absorption or energy loss. Interaction involves entire atom. Constitutes about 10% or reactions at diagnostic energies.

Figure 5.12 plots the probability of photo-electric and Compton interactions for soft tissue represented by the shaded block (Z_{eff} up to ~7.5). Photoelectric events are only common at low photon energies (30kV); most common diagnostic investigations rely to a greater extent on Compton interactions. At higher diagnostic energies (100kV) the photo-electric effect is minimal and attenuation relies almost entirely on Compton Scattering. For equal tissue thicknesses attenuation will now depend on the electron density cm^{-3}.

High kV chest radiographs take advantage of differences in the number of electrons cm^{-3} to give subject contrast. Attenuation increases linearly with an increase in density.

Table 5.5 lists some important materials, their density, electron density and the ratio atomic number to atomic mass (Z:A) remains fairly constant.

5.3.1 Image formation (scatter)

The set of graphs in Figure 5.13(a), (b), (c) indicate the importance of scatter when considering subject contrast. Although the proportion of scatter is most at low energies the amount of scatter leaving the tissue volume is small due to tissue absorption. The scatter component reaches a maximum at about 80keV and then declines as scatter probability decreases.

5.3.2 Image formation (absorption)

Tissue characteristics and x-ray photon energy determine the degree of photoelectric absorption that will occur within the tissue volume. Contrast agents such as barium and iodine increase subject contrast because of their high atomic number (Z^3) and their K-edge absorption falls within diagnostic imaging energies. Air is a negative contrast agent since it attenuates less than tissue.

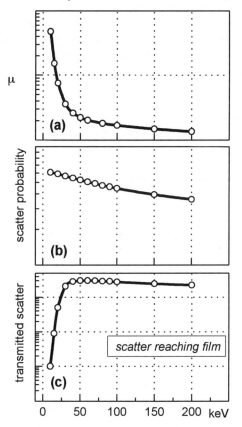

Figure 5.13 (a) Attenuation coefficient for soft tissue and **(b)** the probability of scatter production with photon energy are combined in **(c)** giving an indication of scattered radiation component in the exit beam. The *y*-axes are log scale.

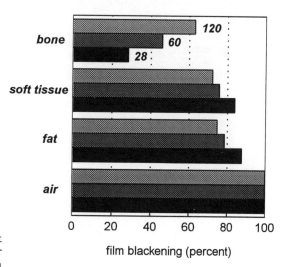

Figure 5.14 Proportion of incident beam reaching image surface (film) through air, fat, soft tissue and bone for three kV settings: 28, 60 and 120kV.

The influence of photon energy on image contrast is illustrated by the bar graphs in Fig.5.14.   Three tissue types and air are exposed to 28, 60 and 120kV x-ray photons used in mammography, conventional and high-kV chest radiographs respectively. The film blackening (which can also be treated as tissue penetration) is represented on the bottom axis. Air gives 100% film blackening for all photon energies but fat and soft tissue show the effect of increased Z and electron density influencing PE and Compton events. The most dramatic difference however is given by bone; at 120kV this becomes more transparent, almost equaling soft tissue and giving a more diagnostically useful chest radiograph.

5.4 RADIATION DOSE

The energy from the incident beam is transferred to the subject in the form of kinetic energy of the recoiling electrons. The largest transfer of energy occurs with the photoelectric effect when all the energy of the incident photon is transferred to the atom. Compton interactions only transfer part of the incident energy; this decreases with increasing photon energy. The units of radiation dose are given in Tab.5.7.

5.4.1 Exposure

The dissipation of energy by ionizing radiation in air is measured as exposure and depends on the number of ion-pairs created. This is defined as radiation exposure X so that:

$$X = \frac{Q}{a} \qquad (5.16)$$

where Q is the sum of all the electronic charges of either sign produced in air when all the electrons released by the ionizing events from a volume of air a are absorbed.

The old unit of exposure was the roentgen R where $1R = 2.58 \times 10^{-4}$ coulomb per kilogram (see Tab.5.7). The SI unit is simply the coulomb per kilogram or C kg^{-1}. The definition of exposure does not specify any time over which the radiation exposure must be received. The energy absorbed from 1C kg^{-1} is calculated in Box.5.6.

Rates of energy deposition are of considerable practical importance when calculating the effect of radiation exposure. These give:

- Exposure rate
- Energy fluence
- Fluence rate or flux density

5.4.2 Absorbed dose

Table 5.7 lists the definitions of exposure and absorbed dose used in radiology. Absorbed dose is expressed in terms of the energy deposited by the ionizing radiation (E_D) in a small volume of material a so that:

$$D = \frac{E_D}{a} \qquad (5.17)$$

Table 5.7 Units of radiation exposure and absorbed dose.

Quantity	Name (non-SI)	Symbol (non-SI)	Name (SI)	Symbol (SI)
Exposure	roentgen	R	coulomb kg^{-1}	C kg^{-1} = 3876R
Absorbed Dose	rad	rad = 0.01 J kg^{-1} μrad, mrad	gray (Gy)	Gy = J kg^{-1} μGy, mGy

The unit of absorbed dose is the gray where $1Gy = 1J\ kg^{-1}$. The gray can be applied to any substance including air and to any type of ionizing radiation (α, β, γ and x- radiation). The non-SI unit is the rad.

Only the energy deposited by photoelectronic events is included in the absorbed dose; scatter events are excluded. Kerma describes both photoelectric and scatter absorption, is also measured in J kg⁻¹ and defined as:

$$K = \frac{E_K}{a} \qquad (5.18)$$

E_K is the sum of the kinetic energy of all charged particles liberated in volume a (by PE, Compton etc.). At diagnostic energies dose approximates to kerma but at energies above 1MeV there may be an appreciable difference. The accurate definition of absorbed dose means the temperature of the absorber must be measured in a precision calorimeter. Since the temperature increase is very small precision instruments are needed so this is not a routine measurement (see Box. 5.6).

Specific gamma ray constant This is a reference dose rate in mSv h⁻¹ due to gamma and x-radiation at 1 meter from a point source containing 1 GBq:

- mSv h⁻¹ m⁻¹ GBq⁻¹ is equivalent to
- μSv h⁻¹ m⁻¹ MBq⁻¹

The dose rates apply to gamma and x-radiation only. Table 5.8 some values of specific gamma ray constant expressed in the above manner. These values are useful when calculating the dose rates received from point sources of radio nuclides used in nuclear medicine.

Table 5.8 Specific gamma ray constant.

Nuclide	Dose rate (see text)
¹³⁷Cesium	8.7×10^{-2}
⁶⁰Cobalt	3.6×10^{-1}
¹²⁵Iodine	3.4×10^{-2}
¹³¹Iodine	5.7×10^{-2}
⁹⁹ᵐTechnetium	1.7×10^{-2}

Box 5.6

Energy given by 1 C kg⁻¹ exposure in air

The energy absorbed from 1 C kg⁻¹ exposure given that the ionization for air is approximately 33.8eV per ion-pair. The charge on the electron is 1.602×10^{-19} C and the energy of 1eV is 1.6×10^{-19}J

The energy produced is 33.8× (1.6×10^{-19})
$$= 5.4 \times 10^{-18} \text{ J}$$
an ion-pair represents a charge of 1.6×10^{-19} C so the energy absorbed is $5.4 \times 10^{-18} / 1.6 \times 10^{-19}$
$$= 33.8 \text{J kg}^{-1}$$

Temperature increase with radiation exposure The temperature rise due to 10Gy exposure is 10Gy = 10 J kg⁻¹.
Specific heat for water is 4190 J kg⁻¹ K⁻¹

The temperature rise is therefore:

$$10/4190 = 2.386 \times 10^{-3} \text{ K}$$

The temperature increase in 1cm³ water for a 10Gy exposure is 0.002386°C

5.4.3 *f*– factor

The deduction of absorbed dose in grays from the exposure in air (coulomb kg⁻¹) is possible since C kg⁻¹ represents the same amount of energy absorbed from the beam, by air, regardless of radiation energy or quality. An energy input of about 34eV from the x-ray beam is required to form an ion-pair. This ionization energy is directly linked to total energy absorption so exposure values measured in air C kg⁻¹ can be converted to expected exposure in tissue (grays) i.e. soft tissue or bone.

Conversion factor The mass attenuation coefficient describes all interactions which lead to the attenuation of photons in matter: photoelectric, elastic and Compton. The mass absorption coefficient (μ_a/ρ), where μ_a is the linear absorption coefficient, only concerns photoelectric absorption since this is responsible for tissue radiation dose:

Absorbed energy per kg tissue
$$= Beam\ energy \times \mu_a/\rho = E\,(\mu_a/\rho)$$

The f–factor is then defined as:

$$\frac{absorbed\ energy\ kg^{-1}\ tissue}{absorbed\ energy\ kg^{-1}\ air} \qquad (5.19)$$

Using a conversion factor expresses eqn.5.19 in grays:

$$f(grays) \quad = \quad 34 \times \frac{\left[\dfrac{\mu_a}{\rho_{tissue}}\right]}{\left[\dfrac{\mu_a}{\rho_{air}}\right]} \qquad (5.20)$$

This is the factor f which converts C kg^{-1} exposure in air to exposure in tissue (grays). So an exposure of 1 coulomb kg^{-1} gives an absorbed dose of 33.85 grays. Box 5.7 uses eqn.5.20 for calculating f–factors for soft tissue and bone at 60keV.

Box 5.7

Calculation of the f–factor for soft tissue at 60keV

$$(\mu/\rho)_{air} = 3.004 \times 10^{-3}$$

Soft Tissue: $(\mu/\rho)_{tissue} = 3.061 \times 10^{-3}$

$$f\text{–factor} = \frac{33.85 \times (3.061 \times 10^{-3})}{3.004 \times 10^{-3}} = 34.49$$

Bone: $(\mu/\rho)_{tissue} = 9.988 \times 10^{-3}$

$$f\text{–factor} = \frac{33.85 \times (9.988 \times 10^{-3})}{3.004 \times 10^{-3}} = 112.54$$

The f–factors for 3 tissue types are plotted in Fig. 5.15

Soft tissue dose   The graph for f–conversion factors in Fig. 5.15 shows that across the diagnostic energy range the exposure in air is very close to the exposure in soft tissue. There

is also a close correlation between soft tissue and water so that water makes an excellent substitute for soft tissue when carrying out dose measurements.

Bone dose   This is a very different case. At diagnostic energies the f–factor values are much higher than for soft tissue. Bone has a higher atomic number (Z = about 13). The absorption coefficient for bone increases rapidly towards the lower energy end due to increasing photoelectric dominance.

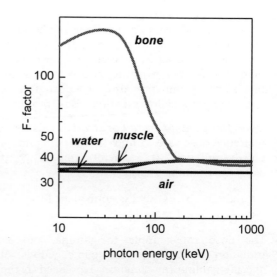

Figure 5.15   The f–factors calculated for photon energy comparing air, water, muscle and bone.

5.4.4   Linear Energy Transfer (LET)

The basic definition of the linear energy transfer is the energy transferred by ionizing radiation to a local volume of absorbing medium (tissue) over its path length expressed in keV µm^{-1}.

The values for LET given in Tab.5.9 shows that heavy charged particles (e.g. alpha particles, protons) have high LET values and as a consequence cause maximum biological damage. Photons and electrons are low LET radiations ranging from 0.2 to 3keV μm^{-1}; photons transfer energy by means of photo-electrons or recoil electrons.

Linear energy transfer is important when considering radiation dose which will be covered in Chapter 22 on radiation protection.

Table 5.9 Linear energy transfer values

Ionizing radiation	LET $keV\ \mu m^{-1}$
X-rays, gammas, electrons (β^-)	0.2 - 3.0
Low energy electrons	3.5 - 7.0
High energy protons, neutrons	23 - 50
Alpha particles	175 - 200

KEYWORDS

absorbed dose: The gray (Gy) 1J kg^{-1} equivalent to 100rads

absorption coefficient: photoelectric absorption

attenuation coefficient: combined attenuation due to photoelectric and scatter effects. Measured as μ m^{-1} (cm^{-1})

Auger electron: electron ejected from K or L shell as an alternative to characteristic radiation emission.

binding energy: the energy associated with an orbital electron. High for K-shell electrons and low for L, M and N.

characteristic radiation: electromagnetic radiation emitted when electrons fill orbital vacancies.

Compton scatter: an interaction between an incident photon and a 'free' electron. The photon loses energy.

elastic scattering: an interaction between an incident photon and the atomic field. There is no loss of energy

electron cascade: filling vacancies in electron orbits (normally K or L-shell vacancies) by electrons in higher (less energetic) orbits. Accompanied by characteristic radiation and Auger electrons.

excitation: energy imparted to an atom without ionization.

f - factor: used for converting exposure in air to exposure in tissue

free electron: in low Z materials (tissue) any electron outside the K-shell.

in-elastic scattering: see Compton scattering

ionization: loss of an orbital electron from an atom forming a charged ion e.g. Na^+ or Cl^-

K-edge: the abrupt increase in photon absorption when the incident photon energy equals the K-orbit binding energy.

mass absorption coefficient: the average energy transferred to the electrons by Compton scattering as a fraction of the total beam energy.

mass attenuation coefficient: the quotient of linear attenuation coefficient and material density μ/ρ .

pair production: the interaction of a photon with an energy exceeding 1.2MeV with the atomic nucleus to produce a positron and an electron.

photoelectric effect: the complete absorption of a photon by interaction with a bound (K or L-shell) electron.

photoelectron: electron ejected from K or L-shell as the result of a photoelectric reaction

recoil electron: the path taken by the free electron after a Compton interaction

scattered photon: the path taken by the incident photon after a Compton interaction.

Interaction of radiation with matter: Detectors

6.1 Radiation detection
6.2 Film as a detector
6.3 Gas detectors
6.4 Luminescent detectors

6.5 Practical detectors
6.6 Semiconductor detectors
6.7 Efficiency and sensitivity

6.1   RADIATION DETECTION

The detection of x- or gamma radiation requires the exploitation of their interaction with matter described in Chapter 5 to produce signals proportional to the radiation energy absorbed.

Three basic reactions in the absorber provide signals for the measurement of radiation energy or activity:

- *Chemical* where radiation causes atomic or molecular excitation of electrons. The prime example is the interaction of film emulsion with x-, γ-radiation or light.
- *Ionization* where atoms lose electrons and become current carrying ions. This reaction forms the basis of gas and semiconductor detectors.
- *Luminescence* (light production): where valency electrons in a crystalline material gain energy from radiation and enter a higher conduction band, from where they eventually move to a lower energy orbit and emit photons in the UV/visible part of the spectrum.

Although these detector materials can be used for detecting most ionizing radiation (α, β, γ and x-rays) they are commonly used as photon detectors in radiology so they will be described in their role as photon (x- or γ-radiation) detectors in this chapter. The type of detector employed in radiology depends on application: whether as a non-imaging or imaging detector.

Non-imaging applications include personnel dosimetry badges, radiation monitoring equipment, isotope dose calibrators or organ uptake probes (i.e. thyroid). These detectors either integrate the radiation signal producing a sum measurement of the total exposure (gray min^{-1} or h^{-1}) or measure the activity as individual photon counts. Activity measurement, which would be required for laboratory estimations (small sample activity) would register individual events of a particular energy. Larger activity measurements can also be provided, again as integrated measurements but this time expressed as becquerels (Bq) or disintegrations per second.

Imaging applications would use large area detectors (film, image plate) or many small detectors as a group (CT gas detectors) or large single crystal detectors (nuclear medicine gamma cameras) in order to give positional information for image construction.

Efficiency and sensitivity of a radiation

detector depends on geometry as well as its ability to absorb radiation. These characteristics will be discussed after the various methods for radiation detection have been described.

6.2   FILM AS A DETECTOR

Photographic effects are widely used as detectors for x and γ–radiation. Chapter 7 deals with photochemical reactions in more detail.   Photon interactions rely on either photoelectric or Compton events to release electrons which then activate the silver halide crystal in the film emulsion.

Both the silver halide and gelatin in the emulsion play an integral part in the photochemical action. The x- or γ–photon ionizes the silver halide (AgBr) into silver and bromine ions. The bromine ion is absorbed by the gelatin and the silver ion migrates to a sensitive region in the crystal. The developing stage, in the subsequent photographic processing, reduces the silver ions to metallic silver whose density is proportional to the initial radiation exposure. This effect can be used to measure radiation dose (film density being proportional to radiation dose) or form a radiographic image.

Film sensitivity   The film as an x or γ–ray detector varies in sensitivity across the photon energy range (Fig. 6.1). Unlike 'tissue equivalent' detectors (see later) AgBr has two K-edges that fall within the diagnostic range of photon energies (Ag is 25.5 and Br is 13keV). Film response (sensitivity) to photon energy decreases at energies lower than 40keV, due to these K-edges as shown by the shaded curve in Fig.6.1.

A typical x-ray film emulsion contains mixed silver halide (Ag(I)Br) and has a density of 1.84×10^{-2} kg m^{-2} (1.84mg cm^{-2}). The mass absorption coefficient at 60keV is typically 0.44m^{-2} kg so the linear attenuation coefficient is 8.1×10^{-2}m^{-2} which gives a quantum efficiency value of $1 - e^{-0.0081}$ or slightly less than 1%.

Film is used as a detector for measuring per-

sonal radiation dose but suffers since it is not tissue equivalent. This will be discussed later.

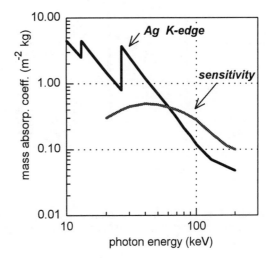

Figure 6.1   Variation of AgBr mass absorption coefficient with photon energy and general film sensitivity with keV.

6.3   GAS DETECTORS

Gas ionization   Only a small amount of energy is required to ionize gas. About 30eV will produce an ion pair. Ion production is proportional to energy absorbed; the charge C (in coulombs kg^{-1}) is:

$$C = \frac{Q}{m} \qquad (6.1)$$

Where Q is the number of ion pairs and m is mass of chamber gas. Gas detectors rely on the ionization of gas atoms and the collection of the induced charge by electrodes as shown diagrammatically in Fig.6.2(a). A high voltage is applied across the electrodes in order to collect the free electrons and gas ions caused by the ionizing event. The signal current is extremely small so amplification is necessary.

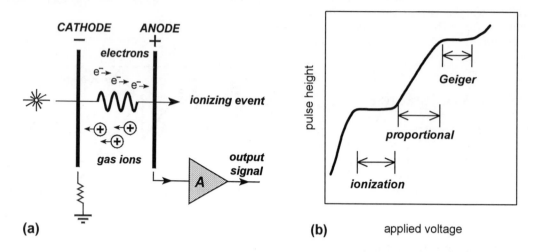

Figure 6.2   **(a)** Simple gas detector design showing an ionization event giving positive gas ions and electrons. **(b)** Increasing the applied voltage alters the characteristic of a gas detector into three regions described in the text.

Gas detector voltage Gas detector action depends on the applied electrode voltage. The following regions can be identified in Fig.6.2(b) :

- The **ionization** region. The first plateau. This is found in the ionization chamber. There is very little change in signal output for change in applied voltage over this range.
- The **proportional** region is found at a higher voltage where the ions are accelerated to cause secondary ionization by collision. This is gas amplification and signal strength is proportional to the energy of the primary radiation and applied voltage. It is energy sensitive.
- The **geiger** region, the second plateau, gives maximum useful gas amplification where each ionization event saturates the chamber with ions giving a peak signal for all energies. It simply registers an ionization event caused by α–, β–, x or γ–radiation as a single electrical pulse.

6.3.1   Ionization detector

The ionization chamber is the simplest form of gas detector and uses the simple design illustrated in Fig.6.2(a). The region between the plates is filled with air or inert gas. Air requires an average energy of 34eV to produce an ion-pair so for a 100keV photon approximately 3000 ions or electrons are formed.

Signals from an ion chamber are very small and need considerable amplification before a useful signal is produced. The amplitude of the signal depends on the number of ions formed and is independent of the applied voltage between the plates. The applied voltage does however influence the speed of ion collection.   The ion chamber has a very slow response and consequently the ion chamber is not used for pulse or event counting. Owing to its slow response radiation energy deposited in the chamber is integrated to give a steady reading of **radiation dose/dose rate** (mGy or mGy s^{-1}) or medium level **radionuclide activity** in disintegrations per second: kBq, MBq. Radiation level is measured as current which is depend-

isotope dose-calibrator

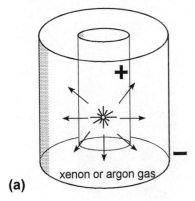

(a)

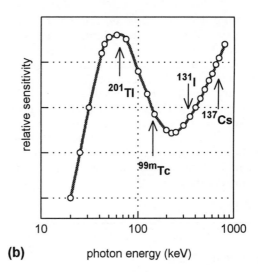

(b)   photon energy (keV)

Figure 6.3 (a) Isotope dose calibrator with almost 4π geometry filled with pressurized gas. (b) The change in response with photon energy for a dose calibrator. Common isotope gamma energies are marked on the curve. Corrections are applied to the readings which allow for this.

dent on both source activity or x-ray intensity and energy of the radiation.

Dose calibrator This design uses a 'well' or 're-entrant' design where a central hollow electrode holds a radioactive sample to be measured (Fig.6.3(a)). Maximum efficiency is achieved by capturing the majority of emissions in a 4π geometry which has been described in Chapter 1. In order to increase efficiency still further a dense gas filling is used: nitrogen, argon or xenon under pressure (>10 atmospheres). The ion chamber does not have a linear response to energy. This is shown in Fig.6.3(b) and corrections for different gamma energies must be applied for each radioactive sample counted.

Xenon gas ion chamber These are commonly found as CT machine detectors. They are manufactured as a single channel divided into many hundreds (700-800) of separate individual chambers with electrodes. The width of each detector is about 1mm, their depth anything up to 20cm. The xenon gas is under pressure to increase density and so efficiency, which is of the order of 50-60%.

Table 6.1 shows the considerable pressure necessary to increase gas density and so improve the detector efficiency.

Table 6.1 Xenon density and pressure

Pressure (atm.)	Density (g cm^{-3})
10	0.056
20	0.121
40	0.26

Survey or monitoring ion-chamber These instruments have a simple construction consisting of flat electrodes and are commonly used in radiology for measuring total dose or dose rates during patient examinations (dose-area product meter) or for quality control measurements (HVL, x-ray room dose rates).

The electrodes are made from air equivalent material (plastic) and air is the detector gas. The chamber can be calibrated in either radiation dose (µGy, mGy) or dose rate (µGy or mGy min^{-1}). The sensitivity of a survey/

monitoring ion chamber is related to gas volume or the size of the chamber itself but very small (thimble) ion chambers are valuable for sampling radiation dose in small volumes (simulated tissue depth dose).

The very small current given by the ionization event is amplified electronically to give a useful signal. Typical signal currents are shown in Box 6.1 for an air chamber. The tiny signals require good cabling and connectors; cable movement can induce noise signals that spoil measurements.

Box 6.1

Ionization current

$1cm^3$ of air weighs 1.3×10^{-6} kg at NTP
$350cm^3$ chamber holds 4.55×10^{-4} kg

$7.5\mu Gy\ h^{-1}$ will give $7.5/34$
$\qquad\qquad\qquad = 0.22\mu C\ kg^{-1}\ h^{-1}$

Exposure $\quad C \quad = \dfrac{Q}{m}$

Charge $\quad\ \ Q \quad = C \times m$

$\qquad\qquad = (2.2\times10^{-7}) \times 3600\ kg^{-1}\ s^{-1}$
$\qquad\qquad\qquad \times (4.55\times10^{-4})$ amps
$\qquad\qquad = 2.78\times10^{-14}$ amp
$\qquad\qquad = 0.0278$ pico-amp

NB: Factors which increase current density:
- Xenon density has $\times5$ that of air (Table 6.1)
- Pressurized gas gives a higher density

Summary of ion chamber detectors

Advantages	Disadvantages
• Walls can be made tissue equivalent	• Small signal currents need very sensitive (expensive) electronic amplification
• All radiation types can be measured	• It has restricted sensitivity
• Can be calibrated for any energy (isotope)	

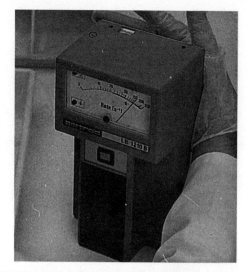

Figure 6.4 Photograph of proportional counter showing large surface area (courtesy of Berthold Inc.)

6.3.2 Proportional Counter

The common gas ion chamber is not fast enough to distinguish individual photon events. Its signal is a result of integrating the many photons interactions happening within its volume. As a consequence this signal is a slowly changing voltage which is proportional to activity level. In order to record individual photon events the detector response time must be improved which can be achieved by increasing the applied voltage to about 1000V. The resulting larger electric field accelerates the electrons in the chamber so their increased kinetic energy can produce secondary ionization (Townsend avalanche) producing about 10^3-10^5 secondary events per original ionization event providing event amplification. The chamber is operated so that the number of secondary events is **proportional** to the number of primary events; this is the origin of the detector's name. Proportional chambers are found as large area radiation monitors (Fig.6.4) and as CT detectors. Both counters use xenon to improve efficiency. The high voltage is between 1000-2000 volts. Since the sensitivity varies with HT proportional chambers need very stable power supplies.

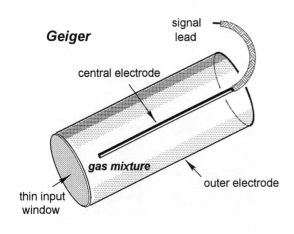

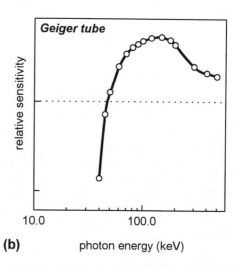

(b) photon energy (keV)

Figure 6.5 **(a)** Basic design for geiger counter showing a cylindrical outer electrode and a central wire electrode. **(b)** The energy response curve for a geiger counter which peaks over the diagnostic range.

Operating voltages depend upon the fill gas which is normally an inert gas such as nitrogen or argon. Krypton and xenon are used for higher energies and higher efficiencies. Gas pressure increases the density of the detector which improves quantum efficiency. Table 6.2 lists some common gas fills for proportional chambers. Butane offers a cheap high density gas but requires frequent replenishment.

Table 6.2   Ion chamber gases

Gas	Density (kg m^{-3} at 20°C)	Application
Air	1.293	x-ray dosimeters
Nitrogen	1.250	dose calibrators
Argon	1.784	dose calibrators
Xenon	5.500	α–, β–, γ– and CT
Butane	5.560	α, β–measurement

A typical large surface area contamination monitor operating at proportional region is xenon filled with a 100cm^2 – 200cm^2 surface detector area with a 6mg cm^{-2} titanium foil

window. Detection sensitivity would be of the order of 3 – 5Bq cm^{-2} for common isotopes (^{125}I and ^{99m}Tc).

6.3.3 Geiger detector

HW Geiger (1882-1945; German physicist) discovered that if the electric field in an ion chamber is increased still further then secondary avalanches can occur giving considerable increase in signal strength for each ionizing event and gas amplification can reach 10^{10}. There is no proportionality as all incident radiation produces the same saturated voltage signal. The construction, shown in Fig.6.5(a), consists of a cylindrical outer electrode with an inner electrode composed of a thin wire which serves to concentrate the electrical field. The operating voltage is much higher, 900-1200 volts, which increases gas amplification considerably. An ion-cascade due to energetic collisions gives a very strong signal for each ionization event. The geiger detector is insensitive to energy, due to the cascade effect, and also insensitive to supply voltage variations since the operating voltage is chosen to be in the center of the plateau.

The discharge produced by an ionization event must be quenched so that the detector returns to its original state, ready for the next event. The GM-Tube is inactive until quenching is complete; this **dead-time** can be 100's of microseconds long so limiting it for high count rates. Chemicals are added to the detector gas in order to quench ion avalanche so that after each ionization the ion-cascade quickly stops; this improves the long count dead-time. The most common additive is bromine and these tubes can be operated at a lower voltage. GM Counters are sensitive to most types of radiation providing the entrance window is thin enough (mica in the case of low β– or α–radiation). GM Counters are excellent cheap contamination monitors or radiation leakage detectors, having peak sensitivity in the diagnostic energy range (Fig.6.5(b)). Their response can be dampened electronically so that radiation levels can be measured in μGy h^{-1} or mGy h^{-1}.

6.4 LUMINESCENT DETECTORS

Röntgen accidentally observed the first interaction of x-rays with matter when activating a luminescent phosphor near his work-bench. Luminescent phosphors still occupy an essential place in diagnostic imaging.

Gamma or x-radiation interacts with the phosphor or scintillator producing a light event whose intensity is proportional to the photon energy deposited. Light production can be instantaneous or delayed and the duration of the light signal can be measured in nanoseconds (10^{-9}s) or tenths of seconds (10^{-1}s). Properties of a good scintillator are:

- Transparency to emitted light
- Large light output
- High photon absorption for γ and x-rays
- Available in large sizes

Figure 6.6 shows the electron bands involved in the general phenomenon of luminescence. Its name is given to a wide range of pheno-mena which result in light being produced after stimulation by either photons or charged particles (electrons).

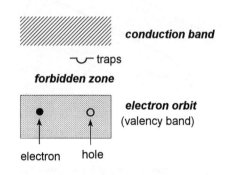

Figure 6.6 Electron bands and the forbidden zone with impurity traps. The valency band shows the presence of an electron and the absence (hole).

The incident photon energy is deposited in the outer valency orbits which causes electrons to jump through the forbidden zone into the conduction zone. At a certain time after this photon event the electrons fall back into the valency band emitting radiation in the form of light.

If impurity traps are present in the forbidden zone the electrons can be caught; their fate then depends on other factors. The term luminescence covers three major phosphor types that are commonly found in radiology and used for both imaging and radiation dose measurement such as counters or storage devices. These are:

- Phosphorescence
- Fluorescence
- Thermoluminescence

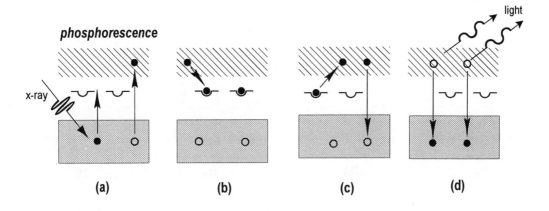

Figure 6.7   Phosphorescence where the impurity traps are empty before interaction with the photon. The sequences **(a)**, **(b)**, **(c)**, **(d)** are described in the text.

Doping   Phosphor sensitivity is improved by doping the pure phosphor material (NaI, CsI) etc. with impurity atoms. Examples of doped crystals, commonly used in radiology, would be NaI:Tl, CsI:Na and Gd_2O_2S:Tb.
The doping materials are responsible for trapping centers in the forbidden zone which give the phosphor its unique properties (light spectrum and wavelength).

6.4.1 Phosphorescence

This is shown diagramatically in Fig.6.7. Radiation ejects electrons from the valency band into the conduction band from where they attempt to return again to the valency band but are caught by trap defects in the forbidden zone. They eventually leave these traps falling into the vacant 'holes' in the valency band and in so doing they emit light. Light output can continue for some time after stimulation by radiation since electrons from the traps are periodically excited into the conduction band.   Summarizing Fig.6.7; the reactions are:

(a)   The phosphor has **empty** traps near the top of the forbidden zone and x-ray photons eject electrons from the valency band into the conduction band.

(b)   After the photon event electrons in the conduction band fall into empty traps in the forbidden zone.

(c)   Intrinsic energy supplied by the crystal again lifts some trapped electrons into conduction band.

(d)   Electrons then fall from the conduction band into vacancies in the valency band (holes) emitting a broad continuous light spectrum. Time between (c) and (d) determines period of emission (10^{-4} to many seconds).

Phosphorescent materials are ideal for video monitor screens or image intensifier output screens yielding a continuous spectrum.

fluorescence

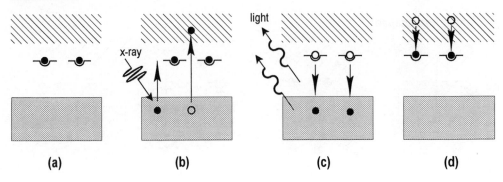

Figure 6.8   Fluorescence principles where the traps are filled at the start. The sequences **(a)**, **(b)**, **(c)**, **(d)** are described in the text.

6.4.2 Fluorescence

This is illustrated in Fig.6.8 where light output stops immediately after photon irradiation; in practice a finite dead-time (after-glow) does exist but this is very short and measured in nanoseconds. Summarizing the reactions associated with fluorescence in Fig.6.8:

(a) The phosphor has full traps near the top of the forbidden zone.

(b) X-ray photons eject electrons from the valency band into the conduction band.

(c) After the photon event the trapped electrons fill holes in the valency band emitting a light pulse (10^{-8} to 10^{-9}s) which has a narrow spectrum.

(d) Electrons from the conduction band then fall into the empty traps in the forbidden zone.

The simplest model for an inorganic scintillator involves crystal impurities and lattice defects providing energy levels in the normally forbidden region. Electrons from the conduction band may enter these centers but there are alternative events that may occur leading to information loss and so reducing the conversion efficiency of the detector.

The **conversion efficiency** for inorganic scintillators can be improved by impurity activation (doping). The added impurity probably occupies interstitial positions in the crystal lattice functioning as luminescence activators. Thallium is a common impurity added in concentrations of 0.8 to 2.0%.

A common fluorescent detector material is sodium iodide which has high density (3.76 g cm^{-3}) and, owing to its high atomic number (Na is 11 and I is 53), has a high photoelectric event absorption coefficient suited for low energy x-ray and gamma ray detection. Cesium iodide is also found as a scintillation material in radiology.

The common applications for fluorescent detectors (scintillators) that are found throughout radiology are:

thermoluminescence

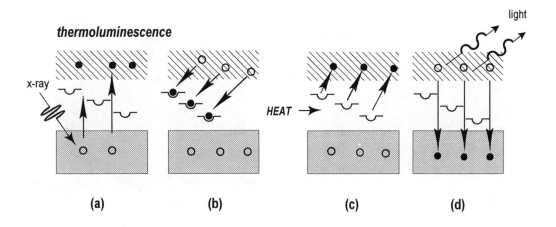

(a)   (b)   (c)   (d)

Figure 6.9   Thermoluminescence principles where the traps are scattered at different energy levels in the forbidden zone. The sequence **(a)**, **(b)**, **(c)**, **(d)** is described in the text.

- Intensifying screens in film cassettes.
- Scintillation crystals in conjunction with photomultiplier light detectors in nuclear medicine, uptake probes and CT detectors.
- Cesium iodide on the face of image intensifiers.

Lithium fluoride, a thermoluminescent material, has an effective atomic number similar to air and soft tissue, showing only a small variation in response to photon energy. It therefore shows **tissue equivalence** making it a valuable radiation dosimeter.

Summarizing the events shown in Fig.6.9 the series of reactions for thermoluminescence are:

6.4.3 Thermoluminescence

This is represented in Fig.6.9. Thermoluminescence differs from the previous examples of phosphorescence and fluorescence since the energy obtained from the radiation exposure is stored indefinitely within the crystal matrix and the output signal (light) is only emitted when the trapped electrons are dislodged by infra-red energy (heat or infra-red laser).

Since the light output is directly proportional to radiation energy input thermoluminescent materials are used as dosimeters and, on a larger scale, phosphor imaging plates.

(a) The phosphor has empty traps in the forbidden zone at different energy levels and during x-ray interaction electrons are ejected from the valency band into the conduction band.

(b) These electrons then fall in to the empty traps where they can stay indefinitely.

(c) Energy (heat) is required to eject the trapped electrons once again into the conduction band.

(d) They fall back into the valency band emitting a broad light spectrum whose intensity is equivalent to the original radiation exposure in (a).

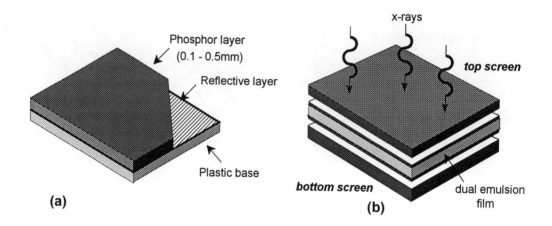

Figure 6.10 **(a)** Construction of an intensifying screen containing a scintillation phosphor. **(b)** A dual emulsion film sandwiched between two intensifying screens to increase efficiency.

6.5 PRACTICAL DETECTORS

A list of practical detectors using luminescent materials and found in radiology is given in Tab.6.3.

Table 6.3 Summary of luminescent detectors

Scintillator	Application
Fluorescence	
NaI:Tl	Scintillator for NM
CsI:Tl	Scintillator for CT
$CaWO_4$	Intensifying screen
Gd_2O_2S:Tb	Intensifying screen
Phosphorescence	
ZnS complex (P4)	Video monitor
ZnCdS:Ag (P20)	Image intensifier
Thermoluminescence	
LiF	Dosimeter
BaF(X) X = F, I or Br	Image plate

6.5.1 Intensifying Screens

Thin sheets plastic impregnated with fluorescent phosphor are incorporated into film cassettes that are used in plain film radiography. They convert x-radiation into visible light which then exposes the film. A large increase in quantum efficiency is obtained and a radiograph can be obtained at a very low patient dose. General construction is shown in Fig.6.10(a) where the intensifying screen consists of phosphor particles bonded within a thin plastic sheet supported on a plastic base. A reflective layer directs the light forward. In order to improve efficiency dual emulsion film is commonly used sandwiched between two intensifying screens, this general arrangement is shown in Fig.6.10(b).

Common phosphor materials used for these fluorescent screens are rare earth materials containing gadolinium and lanthanum; other phosphors use yttrium tantalate or tungstate. All the phosphor materials are doped with impurity elements (terbium, thulium etc.) in order to improve their light output. Intensifying screens are discussed further in Chapter 7.

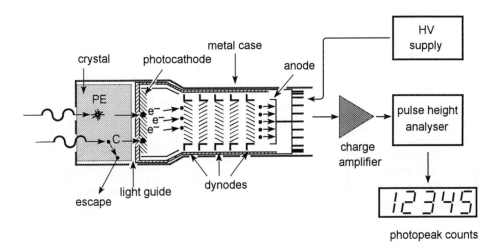

Figure 6.11   Scintillation detector with PM tube and the associated electronic circuits: a stable high voltage, a high input impedance amplifier and a pulse height analyzer. The latter discriminates between signal amplitudes. The final output is shown as a counter display.

6.5.2 Scintillation detector

These are commonly found in nuclear medicine where they are used in gamma cameras and single crystal detectors for uptake studies. Sodium iodide is the scintillator of choice owing to its high quantum efficiency. Photoelectric events within the crystal can be selected by the electronic circuits so eliminating counts due to scatter. The photoelectron output is about 4-12 for NaI:Tl and 1-3 for CsI:Tl. Some plastics are also used as very fast scintillation devices but are not usually seen in radiology.

Scintillation phosphors produce a brief pulse of light for each gamma photon detected; sodium iodide's light output is in the ultraviolet spectrum. The light pulse is detected and converted into an electrical signal by a **photomultiplier** tube. This can multiply the initial light signal by 10^6 or more. Fig 6.11 shows a complete scintillation detector system with its photomultiplier tube (PMT), amplifier, power supply and count display for photopeak events. The photomultiplier consists of a photo-cathode which produces electrons from the light pulse given by the scintillator (usually NaI:Tl) which is in optical contact with its face.

A dynode chain having an increasing positive voltage further multiplies the electrons, achieving in excess of 10^6 multiplication. A very stable high voltage supply to the photomultiplier is essential. The high input impedance (charge) amplifier, shown in the diagram, feeds a pulse height analyzer which sorts the pulses into a storage device depending on their amplitude. In this way scatter events can be discarded and only photo events recorded.

Gamma spectrum (see also **energy resolution**) An ideal scintillation detector (crystal with PMT) converts all the energy of the gamma ray into an electrical signal directly proportional to the gamma energy.

A theoretical spectrum shown in Fig.6.12(a) for [137]Cesium identifies the basic gamma spectrum components. The Compton process shares the incident photon energy between the scattered photon and the recoil electron; the latter decides the intensity of the light output. This depends on whether the collision gives a 180° scatter event (maximum energy deposited) or smaller angle scattering (20° 30° 45° etc.). The variation in the Compton

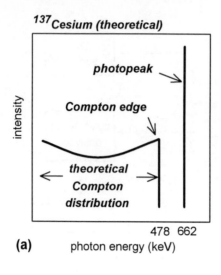

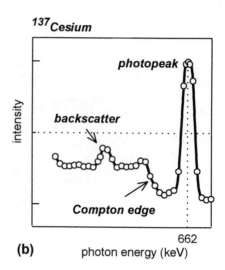

Figure 6.12   **(a)** A gamma spectrum given by a perfect (theoretical) scintillator identifying the Compton event distribution and the photopeak for a gamma photon with a photopeak energy of 662keV from ^{137}Cesium. The Compton edge represents the maximum scatter energy. **(b)** The same spectrum but obtained from a practical NaI:Tl scintillator detector

interactions gives the long Compton scatter spectrum ending abruptly at the Compton edge (180° scatter). The Compton distribution, or Compton valley, represents energy lost in the crystal due to photon scattering events. Only the energy of the recoil electron is transferred to the scintillation crystal; the scattered photon either escapes or is absorbed producing a secondary event. The maximum electron energy which would be given by a 180° scatter can be calculated from eqn.5.9. For a gamma energy of 662keV the scatter photon energy would be:

$$\frac{662}{1+(1.295)\cdot(2)} = 184\text{keV}$$

The electron energy is therefore the incident minus the scattered energy 662–184 which is 478keV; this value defines the Compton edge in Fig.6.12(a). Beyond the Compton edge is a Compton plateau which leads to the **photopeak** representing the energy imparted by the photoelectron, in this case 662keV given by the single gamma photon from the ^{137}Cs decay. Multiple gammas would give a multi-photopeak spectrum.

A real gamma spectrum from ^{137}Cs obtained using a typical single NaI:Tl detector is shown in Fig.6.12(b). Due to statistical fluctuations (caused by thermal effects, non-uniform scintillator response etc.) the photopeak is represented not as a line spectrum but as a distribution. The magnitude of the photopeak distribution is expressed as the **energy resolution**.

Energy resolution   This is measured as the **Full Width at Half Maximum** (FWHM) obtained by measuring the width of the photopeak at half its height (identified by the horizontal dotted line in Fig.6.12(b)); the values for the width are 634 and 690keV, in this example, so the resolution is (690–634)/662 = 0.08 or 8%. The best energy resolution is about 7% for a 662keV ^{137}Cs gamma using a 7.5×7.5cm (3×3″) crystal. Energy resolution is slightly worse for smaller crystal detectors. A gamma camera would have an energy resolution of 10 to 14%. Energy response of the scintillator becomes non-linear for gamma energies below 200keV due to light output variation (about 5%).

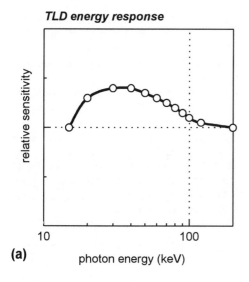

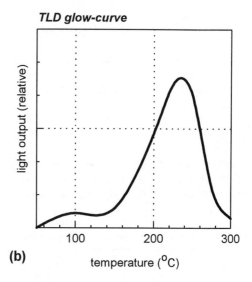

(a)

(b)

Figure 6.13 **(a)** The photon energy response of a thermoluminescent detector and **(b)** The glow-curve showing the optimum temperature for maximum light emission.

Compton scattering causes only a fraction of the deposited energy being recorded since scatter events can escape from the crystal leaving an **escape peak**. This is commonly seen for characteristic x-rays of iodine in an NaI detector. **Back-scatter** from the lead-shield surrounding the detector can also re-enter the crystal causing interference peaks in the Compton part of the spectrum seen in the spectrum of Fig.6.12(b).

The sodium iodide detector NaI:Tl This is the most common scintillator providing very large detector crystals for both portable machines (thyroid monitoring) and fixed multiple detectors (whole body counters). Large thin crystals are used for imaging radio-nuclide distribution in nuclear medicine. Sodium iodide emits short wavelength light in the near UV and requires photomultipliers that are sensitive to this wavelength. This makes them somewhat bulky as portable or small detectors.

Cesium iodide emits visible light and can be operated with a photo-diode. The entire detector can then occupy a very small volume. They are used in CT scanners and certain portable radiation detectors.

6.5.3 Thermoluminescent dosimeter

The number of materials which exhibit the phenomenon of thermoluminescence is considerable but only a limited number find use in radiology. The important properties of a practical thermoluminescent phosphor are photon energy response shown in Fig.6.13(a) and the main trapping center should allow light emission at around 200°C shown as the glow curve in Fig.6.13(b). The material should emit light preferably in or near the blue region of the spectrum. A list of suitable thermoluminescent materials is given in Tab.6.4.

A **personal dosimeter** should absorb radiation with the same sensitivity as soft tissue; these are normally lithium based phosphors in the form of small discs or pellets. The calcium based material is less noisy at low dose rates and is ideal for monitoring low-dose rate areas in laboratories or radiology x-ray rooms. Their dose range is considerable when compared to film dosimeters.

Image plate Thermoluminescent principles are utilized in the construction of the image plate, which has a similar construction to the intensifying screen shown in Fig.6.10(a). This uses a different compound from those used in dosimetry but are in effect large area thermoluminescent dosimeters which carry spatial (image) information. The thermoluminescent material is commonly barium fluorohalide of the type BaFX:Eu^{2+} where X is the halide atom Cl, Br or I. Under x-ray exposure the europium ion changes from the divalent to the trivalent state Eu$^{2+} \rightarrow$ Eu^{3+}. On stimulation by light (laser) of a particular wavelength the trivalent state returns to its original divalent state releasing short wavelength light. This is described further in Chapter 7.

Table 6.4   TLD used for radiation monitoring

Phosphor	Application	Dose range (Gy)
LiF	personal monitoring	10^{-5}-10^3
CaSO$_4$:Tm	environmental monitoring	10^{-7}-10^2
CaF$_2$:Dy	environmental monitoring	10^{-6}-10^4
Li$_2$B$_4$O$_7$:Mn	tissue equivalent	10^{-3}-10^3

6.6   SEMICONDUCTOR DETECTORS

The principle of semiconductor detector has been described in Chapter 2. The amount of energy necessary to create an electron-hole pair is only about 3eV compared to 34eV for a gas ionization detector. Since many more charge carrying pairs are created for each keV absorbed, counting statistics are much improved.

Complex semiconductor detectors using 'hyper-pure' germanium or lithium doped (drifted) silicon are used for spectrometry (identifying gamma emissions). They give superior resolution to all other detector types but are less sensitive and require liquid nitrogen cooling. Hyper-pure germanium detectors show energy resolutions typically less than 1% for the diagnostic energy range: 1keV at 122keV (0.8%) and 2keV at 1.33MeV (0.15%). This FWHM figure is compared to a good sodium iodide detector resolution in Fig.6.14.

Semiconductor diode radiation detectors are simple, robust and do not need cooling. They are used in some kVp meters and for measuring radiation doses in specific locations. Cadmium telluride is a semiconductor material manufactured in the form of small probes for measuring local activity. It gives good energy resolution and can resolve separate gamma energies.

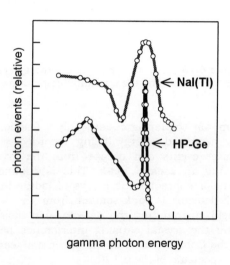

gamma photon energy

Figure 6.14   An NaI:Tl spectrum with an energy resolution of 8–9% and a semiconductor (Ge) spectrum with an energy resolution of <1% compared.

6.7 EFFICIENCY AND SENSITIVITY

If the detector is treated as a simple absorber its clear from the diagram shown previously in Fig.5.1(a) that:

- not every photon will interact within the detector and will be transmitted unchanged.
- some photons will be totally absorbed by the detector.
- some photons will scatter outside the detector volume

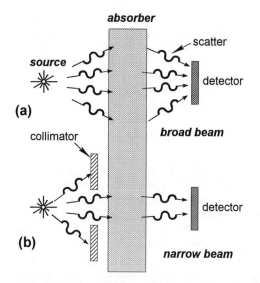

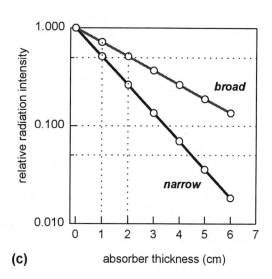

Figure 6.15 **(a)** Broad beam geometry where scatter events can interfere with detection. **(b)** Narrow beam geometry using beam collimation. **(c)** Half value layer for broad and narrow beam geometry. HVL narrow beam is 1cm whereas HVL for the broad beam is 2cm.

The effectiveness as a detector will depend on both its linear attenuation coefficient μ, thickness x and the proportion of the photon beam that the detector surface will intersect and be absorbed within the detector volume. A further measure of a detector's efficiency, not represented in the diagram, concerns those photons that are totally absorbed and their ability to give a useful signal allowing for the detector's dead-time or speed of response and ability to discriminate between a photon event and noise.

A detector's response to radiation is measured in terms of both its efficiency and sensitivity. Efficiency can be separated in to three types:

- **Geometric efficiency**: the area or volume of the detector intercepting the radiation.
- **Intrinsic efficiency**: the absorbing power of the detector for the particular energy radiation.
- **Extrinsic efficiency**: can be identified as the usefulness of the detector signal itself; its light output and light collection (e.g. photomultiplier assembly).

The sensitivity of a detector is a term used here for describing its response relative to photon energy and comparing it to the response given by tissue.

This is a measure of its tissue equivalence and is valuable information when using a detection device for measuring radiation dose and relating detector dose measurement to real tissue dose.

6.7.1 Detector efficiency

Broad and narrow beam geometry Figure 6.15(a) and (b) compare the performance of broad and narrow beam geometry (x or gamma radiation) on a detector surface. In diagram (a) an uncollimated broadbeam allows scattered radiation (whose source originates outside the detector field of view) to reach the detector surface so more radiation reaches the detector than would occur with a narrow beam geometry. A narrow beam in (b) is obtained by using collimators which closely restrict beam dimensions. Collimators are commonly constructed from sheet-lead, 2 to

3mm thick depending on photon energy. A narrow beam ensures that only radiation transmitted in a narrow conic section will be counted. This will be mainly primary radiation with only a small scatter component. Broad beam geometry allows a far greater proportion of scattered radiation to enter the detector field of view. Narrow beam geometry is also improved by positioning the source further from the collimator, making the angle subtended by the detector surface still smaller.

Figure 6.15(c) shows that when the half value layer of two identical source activities is measured, different values are obtained for the broad and narrow geometry. The broad beam appears to have a higher HVL due to the greater proportion of scattered radiation reaching the detector surface. The narrow beam HVL measurement collects less of these scattered photons so gives a smaller value. Broad and narrow beam geometries have important implications in radiology:

- HVL's measured under broad beam conditions are useful for calculating room shielding requirements.
- Narrow beam geometry is important when considering patient examinations.

X-ray field sizes should always be collimated to cover the area of interest so both patient exposure is reduced and scattered radiation reaching the detector surface (film or image intensifier) is reduced. Measuring x-ray equipment HVL should always use narrow beam geometry.

Geometrical efficiency For a point source radiation is emitted isotropically (that is over a spherical surface). Fig.6.16(a) shows it is determined by two parameters: the effective area of the detector (D1, D2, D3) intercepting the beam and the source to detector distance. The geometry is represented diagrammatically in Fig.6.16(b) and the general expression for counting an isotropic source can be stated as:

$$\frac{photons\ reaching\ detector}{photons\ emitted\ from\ source\ (\ 4\pi\ )} \qquad (6.2)$$

For a large detector (D1) there will be more incident photons striking the detector surface than for a smaller detector (D2) and a similar sized detector D3 at a greater distance will intersect fewer photons so size and distance define the solid angle (Ω) subtended by the flat detector, relative to the source:

$$\Omega \propto \frac{A}{d^2} \qquad (6.3)$$

where A is the detector area and Ω is in steradians. For a sphere Ω = 4π or 12.56 steradians and a spherical detector would capture all the radiation; this is referred to as 4π geometry. When the source is on the surface of a flat detector Ω = 2π or 6.28 steradians; this is 2π geometry and gives 50% geometrical efficiency representing a flat surface detector (e.g. gamma camera).

4π geometry An isotropic source emits radiation over a spherical surface of 4π steradians and true 4π detectors would give a geometrical efficiency of 100% so detector efficiency when counting a geometrical source is measured as:

$$E_G = \frac{\Omega}{4\pi} \times 100\% \qquad (6.4)$$

Very few detectors approach anywhere near 4π geometry in radiology. The exception is the dose calibrator where accurate measurement of radioactivity is necessary for patient radiopharmaceutical injections. The detector used is a hollow cylinder which allows the sample to be placed in the center of the detecting volume (gas); the design shown in Fig. 6.3(a)

2π geometry If the radiation source is placed on a large flat detector (e.g. a gamma camera crystal) so that the radiation over a hemisphere is subtended by the detector then this will have 50% geometrical efficiency and show 2π geometry. Clearly, from Fig.6.16(b), a large area detector and a short distance is desirable making Ω large but practical limitations are imposed by the detector encapsulation and shielding etc.

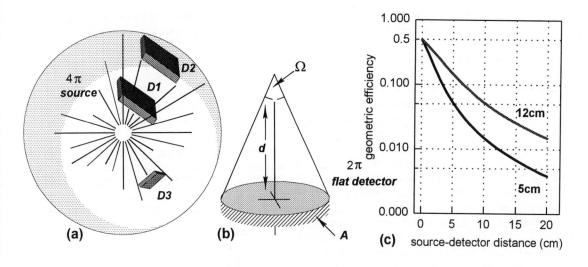

Figure 6.16 **(a)** 4π geometry given by an isotropic source. Two detectors D1 and D2 have the same size but D3 is smaller. **(b)** 2π geometry given by a flat detector subtending the solid angle Ω **(c)** graph plotting 2π geometrical efficiency for two detectors 12cm and 6cm diameter.

A practical formula for calculating geometrical efficiency E_G for a point source with 2π detector geometry is:

$$E_G = 0.5 \times \left(1 - \frac{h}{\sqrt{h^2 + d^2}} \right) \qquad (6.5)$$

where these parameters are identified in Fig.6.16(b). This function is plotted in Fig.6.16(c) for two sizes of detector, both show 2π efficiency (50%) with the source on the detector surface (0cm) but the larger detector (12cm) maintains a higher geometrical efficiency than the smaller (5cm) at distance from the source. At a point 5cm from the source the smaller detector intersects only 5% of the radiation whereas the larger detector intersects approximately 12%

6.7.2 Detector intrinsic efficiency

Quantum efficiency E_Q The ability to absorb incident photons is a measure of detector quantum efficiency and is the fraction of incident photons that are absorbed by the detector. It should not be confused with Detective Quantum Efficiency (DQE) described in Chapter 8. Detector quantum efficiency is measured as:

$$E_Q = 1 - e^{-\mu x_d} \qquad (6.6)$$

where μ is the linear attenuation coefficient and x_d the detector thickness. Since μ is dependent on photon energy, there are three parameters influencing quantum efficiency:

1. Linear attenuation coefficient of the detector material.
2. Detector thickness
3. Photon energy

Overall detector quantum efficiency is also modified by the shielding material surrounding the detector volume such as the input window (aluminium, glass, titanium etc.) and any collimation or grids which would also absorb incident radiation, so E_Q is modified so that:

$$E_Q = e^{-\mu x_w} \times (1 - e^{-\mu x_d}) \qquad (6.7)$$

where μx_w is the attenuation coefficient and thickness of the covering material.

6.7.3 Detector extrinsic efficiency

Conversion efficiency E_C Photons absorbed by the detector must contribute to a measurable signal, either electrical or light. E_C compares the available photon energy with the energy absorbed in the detector. If all the photon energy is utilized (provides a signal) there will be a conversion efficiency of 1.0, however some energy of the incident photon is carried by secondary photons which can scatter outside the detector volume reducing E_C to a value less than 1.0. Compton interactions do not contribute a useful signal but they may end in a photoelectric event which does contribute.

Conversion efficiencies of gas detectors may be quite high particularly if gas amplification takes place (geiger counter). The quantum efficiency of a gas detector is, however, low so a measure of total efficiency is required; this is simply:

$$E_T = E_Q \times E_C \qquad (6.8)$$

Box 6.2 gives some worked examples of total efficiency, comparing various detector types.

Box 6.2

Total efficiency of detectors $E_T = E_Q \times E_C$	
Gas detector with gas amplification E_Q 0.01 E_C 1.0 so E_T is	1%
Scintillation detector (NaI:Tl) E_Q 0.8 E_C 0.5 so E_T is	40%

Intensifying screens (two thickness and different materials)
(a). E_Q 0.4
   E_C 0.5 so E_T is
(b). E_Q 0.25
   E_C 0.8 so E_T is
	
	20%
	
	20%

Although they give identical total efficiencies the first screen is thicker, giving it a higher E_Q but poorer resolution than screen 2, which has a thinner screen but higher E_C

Dead time τ The intrinsic efficiency of a detector decreases with increasing count rate due to the inability to handle high count rates. Consequently there is pulse pile-up due to dead time which can be expressed as:

$$\tau = \frac{detected\ signals}{total\ incident\ photons} \qquad (6.9)$$

The effect of dead-time on detector response is shown graphically in Fig.6.17. The value differs considerably between counter types.

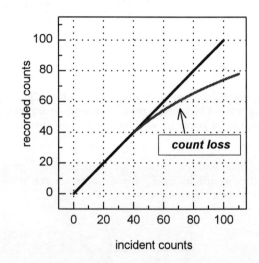

Figure 6.17 A detector with no dead time will give the same detected counts as incident counts for all count rates (straight line). A non-linear response will be seen when fast count events are not resolved and detected counts are less than incident counts above a certain count rate.

The largest dead times are shown by gas detectors where the presence of ionization events from a previous interactions block further signals until these events are neutralized; some gas detectors (geiger counters) have long dead times (300µs) but scintillation detectors have very short dead-times (0.22µs). If a detector with dead time τ indicates a count rate of N then the true count rate N_T is:

$$N_T = \frac{N}{1 - N \cdot \tau} \qquad (6.10)$$

For slow count rates dead-time correction is negligible but as the graph in Fig.6.17 shows at higher count rates significant loss of information is possible. For a Geiger counter with a dead time of 300µs, which indicates a count rate of 1000cps, the true count rate would be: N_T = 1000/1–1000×0.0003 = 1428 so for this count rate a geiger counter would under-estimate the count rate by nearly 50%. On the other hand a scintillation detector with a much shorter dead-time of 0.22µs and an indicated count rate of 100,000cps would give an under-estimation of only 2%.

Energy resolution Detectors that are able to give individual photon event signals such as the proportional counter, the scintillation detector and the semiconductor detector are photon energy sensitive, that is the pulse height is proportional to photon energy. A pulse height discriminator as shown in Fig.6.11 enables a photon energy spectrum to be generated. The energy resolution, as a percentage, is measured as FWHM.

Scintillation detectors give a typical energy resolution of about 8-9% already seen in Fig.6.14. This figure includes crystal and photomultiplier resolution. Non-uniformity in crystal response is due to dispersion within the crystal giving loss of useful light. Spectrometers' resolving power is poorer at lower energies so [137]Cesium (662keV) is commonly used as a standard for resolution measurements.

The **intrinsic peak efficiency** of an energy sensitive detector is the fraction of gamma photons represented within the photopeak distribution. Electrical noise in the photomultiplier amplifier chain also contributes to resolution loss.

The proportional counter gives a similar energy resolution but the semiconductor detector typically gives resolution figures of <1% across the energy range; however since its density is lower than the scintillation crystals its efficiency is much lower, being about 20-30% that of NaI:Tl.

6.7.4 Sensitivity

The absorbed dose has already been defined in Chapter 5. Detector sensitivity is determined by comparing the mass absorption coefficient of the detector material with that of air which is a measure of the energy (radiation dose) absorbed by the detector material per unit of absorbed dose in air (μ_{ab}/ρ for air).

Relative sensitivity or response is measured by comparing this value with the detector's own absorption coefficient (μ_{ab}/ρ for the detector). If these two absorption coefficients are the same for the diagnostic energy range then the detector will have the same sensitivity. Figure 6.18 shows that soft tissue and air have similar sensitivity or response over the diagnostic range. So radiation dose measured by an air ion-detector will be representative of tissue radiation dose. Detector materials that have a mean atomic number close to soft tissue will show **tissue equivalence**.

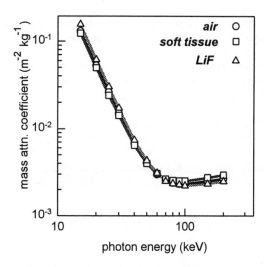

Figure 6.18 Mass absorption coefficient for air, soft tissue and LiF over the diagnostic energy range showing tissue equivalence.

The Z value for soft tissue is 7.64; for air 7.78 and for water 7.51; air and water are therefore tissue equivalent (see Fig.6.18). Lithium fluoride, used as a personal radiation dosimeter, has a Z value of 8.31 and is also treated as tissue equivalent. Film emulsion however has a mean Z value exceeding 35.0 so would have a significantly different sensitivity response to radiation (including K-edge differences) and would not be tissue equivalent (Fig.6.1).

KEYWORDS

2π geometry: relating to a flat detector surface e.g. a gamma camera

4π geometry: relating to a volume detector e.g. dose calibrator

becquerel: a measure of radionuclide activity in disintegrations per second (1dps = 1Bq)

broad beam: an uncollimated radiation beam (x-rays or gamma)

Compton edge: the edge of the gamma spectrum representing 180° scatter

dead time: the speed of response of a detector for counting individual events. Usually measured at a 20% count loss.

efficiency (conversion): The efficiency of signal (e.g. light) production in a detector.

efficiency (geometrical): the fraction of the isotropic emission collected by the detector surface

efficiency (quantum): a measure of photon absorption

energy resolution: measured as FWHM of the photopeak.

luminescence: a general property of some inorganic crystals and plastics involving electron transition between valency and conduction bands.

narrow beam: a collimated radiation beam.

photomultiplier: a light sensitive device for amplifying very small light signals.

photopeak: the part of the gamma spectrum which identifies the photoelectric event. This represents the peak gamma energy.

scintillator: a crystalline or liquid compound which exhibits luminescence.

sensitivity: the response of a detector to different photon energies.

tissue equivalent: having the same sensitivity to photon energy as soft tissue.

7

Photography and the film image

7.1 The photographic principle
7.2 Film sensitometry
7.3 Intensifying screens

7.4 Film processors
7.5 Phosphor imaging plate

7.1   THE PHOTOGRAPHIC PRINCIPLE

Film is the most common hardcopy used in radiology. Although departments are striving to introduce a filmless service with all the theoretical benefits of low cost and security, the demand for an easily portable high quality image will maintain film as the display medium of choice for the next few years.

The film emulsion has been successfully refined for radiology and is used in x-ray imaging with and without screens, video recording, cine-recording and film records from image plates.

7.1.1 The film emulsion

A film emulsion is a mixture of silver halides suspended in gelatin. The silver halide is the light sensitive compound and the gelatin acts both as a supporting material and takes part in the photo chemistry.

Silver halides silver chloride, bromide and iodide are used in various mixtures to alter the sensitivity of the film. The order of light sensitivity is: silver bromide > silver chloride > silver iodide. They have a cuboid crystal structure shown in Fig.7.1(a) and are formed by reacting silver nitrate with alkali halides:

$$AgNO_3 + (KBr \text{ or } NaCl \text{ or } KI)$$
$$\downarrow$$
$$AgBr \text{ or } AgCl \text{ or } AgI$$

Photo-sensitivity This increases with the amount of added silver iodide but rarely exceeds 8% of the silver bromide content. In preparing the silver halide the silver iodide crystallizes first forming nuclei for the silver bromide which then forms the larger crystals (grains)

Gelatin This is the suspending medium for the photochemical mix during the formation of the silver halides (described above). It also separates the crystals or grains. Various control parameters at this stage influence **grain size**. After grain formation the suspension of silver halides in gelatin undergoes a series of ripening processes which introduces a small proportion of silver sulfide from free sulfur present in the gelatin. These Ag_2S crystal defects act as an important **sensitivity centers** in the silver halide crystal and have significant effects on the speed of the film. Their average concentration is about 1:1000000. Greater concentration will increase background darkening or emulsion fog. Modern emulsion uses purified gelatin with controlled amounts of sensitizers (sulfur) added during the course of preparation.

Emulsion construction Overall formation of the film emulsion involves:

- Reacting alkali halides with silver nitrate in the gelatin

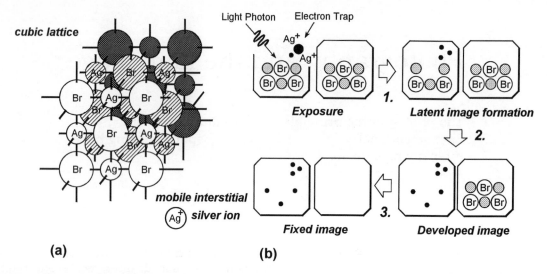

Figure 7.1   **(a)** The construction of the AgBr crystal showing the cuboid structure and a mobile interstitial silver ion. **(b)** The photographic action (1, 2, 3) from light exposure to the fixed image is described in the text.

- Physical ripening: Emulsion stirring to increase grain size
- Chemical or after ripening: Sensitive center formation
- Additional compounds: Optical sensitizers (see below), stabilizers to maintain properties through aging, hardening agents to protect the emulsion surface.

Optical sensitizers   The emulsion in its first stage of manufacture is only sensitive to the blue/ultra-violet part of the light spectrum. Small quantities of optical sensitizers are added to increase sensitivity to the green/yellow/red end of the spectrum.

7.1.2 The photochemical process

The silver halide crystal in its pure form consists of alternate atoms of silver and bromine arranged in a cuboid lattice (Fig.7.1(a)). **Interstitial silver ions** can move within the crystal lattice towards negative electron traps which are positively charged.

The lattice silver and bromine atoms are fixed. Individual silver halide crystals within the emulsion contain:

- Interstitial silver ions which are mobile and positively charged.
- A number of electron traps, defects or sensitivity centers, usually in the form of silver sulfide, which are formed from sulfur in the gelatin during the ripening process. Fig.7.1(b).

Exposure to light   When the emulsion is exposed to light the photon excites a bromine atom in the crystal, which loses an electron (Figure 7.1(b)). The liberated electron is trapped in the crystal defect. The free bromine which is formed escapes into the gelatin and is held there. Neighboring unexposed crystals are unaffected.

All the free electrons produced by light photons are trapped in these centers. The positive charged interstitial silver ions are then attracted to these increasingly negative defect centers, are neutralized by the accumulated negative charges and become silver atoms.

Thus the sensitivity sites become concentrations of silver atoms which are potential **development centers** carrying information in the form of a **latent image;** Stage 1. in Fig.7.1(b) shows these interstitial silver atoms joining the electron trap and forming a complete latent image.

Developing   This process magnifies the latent image by reducing the remaining AgBr in the exposed crystal to silver and giving the developed image as Stage 2. in Fig.7.1(b). Developers usually contain ring compounds of hydro-quinone, amitol or metol. The reaction is:

$$\langle\!\!\!\bigcirc\!\!\!\rangle\text{OH} + \text{AgBr} = \langle\!\!\!\bigcirc\!\!\!\rangle\text{O} + \text{HBr} + \text{Ag}$$

Developer   **Oxidized Developer**

 The AgBr in this reaction is the exposed or activated silver halide which is reduced to silver, leaving the developer in an oxidized state which is no longer active. Latent image silver atoms cause the entire silver halide crystal or grain to be reduced to silver so when the emulsion has been completely developed it will consist of:

- Silver halide crystals reduced completely to silver atoms representing amplified latent image information
- Unexposed and unaltered silver halide crystals.

This is the developed image in Fig.7.1(b).

Fixing   After development the silver halide emulsion is desensitized by fixing the image, this is the final Stage 3 in Fig.7.1(b).   The fixer compound is ammonium thiosulfate $(\text{NH}_4)_2\text{S}_2\text{O}_3$ which removes the unexposed, unaltered silver halide as a soluble complex:

$$\text{Ag}^+\text{Br}^- + (\text{S}_2\text{O}_3)^{2-} \rightarrow \text{Ag}(\text{S}_2\text{O}_3)^- + \text{Br}^-$$

The silver thiosulfate complex is carried out of the emulsion when the film is thoroughly washed with clean water. This complex is still light sensitive and will slowly decompose leaving a silver deposit on the film image in poorly washed films which is the main cause of darkening and consequent deterioration of archived films.

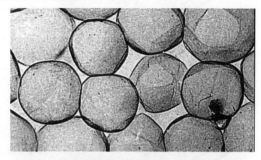
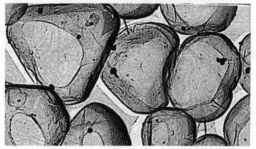

Figure 7.2   Irregular grain sizes giving a wide latitude low contrast emulsion and uniform grain size giving a high contrast emulsion.

Grain (crystal) size   An enlarged picture of silver halide grains is shown in Fig.7.2. The grain affects the film image in four ways:

1. Large grain size increase **film sensitivity** since more silver atoms are produced from each light photon
2. **Resolution** is degraded by large grain sizes since the large area will intercept more photons, fine image detail will be lost.
3. The **contrast** of the film is influenced by the variety of grain sizes: mixed grain size will give a low contrast: single grain size will give a high contrast.
4. Large grains are visible as **mottle** on the final image.

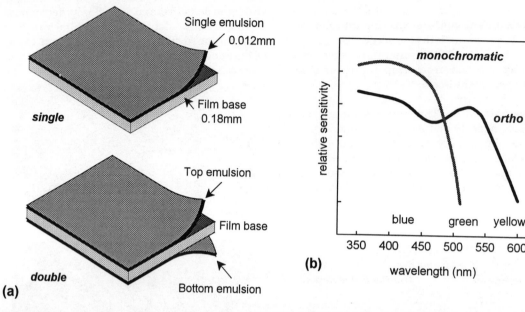

Figure 7.3 **(a)** Film structure of single and double sided emulsions. Only the film base and emulsion are shown; the two coatings are omitted for clarity. **(b)** Film response to different light wavelengths for monochromatic (blue) and orthochromatic (green) light.

7.1.3 Film structure

Films used for radiography usually consist of a polyester base onto which the silver halide emulsion is spread. **Single** or **double sided** emulsion layers can be provided for different applications. Figure 7.3(a) shows a four layer single sided emulsion and a seven layer double emulsion film. The four layers of a single emulsion film are:

- The supporting polyester **base**
- The **sub-coating** which ensures the emulsion adheres to the film base
- The halide **emulsion** itself
- The **protective-coating** which protects emulsion from mechanical damage.

The single emulsion film is used for recording high definition images such as mammographs or electronic displays (CRT or laser imagers). Double-sided film is designed for cassettes that have dual intensifying screens. It increases efficiency but has poorer resolution.

The polyester base offers important properties:

- Strength and tear resistant
- Waterproof
- Dimensional stability and flatness
- Non-flammable
- Good aging properties for archiving

Conventional **screen film** has a thin emulsion layer designed for automatic processing. The thinner emulsion gives:

- Shorter development and fixing times,
- More efficient washing (removing practically all of the resident chemicals).
- Rapid drying.

Non-screen film has thicker emulsion which is more sensitive to x-radiation. It is sometimes used for very high resolution work (bone imaging) and should not be used in automatic processors, since this will damage its thicker emulsion layer.

Optical sensitizers These are added to film emulsion in order to extend the sensitivity to longer wavelength light, so that the film type can be manufactured closely matching the light output from intensifying screen phosphors used in the cassette.

The spectral sensitivity for two film types, **monochromatic** (blue) and **orthochromatic** (blue/green) are shown in Fig.7.3(b).

Monochromatic film The natural sensitivity of silver halide emulsion, without sensitizer, is for UV and blue part of the light spectrum. This film type is used for blue emitting intensifying screens i.e. tungstate, lanthanum, barium or yttrium based screens.

Orthochromatic The film response is extended into the green portion of the spectrum by adding optical sensitizers to the film emulsion. Rare earth gadolinium intensifying screens require orthochromatic film since they emit green light. Mixed screens of lanthanum and gadolinium use the full sensitivity of ortho-film by supplying both green and blue light; this increases sensitivity.

Panchromatic This film type is sensitive to the entire visible spectrum and is not commonly met in radiology except in cine-fluorography which uses commercial panchromatic 35mm cine-film.

Film storage As unexposed film ages certain chemical and thermal changes occur in the emulsion which increase background fog levels. Ideal storage conditions for unexposed film are a maximum temperature of 20°C with a relative humidity of 50%. Cold storage can lengthen the useful life of a film which can have significant effects in hot climates. Exposed but unprocessed film deteriorates gradually, losing low contrast detail, unless placed in cold storage.

If either unexposed or exposed film is kept in a cassette its sensitivity to background radiation will be increased considerably (due to light emission from the intensifying screen) and its fog level will increase over time. Cassettes loaded with film for immediate use should be shielded from x-ray scatter or placed at some distance from the x-ray machine.

Exposed and processed film is stable and providing it has been processed properly (adequately fixed and washed) and stored under the same conditions as unexposed film it should retain its image detail for 2-3 decades before low contrast information is lost.

Summary

- Film emulsion consists of AgBr + AgI in gelatin. AgBr is the major ingredient.
- AgI enhances sensitivity (8% maximum concentration)
- Gelatin base keeps silver halide as separate crystals. Small sulfur impurities in gelatin form silver sulfide sensitivity centers or defects which increase sensitivity.
- Gelatin acts as a bromine receptor.
- Emulsion ripening: Increases grain size and sensitivity.
- Exposure to light forms free electrons:
  $$hf \rightarrow Br^- \rightarrow Br + e^-$$
- Sensitivity centers absorb the free electrons forming regions of negative charge within the exposed crystal.
- Mobile silver ions migrate to these negative sensitivity centers where they are neutralized and form silver atoms.
- Defects holding the silver atoms contain latent image information and become development centers
- Developing amplifies latent image by reducing all the remaining AgBr in the silver halide grain to silver.
- Fixing removes unexposed silver halide as soluble complex.
- Grain size affects sensitivity; large grains are more sensitive (contrast) but reduce resolution (graininess).
- Mixed grain size has greater latitude (low contrast).

7.2 FILM SENSITOMETRY

Film was originally constructed for recording changes in light intensity (L.J. Daguerre 1789-1851; French and W.H. Fox-Talbot 1800-1877, British scientists).

Film is not very sensitive to x-rays; its relative sensitivity to light and x-rays is shown in Fig.7.4. Film is shown to have a sensitivity to very low light levels but is relatively insensitive to x-ray exposure, however it does have a useful linear response to x- and γ–radiation exposure which is utilized for measuring radiation dose as a film-dosimeter.

Film's most sensitive region is in the blue spectrum; optical sensitizers extend the response toward green as already described.

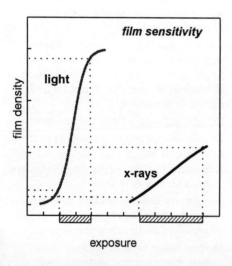

exposure

Figure 7.4 Film's high sensitivity for light as compared to the low sensitivity for x-ray photons; however the x-ray response is linear which is useful for measuring radiation dose.

Intensifying screens   In order to improve the efficiency for recording x-ray information a phosphor intensifying screen which converts x-rays to light is interposed between x-ray beam and film. The screen is a phosphor scintillator and converts high energy x-ray photons into lower energy visible light photons; the light wavelength depends on the phosphor type.

7.2.1. Film characteristics

The **characteristic curves** plotting film response (or density) against exposure, shown in Fig.7.4, compare the sensitivities between an x-ray exposure made with and without intensifying screens. A significant increase in sensitivity is obvious when screens are used and the film exposed to light, however only a section of the curve retains linearity.

Although Röntgen first observed the effect of x-rays when they reacted with a phosphor (barium platino-cyanide), the introduction of practical phosphor intensifying screens to radiography was made in 1896 by TA Edison (1847-1931; USA, inventor). His intensifying screens were responsible for increased sensitivity and a significant reduction in patient dose during radiological investigations.

Light sensitometry   Film characteristics are best obtained by illuminating the film with a calibrated gray scale from a sensitometer, an example is shown in Fig.7.5(a). If the gray scale densities are plotted against exposure then a film **characteristic curve** is obtained. The characteristic curve for a film or film/screen combination is shown in Fig.7.5(b). The different steps are measured using a calibrated spot densitometer. The densitometer calculates each optical density OD as:

$$OD = \log_{10} \frac{I_O}{I} \qquad (7.1)$$

I_O being the reference intensity of the incident light source and I the intensity through the exposed section of the film (wedge-step). If the log relative exposure level is plotted on the x-axis and the resultant optical density (D) plotted on the y-axis then a characteristic curve is obtained which describes the film quantitative response to light and reveals many important film qualities.

An early name for the characteristic curve was the H and D Curve after the Swiss F. Hurter 1844-1898 and the American V.C. Driffield 1848-1915. The curve is now commonly called the $D/\log E$ curve. Fig.7.5(b) shows the distinguishing parts:

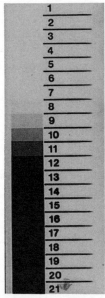

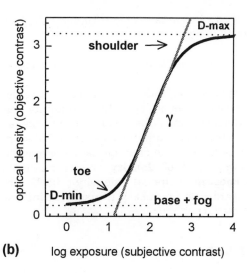

(b) log exposure (subjective contrast)

Figure 7.5 **(a)** A sensitometric gray scale obtained from a calibrated sensitometer directly exposing film to either blue or green light. **(b)** The characteristic response of a film to light shown by plotting log. exposure against optical density measured with a densitometer. The features are identified in the text.

- The **fog level** is a density reading of the background noise caused mainly by thermal effects; it can also result from high radiation background levels (unshielded storage conditions).

- The **threshold value** marks the lowest exposure that gives a density value above the fog-level.

- The **toe** region is the low exposure non-linear portion of the curve seen in the radiograph in denser tissue: bone, heart shadow and diaphragm.

- The straight line or **slope** of the curve describes the most important property of the film since it carries most information about soft tissue detail as seen in the lung fields and most clearly in mammography. The steeper this portion of the curve the more **contrast** will the film image have.

- The **shoulder** region enters another non-linear response where all the film grains have been saturated and maximum density is seen (black); hollow regions of the anatomy (gut) and gas (pneumothorax) are radiographic examples.

X-ray sensitometry In order to measure the response of a **film/screen** combination to radiation it is necessary to expose it to a graded radiation intensity. This is commonly achieved by using an x-ray source and a stepped aluminum wedge but this is not ideal since the x-ray beam undergoes non-uniform filtration through the increasing thicknesses of aluminum. This can be solved to some extent by hardening the beam with added filtration but a more consistent x-ray exposure is made when (for a fixed value of kV and mAs) a lead-screen is moved a fixed series of distances over the cassette creating a stepped series of exposures. At the end of the exposure sequence the first strip has seen the most radiation and the last strip has seen one exposure. Beam quality remains constant throughout this method.

As with light sensitometry exposure is represented on the *x*-axis of the characteristic curve as the radiation intensity per unit time:

$$E = I \times t \qquad (7.2)$$

The value E is usually a relative measure of exposure. Optical density is directly related to x-radiation exposure E from eqn.7.2 measured in mAs ($I \times t$). Under film/screen conditions:

Optical Density ∝ Exposure (mAs)

Exposure on the characteristic curve is represented as a logarithmic quantity $\log_{10}E$ which encompasses a wide range of exposure levels representing the exponential absorption of radiation. The characteristic curve is therefore a plot of **density** versus relative **log. exposure.** Optical density itself is a logarithmic product of transmitted intensities (eqn.7.1).

7.2.2 Film optical density (OD)

Optical density   If I_0 is the light intensity of the film viewing box and I is the intensity transmitted by an area of exposed film then this optical density, already described by eqn.7.1, will be:

$$OD = \log_{10} \frac{I_0}{I}$$

Allocating a value of 1000 for I_0 and 100 for I then the film's optical density is $\log_{10}$ or 1.0. An optical density equal to 1.0 represents a medium gray level.

The optical density measurement is independent of the incident (viewing box) intensity. Table.7.1 gives examples of the logarithmic scale of light intensity transmitted through a gray-scale film image and Fig.7.6 plots image brightness against optical density showing the logarithmic response.

The response of the eye to different light intensities is also logarithmic so the objective measurement of density agrees with the subjective assessment by the eye. This table shows that an increase in density of 0.3 reduces the transmitted light intensity by half.

Useful densities seen in radiographs range between 0.2 and 2.0. Lung areas where little absorption has taken place are between 2.5 and 3.0; densities higher than this carry little information. Denser areas of the mediastinum are between 0.2 and 1.0.

Table 7.1   Optical density and log intensity.

Fraction transmitted I_1	$\log_{10}$ value	Optical density
1.0	log 1.0	0.0
0.5	log 0.5	0.3
0.1	log 10	1.0
0.01	log 100	2.0
0.001	log 1000	3.0
0.0001	log 10000	4.0

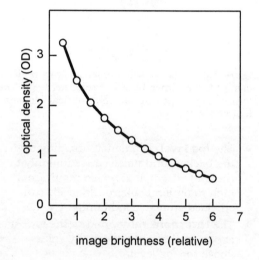

Figure 7.6 The logarithmic relationship between image brightness and film optical density.

7.2.3 Exposure latitude

Figure 7.7(a) and (b) shows two characteristic curves. Film (a) is a high contrast film requiring only a narrow exposure range to achieve this optical density difference whereas the film in (b) requires an increased exposure range.

The film in (a) has a steeper straight line or slope and so will give more rapid density changes for a given narrow range of exposures.

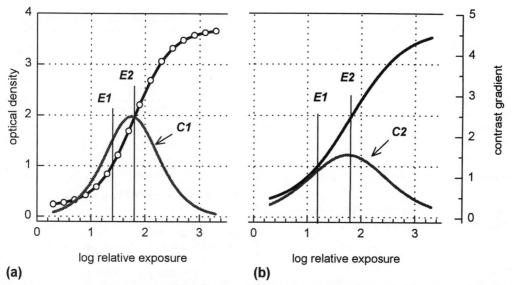

Figure 7.7 **(a)** An example of a high contrast film having narrow latitude. The contrast gradient curve has a peak value of 2.5 (right hand *y*-axis). Points E1 and E2 are used in Box.7.1 **(b)** a low contrast film having a wider latitude. The contrast gradient peak value is 1.6.

The film in (b) has a longer slope and has less contrast than film (a) for the same exposure; it has a wider **latitude** than (a).

The slope of the straight portion of the characteristic curve gives a measure of the film contrast. The steeper this slope the greater the range of optical densities for a small change in exposure levels. This slope is measured as the gamma (γ) and can be defined:

$$\gamma = \frac{D2 - D1}{\log E2 - \log E1} \tag{7.3}$$

D1 and *D2* are the film densities obtained from exposures *E1* and *E2* represented in Fig.7.7(a). A large γ has a high contrast useful for imaging a narrow range of tissue densities and so accentuating any small differences between normal and abnormal states e.g. mammography. Film (b) with a wider latitude (smaller γ) is useful for imaging mixed tissue types with a broader range of attenuation coefficients such as chest radiography. So high contrast film will image small differences in tissue attenuation while low contrast (wide latitude) film will image a wider variety of tissue densities. Film latitude is therefore a measure of the film's **dynamic range**.

Film contrast differs depending on the position along the slope; this can be seen from the change in symbol positioning on the slope in Fig.7.7(a); the most separation between symbols is in the middle of the curve.

Contrast gradient curve This gives the film contrast value for all parts of the characteristic curve by taking the contrast differential of the slope. Its peak value corresponds to the center of the characteristic curve.

Contrast gradient curves (C1 and C2) indicate the magnitude of film contrast in Fig. 7.7(a) and (b). The first characteristic curve is steep so has a larger peak value for C1. The second curve has a wider latitude and a smaller peak contrast value C2. The peak values of C1 and C2 correspond to the γ values calculated in Box.7.1 (allowing for rounding errors).

Box 7.1

Contrast differences in Fig.7.7(a)

For the same density difference ΔD of
$$D2 - D1 = 2 - 1 = 1$$

High contrast film Fig.7.7(a) requires an exposure difference $\Delta logE$: $logE1$ of 1.4 and $logE2$ of 1.8

$$\text{Contrast } (\gamma) = \frac{\Delta D}{\Delta \, logE} = \frac{1}{0.4} = 2.5$$

Low contrast film Fig.7.7(b) requires an exposure $logE1$ of 1.2 and $logE2$ of 1.8, so:

$$\text{Contrast } (\gamma) = \frac{\Delta D}{\Delta \, logE} = \frac{1}{0.6} = 1.66$$

Therefore the high contrast film gives a contrast range of almost ×1.5 that of the low contrast film.
 The contrast gradient peaks C1 and C2 in Fig.7.6(a), (b), reflect these calculated values. (right hand y-axis)

Film and visual contrast The film gamma or slope is a measure of film contrast, a typical value being about 3. Since contrast difference C is $D2 - D1$ this can be rewritten from eqn.7.3 as:

$$C = \gamma \, (\log E2 - \log E1) \qquad (7.4)$$

Visual contrast between two light intensities $I1$ and $I2$ is appreciated as a logarithmic scale:

$$Visual\ Contrast = \log I2 - \log I1 \qquad (7.5)$$

Since the two exposures $E1$ and $E2$ were obtained from two x-ray intensities the visual contrast can be expressed as:

$$Visual\ Contrast = \gamma(\log I2 - \log I1) \qquad (7.6)$$

This demonstrates that film contrast has a similar logarithmic response to visual contrast.
 Table 7.2 lists the four major types of contrast which influence image quality:

subject, radiographic, objective, and subjective contrast. These all influence the visibility of low contrast detail in a diagnostic image.

Table 7.2 Divisions of image contrast

1.   **Subject Contrast**
• Kilovoltage
• Attenuation Coefficient (μ)
• Scatter (tissue thickness x)
• Beam filtration
2.   **Radiographic Contrast**
• Film type (emulsion, grain size)
• Film gamma (γ)
• Film processor (developer temperature, processing time)
• Screen type (rare earth etc.)
• Grid type
3.   **Objective Contrast**
• Optical Density
4.   **Subjective Contrast**
• Film viewer
• Light color
• Masking

From the characteristic curves shown in Fig.7.7(a) and (b) the x-axis represents log exposure values $\Delta logE$ and is influenced by **subject contrast**, in other words those factors which control the exit radiation dose (kV, μ, thickness etc.) and ΔD (y-axis) represents **objective contrast**, the quantitative measure of film optical density.

7.2.4 Sensitivity (film-speed)

Figure 7.8 shows two characteristic curves A and B having identical gammas but the curve for film B is displaced further to the right. Since film A responds to lower exposure levels it is more sensitive than film B; it is a **faster** film.
 Fast films will be displaced to the left; slow films to the right on the x-axis. A mid-point density value of 1.0 is usually chosen to

measure relative film speeds. Box 7.2 calculates the increased exposure necessary for higher film densities and film speed. The faster film in Fig.7.8 will require less radiation to achieve the same optical densities as the slower film.

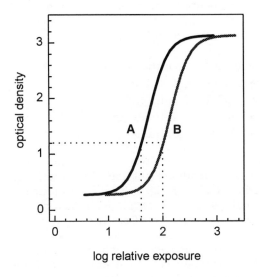

Figure 7.8 The films A and B have different speeds; film A is more sensitive or faster than B.

Box 7.2

Film sensitivity

The film in Fig.7.7(a) requires an exposure level of 1.4 to obtain an OD of 1.0 and an exposure of 1.8 for an OD of 2.0. The $\Delta logE = 0.4$. The anti-log of this is $10^{0.4} = 2.5$ so an optical density of 2.0 for this film will require ×2.5 increased exposure over OD 1.0 (e.g. from 20 to 50mAs).

Film speed

Films A and B in Fig.7.8 require an exposure $logEA$ is 1.6 and log EB of 2.0 for the same reference density (OD = 1.0).
Difference log EB – log EA = 0.4
Converting from log values $10^{0.4}$ = 2.5
So Film A is ×2.5 faster than Film B

7.2.5 Film processing

Developing time and developer temperature The characteristic curve changes for different developer times and temperatures. The change for developing temperature is shown in Fig.7.9(a). Both the slope (contrast) and position of the curve (speed) alters along with an increase in the level of base + fog. There are optimal conditions for each film type and in order to maximize film contrast and speed the manufacturer's recommended temperatures and processor timing should be adhered to. Most daylight film processors have their timing fixed to suit either 90s or 3min processing cycles but the temperature can be easily adjusted; the optimal setting is typically between 33° and 36°C.

Higher developer temperature increases film contrast sensitivity (speed). As a consequence x-ray exposure can be reduced so the patient **radiation exposure** is similarly reduced. This is a most important factor particularly in mammography and pediatric examinations where patient dose must be held at minimum levels. There is a limit to these increases however since the graph in Fig.7.9(b) shows that base + fog levels increase significantly if temperature is increased excessively.

Quantitaion of film response To produce a characteristic curve a series of film densities are produced by known exposures (already described in 7.2.1). These can be a series of stepped exposures on the film using a sensitometer as shown in Fig.7.5(a); a similar exposure wedge can be obtained from x-rays using an aluminum wedge placed on the film cassette. This is x-ray sensitometry, described previously and although it provides an easy method for judging film response, it suffers from inaccuracies due to x-ray spectrum filtration by the individual aluminum steps.

Practical sensitometry Figure 7.10(a) is a characteristic $D/logE$ curve similar to the ones already given in Fig.7.7(a) and (b). This curve was obtained by using a 21 step (0 to 20) density wedge using a light-sensitometer.

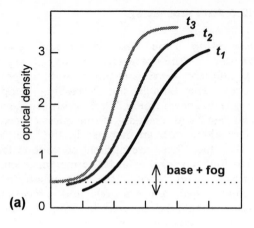

(a)

log. exposure

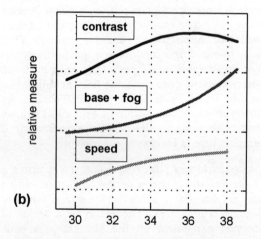

(b)

Figure 7.9 **(a)** The change in the characteristic curve with developing conditions; as the developer temperature is increased from t_1 to t_3 the characteristic curve becomes steeper and displaced to the left (speed increased). **(b)** The variation of film contrast, base+fog and speed (sensitivity) with developer temperature.

The sensitometer is a stable light source illuminating an optical step wedge. Blue or green light is used, depending on film type. Each step on the wedge represents a $logE \sqrt{2}$ or 0.15 incremental change in light intensity

(exposure) which spans the typical density range of a radiographic film. The 21 steps will therefore cover a $logE$ range from 0 to 3.

The curve obtained from a sensitometry step wedge can be used routinely for testing film processing quality for the same film type or the differences between different film types under identical processing conditions. The following parameters can be measured from the curve shown in Fig.7.10(a):

- Base + Fog or the Gross Fog
- Maximum density or D-max
- The Speed Index (SI)
- The Contrast Index (CI)
- The Average Gradient (γ)

The calculations in Box 7.3 explain how these measurements are obtained from the characteristic curve of Fig. 7.10(a). The precise calculations differ between manufacturers but the Speed Index and Contrast Index are useful warning measures for changes in film processor performance such as developer chemical changes or temperature conditions, providing that one manufacturer's instrument is used.

The sensitometric strip can be read either automatically when the results are produced on a print-out or the strip can be analyzed manually. Both methods rely on a **densitometer** which is an illuminated photoelectric cell calibrated directly in optical density units.

Figure 7.10(b) is an example of a quality control sheet for a film processor plotting the values for SI, CI and base + fog on a daily monitoring routine.

Summary:

- **Characteristic Curve**: is a plot of density against log exposure
- **Density**: Represents objective contrast and is a quantitative measurement
- **Exposure**: is influenced by Subject Contrast (attenuation coefficient, kV, filtration etc.)

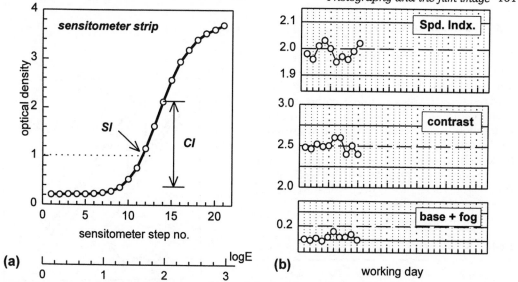

Figure 7.10 (a) A characteristic curve obtained from the sensitometric strip shown in Fig.7.5(a). The speed index and contrast index range are indicated. **(b)** quality control sheet used for daily routine film processor checking .

- **Gamma**: the slope of the characteristic curve is a measure of film contrast (a component of radiographic contrast) and is inversely proportional to latitude
- **Sensitivity**: is measured as film speed

Box 7.3

Sensitometry results (Figure 7.10(a))

Base + fog (BF): 0.20

Dmin:	Step 6:	*LogEmin*	0.90
D1:	OD 1.0 + BF: Step 12	*LogE1*	1.80
D2:	OD 2.0 + BF: Step 14	*LogE2*	2.1

Speed Index = *D1* =1.80

Contrast Index = *D2* – *Dmin* = 1.2

Average gradient (γ) $\dfrac{D2 - D1}{E2 - E1}$ = 3.3

NB Calculations may vary between manufacturer's of printing densitometers.

7.3 INTENSIFYING SCREENS

Film responds to light far more efficiently than x-rays so phosphor intensifying screens are interposed between the x-ray beam and the film emulsion in the cassette. Phosphors emit light due to **luminescence** where short wavelength radiation is absorbed and longer wavelengths are emitted (ultra-violet and visible). Two kinds of luminescence play an important role in intensifying screens:

- **Fluorescence** light emission stops when the exciting radiation ceases.
- **Phosphorescence** light emission continues for a time after the exciting radiation has stopped giving after glow. This is an undesirable property for intensifying phosphor screens and substances are added during manufacture to quench phosphorescence.

An x-ray film alone absorbs about 1-2% of the incident beam but intensifying screens using elements that have Z values from 57 to 74 are effective absorbers of x-radiation (30-50%).

7.3.1   Phosphor materials

An early phosphor material used for intensifying screens was calcium tungstate, but this has been superseded by other materials such as complex compounds of yttrium and rare earth elements lanthanum and gadolinium.   The increased attenuation coefficients for these elements (K-edges) and peak light production are important parameters which contribute to their efficiency. Table 7.3 lists the properties of these phosphor compounds.

Table 7.3 Common intensifying screen phosphors

Phosphor	λ (nm)	K-Edge
$CaWO_4$	Main peak 420	69.5 (W)
Gd_2O_2S :Tb	545	50.2 (Gd)
La_2OBr :Tb	360, 475	38.8 (La)

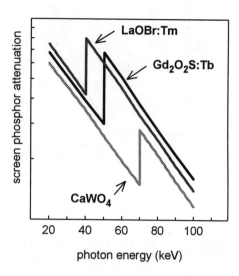

Figure 7.11   Relative absorption curves for lanthanum, gadolinium and tungsten showing the position of the K-edges

The screen phosphor absorption over a range of x-ray energies is shown in Fig.7.11. The K-edges for lanthanum, gadolinium and tungsten occur within the diagnostic energy band from 20 to 120kV which change their quantum efficiency with photon energy as shown in Tab. 7.4.

Ideal properties   The ideal phosphor for intensifying screens should have the following properties:

- A single line emission: The light spectrum should not be too broad. The film can then be designed to respond to a specific wavelength reducing light scatter within the phosphor.
- A medium energy K-edge: so that higher energies (primary beam) are absorbed more efficiently than lower energies (scattered radiation).
- Long-wavelength light which gives more light photons for each x-ray photon.
- High conversion efficiency of x-ray to light photons.

Calcium tungstate   This was an early choice for phosphor screens. Its light emission is in the UV/blue part of the spectrum (Table.7.3) which complements the blue sensitivity of silver halide in the basic film. It has a continuous spectrum, which is a disadvantage, having a maximum peak at 420 to 450nm.   Pigment added to the calcium tungstate phosphor reduces light scatter within the intensifying screen but this also affects overall light output. Calcium tungstate has rapidly been replaced by rare-earth phosphor materials which are up to 5 times more efficient (Table 7.4).

Table 7.4 Phosphor absorption and efficiency

Screen	40keV	60keV	80keV	*IE %
$CaWO_4$	33	13	27	5
Y_2O_2S:Tb	32	12	5	24
LaOBr:Tb	62	38	19	18
Gd_2O_2S:Tb	37	51	28	20

*IE - Total intrinsic efficiency

Rare earth materials Table 7.4 lists intensifying screen phosphors that are based on the rare earth elements lanthanum and gadolinium. Other compounds using yttrium tungstate and tantalate are also available.

These intensifying phosphors are a precise mixture of phosphor and activator material. The activators give peaks or emission lines to the fluorescent spectrum; common doping materials used as activators are:

- Europium (Eu),
- Thulium (Tm)
- Terbium (Tb)

Calcium tungstate has no added activator and gives a continuous spectrum. The spectra for rare earth phosphors and calcium tungstate are compared in Fig.7.12(a), (b).

Lanthanum phosphors Lanthanum oxybromide LaOBr doped with terbium was one of the first rare-earth phosphors to be used for intensifying screen material. Its great advantage was that it emitted blue light which matched available film stock still being used for calcium tungstate screens. Lanthanum gives two light emissions at 360nm and 475nm. The spectrum shown in Fig.7.12(a) compares its relative light output with calcium tungstate.

Gadolinium phosphors Gadolinium oxysulfide doped with either terbium or europium is a more efficient phosphor than lanthanum and gives greater light output. Although several small peaks are seen in the spectrum a single dominant peak occurs at 540nm which corresponds to the green part of the visible spectrum; calcium tungstate is shown here for comparison (Fig.7.12(b)). Gadolinium is more sensitive than either calcium tungstate or lanthanum and as a consequence is the most common phosphor material used in film/screen radiology. Table 7.4 shows the relative absorption for differing x-ray energies and phosphor type. The overall intrinsic efficiency is a combined figure for both quantum and conversion efficiency.

Lanthanum and gadolinium are sometimes mixed to produce a comprehensive intensifying screen combining the benefits of both K-edges giving increased absorption from 40 to 100 kV and light output in the blue and green spectrum: this increases film sensitivity.

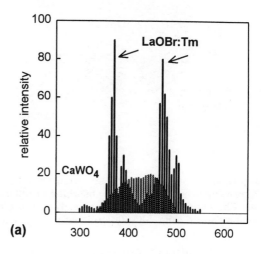

(a)

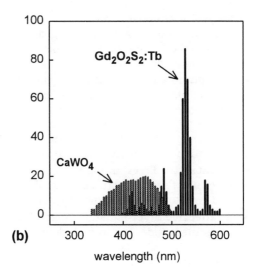

(b)

Figure 7.12 (a) Lanthanum and (b) Gadolinium light spectra compared to CaWO$_4$ showing peaks rather than a broad wavelength spectrum.

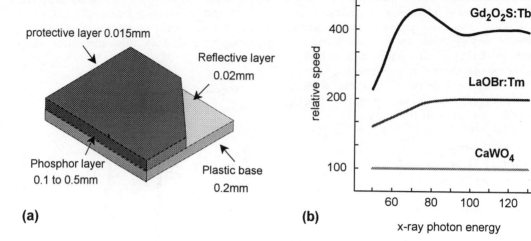

Figure 7.13 **(a)** Screen construction showing waterproof protective layer, the phosphor layer and supporting layers. There is an absorbing or reflective layer depending on application (detail or speed). **(b)** The change of sensitivity (speed) with x-ray energy for three screen types. Par-speed is 100, medium speed from 200-300 and fast screens above 400.

7.3.2 Practical intensifying screens

Construction The construction of a phosphor screen (Fig.7.13(a)) consists of four layers:

- **Polyester support** is made from plastic (0.2mm); a thin light-absorbing layer can also be present on which the phosphor is deposited.
- **Phosphor coating** which is the uniform layer of phosphor crystals in a binder substance sometimes containing pigment. The thickness of this layer, 0.1 to 0.5mm, is critical to the speed and resolution of the intensifying screen.
- A **protective layer** on top prevents build up of static electricity, abrasion and is waterproof so allowing cleaning.
- A **reflective layer** is usually made from titanium dioxide, but in high detail screens this layer is replaced with an absorbing layer.

Light output Knowing the wavelength of the emitted light (Table 7.3) and the intrinsic efficiency of the phosphor (Table.7.4) then the number of light photons generated by the phosphor can be calculated. This is demonstrated in Box 7.4 showing that the rare-earth phosphors can give 4 to 5 times more light than $CaWO_4$

Intensification Factor If a film is exposed to give the same density with and without screens then intensifying screen properties can be compared as:

Intensification factor
$$= \frac{Exposure\ without\ screens}{Exposure\ with\ screens} \quad (7.7)$$

This is a measure of screen speed. The three general categories for screen speed in conventional radiology are:

- Speed 25: slow high resolution detail screens.
- Speed 100: medium speed (par-speed)
- Speed 200-400: fast/very fast for low patient dose examinations e.g. lumbar spine.

X-radiation energy The K-edge of the phosphor element determines absorption already seen in Fig.7.11. The overall sen-

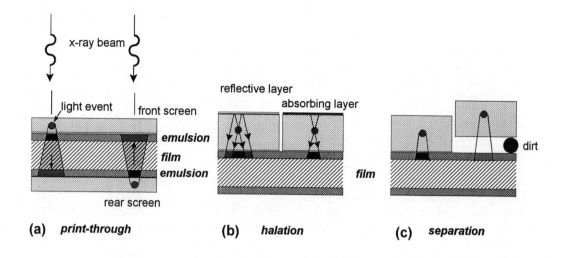

Figure 7.14 Film screen artifacts, **(a)** print-through, **(b)** halation, **(c)** separation.

sitivity (light output) also varies with energy. The set of graphs in Fig.7.13(b) for three screen speeds shows that the sensitivity for each screen peaks at about 70-80keV. The calcium tungstate par-response (speed 100) is shown as reference.

Efficiency Screen efficiency is the product of absorption and conversion efficiency. Major factors playing a part are:

- **Phosphor type** (conventional or rare earth): a higher atomic number increases absorption and conversion (intrinsic) efficiency influences light output.
- **Phosphor thickness**: x-ray absorption increases with increased thickness, light output also increase but resolution decreases substantially so there is a compromise between speed/ sensitivity and resolution. Light reaching film is also reduced due to internal absorption.
- **Phosphor crystal size**: in the same way as thickness larger phosphor grain size increases fluorescent emission. High

speed screens have larger crystal sizes.
- Phosphor **pigments** used in conventional screens (calcium tungstate) reduce lateral spreading improving resolution, but also block some light emission.
- Photon energy is an important factor influencing overall screen efficiency seen in Fig.7.13(b).

Screen thickness The absorption of x-rays by the screens depends on the x-ray energy. Low energy x-rays are absorbed mostly by the front screens, so a mammography cassette needs only one screen. At higher energies the x-rays are equally absorbed by a twin screen cassette. High detail screens give the best resolution and use thin screens. The increased efficiency of the rare-earth phosphors gives improved efficiency even with thin phosphor thickness. These screens have below-par (<100) speed.

Low dose fast screens are more efficient and give the lowest patient dose. They have thicker phosphor layers and absorb more x-radiation but their resolution and low contrast detail are compromised

They can also give significant image mottle since they require less x-ray photons (quantum noise). These features are less important in some investigations (lumbar spine, pregnant patients) since screens with speeds from 200 to 800 require very low x-ray exposure so the patient dose is correspondingly smaller.

Film-screen artifacts image unsharpness is made up of geometric unsharpness (focal spot and source, object, film distances), movement unsharpness and radiographic unsharpness. Film-intensifying screen contact is a major contributor to radiographic unsharpness. The three main factors are illustrated in Fig.7.13(a), (b) and (c). Cross over or print-through effects (a) are caused by light penetrating across the film base and scattering into the opposite emulsion; pigmentation is added to the polyester layer to prevent this.

Halation is caused by reflection (b) and this is prevented by applying a black absorbing layer.   Separation of the intensifying screen (c) from the film surface by dust or grit causes major distortion so the screens should be cleaned regularly. A too thick protective layer can also add to this type of distortion.

Summary

- Intensifying screen: A scintillation phosphor converting x-rays to light
- Phosphor materials: Early phosphor calcium tungstate (5% efficient) replaced by rare earth compounds lanthanum and gadolinium (nearly 20% efficient)
- Light spectrum: lanthanum blue, uses monochromatic film; gadolinium green uses orthochromatic film.
- Intensification factor a measure of screen speed ranges from 25 (detail) up to 400 (low dose)
- Screen thickness influences screen speed.
- Radiographic contrast influenced by film gamma and intensifying screen type

Box 7.4

Conversion efficiency of intensifying phosphors.

The ability of the intensifying screen to convert x-ray photons to light photons can be calculated for any particular phosphor type if the light output is known. For an x-ray photon energy of 60keV:

Calcium tungstate emits most light at 430nm with approximately 5% efficiency

$$= \frac{1240}{\text{wavelength}} = \frac{1240}{430} = 3\text{eV}$$

$$\text{Light output} = \frac{60000 \times 0.05}{3} = 1000 \text{ photons.}$$

Lanthanum oxy-bromide emits two peaks at 360nm (3.4eV) and 475nm (2.6eV) with approximately 20% efficiency.

$$\text{Light output} = \frac{60000 \times 0.2}{0.5 \, (3.4 + 2.6)} = 4000 \text{ photons}$$

Gadolinium oxy-sulfide emits light at a major peak of 530nm (2.3ev) also with approximately 20% efficiency.

$$\text{Light output} = \frac{60000 \times 0.2}{2.3} = 5200 \text{ photons}$$

7.3.3 Cassette design

A number of designs are offered by manufacturers but they all combine the following basic components.

Dual screen cassettes For a dual-screen cassette, used at conventional kilovoltages (~60kV and above), the front screen stops contributing useful light to the film at quite low densities but the rear screens continue to contribute useful light. The dual screen cassette is the most common design in radiology and gives a significant increase in quantum efficiency.

Single screen cassettes At lower kilovoltages (mammography) light output comes almost entirely from just below the screen

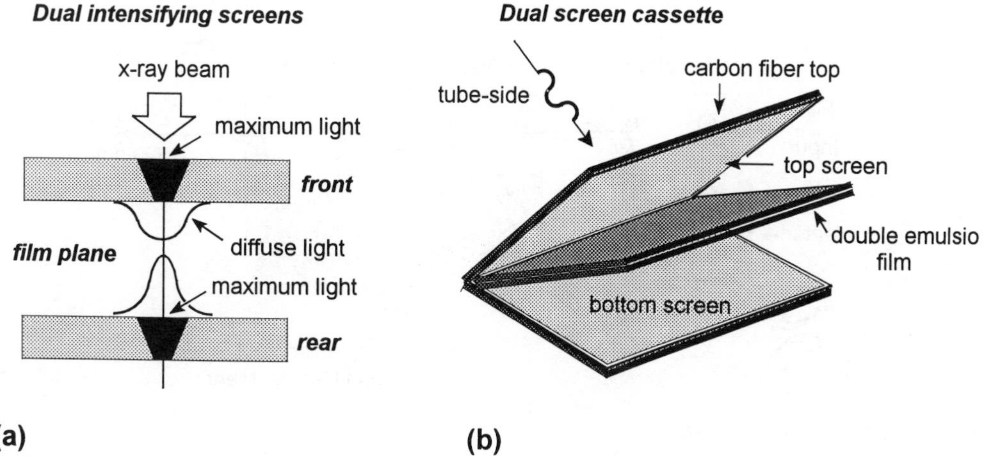

Dual intensifying screens

Dual screen cassette

(a)   **(b)**

Figure 7.15 (a) Screen thickness and the diffusion of light (b) A typical cassette design for a double emulsion film. The entrance face is made from carbon fiber for minimum losses.

surface so light from the front screen is quickly absorbed and does not reach the film. This is shown in Fig.7.15(a) where the light from the front screen undergoes diffusion giving a blurred image but the rear screen contributes surface light and a sharper image. Figure 7.15(b) shows the design for a typical dual screen cassette where the x-ray beam passes through the top screen exposing the first emulsion layer. Other x-rays are absorbed in the bottom screen when the second emulsion is exposed; quantum efficiency is thereby increased quite considerably.

Different screen thicknesses in dual screen cassettes are used depending on the investigation. In some instances screen asymmetry is an advantage:

- For low kV work thin front and rear screens are most efficient.
- For medium kV work an advantage can be achieved by having thin front screens and thicker rear screens (screen asymmetry)
- For high kV work (fluoroscopy and chest) a medium thickness front screen and maximum thickness rear screen would be the best choice.

Mammography This poses a special problem since all the light is produced in the first few microns of the screen surface. A single emulsion film is used and a single thin screen applied. The x-ray beam is directed through the back of the film where some of the low energy photons interact with the emulsion. The rest of the photons interact with the surface of the phosphor so exposing the emulsion.

Table 7.5 Dose reduction using faster screens

Investigation	par-speed (mGy)	fast (mGy)
Lumbar spine	22.0	7.0
AP abdomen	14.8	7.3
AP pelvis	11.2	6.0
IV urogram	4.0	1.5
Mammography	5 - 10	0.12 - 0.2

Radiation dose reduction Patient dose reduction can be significant with the careful application of fast screens to x-ray investigations. The fastest screens are reserved for those studies where maximum

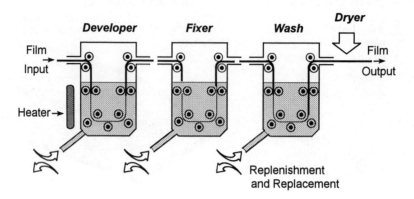

Figure 7.16   The basic components of a film processor showing separate tanks holding developer, fixer and washing water. Developer and fixer are replenished continuously

detail is not required: some barium/iodine contrast studies and dorsal/lateral and pelvic studies fall into this category. Table 7.5 demonstrates the magnitude of dose reduction possible by increasing screen speed from par-speed which is given as reference. For studies requiring a wide gray scale capability such as chest radiography and mammography, quantum mottle becomes a serious objection to increasing screen speed further above 200; valuable diagnostic detail could be lost.

7.4   FILM PROCESSORS

The diagram of an automatic film processor commonly found in diagnostic radiology departments is shown in Fig.7.16. There are three baths containing developer, fixer and water (used as the film washing bath). The chemicals in the developer and fixer are gradually exhausted so a method of replenishment is necessary.   The temperature of the developer is critical and influences image quality; its influence on film speed, contrast and film fog have been seen already in Fig.7.9(b).

Replenishment   The developer activity gradually diminishes so concentrated developer solution is added from time to time to the tank so maintaining effectiveness. Replenishment can be continued for some days before the tank requires complete emptying and renewal. The replenishment cycle is controlled by monitoring film throughput. Exhausted fixer goes into a silver recovery unit so that the soluble silver compound is decomposed to give pure silver which is recovered before the fixer is disposed via the drain. Tab.7.6 lists the parameters and performance of a common processor.

Table 7.6 Typical film processor specifications

	Developer	Fixer
Temperature	32 - 37°C	
Tank Capacity	20 liters	20 liters
Film Treated (m^2)	400ml/m^2	600ml/m^2
Processor Speed	92cm/minute (2 minutes)	
	46cm/minute (4 minutes)	
Capacity	240 films/hour	
	120 films/hour	

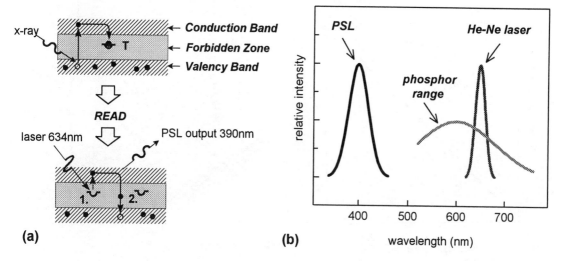

(a) **(b)**

Figure 7.17 **(a)** The principle of image plate thermoluminescence. X-ray photons excite electrons from the valency into the conduction band; they are trapped in the forbidden zone where they are held indefinitely. An infra-red laser liberates the trapped electrons emitting PSL whose intensity is proportional to the initial x-ray exposure. **(b)** The light spectra associated with the image plate showing the stimulated illumination in the visible/infra-red region and the photo-stimulable luminescence in the ultra-violet range.

7.4.1   Silver recovery

The silver content of radiography films varies between 3000-6000g 1000 m^{-2} depending on film type. A surface area of 1000 m^{-2} is equivalent to 6000 films size 14″×17″ or 36×43cm. Scrap processed film contains about 7-26g silver per kilogram. The limit of silver concentration in fixer is 4-6g per liter before replacement. Most regulations require that the silver recovery effluent for discharge to the public sewer should be less than 0.2g silver per liter.   Three methods are available for silver recovery:

1) ***Electrolyte method*** Uses a carbon anode and stainless steel cathode:
   $Ag^+ + e^- \rightarrow Ag$ precipitated on cathode.
   A good recovery is possible and the fixer can be reused.   The current density of the equipment is critical; too high and silver sulfide is formed, too low and efficiency is lowered.   The optimum pH is 5. This is the common method for silver recovery attached to automatic processors in radiology departments.

2) ***Metal replacement***   This uses steel wool to precipitate silver. The iron goes into solution and the fixer cannot be re-used. It is 98% efficient.

3) ***Chemical method***   Uses sodium sulfide to precipitate silver sulfide from solution. It removes 100% of the silver but produces hydrogen sulfide which is hazardous.

7.5 PHOSPHOR IMAGING PLATE

In 1983 researchers at Fuji laboratories developed an erasable x-ray imaging device based on the x-ray excitation of a phosphor layer and subsequent reading the stored image data with an infra-red laser (photo-stimulable luminescence). Results showed that the imaging plate was more sensitive than conventional x-ray film with intensifying screens.   Thermoluminescence   has   been described for x-ray detection in Chapter 6 where x- or γ–radiation elevates valency electrons into the conduction band.

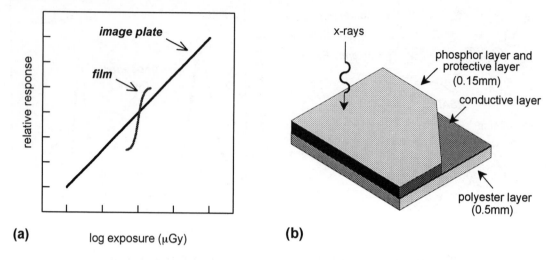

Figure 7.18   **(a)** Image plate dynamic range compared to film **(b)** The sandwich construction of the image plate showing the phosphor layer placed on an antistatic conductive metal film.

This energy is then released by the application of heat (thermoluminescence). The basic principles are shown in Fig.7.17(a) where infra-red irradiation by laser gives the photo-stimulated luminescence (PSL) which carries the data used by the imaging plate.

7.5.1 Photo-stimulated luminescence (PSL)

The phosphor material used for the imaging plate is a complex barium halide doped with europium. The principle of recording and reading the x-ray information stored after exposure involves a writing (exposure) and reading (image formation) cycle.

X-ray absorption   When the imaging plate absorbs x-ray energy some of the Eu^{2+} ions are ionized to Eu^{3+} liberating electrons to the conduction band of the phosphor crystals :

$$Eu^{2+} \rightarrow (\text{x-ray irradiation}) \rightarrow Eu^{3+} + e^-$$

The free electrons are ejected into the conduction band where they can move throughout the crystal lattice. The presence of impurities (e.g. bromine) introduces energy levels in the forbidden zone called F-centers. The free

electrons are trapped into a meta-stable state in these F-centers.

Readout   This stored energy, which represents the original x-radiation, and is released by stimulating the lattice again but this time with radiation of a much lower energy band; the bandwidth of the stimulation radiation is shown by the broad graph of Fig.7.17(b) ranging from 500-750nm which releases the electrons from their traps. The wavelength of the infrared helium-neon laser (633nm) conveniently sits within this bandwidth and is therefore an ideal energy source for stimulating the crystal lattice and causing the luminescence (PSL) which occupies the shorter wavelength of 400nm. Its intensity is almost exactly proportional to the original x-ray exposure. There are very small losses due to some excited electrons missing the traps and returning immediately to the valency band.

Sensitivity   The image plate sensitivity is far superior to film/screen. Fig.7.18(a) plots exposure versus response (dynamic range) and shows the increase in sensitivity and the extended response of the imaging plate for very low radiation dose. The practical dynamic range is 1:10000 compared to film-screen of 1:1000. The response of the luminescence is linear from 8 x-ray photons per pixel to 4×10^4 photons per pixel: a range of 1 to 5×10^3.

Practical device   The typical commercial imaging plate is a 0.5mm flexible plastic plate coated with phosphor crystals, such as $BaFBr:Eu^{2+}$, in a plastic binder. Europium, as the Eu^{2+} ion, acts as an activator. Fig.7.18(b) shows the basic construction for a high resolution imaging plate with a phosphor thickness of 150μm. Routine image plates can have a phosphor up to 0.4mm thick. Other halide mixtures such as BaFCl and BaF are also available.   The plate is capable of storing energy not only from x-rays but also from UV light or electrons.

When the phosphor is stimulated by visible or infra red illumination it emits photo-stimulated luminescence (PSL), the intensity of which is proportional to the absorbed radiation energy.   Exposure to visible or infra-red light releases the trapped electrons from the F-centers in the crystal back to the conduction band   where they convert the Eu^{3+} back into Eu^{2+}, emitting characteristic radiation of europium at 390nm, as luminescent light:

$$Eu^{3+} + e^- \rightarrow \text{influenced by IR laser}$$
$$\rightarrow Eu^{2+} + hf \text{ (PSL at 390nm)}$$

The response time of the PSL is fast (0.8ms) so it is possible to read many megabytes of image data within a few seconds using a scanning laser beam. The PSL has a wavelength of 390nm (ultra-violet) and the laser wavelength is 632.8nm (infra-red). The PSL with a wavelength of 390nm (UV) has a FWHM of 150mm giving a possible 10 pixels mm^{-1}, the laser scanning pitch is 5-10 pixel mm^{-1}.   Since the PSL decay is 0.8ms a 5000×4000 pixel matrix will take:

$$(2 \times 10^7) \times (0.8 \times 10^{-6}) = 16 \text{ s}$$

Each reading is digitized to 10 bits and the image plate has a 80% photon capture efficiency.

The component parts required for reading an exposed image plate is shown in Fig.7.19 where the He-Ne laser beam scans the image plate by means of a rotating mirror. The shorter wavelength PSL is collected by a photomultiplier tube (PMT) and fiber optic light guide.   The PMT signals are log-arithmically amplified and stored in a digital matrix which can be used to give a film image or be part of a digital image display system. The screen is then completely erased with an intense light source before reuse.

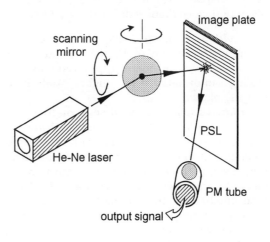

Figure 7.19   Image plate readout procedure using an infra-red He-Ne laser beam scanning the plate using a rotating mirror. The PSL is picked up by a photomultiplier tube and its signal fed into a digital imager.

Image quality   Current commercial image plate systems offer matrix sizes of 1760×2140 for standard resolution (ST) and 2000×2510 pixels for high resolution (HR). These are digitized to 10 bits.   The effective resolution is 2.5Lp mm^{-1} for 35×43cm ST plates and approximately 5Lp mm^{-1} for 18×24cm HR plates. Chest x-ray systems commonly employ a 3584×4096 by 12 bit deep matrix having 5-10 pixels mm^{-1} resolution. When reading the image from the plate the computer builds a density histogram of the picture so that optimum gray scale can be allocated to the available count density (histogram equalization).

Image display   The x-ray images recorded on the imaging plate are scanned by a narrow He-Ne laser beam and the issuing light collected by a photomultiplier whose signal output is digitized to either 10 or 12 bit accuracy and stored in the memory of an image processor (dedicated computer).

The image processor enhances the information (smoothing, edge enhancement etc.) before display, which can either be a high resolution video display or hard-copy film.

The video display   This should give a minimum resolution of 1024 lines but 2048 or more would be more appropriate for revealing information in higher definition imaging plates.

Film hard-copy   A second semiconductor or helium-neon laser is used for transferring the image information from the array processor memory onto film. The array processor feeds the image information from its memory into a digital to analog converter. This analog signal then modulates the intensity of the laser while scanning the film. The film is a single emulsion with a peak sensitivity at 633nm to match the laser output. Two images can be printed onto a single sheet of film; one can be unaltered image data, the other can be edge enhanced.

Comparison with film/screen   Compared to other integrating image detectors (film and video cameras) the dynamic range of the imaging plate system is much wider; approximately $1:10^5$. The noise level is equivalent to 3 x-ray photons per pixel which compares to the film fog-level of 1000 x-ray photons per equivalent area. The plate yields reproducible results over many repeated uses. Particular radiology advantages:

- Broad dynamic range showing low contrast differences
- Digital manipulation of the image (edge enhancement)
- Electronic storage and retrieval of image

- Patient dose reduction.

The limitations of film recording, compared to image plate are:

- Expense
- Poor contrast ~5% difference visible
- Absorbs only 30-50% of available x-ray photons
- Not easily transferable to digital storage

7.5.2 Selenium image plate

Virtually all radiology imaging devices depend on the process of luminescence e.g. intensifying screens, image phosphor plate, image intensifier screen, which either exposes a film directly or provides a signal that can be converted into an electrical signal for further processing.

The selenium image plate uses electrostatic charges to build up picture information from x-ray exposure. The principle has been used earlier in the form of xero-radiography where an electrostatically charged selenium plate is exposed to x-rays whose ionizing events discharge the plate locally so building up image detail. The xero-radiographic plate was then dusted with fine toner powder which clung to the remaining charged areas. The powder pattern was then transferred to paper and fixed by heating. The whole process was not very reliable but gave excellent resolution pictures with edge enhancement although the contrast information was poor.

The xero-radiograph soon lost favor in the face of new rare-earth screens and digital image techniques.

The selenium image plate   Selenium has now reemerged as a promising image device as an electronically scanned selenium image plate. The image quality is good for both resolution and contrast. Figure 7.20(a), (b) and (c) illustrates the preparation, exposure and readout of a selenium image plate The selenium is about 0.5mm thick deposited on a metal surface and is used in the following manner, illustrated in Fig.7.20:

(a) The plate is first prepared by applying a uniform electrical charge (1500V) on its surface.
(b) The charged plate is then exposed to the x-ray source (most commonly from a chest unit) when free electrons generated from the ionizing events discharge the plate locally.
(c) The plate is then scanned with a small electrode assembly at about 0.1mm from the plate surface in a scan-line pattern similar to the image plate laser. The surface is scanned in approximately 10 seconds.

After read-out the plate is recharges ready for the next exposure. The electrical image signals are collected and form an image matrix of typically 2000×2000 pixels each pixel representing about 0.2mm and 14 bits deep.

The selenium image has a dynamic range equivalent to the image phosphor plate. Since the image is carried by surface charges it does not suffer from the same disadvantage of light diffusion with depth as luminescent phosphors. Selenium is a low density material and therefore is a poor x-ray absorber and detector efficiency consequently suffers. DQE is 0.25 at 2Lp mm^{-1} for a dose of 3.3µGy

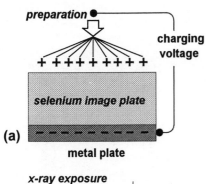

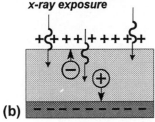

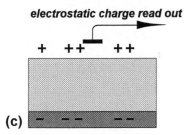

Figure 7.20 The selenium image plate: **(a)** preparation **(b)** exposure **(c)** data extraction; details are given in the text.

KEYWORDS

base fog: background density film reading

densitometer: measures film density in comparative optical density units

developer: a reducing compound of hydroquinone or metol variety which magnifies the latent film image.

emulsion: a complex of silver halides

exposure: a timed exposure to light or x-rays

film: mono-chromatic: blue light sensitive

film: ortho-chromatic: blue/green light sensitive

film: pan-chromatic: sensitive to the complete visible spectrum

film base: a polyester material supporting the emulsion, sometimes colored blue.

film speed: film sensitivity to exposure

fixer: a thiosulfate compound which removes unexposed silver halide

gamma: slope of film characteristic curve. a measure of film contrast.

gelatin: the suspending medium for the silver halides.

image plate: film-less recording using either phosphor material or selenium.
latitude: film contrast

objective contrast: optical density

optical density: a logarithmic measure of intensity transmission

optical sensitizers: dyes added to film emulsion to increase spectrum response.

photo-stimulated luminescence: light emitted by phosphor plate when stimulated by infra-red laser.

screen pigment: pigment added to intensifying screen to prevent light diffusion.

screen activators: mainly rare earth trace elements added to phosphors to increase efficiency of emission.

sensitometer: a calibrated light source for exposing a stepped gray-scale.

shoulder: the non-linear region of saturated exposure.

silver halides: film emulsion components of silver iodide, bromide and chloride.

slope: the straight-line portion of the film characteristic.

subject contrast: factors influencing the emerging x-ray beam and film exposure. The x-axis on the film characteristic.

threshold value: the lowest density measurement above base + fog level.

toe: the non-linear minimum recorded density.

8

The Analog Image : Film and Video

8.1 Vision

8.2 Image detector surface

8.3 Image quality factors

8.4 Scatter and grids

8.5 Image quality measurement

8.6 Hardcopy devices

8.1 VISION

There are two light sensitive receptors in the eye - the cones and the rods. The cones (~6.5million in each eye) are primarily used for photopic or daylight vision. Cones see fine detail and are color sensitive (maximal sensitivity 550nm: yellow-green). Each cone is directly connected to the brain. The rods are used for poor light conditions (scotopic vision), each eye having about 120million. Several rods share their signals along a common nerve fiber, unlike the cones, and are most sensitive to 510nm or blue-green. If a typical clinical radiograph is considered that is recorded on film the clinician is mainly concerned with:

- The ability to see small detail i.e. hairline fracture, micro-calcifications
- The recognition of low contrast differences that may indicate pathology i.e. pneumo-thorax, breast cancer, TB lesions etc.
- The image quality (signal to noise ratio) sufficiently high to inspire confidence in the diagnostic accuracy.

The human eye has limitations in resolution and contrast levels that must also be considered when viewing diagnostic information in a radiograph. The critical factors are:

- Image brightness level
- Low contrast differences within the image
- Image detail

8.1.1 Visual sensitivity

Luminance The units commonly used to describe light intensities depend on the source. For example when measuring the amount of light emanating from a view box or a video monitor the luminance is measured in SI units of nits or candela m^{-2}. A table of values is give in Tab.8.1 comparing SI and non-SI values.

Tab.8.2 shows the range of luminance intensity that the human eye is exposed in the environment, showing that the dynamic range of the eye is about 1:10^6. Fig.8.1(a) plots the relative sensitivity of cones and rods to the visible spectrum; the eye is most sensitive to green/yellows.

Table 8.1 Units for luminance and illuminance

Luminance	
SI unit	1 candela m^{-2} (cd m^{-2})
Non-SI unit	1 Lambert = cd cm^{-2}
Conversion factor	1 milliL = 3.183 cd m^{-2}
Non-SI unit	1 foot Lambert = cd ft
Conversion factor	1 nit = 1/3.426 ft L
Illuminance	
SI unit	1 lux = 1 lumen m^{-2}
	1 lux = 10.746 ft candles

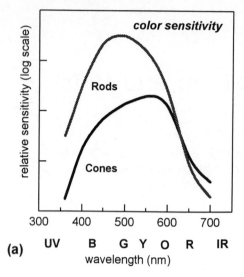

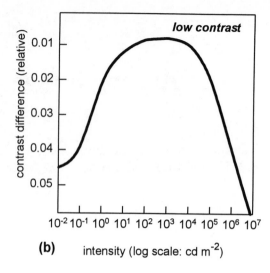

Figure 8.1 **(a)** The relative sensitivity of rods and cones to the color spectrum. Rods are more sensitive to low light levels **(b)** The loss of visible contrast with intensity of illumination. Low contrast difference is toward the top of the y-axis.

Illuminance When measuring the illumination of objects in a room such as the light level at a desk top, or light level incident on a video screen (glare), the illuminance is measured in SI units of lux. The old units were foot-candles or lumen m^{-2}.

The effect of object brightness on visible contrast differences is shown in Fig. 8.1(b) where the ability to see low contrast differences increases toward the top of the y-axis. Loss of visual contrast occurs at high and low illumination levels. Peak sensitivity occurs at levels equivalent to radiograph viewing boxes and video screens; levels are listed in Tab.8.2

Table 8.2 Approximate luminance levels

Object	Luminance cd m^{-2}
White Surface-sunlight	3×10^4
Viewing Light Box	2×10^3
White level video screen	200
Reading Light	30
Black level video screen	0.1
White surface-moonlight	0.03

8.1.2 Visual contrast

The eye has a very large dynamic range achieved by adapting to a given luminance level. In order to show a video monitor which is operating in the range of 0.1 to 100cd m^{-2} the eye must adapt to a lower level of illumination than it would when viewing a hard copy text in bright daylight.

Visual contrast sensitivity can is described in terms of the log. difference between intensities. Visual contrast between two intensities I_a and I_b would have a contrast difference of:

$$C = \log I_a - \log I_b \qquad (8.1)$$

An eye that is adapted to the average light intensity of a video-screen can accept a brightness range of about 1:30 (30dB) so a gray scale range of about 35 shades can be appreciated.

The signal amplitudes that are visible are evaluated logarithmically in compliance with Weber's Law, which states that visible differences in light intensity are separated by fixed logarithmic values. The signal dynamic range of 30dB is resolvable in contrast differences of about 1dB; this has a significant influence on the eye's spatial resolution. A wider range of contrasts can be distinguished if the image is digitally 'windowed' which selects a narrow range of image data for display (discussed further with computed tomography).

Integration time This is the time taken by the eye to accumulate visual information and varies according to viewing conditions. It depends on the state of adaptation to lighting conditions and intensity of the light stimulus. Integration time has values from 100 to 300ms in the dark adapted (scotopic) eye and 15-100ms in the light adapted eye (photopic). More detail cannot be extracted from the image by extending viewing time so optimum image quality (contrast, density) is essential if visual detail is to be distinguished particularly in moving (real-time) fluoroscopic images.

8.1.3 Visual resolution

Line pairs A common method for measuring visible resolution uses a line-pairs grating as illustrated in Fig.8.2. The grating has bars, one black and one white which represents one line-pair. A line-pair is equivalent to 1 cycle. The grating shown in the diagram has 10 black and white line pairs over a 1mm distance; gratings are available for radiography having line spacing up to 20 Lp mm^{-1}. The resolution limit is reached when the system will just resolve 2 lines spaced $1/x$ mm apart; this will represent x Lp mm^{-1}. A 0.5mm line separation would be represented by 2Lp mm^{-1} (each line pair covers 0.5mm) and 0.1mm line spacing would be 10 Lp mm^{-1}. Five line-pairs per mm (5Lp mm^{-1}) would be represented by 10 black and white bars on the film image; each bar being 0.1mm thick. This is the typical resolving power of a conventional radiograph, correctly exposed and developed.

Maximum visual resolution, determined by the cones, is just about 30Lp mm^{-1} under optimal conditions. Doubling the distance reduces this figure to 15 line pairs. Res-

olution in a film/screen system is limited by the intensifying screen and varies from 3 to 8 Lp mm^{-1} depending on screen type (speed and phosphor). Resolution is sometimes expressed in larger units of line pairs per centimeter Lp cm^{-1} (nuclear medicine).

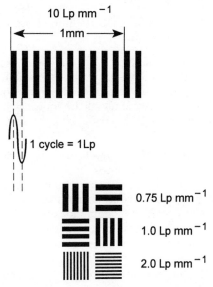

Figure 8.2 A 10Lp mm^{-1} grating. A line pair is equivalent to 1 cycle mm^{-1}. Line pair patterns in radiology sometimes take the form of blocks as shown here which test resolution in both x and y-axes.

8.2 IMAGE DETECTOR SURFACE

The separate factors and devices making up the radiographic image have been described earlier in Chapter 7 identifying the film/screen detector as the most common form of analog image.

Image quality There are three major parameters that describe image quality:

1. **Resolution** is influenced by the machine itself (x-ray tube), movement (patient) and recording medium (film, image plate, video, computer digitization).
2. **Contrast** is also influenced by system performance but also by the physical

attributes of the different tissues, kV and detector sensitivity. The dynamic range of a recording medium (film, video display) decides the contrast range that can be represented.

3. **Noise**, a component of all images, is introduced either by quantum effects (photon density), mottle, film graininess or electronic noise.

Several factors also play an important role in forming the radiographic image sensitivity (speed). Acceptable image quality depends on the absorption efficiency of the image detector and its response (blackening or light output).

Diagnostic quality Image quality varies in the separate disciplines of radiology (i.e. conventional x-ray, nuclear medicine, ultrasound etc.); all show limitations in resolution, contrast and noise. This does not detract, however, from their diagnostic usefulness. An image acceptable as diagnostic quality in nuclear medicine and ultrasound would be rejected as sub-standard in conventional radiology

Diagnostic quality of an image is a subjective measurement and indicates the ability to demonstrate an abnormality. An inherently photon poor imaging system (nuclear medicine) is equally able to give a diagnostic quality image as well as a high resolution system where increased photon density gives finer pathological detail (chest radiograph or mammography). This can be demonstrated by ranking the contrast and resolution capabilities of the common imaging procedures from 1 (poor) to 3 (excellent) in Tab.8.3. Nuclear medicine and ultrasound, in spite of their intrinsic poor image quality, give adequate diagnostic information.

Improvements in display performance (increased resolution and contrast) would probably not influence this ranking since image quality is limited by other factors (quantum noise). So increasing the resolution of nuclear medicine displays from 1 Lp cm^{-1} to 4Lp cm^{-1} will have no effect if the gamma-camera imaging device can only resolve 2 Lp cm^{-1}

Table 8.3 Ranking diagnostic image quality

Image	Resolution	Contrast	Noise
Mammogram	3	3	3
Chest film	2	2	2
Extremity film	3	2	2
CT	2	3	3
MRI	2	3	2
Ultrasound	2	1	1
Nuclear med.	1	1	1

8.2.1 The film image

Film speed (sensitivity) It has already been shown that film alone is a very insensitive medium for x-ray imaging; radiographic film is specially designed to be used in combination with intensifying screens. The list in Tab.8.4 compares the performance of x-ray film with conventional 35mm black and white camera film. Generally x-ray film offers a much higher contrast for a reduced resolution. Film resolution is usually limited, in radiology, by other factors than the film itself (intensifying screens).

Table 8.4 Medical and conventional film compared

Performance	Medical X-ray film	Conventional B/W film
Speed (ASA/DIN)	60/19° to 80/20°	100/21°
Contrast	2.5 - 3.0	0.7 - 0.9
Tonal value	black	mid-gray/black
Grain size	2.0 - 2.3μm	0.6-0.8μm
Resolution	40Lp mm^{-1}	70-120Lp mm^{-1}

Contrast: The contrast offered by the film emulsion has been discussed in Chapter 7. Peak contrast is measured as the film's gamma and this is shown to be high in radiological film compared to conventional film stock (Table 8.4). The dynamic range can be tailored to the application: film used for video screen recording has a wide latitude (large dynamic range) while mammography film has a narrow dynamic range so that close tissue characteristics can be separated

Resolution Conventional radiographic film can resolve 5-8 Lp mm^{-1} and this is sufficient for most clinical studies. Since mammography demands a higher resolving power film resolution is increased although film resolution is not a limiting factor even in this examination since the intensifying screens themselves have a poorer resolving power and these are the limiting factor.

8.2.2 Intensifying phosphors

The mechanism causing phosphorescence (described in Chapter 5) is found in several types of imaging devices in radiology:

- Intensifying screens in film cassettes
- Image intensifier input and output screens
- Large single crystal detectors for nuclear medicine gamma cameras
- Image plates used in computed radiology

The first three phosphor imaging devices translate x- or gamma-radiation directly into light photons, however the image plate requires a secondary energy source (infra-red laser) in order to release stored energy in the form of light which can then be used for image formation.

Phosphor materials Intensifying screens predominantly use rare earth phosphors containing gadolinium or lanthanum but newer materials containing yttrium offer improved efficiency. Image intensifier tubes use sodium doped cesium iodide (CsI:Na), since this material has a good absorption for x-ray photons and its needle-like crystal structure reduces light scatter which maintains resolution. Image plates use complex barium fluoro-halide compounds.

Sensitivity In all cases the light output varies according to x-ray intensity and energy so the continuous x-ray spectrum gives a range of light intensities. Phosphor detectors are most commonly seen as intensifying screens in film-screen cassettes and conventional radiology uses a double emulsion film sandwiched between two intensifying screens whose thickness is chosen for the particular investigation. Screen thickness (from 100-500μm) is normally quoted as a weight per unit area: 100 to 165mg cm^{-2} is a typical range. Sensitivity increases with thickness due to improved absorption but resolution becomes poorer.

In general intensifying screens contribute 97% to film blackening, the x-radiation itself contributing only 3%. The increased sensitivity achieved by using intensifying screens decreases patient radiation dose by a factor of 15 to 20 and the consequent shorter exposure times reduce movement unsharpness.

Resolution Radiographic unsharpness is introduced by all phosphor screens since the light production occurs at some depth within the phosphor depending on the photon energy (Fig. 8.3(a)). As the x-ray photon energy increases it penetrates further into the phosphor causing diffusion of the deeper light event so there is a significant geometrical broadening when it reaches the film emulsion at the phosphor surface. As a consequence conventional film-screens have a typical resolution of 5 to 8Lp mm^{-1}. Image plates can also be treated as intensifying phosphors but they store information using thermo-luminescent principles; their light emission occurs at depth within the phosphor so degrading image resolution which is typically 5Lp mm^{-1}.

Light diffusion can be controlled by using thinner phosphor screens (Fig.8.3(b)) but sensitivity is greatly reduced since only a fraction of the beam is absorbed. Low keV photons react at the surface so the light event undergoes minimal diffusion giving a sharp film image (usually 10-15Lp mm^{-1} for single screen mammography). For this reason the beam enters the film back so photon interaction occurs near the film emulsion.

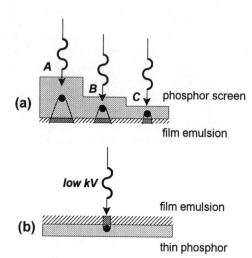

Figure 8.3 An image phosphor surface (intensifying screen or image plate) showing shallow and deep light events depending on photon energy. These cause radiographic unsharpness. Thinner phosphors are used for mammography.

Summary

In general intensifying screens:

- Increase radiographic unsharpness
- Reduce movement unsharpness
- Reduce patient dose

The properties of an intensifying screen are influenced by:

- Phosphor compound (density and light conversion efficiency)
- Phosphor thickness (mg cm^{-2})
- Proportion of light diffusion
- Phosphor grain size
- Phosphor transparency
- Radiation energy

Screen resolution can be increased by having:

- A thin phosphor
- Small phosphor crystals
- A light absorbent layer on the phosphor

base preventing reflection.
- A very thin protective layer

Optimum phosphor performance is obtained by:

- Maximum absorption
- Maximum x-ray to light conversion efficiency
- Matching phosphor light wavelength to film sensitivity.

8.2.3 The Video image

The principles of television using a scanning electron beam were simultaneously developed by L. de Forest (1873-1961, American physicist) and A.D. Blumlein (1903-1942, British engineer). The television or video display is an analog image but, unlike film, breaks up image information into a sequence of scan lines which degrades the original x-ray image data, particularly resolution.

Video waveform   The basic video waveform is shown in Fig.8.4(a) for a single scan line with black and white levels and synchronization pulses which indicate the 'end-of-line'. The time per scan line will differ according to the video standard.
The scanning pattern is identical between camera and display maintaining overall synchronization.

Interlacing   In the early development stages of television the requirement for high speed electronics was reduced by employing a method of scan-line interlacing. Half the image was transmitted at a time as alternate fields (odd then even-line numbers). Combining each field gave a complete interlaced frame at 25 or 30 frames per second, depending on the supply frequency (50 or 60Hz). Domestic tele-vision is still broadcast in an interlaced format. Since 25 or 30 frames s^{-1} (fps) are adequate it is only necessary to transmit this rate so the complete line count (525 or 625) is

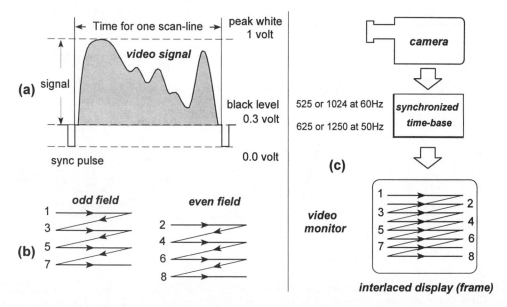

Figure 8.4　(a) A single video scan line showing the extreme signal levels associated with black and white and the synchronization pulses for end of line. (b) video interlacing pattern showing odd and even fields combined to form a video frame. (c) camera and display with a common time-base giving a synchronized scan rate.

transmitted in 2 halves, odd lines then even lines as shown in Fig.8.4(b). The interlacing patterns shown in Fig.8.4(b), have odd and even line fields at 50 or 60 fields per second which are combined to give a complete video picture frame at 25 or 30 frames per second. Frequency restrictions in domestic television are not a serious problem in radiological imaging; non-interlaced high resolution displays having increased scan lines and line densities greater than 1000 have become standard. The line scanning for a video system (as transmitted or using a closed-circuit) is synchronized between camera and display with a common time-base, shown in Fig.8.4(c).

Bandwidth　The frequency necessary to transmit video display data is the product of the display resolution, the number of scan lines in the display and the frame rate. Box 8.1 gives some examples.

Line standards　The number of horizontal scanning lines used for domestic television has 525 lines in the Americas and Japan and 625 lines in Europe. For moving pictures it is necessary to display a frame rate which takes advantage of vision persistence and high enough to prevent flicker. Figure 8.5(a) shows the sensitivity of the eye to frame frequency and flicker.

For historical reasons the frame rate is dictated by the mains line frequency; 525 lines uses a frame rate of 60 fps, 625 lines uses 50 fps. Increasing scan line numbers (up to 2000 to 3000 in some high definition displays) require a much higher frame rate in order to prevent flicker problems.

Video standards for radiology　In order to achieve acceptable sharpness video displays in radiology have a higher resolution standard than those offered by domestic television. Original radiology display systems used domestic television standards but most recent video displays now utilize high definition line standards of 1024, 1249 and 2048 lines using a non-interlaced format.

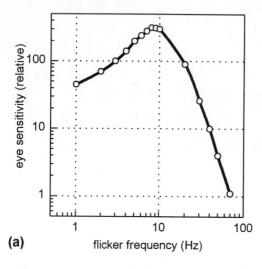

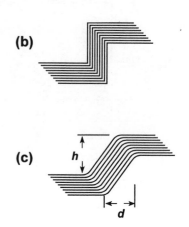

Figure 8.5 **(a)** Flicker sensitivity of the human eye peaks at about 10Hz but is still apparent at 20Hz. **(b)** A sharp change across an image boundary (tissue difference) giving optimum visibility **(c)** The overall effect of unsharpness which smoothes the boundaries reducing both resolution and contrast difference. Visible contrast is lost as *d* increases although *h* is the same.

These display systems use 70 to 100 frames per second eliminating flicker. High definition radiology displays can use 3000 scan lines in order to give film-like image quality.

Box 8.1

Video bandwidth

Video bandwidth can be calculated from the formula: $r \times s \times f$ where r = resolution along the line (normally symmetrical with the line standard), s = line standard and f = frames per second, this is 30 fps (USA) and 25 fps (Europe). So video bandwidth for:

USA: $500 \times 512 \times 30 = 7.6\text{MHz}$
Europe: $600 \times 625 \times 25 = 9.3\text{MHz}$

Video and film image resolution is compared in Tab.8.5. A good chest radiograph can achieve 5Lp mm^{-1} and a detail screen about 8Lp mm^{-1}. The best film resolution is given in mammography where 15 to 20Lp mm^{-1} is routinely obtained. High resolution, progressive scan (non-interlaced) 2000 to 3000 scan line monitors can achieve in excess of 5Lp mm^{-1} but film/screen is still able to offer the best image quality in terms of resolution.

Table 8.5 Resolution of film and video compared.

Analog Image	Resolution Lp mm^{-1}
Film	
Chest (35 × 43cm)	5
Mammography (24×18cm)	20
Video (scan lines)	
1024	3.0
1249	3.5

8.3   IMAGE QUALITY FACTORS

The three factors which define image quality are:

- resolution
- contrast
- noise

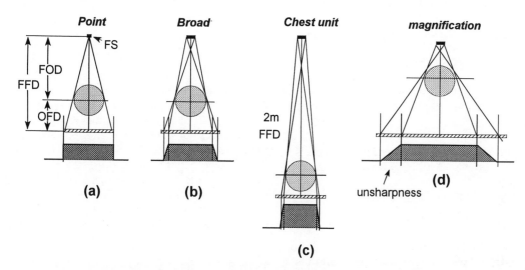

Figure 8.6 (**a**) for a small (point) focal spot giving no geometrical unsharpness (**b**) a broad focal spot causes a penumbra to be formed which results in sloping edges and unsharpness and (**c**) a chest unit minimizes the unsharpness by maintaining a large FFD (**d**) magnification views require a reduction in the focal spot size.

All images whether analog, video or digital can be analyzed using these parameters. Image quality should be able to reproduce faithfully the machine's capabilities i.e. its own potential resolution (focal spot size), contrast (attenuation coefficients) and noise (dictated by the photon density). An image system which is unable to record all the x-ray image information will miss important diagnostic detail, conversely an image that exceeds the performance figures of the machine will only serve to emphasize noise.

8.3.1 Resolution

Figure 8.5(b) shows an image density change as a step which can represent contrast between two structures or fine detail (resolution). Image spatial resolution in the radiographic image is influenced by two factors which degrade resolution giving overall 'image unsharpness'; this is shown in Fig.8.5(c). The ability to distinguish a step change in image density depends on the magnitude of the change h and the distance over which the change occurs d. Although the intensity change across the boundaries are the same in Fig.8.5(c) the sharp boundary in the top step is easily visible whereas the gradual intensity change in the bottom step becomes less visible as distance d increases although the height h remains the same. Objects having a gradual change must be larger in order to be visible. The combined unsharpness of a radiograph is made up from geometric unsharpness, movement or kinetic unsharpness and radiographic unsharpness (i.e. film/ screen)

- **Geometrical unsharpness U_g** is influenced by distances between x-ray tube, patient and image surface as well as x-ray focal spot size.
- **Movement unsharpness U_m** is due simply to patient and organ movement.
- **Radiographic unsharpness U_r** causes image blurring due to poor film/screen contact and diffusion of light within the phosphor material.

The total unsharpness figure is then the geometrical mean of these values:

$$U_{total} = \sqrt{U_g + U_m + U_r} \qquad (8.2)$$

Geometrical unsharpness U_g   There are three parameters which influence geometrical unsharpness:

- Focus to Film Distance (FFD), which is the same as Source to Image Distance (SID)
- Object to Film Distance (OFD)
- Focal Spot size (FS)

Fig.8.6(a) to (d) shows the relationship between these parameters and **penumbra** size which causes edge smoothing and consequent loss of resolution. The central area, called the **umbra**, has this shadow penumbra whose size is determined by geometrical factors; this is similar to a light penumbra described in Chapter 2.

Loss of image detail is primarily caused by the x-ray tube focal spot size, but the choice of focal spot size is a trade off between image sharpness and tube heat dissipation. The point source in Fig.8.6(a) gives the sharpest image with no geometrical unsharpness regardless of beam distances. However x-ray tubes do not have a point source; the target always has finite dimensions as shown in (b). Optimum resolution is therefore achieved by keeping FS small, FFD large and OFD small.

Table 8.6 shows the relationships between the different geometrical parameters which cause unsharpness. They can be related with geometrical unsharpness as:

$$U_g = \frac{FS \times OFD}{FFD - OFD} \qquad (8.3)$$

So a large focal spot (FS) and increased distance between object and imaging surface (film) OFD increases unsharpness, conversely increasing the distance between x-ray tube and image surface (FFD) decreases unsharpness, as seen in Fig.8.6(c).

Image magnification m   This is controlled by altering FFD and OFD as illustrated in Fig.8.6(d), then:

$$m = \frac{FFD}{FFD - OFD} \qquad (8.4)$$

If the object is on the cassette surface then OFD = 0 and magnification is 1.0 (real size). For an FFD of 60cm (mammography) if the breast is 20cm offset from the cassette then magnification will be 60/50 or ×1.5. Equation 8.4 shows that increasing the distance between object and image surface will magnify the image but this is incompatible with minimum geometrical unsharpness (eqn.8.3) so the focal spot size is reduced e.g. from 0.4 to 0.1mm in mammography.

Table 8.6   Parameter change

	increase unsharpness	decrease unsharpness
Focal spot	large	small
FFD	small	large
OFD	large	small

Chest radiography   A large FFD is commonly used in chest radiography (Fig.8.7(c)) and Box 8.2 gives a worked example showing the benefits of large focus to film distances. The examples given demonstrate that the large FFD employed in chest radiology reduces the importance of focal spot size and its effect on determining image resolution but focal spot sizes are critical for closer FFD's such as those used in mammography.

Figure 8.8(b) illustrates how a large FFD overcomes differing resolution with depth. The 2m FFD used in a chest unit allows image detail to be retained throughout the depth of the lung fields, whereas shorter FFD's cause unsharpness: Fig.8.8(a).

At large FFD's the beam intensity is much reduced due the inverse square law and since

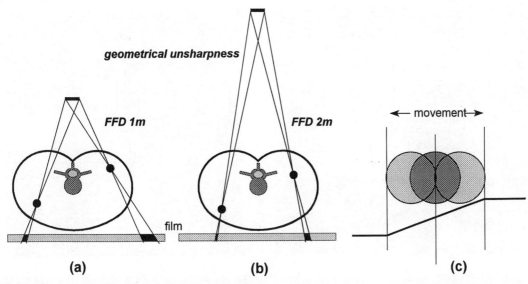

geometrical unsharpness

FFD 1m

FFD 2m

← movement →

film

(a)   (b)   (c)

Figure 8.7   **(a)** An example of the benefits of a large FFD used in chest radiography. **(b)**The change in unsharpness for surface and mid-field lesions, by changing FFD from 1 to 2m **(c)** An example of movement unsharpness caused by a moving blood vessel which destroys the sharp boundary which would otherwise be given by a static vessel.

the exposure timing is also short the tube rating must be high.

Movement unsharpness U_m   Major factor is patient or organ movement and Fig.8.7(c) shows how a sharp edge can be degraded by patient or organ movement. Machine movement or vibration can also play a significant part. Movement unsharpness is kept small by using high kV.

Due to the increased efficiency of x-ray production at high kV's a reduction in mAs can be made giving a faster exposure time for the same tube current. Faster intensifying screens can also be used.

Cardiac movement and large vessel movement in chest radiography are examples of movement unsharpness. It is necessary to give an exposure time of 0.01 seconds to overcome movement and maintain a 1Lp mm^{-1} resolution in the final image. Movement can also be controlled if respiration or EKG signals are used to gate image data acquisition but this requires digital data acquisition that will be described in subsequent chapters.

Box 8.2

Image resolution FS and FFD

Focal spot size: (eqn.8.3) The fixed FFD in mammography is 60cm and the focal spot is 0.4mm. If the center of the breast is 3cm from the film plane (OFD) then:

$$U_g = \frac{0.4 \times 3}{60 - 3} = 0.02\text{mm}$$

For ×2 magnification the OFD is increased to 30cm and the focal spot changed to 0.1mm, to maintain sharpness then U_g = 0.1mm

Conclusion: In order to resolve microcalcifications of ~130µm a smaller focal spot is essential.

Focus to film distance: (chest radiography) Using a focal spot of 1.2mm, FFD of 1m and a chest depth 25cm (mid lung-field OFD 12.5cm). Surface lesions : U_g = 0.4mm Mid field lesions give U_g of 0.17mm. For an FFD of 2m surface lesions are shown with a U_g of 0.17mm and mid-field lesions with a U_g of 0.08mm.

Conclusion: At a FFD of 2m lesions are shown sharply at all volume depths.

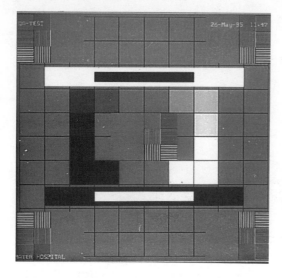 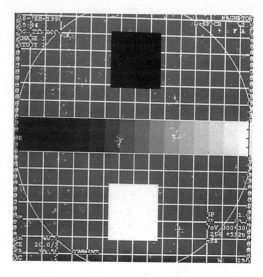

Figure 8.8 Contrast and resolution test patterns for both **(a)** film display and **(b)** equipment performance such as CT or DSA. These low contrast images are also used for quantifying contrast.

Radiographic unsharpness U_r This is associated with the imaging surface itself including the intensifying screen and anti-scatter grid. The film usually has a greater resolution capability than most radiological applications demand so radiographic unsharpness is caused almost entirely by the intensifying screen. This can be single (in the case of mammography) or double (conventional screen film radiology). Single screens used in detail radiography and mammography give the highest resolution since light diffusion is minimal (see Chapter 7). Grid strops may be visible when using static grids (chest radiography) either as lines on the film or moiré fringes on a video display.

8.3.2 Contrast

Image contrast is measured in practice by viewing specific test patterns; examples are shown in Fig.8.8. The strict definition of contrast (the difference between two areas as ΔC) varies depending on conditions:

- **Subject contrast**, which concerns beam intensity differences within the subject (patient) is described as:

$$\Delta C = I2 - I1 \qquad (8.5)$$

- **Radiographic contrast**, which concerns an image density difference is:

$$\Delta C = \frac{D2 - D1}{D1} \qquad (8.6)$$

- **Film contrast**, which relates film exposure to density is:

$$\gamma = \frac{D2 - D1}{\log E2 - \log E1} \qquad (8.7)$$

- **Visual contrast**, the perception of the image, concerns itself with intensities in the same way as subject contrast but using a logarithmic scale in eqn. 8.5:

$$\Delta C = \log I2 - \log I1 \qquad (8.8)$$

The difference between intensities ($I1$ and $I2$) is given by an absolute difference (subject and visual contrast). As an example of eqn.8.5 intensity contrasts: $100-20=80$ and $25-5=20$ whereas radiographic and film contrast are **relative** differences. If the above values now relate to $D1$ and $D2$ as in eqn.8.6 and 8.7 then the relative contrasts will be the same i.e. 4.0. So the contrast between signal and background is calculated differently depending on whether we are considering intensities or image densities.

Subject and visual contrast. Substituting I_a and I_b for $I1$ and $I2$ in eqn.8.5 then the difference in subject contrast C between two intensities is simply $C = I_a - I_b$ however since the eye has a logarithmic response (Weber law) the visual contrast difference (restating eqn.8.8) is:

$$C = \log I_a - \log I_b \qquad (8.9)$$

Applying the exponential law formula derived in Chap.2 to the incident beam I_o:

$$I_a = I_o\, e^{-\mu_a x} \text{ and } I_b = I_o\, e^{-\mu_b x} \qquad (8.10)$$

the two tissues of thickness x have attenuation coefficients of μ_a and μ_b. Visual contrast can now be expressed as:

$$C_v = \log (I_o\, e^{-\mu_a x}) - \log (I_o\, e^{-\mu_b x})$$

Box 8.3 shows that this can be simplified since:

$$I_a = \log I_o - 0.4343\mu_a\, x$$

So the visual contrast varies as:

$$C = 0.4343x \times (\mu_b - \mu_a) \qquad (8.11)$$

which indicates that contrast increases with tissue thickness x (giving more attenuation) and with the increasing difference in the attenuation coefficients $\mu_a - \mu_b$.

Box 8.3

Derivation of visual contrast parameters.

Rearranging equations in 8.10 to remove the negative sign:

Since $\quad \dfrac{I_a}{I_o} = e^{-\mu_a x}$ then $\quad \dfrac{I_o}{I_a} = e^{\mu_a x}$

taking common logs

$\log \dfrac{I_o}{I_a} = \log (e^{\mu_a x}) = \log e \times \mu_a\, x = 0.4343\mu_a\, x$

(since $\log_{10} e = 0.4343$)

Then from the general eqn.8.8

$C = (\log I_o - 0.4343\mu_a\, x) - (\log I_o + 0.4343\mu_b\, x)$

$\quad = 0.4343x \times (\mu_b - \mu_a)$ which is eqn.8.11

Subject contrast This has been described in Chapter 4 and in general concerns interaction of x-rays with matter, x-ray beam quality together with machine and tissue characteristics. In detail these are :

- Tissue thickness x
- Tissue density (kg L^{-1} or kg m^{-3})
- Tissue electron density
- Tissue effective atomic number Z
- Tissue attenuation coefficient μ
- X-ray energy kV
- X-ray filtration (spectrum quality)
- Scatter within the tissue.

Subject contrast and kilovoltage The effect of atomic number on photoelectric absorption and electron density on Compton scattering has already been described in Chapter 4. As x-ray energy (keV) increases subject contrast becomes more dependent on electron density as the probability of Compton reactions increases.

image contrast

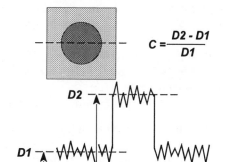

$$C = \frac{D2 - D1}{D1}$$

Figure 8.9 A profile through a dual density image (upper sketch) demonstrating radiographic contrast measurement using *D1* as the background mean value and *D2* the signal mean value. Noise is superimposed on both the background and object.

188 *Physics of Diagnostic Imaging*

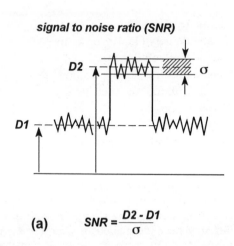

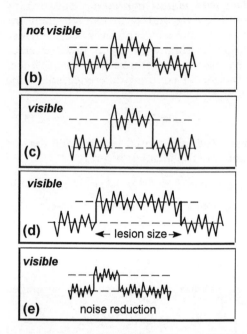

Figure 8.10 (a) The measurement of signal to noise ratio compares the standard deviation of the noise with the difference between background and signal amplitude. (b) Signal noise obscures lesion visibility, (c) signal strength increases making lesion visible, (d) a larger lesion size influences visibility or (e) noise reduction renders small lesions visible.

Radiographic contrast This concerns image forming properties of the detector which are :

- Film and Screen characteristics
- Detector performance (image intensifier, gamma camera etc.)
- Scatter rejection (collimator and grids)

Figure 8.9 illustrates radiographic contrast as an intensity profile taken through two densities on the film $D1$ and $D2$. The profile is a step change complete with image noise. The densities are measured as the mean level of the noise variation.

Objective contrast This is a quantitative measure of the optical density of the image This has been described in Chapter 7 in conjunction with the film characteristic curve and depends on image density difference (film, video) or the windowing level (CT or DSA).

Subjective contrast This depends on image viewing conditions and covers all external factors:

- Room viewing conditions (background lighting, viewing distance)
- View-box characteristics (intensity, light-color)
- Magnification and minification

The two test phantoms in Figure 8.8 are used for measuring the low contrast capability of a film/screen and a video display and the low contrast measurement of a CT machine.

8.3.3 Image noise

Signal to noise ratio (SNR) This is illustrated in Fig.8.10(a). The noise component of the signal is the standard deviation (σ) of the signal level $D2$.

The signal strength ΔS is first measured:

$$\Delta S = D2 - D1 \qquad (8.12)$$

Where $D2$ is the target intensity and $D1$ background intensity (as before), measured by taking a profile through the object. The standard deviation σ of the noise is measured and the signal to noise ratio is then calculated as:

$$SNR = \frac{\Delta S}{\sigma} \qquad (8.13)$$

The SNR should be as high as possible (keeping σ small) in order to achieve good low contrast recording and Fig.8.10(b) to (e) explores the problem of lesion visibility in the presence of noise. The examples show that for a given background noise lesion visibility is achieved by either increasing signal levels or lesion size. The best solution however is to decrease the noise itself.

Quantum noise When a screen/film is exposed to a uniform x-ray exposure the film density, on processing, shows microscopic fluctuations. This is **mottle** and varies according to 3 major parameters:

- Graininess of the film (this is not usually a problem)
- Phosphor thickness (sensitivity)
- X-ray photon density

These random fluctuations become more obvious if the photon number is small: this causes quantum noise or mottle on the image. Since this depends on photon density quantum noise is inversely proportion to patient dose. Quantum noise is influenced by:

- Fast intensifying screens using far fewer x-ray photons for image formation so $\sqrt{N}$ becomes significant. This stage in image formation and loss of photon density is called the quantum sink
- Enlargement of the radiograph by altering the Object to Film Distance decreases photon density and increases noise.

- Patient dose; increased photon density increases patient dose.

Quantum noise reduces the level of low contrast detectability and will affect resolution since it reduces the sharpness of intensity change.

A typical radiographic density would be 1×10^5 photons mm^{-2}. Quantum noise at this level would be minimal. However noise is most evident on nuclear medicine images where densities are of the order of 12 to 15 photons mm^{-2}. The performance of intensifier screens and film is given in Tab. 8.7. The relative noise figures and sensitivity in terms of dose is given.

Table 8.7 The properties of analog images

Film/Screen	Resolution (Lp mm^{-1})	Noise	Dose (mGy)
CaWO$_4$			
High Speed	4.5	31	5.0
Universal	5.6	26	13.0
Detail	8.0	24	24.0
Gd$_2$O$_2$S:Tb			
High Speed	4.7	26	2.0
Universal	5.5	24	3.0
Detail	7.5	22	8.0
Mammography	11.0	20	3.0
Cut Film	5.0*	30*	1.0
Cine Film	5.0*	High	Low
Image Plate	6.0	v. low	v. low

* Limited by Image Intensifier

Dynamic range The need to represent a wide range of anatomical detail on a film image is an important diagnostic requirement; the wider the range the greater image information. The dynamic range of the signal itself is the ratio of x-ray intensity with no attenuation to x-ray intensity at maximum tissue attenuation. A calculation for dynamic range in Box 8.4 shows a the dynamic range of radiographic film as 1:100 which covers an optical density of about 0.5 to 2.5. The video dynamic range is the maximum video signal (typically 1V) divided by the RMS of the noise. Noise values are typically 1mV, so the dynamic range of an image intensifier video

$$contrast\ (C) = \frac{D2 - D1}{D1}$$

$$contrast + scatter\ (Cs) = \frac{D2 - D1}{D1 + S}$$

D1 = 12 D2 = 3   D1 = 12 D2 = 3   S = 2

$$C = \frac{12 - 3}{3} = 3.0 \qquad Cs = \frac{12 - 3}{3 + 2} = 1.8$$

(a)

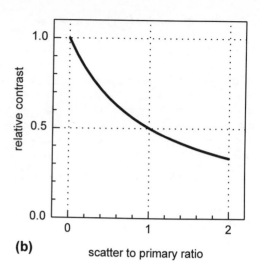

(b)   scatter to primary ratio

Figure 8.11   **(a)** The loss of image contrast by scattered radiation from adjacent areas. This is further investigated in Box 8.4. **(b)** The scatter to primary ratio influencing image contrast. A scatter to primary ratio of 1.0 reduces contrast by 50%

system is given by the system signal to noise ratio (SNR) and a dynamic range of 1:1000 would be expected.

Box 8.4

Dynamic ranges required

Overall attenuation of beam through patient is
$$I_{out} = I_{in}\ e^{-\mu x}$$
Dynamic range required to register full attenuation information is
$$I_{in}/I_{out}\ where\ I_{in} = 1.0$$

Example A.
Mammography where E_{eff} = 20keV, x = 5cm and μ = 0.7613

Dynamic range $= \dfrac{1}{e^{-(0.7613 \times 5)}} =$ **50:1**

Example B
Abdomen where E_{eff} = 60keV, x = 20cm and μ = 0.2046 dynamic range   **60:1**
Example C
Chest where E_{eff} = 125keV
x = 30cm and μ = 0.160 dynamic range   **120:1**
The film latitude must match these dynamic ranges to capture the entire contrast range.
Typical film dynamic range is from **10:1** to **100:1** depending on film latitude
Image plate displays have a very wide dynamic range of about **10,000:1**

The SNR decreases with video bandwidth so very high quality components are essential with high definition video displays (1024 and 1250 line) and consequently these units have SNR values at least ×2 higher (1:2000 and up to 1:6000). Since fluoroscopy uses low x-ray exposures the video signal is small so the dynamic range is an important parameter.

8.4   SCATTER AND GRIDS

The influence of scatter on contrast is simplistically demonstrated in Fig.8.11(a) where areas outside D1 and D2 contribute scattered photons so significantly decreasing subject contrast.   This scatter within the patient appears on the image detector as a misplaced event, adding to image noise.

8.4.1 Scatter to primary ratio

The scatter component S degrades maximum subject contrast C giving a final scatter contrast C_s so:

$$C_s = \frac{\Delta D}{D1 + S} \qquad (8.14)$$

Box 8.5 shows that this is equivalent to:

$$C_s = \frac{C}{(1 + R)} \qquad (8.15)$$

where R is the scatter to primary ratio. The values given in Fig.8.11(a) are recalculated in the Box 8.5. The scatter to primary ratio is plotted against contrast degradation in Fig. 8.11(b) and shows that when this ratio has a value of 1:1 then contrast is reduced by 50%.

Box.8.5

Scatter component and scatter to primary ratio.

From the values given in Fig.8.12(a)

Contrast without scatter: $C = \dfrac{D2 - D1}{D1} = 3.0$

Contrast with scatter $(C_S) = \dfrac{(D2 + S) - (D1 + S)}{D1 + S}$

since $(D2+S) - (D1+S) = D2 - D1$ then

$$C_S = \frac{D2 - D1}{D1 + S} \qquad = \qquad 1.8$$

introducing the *scatter : primary* ratio R (2:3)

then $\quad C_S \quad = \dfrac{C}{(1 + R)} \quad = \dfrac{3}{1.666} \quad = \quad 1.8$

Chapter 7 has already shown that the probability of Compton scatter is highest at low photon energies but the greatest proportion of low energy scatter is absorbed within the patient. So the amount of scatter reaching the imaging surface increases with energy, peaking at about 80kV; since the scatter is in the forward direction it travels toward the film.

Tissue type also influences scatter production since the probability of a scatter event (σ/ρ) is proportional to electron density but inversely proportional to energy so:

$$\frac{\sigma}{\rho} \quad \propto \quad \frac{Electron\ Density}{Photon\ Energy} \qquad (8.16)$$

Various factors also reduce the effect of scatter on the image. The intensifying screen phosphor sensitivity is much less for low energy scatter photons and K-edge filtration precisely shapes the x-ray spectrum reducing the intensity of higher energy photons from the x-ray beam that are not required (e.g. mammography) so reducing the amount of scattered radiation reaching the film.

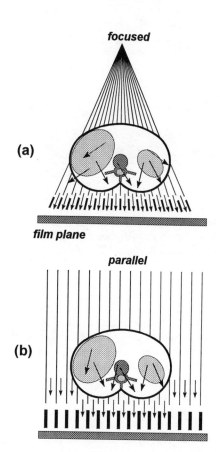

Figure 8.12 **(a)** The design and operation of focused and **(b)** parallel anti-scatter grids. The focused grid gives increased efficiency since it mimics the beam geometry.

8.4.2 Grid design

The problem of separating scatter from primary radiation was addressed by Bucky in 1913 when he introduced a grating or grid of thin lead strips which collimated the emerging radiation from the patient allowing the un-

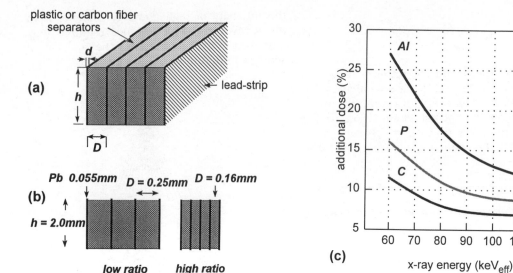

Figure 8.13   **(a)** Antiscatter grid showing sandwich construction with lead strips (thickness d) with interspace material (thickness D). The grid assembly has a height h and it is protected by a thin plastic or metal cover. **(b)** The difference in interspace gap between a low and high ratio grid **(c)** Dose reduction over the diagnostic x-ray range by using carbon fiber (C) instead of aluminum (Al) or plastic (P) spaced grids.

scattered primary beam to reach the film, blocking most of the off-axis scatter radiation which approached the lead-strips at an angle.

Scatter is significantly reduced by placing a grid between the patient and the film cassette or imaging surface (image intensifier).

Focused or parallel grids   A focused and parallel grid design is shown in Fig. 8.12(a) and (b). Focused grids follow the sector geometry of the x-ray beam more closely so are more efficient in accepting the primary beam at shorter FFDs. Common focal distances for these grids are 80, 100, 140, 180cm for conventional radiology and 60cm for mammography.

If larger FFDs are used than those recommended then the x-ray beam is cut off at the image periphery. Off center beams also give image artifacts. This is discussed later. Parallel grids have their lead-strips arranged in a parallel fashion (they are not focused). Since the x-ray beam radiates at an increasing oblique angle toward the edge of

the grid there will be increasing cut-off with a parallel design so they are only suitable for FFDs exceeding 2m when the x-ray beam itself approximates to parallel lines; this is the case in chest radiography where static high ratio parallel grids are used.

Lead strip thickness d   The grid has very thin strips of metal sandwiched between radiolucent material (plastic or carbon fiber) which forms a composite grating (Fig. 8.13(a)) Metals used in the construction of grids are Lead ($Z=82$), Tungsten ($Z=74$) and Tantalum ($Z=73$); lead is the most common material. The quantity of lead (g cm^{-2}) of a grid is a measure of its contrast improvement capability since this is a rough measure of lead-strip density per unit area of grid surface. Thick lead strips, however, remove a significant proportion of the primary radiation which is required for image formation so the lead strips should be thin enough to stop scattered radiation at the intended kVp at the same time blocking minimal primary beam photons. Typical thicknesses for general radiology are between 0.036 and 0.07mm, thinner strips can be obtained by using tungsten or tantalum. Example dimensions are given in Fig.8.13(b) for a low and high ratio grid.

Interspace material thickness D The lead strips are supported and separated by low density material, transparent to x-rays. This can be aluminum in the finer grids (high strip density) but is more usually paper, plastic or more recently carbon fiber; the thickness is normally limited to 0.150mm

The interspace material will remove a small proportion of the primary beam so its density should be as low as possible particularly in low dose investigations such as mammography and pediatric studies. Figure 8.13(c) shows the percentage dose reduction that can be achieved by using carbon fiber instead of aluminum or plastic/paper. The carbon fiber interspace material achieves dose reduction by up to 30% depending on kV and grid ratio.

Line density   lines cm^{-1} Very thin lead strips or lamellae stop less primary radiation and in high ratio grids line density is increased by decreasing the strip thickness d. This is calculated as:

$$L = \frac{10}{D+d} \quad \text{L cm}^{-1} \quad (8.17)$$

Common line densities are 22 to 77L cm^{-1}. High line density grids are less selective than low line density at higher kVp. Box 8.6 calculates the different line densities and x-ray transmission for three grid types: conventional (A), high resolution (B) and mammography (C).

These calculations demonstrate that primary transmission is typically 75% for common grid types and increases to over 80% for mammography where it is important to reduce patient radiation dose by utilizing the maximum proportion of primary beam.

Moving and stationary grids Although the use of anti-scatter grids in diagnostic radiology prevents scattered radiation reaching the film surface one of the disadvantages is the shadows of the metal strips can be seen on the resulting image. A moving grid (developed by Potter in 1920 and called the Potter Bucky Diaphragm) eliminates the grid patterns on the image.

These were introduced first as a spring operated device but modern Potter Bucky diaphragms are now motor driven giving a more uniform oscillating movement during exposure. They can produce a stroboscopic artifact with very short exposure times.

Fluoroscopy has a lower visual resolution than film so stationary grids are used. Very fast exposures of about 20milliseconds (high kV chest x-ray) also use stationary grids since grid movement would be too slow. It is important to have effective grid movement in mammography since this procedure has the highest resolution.

Box 8.6

Grid specifications

Grid parameters that are used are: strip thickness d interspace thickness D grid height h; the latter give the grid ratio r

	r	d	D	h
Grid A	8:1	0.07	0.18	1.4
Grid B	12:1	0.035	0.10	2.1
Grid C	3.5:1	0.035	0.28	1.0

Line density$=\dfrac{10}{d+D}$ lines per cm

Transmission of primary radiation

$$T_p = \frac{D}{d+D} \quad \text{percent}$$

Grid A (conventional)
 Line density = 40 L cm^{-2}
 Transmission = 72%
Grid B (chest x-ray)
 Line density = 74 L cm^{-2}
 Transmission = 74%
Grid C (mammography)
 Line density = 32 L cm^{-2}
 Transmission = 88%

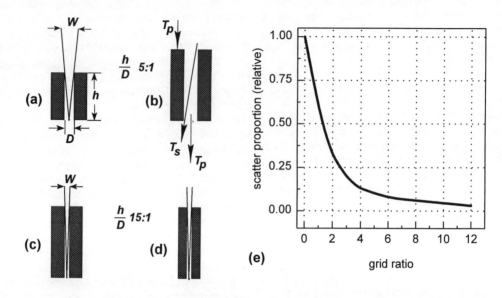

Figure 8.14 **(a)** Grid ratios of 5:1 showing acceptance angle and **(b)** identifying primary and scattered beams. **(c)** 15:1 ratio grid demonstrating that lead-strip thickness does not alter grid ratio values in **(d)**. **(e)** Scatter transmission reduction with increasing grid ratio

Multiline grids Advances in the manufacture of grids have produced line densities up to 60 to 70 L cm^{-1}. The advantages are that these grids can be stationary since 70 L cm^{-1} can only be detected by magnifying the image. Image contrast is similar to a moving 40 L cm^{-1} grid.

Cross grids these consist of two focused grids lying on top of one another. Crossed grids give a high reduction of scattered radiation in both x and y planes but beam alignment must be exactly perpendicular if they are not to introduce artifacts.

8.4.3 Grid specifications

Various parameters are used for describing grid performance. These are:

- grid ratio
- line density
- grid factor/Bucky factor
- contrast improvement factor
- selectivity

Figure 8.14(a) to (d) shows the general grid construction and the dimensions that take part in the various specifications. Grid performance, in general, can be described in terms of contrast improvement factor (CIF) and exposure (or radiation dose) increase factor (grid factor). Both are strongly dependent on exposure conditions (kVp, field size, tissue type etc.).

Grid Ratio r This is the ratio between grid height h and interspace distance D so that:

$$r = \frac{h}{D} \qquad (8.18)$$

Common values are 3.5:1 or 5:1 for mammography, 15:1 up to 20:1 for conventional radiography and 30:1, 40:1 for high kV chest radiography. The ratio for both grids Fig.8.14(a) and (b) is 5:1; the height and spacer thickness have been altered proportionately. The grid ratio for (c) and (d) is 15:1, the thickness of the lead-strip has not altered this but the proportion of available primary radiation T_p would have increased due to the thinner lead septa. The width W of the acceptance angle θ is related to h and D as:

$$\tan \theta = \frac{D}{h} \tag{8.19}$$

Grid ratio determines the scatter to primary ratio that reaches the image detector. High ratio grids pass less scatter and give better image contrast component but need more careful alignment with beam geometry. The graph in Fig.8.14(e) shows the reduction of scatter transmission as the grid ratio is increased, for the same kV. Both axes are logarithmic so the straight line relationship shows that scatter reduction follows a square law relationship. The grid ratio and line density are used for describing grids in terms of ratio and density. The combination is shown in Tab.8.8.

Table 8.8   Grid specifications

Term	Definition	Typical value
Grid ratio	h/D	12:1 5:1
Line density	$1/(d+D)$ L cm^{-1}	28-60L cm^{-1}
General specification	small field	Pb 12/40
	large field	Pb 5/28
	mammography	Pb 3/28
	fluoroscopy	Pb 12/36

The parameters associated with radiation incident on the grid I_0 and transmitted by the grid, identified in Fig.8.14(b), are defined as:

- The primary radiation transmitted through the grid T_p
- The scattered radiation transmitted through the grid T_s
- The total radiation transmitted through the grid $T_t = T_p + T_s$

The fractional transmission for a grid can be simply measured by noting the exposure values with and without the grid in place:

$$\text{Transmission } T_t = \frac{mAs \text{ with grid}}{mAs \text{ without grid}} \tag{8.20}$$

This value has already been calculated for the grids in Box 8.6 using the various thicknesses of the lead and interspace material. However this calculation does not allow for absorption by the interspace material itself.

Grid exposure factor GF   This is also known as the grid factor or Bucky factor. It is a measure of the increased dose required when using a grid.

GF is the exposure multiplication factor in order to achieve the same film blackening when using the grid at the same kVp. It is usually obtained by measuring the transmitted radiation T_t and incident radiation I_0 and is a direct measure of absorption of both primary and secondary radiation by the grid:

$$GF = \frac{\text{Incident radiation } I_o}{\text{Transmitted radiation } T_t} \tag{8.21}$$

The grid factor is an indication of the grid's ability to stop both primary and secondary radiation but decreases with increasing kVp due to penetration of the lead strips as shown in Fig.8.15(a).

Contrast Improvement Factor CIF   An x-ray grid has only one function and that is to improve the contrast of the x-ray image by preventing scattered radiation reaching the image surface. The effectiveness of this operation is indicated by the contrast improvement factor (*CIF*):

$$CIF = \frac{\text{contrast with grid}}{\text{contrast without grid}} \tag{8.22}$$

Two densities are chosen (on an aluminum step wedge) and their differences measured with and without a grid. If the total transmitted radiation were $T_t = T_p + T_s$ then eqn.8.22 can be expressed as

$$CIF = \frac{T_p}{T_t} \tag{8.23}$$

Contrast degrades as the scatter component of T_t increases. A typical grid can improve

196 *Physics of Diagnostic Imaging*

contrast by a factor of ×3 to ×4 but depends a great deal on size and tissue type as well as the kVp being used. The CIF value degrades as kVp is increased due to penetration of the lead-strips Fig.8.15(b) and a steady decline in contrast is seen.

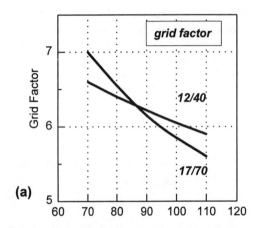

(a)

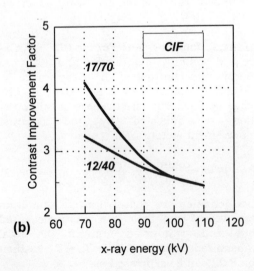

(b)

x-ray energy (kV)

Figure 8.15   **(a)** Grid factor decreasing with increased kV. **(b)** CIF factor decreases with increasing kV. The higher ratio/line number grid has a superior CIF at low energies but this is lost for higher energy x-ray imaging.

Selectivity Σ   This depends on grid ratio and lead strip thickness. It measures transmitted scatter T_s as a percentage of the primary beam T_p reaching the film.

$$\Sigma = \frac{transmitted\ primary}{transmitted\ scatter} = \frac{T_p}{T_s} \quad (8.24)$$

An efficient grid would stop all scattered radiation and pass all the primary so making $\Sigma = \infty$. If 20% of scatter is transmitted then Σ is 5 which would seriously degrade image quality. A more acceptable figure would be a Σ value of 6 to 8. More efficient grids will have still higher values.

Table 8.9 lists a series of grids with various ratio/line density values with their GF, CIF performance figures. These last two parameters can be combined to give a quality factor. Since the CIF value should be large and GF small the quality factor value should be as high as possible.

Table 8.9 Summary of grid terms, the ratio of GF with CIF gives an overall quality factor.

Grid	CIF	GF	Σ	Quality factor CIF:GF
General				
8/28	3.3	4.7	5.5	0.70
12/28	3.9	5.7	7.9	0.67
High Contrast				
8/36	2.9	3.9	4.3	0.74
12/36	3.6	5.1	6.4	0.72
Mammography	2.4	3.0	6.2	0.8
Image intensifier				
12/44	3.6	5.2	6.6	0.70

Grid misalignment   Figure 8.16(a) and (b) illustrates two common faults that are found when using either parallel or focused grids. The focused grid must be used at a recommended distance from the focal point since bringing the focal spot (x-ray tube) nearer will cause shadowing, seen as thick bars on the image.

Similarly if the x-ray tube is used too near a parallel grid shadow bars will be seen. High ratio parallel grids are commonly used in high voltage kV chest radiography; a distance of at least 2m should be maintained in order to prevent these artifacts.

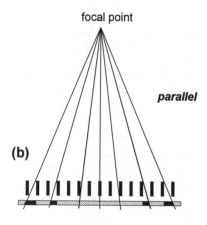

(a) focused

(b) parallel

focal point

focal point

Figure 8.16 Misalignment for both **(a)** a focused and **(b)** a parallel grid showing how grid shadow is caused by the lead-strips

8.5   IMAGE QUALITY MEASUREMENT

Previous sections have described simple methods for expressing resolution and contrast as well as signal to noise ratio. More complex analyses are necessary to give a comprehensive value of image quality, some combining the 3 major parameters of resolution, contrast and noise. These are

- Point Spread Function (PSF)
- Line Spread Function (LSF)
- Modulation Transfer Function (MTF)
- Wiener Spectrum
- Contrast Detail Diagram (CDD)
- Detective Quantum Efficiency (DQE)

A Receiver Operator Characteristic (ROC) curve is a subjective measurement of the effectiveness of an image to convey information. This requires resolution, contrast and noise to be optimum for the clinical detail studied.

8.5.1 Point spread function

The point spread function (PSF) is the simplest test of spatial resolution in an imaging system. The x-ray image surface (film cassette) is covered with a lead sheet pierced with 10 μm (micron) holes. This size is critical since they must be smaller than the resolution limit of the system.

Sufficient exposure is given to achieve a point image on the film and then a microdensitometer is used to measure a profile density through the point center. This profile is the point spread function (PSF). An example is given in Fig.8.17. In practice it is difficult to measure since a very small point needs to be displayed requiring considerable exposure time under very steady conditions.

The PS profile in Fig.8.17 gives a full-width-at-half-maximum value. The effect of scatter reaching the image detector (grid or collimator having septa penetration) broadens the 'skirt' or 'tail' of the curve giving a larger value for the Full-Width at Tenth-Maximum (FWTM). Long 'tails' cause spreading beyond the source boundaries which contributes to the total unsharpness (geometrical and radiographic).   This is an indication of the radiation penetrating the lead-strips in an anti-scatter grid or collimator on a gamma camera.

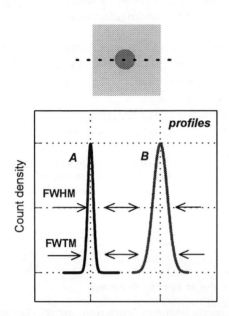

Figure 8.17   A point source of radiation on a detector surface yielding the Full Width at Half Maximum (FWHM) and tenth maximum (FWTM).

Resolution   Two point sources can be used to measure the resolving power of a display. The point sources can theoretically be resolved if the separation is greater than the FWHM of the PSF. This is demonstrated in Fig.8.18. A distance less than the FWHM in (a) displays the points as a single entity. In (b) the point source separation equals the FWHM; this is the threshold point when two separate points can just be resolved. The two point sources in (c) are separated by a distance that is greater than the FWHM, the overall envelope clearly resolves the two separate points.

A film screen can resolve approximately 50 to 100µm point sources, CT 0.3mm and MRI 0.7mm. Ultrasound resolves about 1mm and nuclear medicine 3mm, depending on the field of view.

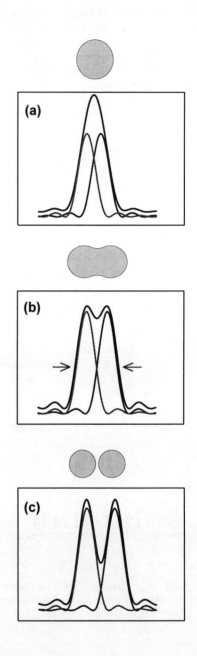

Figure 8.18   **(a)** shows complete merging of the point sources when their separation is <FWHM. **(b)** resolvable points are displayed when distanced by their FWHM value, **(c)** points clearly resolved when separation is >FWHM.

8.5.2 Line spread function (LSF)

A point spread function has limitations as an image test tool since it only represents discrete points on the image surface. A line source in the form of a 10μm metal slit (usually made from platinum) provides a measure along a complete axis of the imaging surface as shown in Fig.8.19(a). This is measured as the line spread function (LSF).

The LSF is a better measure since it is easier to make a line source using two knife edges with a 10μm (microns) gap. The density of the line profile, recorded by the image, is then read with a micro-densitometer as before.

The LSF example in Fig.8.19(b) shows a more comprehensive measure of image detector performance. The resolving power of a complete image axis is demonstrated in one measurement.

The principle of MTF is shown in Fig.8.20 where an input signal, usually in the form of fixed amplitude but varying frequency sine waves, is recorded by the imaging medium: film, television monitor, image intensifier, gamma camera etc.

As the frequency of the input signal increases the ability of the recording system to faithfully follow the signal begins to fail. The recording system modulates, or degrades, the signal so that the output amplitude is reduced. The ratio of the output signal amplitude to the input signal amplitude at each frequency is the MTF. The transfer of frequencies from source to the imaging system defines the MTF as:

$$\text{MTF} = \frac{recorded\ signal\ frequencies}{original\ signal\ frequencies} \quad (8.25)$$

A perfect system would have an MTF of 1.0 and this value is given by most imaging systems for very low frequency signals. The MTF value then falls off as higher frequencies are recorded.

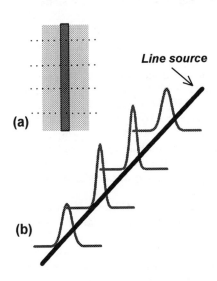

Figure 8.19   (a) A line source placed on an imaging surface and yielding a series of profiles (b) as a line spread function (LSF).

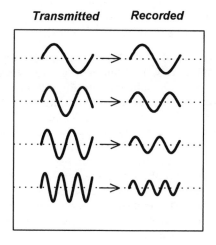

Figure 8.20   Transmitted signal frequencies and recorded image signals showing loss of signal strength with frequency. The loss of frequency information (resolution) is plotted as the MTF

8.5.3 Modulation transfer function

A quantitative analysis of an imaging systems resolution capability and the degradation it gives to the image data is given by the modulation transfer function (MTF).

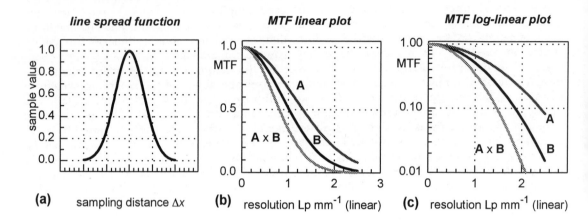

Figure 8.21 **(a)** The LSF used as a data source for computing the MTF. **(b)** The MTF plotted on linear axes and **(c)** the MTF values are plotted on a log scale for the same two film screen systems

The MTF is extremely useful since it allows the resolving power of each image component to be quantified e.g. intensifying screen, film and the combination of both. A complete fluoroscopy imaging chain can be studied: the image intensifier input phosphor, the photocathode, the output screen, the video camera and the final video display, so that weak points can be identified and corrected.

Derivation of the MTF Individual readings are taken from the line spread function at fixed intervals shown in Fig.8.21(a). The formula which is used for calculating the MTF involves a Fourier analysis (Chapter 7). The resolution of each factor in the LSF can be described in terms of spatial frequency response and those frequency dependent variations (amplitude losses) are combined in the modulation transfer function. The following MTF equation which extracts the frequency components from the LSF uses the Fourier transform:

$$\frac{\sum\limits_{j=1}^{m} L(x_j, z) \times (\cos 2p\upsilon x_j - i \cdot \sin 2p\upsilon x_j)}{\sum\limits_{j=1}^{m} L(x_j, z)} \quad (8.26)$$

Where $L(x_j, z)$ represents m individual line spread values at Δx sampling interval using a spatial frequency of υ Lp mm^{-1} shown taken from the readings in the figure.

The MTF is easily calculated by digitizing the PSF or LSF measurements and using a computer program for calculations, using eqn.8.26. A sub-routine program for calculating the modulation transfer function is given in the Appendix. This is written in GW-BASIC and can be incorporated into a main program.

The individual MTFs for film A and intensifying screen B are shown in Fig.8.21(b) and (c). Multiplying the individual MTF's gives the expected MTF of the final display A×B shown in the linear-linear and semi-log of the same MTF data in Fig.8.21(b),(c).

An imaging system having perfect reproduction of its transmitted frequencies gives an MTF value of 1.0. However all imaging systems show a limitation; the limit of visual detail is normally taken at an MTF of 0.1 (10%) which is the **cut-off frequency**. Others quote the resolution limitation to be nearer 4% The area under the MTF curve, up to the cut-off frequency, gives a value of the overall system resolution. Manufacturers sometimes quote 50%, 10% and 2% values.

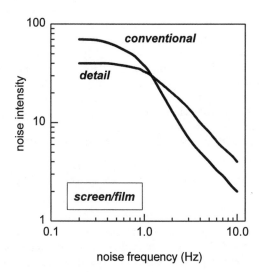

Figure 8.22 Wiener spectrum for detail and conventional screen/film. Although the detail screen will give a higher resolution it will also give most noise in the higher frequencies.

8.5.4 Wiener spectrum

Noise can be measured quantitatively by using the Wiener Spectrum which plots the noise of a system as a function of its frequency content; high and low frequency noise can be readily identified. It is generally agreed that the frequency range of 0.2 to 1Lp mm^{-1} is relevant to radiology since these frequencies are easily visible and their effect noticed. For film/screen systems the relationship between the modulation transfer function (MTF) and the Wiener spectrum WS is:

$$WS = \frac{G^2}{n} (MTF)^2 \qquad (8.27)$$

Where n is the number of photons absorbed and G is the film gamma. For a given x-ray exposure the film γ (contrast) is proportional to the Wiener spectrum. A change in the speed (sensitivity) alters n since noise increases with sensitivity.

The Wiener spectrum shown in Fig.8.22 shows a typical noise spectrum from a film/screen combination. The background noise is predominantly low frequency, identified as film grain and phosphor structure. High frequency noise is increased when detail (thin) intensifying screens are used and is related to poor photon absorption (quantum efficiency).

8.5.5 Contrast detail graph

The results from the low contrast phantom shown in Fig.8.8 can be expressed as a Contrast/Detail Diagram which indicates the threshold contrast needed to detect an object as a function of its diameter. Contrast detail analysis is a graphic representation which relates the minimum (threshold) contrast necessary to visualize an object of a certain size in a noisy image. The basic components of a contrast detail curve obtained from the low contrast phantom are shown in Fig.8.23(a).

Contrast is displayed on the *y*-axis and object size on the *x*-axis. The curve shows that larger objects can be seen more easily at low contrast levels while smaller objects require much higher contrast differences before they become visible in the same noisy image. This has already been demonstrated in Fig.8.10(b) to (e) when discussing signal to noise ratio. The contrast-detail curve in Fig.8.23(a) starts at the upper left corner at an object size which is the resolution limit of the system and declines asymptotically. Above the curve the conditions (image noise) satisfy visibility of the object; below the curve conditions prevent visibility.

Contrast detail curves are constructed using results obtained from a group of observers, viewing a test image containing a set of precisely sized objects and varying contrast levels. The test image is obtained from an imaging system under different conditions (kVp, mAs, screen types, film types, etc.). Figure 8.23(b) gives an example of a set of contrast detail curves obtained for two exposure (mAs) settings.

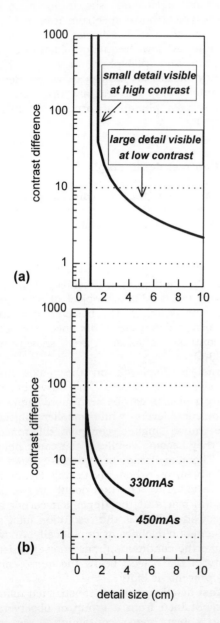

(a)

small detail visible
at high contrast

large detail visible
at low contrast

(b)

330mAs

450mAs

detail size (cm)

Figure 8.23 **(a)** Contrast Detail diagram showing small object size visible at high contrast levels but as the object detail loses contrast then these are only visible if their sizes increase. Contrast levels above the curve are not visible. **(b)** Contrast-detail improvement with increasing exposure levels (mAs) allowing smaller low contrast objects to be seen at 450mAs.

8.5.6 Detective quantum efficiency (DQE)

The DQE of an imaging system describes the system accuracy of response to information (emerging x-ray beam, gamma radiation, light etc.). Signal to noise ratios vary at every stage of image production and will increase overall. If the SNR variation in the photon beam (subject contrast) is SNR_{in} and the SNR of the detection process (radiographic contrast in the intensifying screen, image intensifier phosphor or image plate, etc.) is SNR_{out} then the DQE compares input and output SNR as:

$$DQE = \left(\frac{SNR_{out}}{SNR_{in}}\right)^2 \qquad (8.28)$$

The SNR of an incident photon flux N is $\sqrt{N}$ which is due to quantum noise variations. The SNR of the detector is dependent on absorbed photon number N_{ab} its noise being $\sqrt{N_{ab}}$. The value of N_{ab} is closely dependent on photon absorption which is influenced by both μ and screen thickness. Conversion efficiency (e.g. light production) is also crucial.

The DQE for film (Fig.8.24(a)) shows how critical film processing is so that optimum film density between 1 and 2 is maintained for the image density likely to represent pathology in the image. The comparison between film/screen and image phosphor plate DQE values in Fig.8.24(b) indicates the change of DQE value with system resolution since in order to improve resolution the phosphor screen thickness must be reduced, increasing noise and so reducing SNR_{out}.

The limiting spatial resolution for CR at present is 5Lp mm^{-1} compared to film screens which can extend to 15Lp mm^{-1}; the smallest detail resolvable with present film screens (mammography) is about 130μm.

8.5.7   ROC curves

Receiver Operating Characteristic curves provide an objective assessment of an imaging chain, whether it be a simple string such as:

film-screen → film processor → film quality

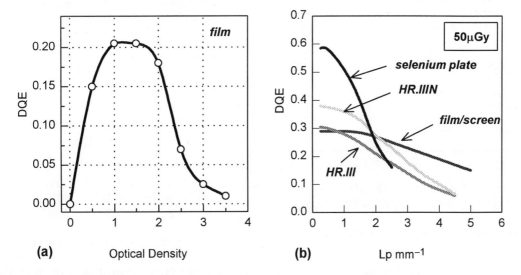

Figure 8.24 **(a)** DQE for film has a maximum value when the image detail has an optical density between 1 and 2. Film processing quality is important in order to maintain this. **(b)** The decrease with resolution of DQE for film/screen and image plate exposed to 50μGy. HRIIIN is a high resolution version of HRIII phosphor image plate. The performance of a typical selenium image plate is included.

or a more complex string such as:

image plate →image digitization
→ data manipulation → color video display

It enables display sensitivity, specificity and overall accuracy of a particular display system to be compared with another system so that decisions can be made regarding the success or improvement that the new system may give and a measure of its diagnostic sensitivity and specificity.

Sensitivity and specificity The final test for any display system is its clinical success for detecting disease. This is purely subjective and depends not only on the quality (resolution, contrast, noise) of the image but also the viewing conditions and the skill of the observer in discriminating between a true and a false uptake or lesion on the display.

Detecting a positive lesion (true positive) or reporting a negative finding (true negative) becomes more difficult as either contrast or size diminishes. A procedure for estimating the accuracy of visual image analysis considers also the reporting of mistaken lesions (false positive) and missed lesions (false negative) and gives a measure of **sensitivity**, which is the ability to detect abnormality and **specificity** or the ability to report a negative finding or detect a normal result. A 2×2 table format for this analysis is shown in Tab.8.10.

Applying this test to an imaging system requires a series of images to be recorded which contain lesions/objects of varying size and contrast. These are either radio-opaque objects in the case of x-ray images or radio-active sources in the case of nuclear medicine. They can also be computer derived 'lesions'. Certain images in the series are completely clear and contain no lesions. A noisy image background is present to a fixed degree in all the images. About a 100 images make up the series and these are given to a panel of observers for judging. Table 8.10 shows how the results would be set out comparing the known lesion number (master copy) with the reported lesion number (test result).

Table 8.10 Result table

Test result	Master +	Copy −	Total
Positive test image	TP	FP	TP+FP
Negative test image	FN	TN	FN+TN
Total	TP+FN	FP+TN	TP+FN+FP+TN

TP = true positive; TN = true negative
FP = false positive; FN = false negative

The results from the table give three measurements:

Sensitivity $\dfrac{TP}{TP + FN}$ (8.29)

Selectivity $\dfrac{TN}{TN + FP}$ (8.30)

Overall accuracy $\dfrac{TP + TN}{Grand\ total}$ (8.31)

For a dual series of 200 images, one with a 50% incidence of lesions and the other with a 10% incidence the following results were obtained:

(1) Series total 200 images with a 50% incidence:

Test result	Master +	Copy −	Total
Positive test image	75	30	105
Negative test image	25	70	95
Total	100	100	200

From eqns. 8.29, 8.30, 8.31:

Sensitivity = 75/100 = 75%
Specificity = 70/100 = 70%
Accuracy = 145/200 = 72.5%

(2) The second series of 200 images have a 10% incidence:

Test result	Master +	Copy −	Total
Positive test image	10	30	40
Negative test image	10	150	160
Total	20	180	200

Sensitivity = 10/20 = 50%
Specificity = 150/180 = 83%
Accuracy = 40/200 = 20%

These two examples demonstrate the real effect of disease incidence in the population being studied on the sensitivity and specificity of a test. A high incidence of disease (or a high number of lesions in the image) gives a test with a higher sensitivity than a population with a low incidence of disease (lower number of lesions in the image data set). The specificity shows the opposite effect.

The diagnostic image If two investigations (Test A and Test B) are performed on the same patient then the separate sensitivity and specificity figures for each test can be combined to give improved accuracy. For instance the sensitivity/specificity for a nuclear medicine and CT investigation are known to give the following precision:

Investigation	Sensitivity %	Specificity %
Test A	80	60
Test B	90	90

Then the combined sensitivity/specificity figures for the first case when:

- A and/or B are positive,
- A and B are negative

Combined Sensitivity =

$$\frac{Sensitivity\ A + (100 - Sensitivity\ A) \times Sensitivity\ B}{100}$$

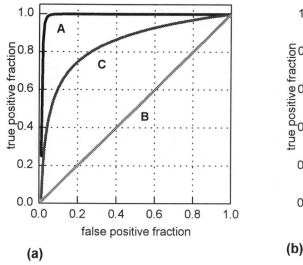

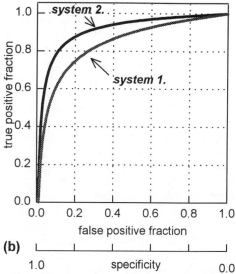

Figure 8.25 **(a)** A set of ROC curves. Curve A would be given by a perfect system, Curve B by a system giving a purely random result (50:50) and Curve C by a practical display system offering diagnostic advantages. **(b)** A set of two curves from two separate display systems showing that Display 2 has a superior performance to display system 1 for detecting a particular pathology.

Combine Specifity =
$$\frac{Specificity\ A \times Specificity\ B}{100}$$

The combined Sensitivity/Specificity figures for the second case when:

- A and B are positive
- A and/or B are negative

are:

Combined Sensitivity =
$$\frac{Sensitivity\ A \times Sensitivity\ B}{100}$$

Combined Specificity =
$$\frac{Specificity\ A + (100 - Specificity\ A) \times Specificity\ B}{100}$$

For the combined nuclear medicine and CT investigations the first case will present a sensitivity of 98% and a specificity of 54% and the second case will present a sensitivity of 72% and a specificity of 96%. So combining the results from carefully chosen investigations markedly improves overall sensitivity and specificity.

A test with a high sensitivity is good for detecting disease in a population where the incidence of disease is low: it will give few false negatives. This will exclude disease which should be the object with screening tests. A test with a high specificity is good for detecting the absence of disease in (say) a patient group where there is a high probability of the disease since there are few false positives so preventing unnecessary treatment, particularly if the treatment carries its own risk. Double viewing the same images from one investigation (mammography) will similarly improve sensitivity and specificity in a population with low disease incidence and improve significantly on the figures demonstrated in the second group having only 10% disease.

The Receiver Operating Characteristic Curve This plots the true positive fraction (TPF) of an observer response against the false positive fraction (FPF). It allows a quantitative comparison between imaging systems (CT, MRI, film radiology etc.) for detecting various pathology.

A typical ROC curve is shown in Fig.8.25(a) The TPF, on the *y*-axis, is the percentage of patients correctly identified having positive findings. The FPF score is the percentage of patients who were called positive but were really normal. A move toward the right is a less sensitive diagnostic test. A move toward the left denotes a more sensitive test: i.e. increase in specificity but decrease in sensitivity. The upper right corner shows a 100% sensitivity and 0% specificity i.e. all the findings deemed abnormal. The lower left corner shows 0% sensitivity but 100% specificity: all the findings are normal.

Since FPF is 1–Specificity, reversing the values on the *x*-axis directly converts it to specificity. In order to judge effectiveness of a new film/screen, video or digital imaging system for the improvement (if any) in sensitivity, a series of test images (usually 100) containing objects with a range of contrast, corresponding to a range of detection difficulty, are viewed by a group of observers who report their confidence at detecting the object. Roughly half the cases in the image set have no objects.   A ranking/scoring system from 1 to 5 would be:

1) Definitely Normal (only obvious normals scored) where false positive rate would be high and the false negative low
2) Probably Normal (probably no lesion)
3) Maybe Normal (don't know)
4) Probably Abnormal (probably a lesion)
5) Definitely Abnormal (only obvious lesions scored) where the false positive rate would be low and false negative would be high

The ROC curve shown in Fig.8.25(b) shows such a result and demonstrates quite convincingly that System 2 has a better detection performance than System 1.

8.6   HARDCOPY DEVICES

The eventual film record from a clinical study can originate from 3 sources:

• Cassette with intensifying screens.

• A video screen through a system of lenses.
• A laser imager

The first has been described in Chapter 7 and is the simplest method of recording x-ray images.   The second and third methods require electronic handling of the image information to produce a video signal which is then transferred to either a CRT screen or laser optical system which eventually produces the light which exposes the film.

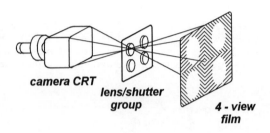

camera CRT
lens/shutter group
4 - view film

Figure 8.26 A video multi-format camera

8.6.1 Video film formatter

This method uses a cathode-ray tube (CRT). The image is directed by a series of mirrors and lenses onto a film surface. Since it can provide single or multiple images on a single sheet of film it is often referred to as a multi-format camera. Fig.8.26 shows a simplified diagram of a multi-format camera.

It can handle low or high resolution video signals (512/625 or 1024/1249 lines). Each image contains the full complement of scan lines so resolution is unaffected even for small(35mm slide) images.   Since a video camera is commonly restricted to an 8×10 film size it is not possible to hold more than about six images on each film for routine clinical in-spection and the CRT screen must be optically flat to give perfectly rectangular film images without rounded verticals.

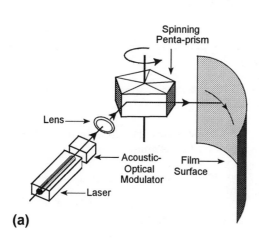

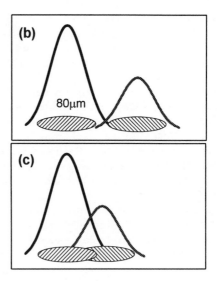

Figure 8.27 **(a)** The basic components of a laser imager. **(b)** Laser dot dimensions which are critical for accurate dot placement **(c)** overlapping dot placement degrades image quality

8.6.2   Laser Imager

The main action of a laser imager is to capture the incoming digitized video signal which then modulates a laser beam scanning a film surface. Several machines (CT, MRI, nuclear medicine etc.) can share a single laser imager.

The diagram in Fig.8.27(a) identifies the major component parts of a laser imager. The critical design concerns the prism and mirror scanning assembly which moves the modulated laser beam over the film surface. The film scanning is achieved by a constantly rotating prism in the laser light beam which traces a path on the film which is held in a semi-circular drum. At the end of each scan line the beam is shifted down until the entire sheet of film has been exposed.

Size of image   The laser scans a 14×17 inch film producing an area of 4096×5120 pixels; a total of 21 million pixels. This would accommodate about twenty 1024×1024 images from a CT, MRI etc. Each line of pixels (4096) is exposed in approximately 3.8ms so

the time required to expose the complete film area is about 20s. The He-Ne laser produces red light (630nm) so special red-sensitive film is necessary. Dry laser imagers which do not rely on photographic principles use opaque carbon or silver based film stock. The laser removes small areas of this opaque material forming an image equal to or superior than the quality of a wet (photographic) laser film imager.

Gray scale   the exposure density of each pixel is determined by the signal strength at that point. The image signal modulates the intensity of the laser beam through an Acoustic Optical Modulator (AOM) which contains a crystal transducer. An electrical signal is converted into an acoustic signal which changes the refractive index of the crystal scattering the light at different angles from the main beam, so reducing the main beam intensity. The scatter intensity depends on the size of the acoustic signal. The main beam passes through a small slot which blocks the scattered light from reaching the film surface. The AOM operates with a 12bit resolution.

Laser beam diameter The size of the laser dot which exposes the film is critical for producing good spatial resolution (Fig 8.27(b)) and misplacement of the spot leads to lost image detail (Fig.8.27(c)). The laser beam passes through a lens system which gives a typical beam diameter of 85μm giving an image matrix size of typically 4096× 5120 pixels, representing 12 pixels mm^{-1}.

A line error deviation of 3% requires a laser beam placement accuracy of ±1.3μm. The mechanical precision is therefore very high and vibration must be prevented over the exposure 20s exposure time. Look-up tables within the digital control can give a truly linear or various non-linear scales.

The disadvantage of the laser imager is the fixed image matrix size. Multiple images would share the total 4096×5120 matrix. High definition (1024/1249 line) video images in multi-format (4×5 image set) would only just be faithfully recorded. Specifications for a typical laser imager are given in Table 8.11

Table 8.11 Laser imager specifications

Laser type	Helium/Neon
Film	Red Sensitive
Film sizes (inches)	8×10, 11×14, 14×17
Modulation depth (gray scale)	12 bits
Pixels on 14"×17" film	4096× 5120
Processor cycle	48 - 60s
Number of inputs	4

KEYWORDS

anisoplanasy: resolution varying over the tube face.

Bucky factor: exposure increase factor when using a grid.

contrast: film: the slope of the characteristic curve: film gamma.

contrast: image: relative measure of density differences

contrast: subject: absolute measure of intensity differences.

contrast: visual: absolute measure of log intensity differences.

contrast detail diagram: graphic display comparing contrast and resolution.

contrast improvement factor: improvement of contrast when grid is used.

detective quantum efficiency (DQE): comparison of input and output signal to noise ratios.

dynamic range: range of exposure levels that can be displayed or recorded.

film speed: film sensitivity measured for an optical density =1.

grid factor: increase in exposure when grid is used (see also Bucky factor)

grid line density: number of lead strips in an anti-scatter grid per centimeter.

grid ratio: ratio of grid height to interspace distance.

illuminance: reflected light intensity in *lux*.

interlacing: a method for reducing the bandwidth necessary to give a video display. Fields are interlaced to give each frame.

line pairs: resolution measurement using a grating of paired light and dark lines

line spread function: a count profile taken through a line strip on a display.

line standard: the standard number of video lines in a display i.e. 525, 625,1024, 1249 etc.

luminance: the light intensity given by a source measured in candela.

modulation transfer function (MTF): a complete description of the display resolution Derived from the PSF or LSF.

Nyquist frequency: the minimum frequency at which a signal must be sampled to prevent signal distortion.

phosphor: a compound exhibiting luminescence

point spread function (PSF): the count profile through a displayed point source.

quantum mottle: random noise exhibited by a display system.

resolution: spatial: the minimum distance required by a display to resolve two point sources

resolution: temporal: the ability to separate two events in time

selectivity: ratio of transmission of primary and scatter radiation

signal to noise ratio (SNR): the displayed signal divided by the standard deviation of signal noise.

spatial non-uniformity: irregular response to radiation across the input field of view.

unsharpness: geometric: penumbra associated with an edge or point source due to geometrical factors: focal spot or source to object or source to detector distances.

unsharpness: movement: display penumbra due to movement.

unsharpness: radiographic: display penumbra due to image detector properties

vignetting: reduced energy transfer on the periphery of the field of view

9

Special procedures: Low kilovoltage, high kilovoltage imaging

9.1 Low kilovoltage imaging
9.2 High kilovoltage imaging

9.1 LOW KILOVOLTAGE: IMAGING

Radiography commonly employs x-ray energies between 50 and 80kVp but special imaging requirements sometimes utilize the particular properties offered by lower (25-40kVp) and higher (125-140kVp) x-ray photon energies. Lower energies ensure that photoelectric events are dominant, even in soft tissues, giving maximum subject contrast. It is very effective for differentiating soft tissue detail but is only practical for tissue thick-nesses of a few centimeters; its most impor-tant application is mammography.

The practical x-ray energy for mammo-graphy is 25 to 30kV which ensures photo-electric events are dominant. Although the spectrum embraces lower photon energies of ~15kV these are preferentially absorbed with-in the tissue. Higher energies (>30kV) do not contribute to image contrast so are not util-ized. Higher kV imaging energies rely on Compton interactions which allow a broad range of tissue types (bone and soft tissue) to be represented on the image. Fig.9.1 shows relative contributions from photoelectric and Compton events for mammography (shaded column). The double hatched region is the voltage range 100-120keV which relies almost entirely on Compton reactions for image formation.

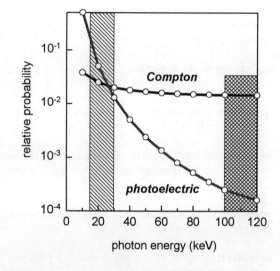

Figure 9.1 The probability for photoelectric and Compton reactions changes with photon energy. At mammography energies (single hatching) the photoelectric dominates but at high kV's (double hatching) image formation depends on Compton events.

9.1.1 Low kV interactions

It has been seen from Chapter 5 that the major factors which emphasize photon ab-sorption differences in tissue (subject contrast) are kilovoltage, linear attenuation coefficient and tissue thickness. Very similar soft tissues in the breast require low kilovoltage imaging so maximizing photoelectric effects (PE) which are most sensitive to even small tissue differences.

Photoelectric absorption τ is influenced by tissue density, atomic number ($Z \sim 7.4$) and photon energy E. Photoelectric absorption for soft tissue decreases rapidly with increasing energy, this can be seen over the shaded portion of Fig.9.1. The steep portion of the linear attenuation coefficient curve is predominantly due to photoelectric interactions where:

$$\tau \propto \frac{Z^3}{E^3} \qquad (9.1)$$

Tissue absorption Tissue thickness considerably influences photon transmission at low kilovoltages. The photon transmission for a tissue thickness of 5cm is plotted in Fig.9.2 and shows that for photon energies between 20 and 30kVp the transmitted photon fraction is between 3 and 35%, being about 20% at practical kilovoltage levels of 28kVeff.

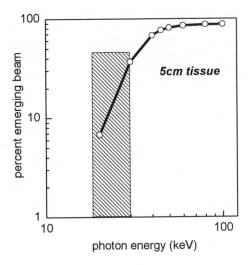

Figure 9.2 Photon transmission through 5cm soft tissue. The shaded area identifies the mammography energy range.

Dense breasts would have even less transmission. Tissue thickness plays a very important part in mammography and tissue (breast) compression significantly improves photon transmission. It also reduces scatter radiation which increases significantly with tissue thickness degrading subject contrast.

9.1.2 Mammography x-ray systems

In order to achieve the best image quality at low kV, for minimum patient dose, all aspects of machine design must be optimized to give the best quality image for minimum patient radiation dose. Important design points are:

- x-ray tube construction
- efficient generator supply
- tissue compression
- automatic dose control

The overall design for a mammography x-ray tube is shown in Fig.9.3(a). Cooling problems are not as serious as conventional x-ray tubes and a surrounding oil bath is not necessary since forced air cooling is adequate. A list of x-ray tube specifications is given in Tab.9.1 for two common types.

The x-ray tube window must be made from low density material in order to transmit the low energy photons. A glass window would be too dense and be a significant absorber so a beryllium insert is commonly used. Tubes having a metal construction (stainless steel and glass) are now common.

Focal spot The mammography x-ray tube gives two focal spot sizes 0.4mm for surface and 0.1mm for magnification imaging. The effective dimensions vary across the beam width and Fig.9.3(a) shows the focal spot can be quite broad at the edge of the beam near the cathode (chest wall) but improves toward the tube-anode (central area of the breast).

Anode Anode construction is shown in Fig. 9.3(b) The common form of x-ray tube design uses a molybdenum anode to give useful K-edge peaks in the spectrum at 17keV

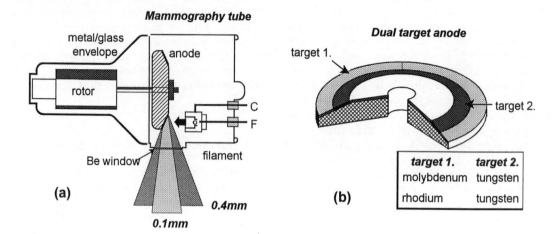

Figure 9.3   **(a)** General x-ray tube design showing very close positioning of cathode and anode. Dual focal spots are achieved here by cathode focusing. The beryllium window has a very low absorption factor for these low kV x-rays. **(b)** A dual target anode giving both molybdenum and tungsten targets which gives optimum image quality for different breast thicknesses.

and 20keV as shown in Fig.9.4(a), however more efficient x-ray production is obtained from a tungsten anode which is shown for comparison. (efficiency for Mo = 0.09% and W = 0.16% at 20kV; see Chap.3)

X-ray spectrum   The spectral shapes of molybdenum and tungsten are compared in Fig. 9.4(a); both have useful properties. Molybdenum anodes have characteristic radiation at 17 and 20keV which comprise 19 to 29% of the output intensity giving peak output in the most valuable part of the spectrum. Tungsten, having a higher atomic number, improves x-ray intensity overall.

Table 9.1 shows that a molybdenum target has lower ratings than tungsten but since it provides useful characteristic line spectra it is retained by some manufacturers who provide a twin anode design having targets of both molybdenum and tungsten.

Cathode - filament   Designs for the filament cathode assembly are shown in Fig.9.4(b) to (d). These use either a double wound filament to increase the electron density (b) or a flat ribbon filament (d). Circular filaments at short distances from the anode can give an unfocussed beam of electrons causing penumbra formation on the target.

Since the electron cloud tends to concentrate on the edges of the filament the cross section of the electron beam is not uniform but has a 'camel's hump' profile shown in Fig.9.4(c). This shape forms two areas of high intensity on the anode surface instead of just one which effectively gives two focal spots side by side. These mutually interfere giving another source of geometrical unsharpness and seriously limiting image resolution. A flat section filament minimizes this problem.

Different focal spot sizes are selected by either a negative bias on the cathode which re-focuses the electrons, or by using dual filaments focused on two target areas.

Space charge effect   Space charge problems at low kilovoltage reduce the maximum available tube current regardless of extra filament heating. As a consequence filament design is optimized to give sharp electron beam shapes already seen in Fig.9.4(d).

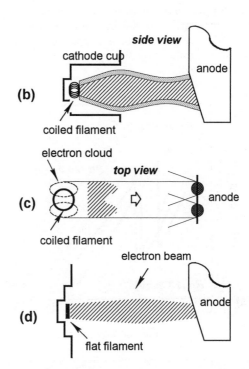

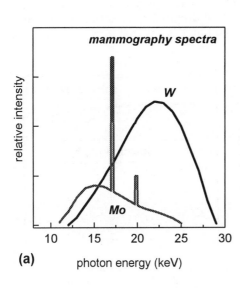

(a)

Figure 9.4 **(a)** X-ray beam spectra for molybdenum and tungsten targets used in mammography. The characteristic x-rays of molybdenum are a significant part of the spectrum. Tungsten gives more intensity at a higher effective energy. **(b)** Cathode assembly with coiled filament giving a broad electron beam with shadowing **(c)** this also gives a 'camel-hump' profile generating two focal areas **(d)** the flat filament gives a more tightly focused uniform beam.

Electrical compensation circuits are necessary for adjusting the filament current when changing low kVp settings, this overcomes space charge effects on tube current for different kV settings.

Table 9.1 Mammography tube specifications.

Specification	Molybdenum	Tungsten
Anode diam. (mm)	100	100
Target Angle	22°	22°
Focal Spot (mm)	0.15/0.4	0.1/0.4
Loading (kW)	0.9/6.5	1.3/9.5
Maximum mA at 30kV	Fine 26	36
	Broad 185	250
Heat Storage	200kJ	300kJ
	(270kHU)	(400kHU)

Filters (K-edge) Beam quality (HVL) incident on the breast depends on the thickness and composition of the compression paddle and the fixed filtration employed. The HVL of a 30kV x-ray beam should lie within 0.3 to 0.4mm. Higher HVL's indicate a higher effective kV, which is not useful since it will reduce overall photoelectric effect resulting in loss of image contrast. Employing suitable filters whose K-edges fall within the mammography kV range (Rh 23.2, Pd 24.4, Mo 20.0keV shown in Fig.9.5(a)) effectively reduces higher photon energies from the x-ray beam. The use of K-edge filtration is shown in Fig.9.5(b) where molybdenum and rhodium give a spectrum shape which restricts the higher energies above the K-edge, so reducing patient dose.

Generator kV plays a minor role in deciding effective energy. So K-edge filtered spectra offer precise energies over a narrow spectrum range and significantly reduce the less useful high kV energies.

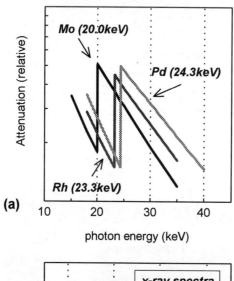

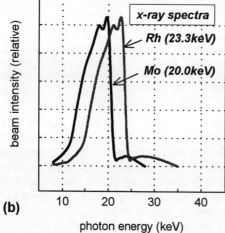

Figure 9.5 **(a)** Attenuation curves for molybdenum, palladium and rhodium showing their K-edges. **(b)** Two K-edge filtered spectra for molybdenum and rhodium commonly employed in mammography machines

Generator (high frequency) Due to space charge effects adequate tube current is a problem in low kV studies. Low power

generators (single or 3-phase) with limited tube current (<200mA) overcome this limitation by increasing exposure time to achieve the required mAs value. This has two serious disadvantages, the loss of image resolution due to movement unsharpness and reduced film density due to reciprocity loss.

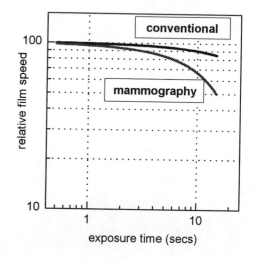

Figure 9.6 Reciprocity losses in the film image for extended exposure times.

Reciprocity losses Figure 9.6 compares loss of film speed due to reciprocity effects in mammography and conventional radiography. For exposure times longer than 2s reciprocity losses become serious. These losses are not so evident in conventional work. When higher tube currents are required at low kVp's the filament must be raised to much higher temperatures to maintain the mA value. This is the rating restriction seen previously (Chapter 4) as the flattened curve at 20, 30, 40kV.

At low anode kV's especially for strongly focused small focal spots (0.1mm magnification) tube current is essentially space charge limited which can be improved by increasing filament area (double filaments) and decreasing the cathode anode distance. Alternative filament designs have already been seen in Fig.9.4. Tube current cannot be

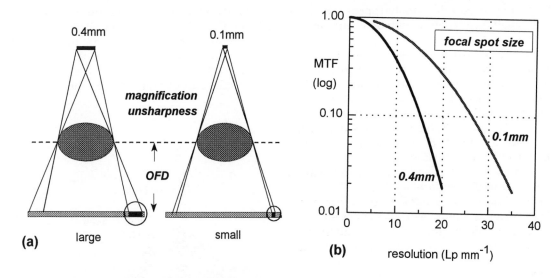

Figure 9.7 **(a)** Geometrical unsharpness for 0.4mm and 0.1mm focal spots showing loss of resolution for magnification views (large object to film distance). **(b)** The MTF curves for 0.4 and 0.1mm. The 20% cutoff is at 10 and 22Lp mm^{-1} respectively.

increased by raising the filament temperature and attempting to increase available electrons. Modern high frequency generators (5-10kHz) are able to deliver tube currents up to 300mA, allowing much shorter exposures.

Summary of low kilovoltage techniques
Disadvantages

- Conflicts with the practice of high kV to reduce patient dose.
- X-ray tube operates inefficiently at low kV's
- High filament current
- Low tube current
- Extended exposure times
- Heel effect for small anode angles.
- Image non-uniformity (resolution and contrast)
- Scatter radiation problems
- Intensifying screen low sensitivity
- Primary beam absorption by cassette

Advantages:

- Scatter radiation easily absorbed
- Very high resolution

- Good contrast between soft tissues
- Staff radiation dose low

9.1.3 Mammography image quality

Although photoelectric reactions are dominant in mammography some weak Compton scatter is present (Fig. 9.1(a)). Very few of these low energy scatter events reach the film surface since they are easily absorbed within the tissue. This has been discussed in Chapter 5. Scatter photon attenuation over the diagnostic range is very effectively absorbed by tissue at low energies giving only a small scatter component at the film/image surface. The scatter photons reaching the film increase above 30kV as tissue attenuation coefficient plays a less important role.

Unsharpness and magnification Magnification is commonly used in mammography to increase resolution for equivocal regions. This is achieved by decreasing FOD. The increased unsharpness can be minimized if the focal spot size is reduced from 0.4 to

0.1mm. Comparative unsharpness for large and small focal spots is demonstrated in Fig. 9.7(a).

The improvement in image resolution can be measured by comparing the MTF for the two focal spot sizes 0.4mm and 0.1mm Fig. 9.7(b). Since the anode loading increases for 0.1mm the tube rating is smaller for magnification views (as seen in Table 9.1 for maximum mA at 30kV for fine and broad focal spots) and fine focus is not used routinely. Box 9.1 estimates the smallest visible detail with a 0.4mm and 0.1mm focal spot.

Patient dose also increases due to decreased FOD (inverse square law). Focal spot size does not visibly influence resolution with surface contact (non magnification) imaging.

Box 9.1

Unsharpness for mammography

$$FFD = 60\text{cm}$$
$$d = 28\text{cm (magnification)}$$
$$F = 0.4\text{mm}$$

$$\frac{s}{F} = \frac{d}{FFD - d}$$

$$s = \frac{F \times d}{FFD - d} \qquad (9.2)$$

$$s = (0.4 \times 280)/(600{-}280) = 0.35\text{mm}$$

The 350μm penumbra would seriously reduce the ability to see 100 μm micro-calcifications.
A focal spot of 0.1mm reduces this unsharpness to 0.08mm (80 μm) so surface imaging uses 0.4mm and magnification 0.1mm focal spots.

Cassette design The cassette design used for mammography is shown in Fig. 9.8. Since the x-ray photon, at low kVs is preferentially absorbed within the first few microns of the screen surface it is important that very close contact is made between the single film emulsion and the screen. In some instances

the film and screen are vacuum packed to achieve this. The illustration shows that the x-ray beam is directed through the back of the film, passing first through the emulsion before interacting with the screen surface whose light output then exposes the film.

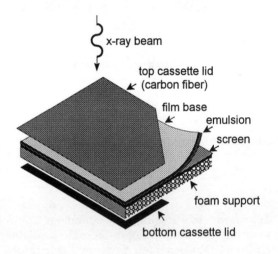

Figure 9.8 Film screen cassette construction showing single emulsion film lying face down on the intensifying screen phosphor.

Scatter and grids Low energy photons are scattered isotropically so the anti-scatter grid used in mammography has a low ratio; $h/D = 4$ or 5. Efficiency is improved by using a grid focused to 60cm with lead septa density 27-50 lines cm^{-1}. Its construction is shown in Fig.9.9(a).

The grid factor (the ratio between incident and transmitted radiation) is kept as low as possible (approximately 2) by using thin septa; these are typically <20μm thick. The grid height h is typically <1mm. Specifications for two mammography grids are given in Tab.9.2 where septa thickness d, grid height h and spacer thickness D are compared.

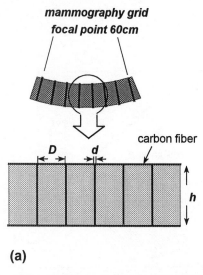

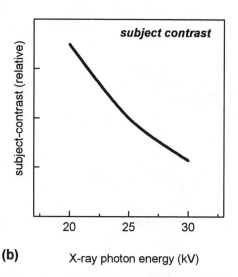

Figure 9.9 **(a)** Focused grid and construction used for mammography showing lead-septa thickness d, carbon fiber dividers D and carbon fiber top and bottom plates. The height h is typically 0.7 to 1.0mm **(b)** The change in subject contrast with kV between soft tissue and fat from the difference in linear attenuation coefficient values.

Table 9.2 Two grid specifications (in mm)

Grid	d	h	D	Pb%
4/27	0.05	1.2	0.32	13.5
5/44	0.016	1.0	0.21	7.0

Contrast Subject contrast can be estimated by subtracting the attenuation coefficients for soft tissue and fat; the result is plotted in Fig.9.9(b). Differences between like tissues can be best distinguished at low photon energies but Fig.9.2 has already demonstrated that transmission is poor at low energies so a compromise energy must be chosen at about 28kV giving good transmission while retaining sufficient image contrast for diagnostic quality images. Atomic number Z, tissue density and thickness all play an important part in subject contrast.

The heel effect This is more pronounced in mammography where small anode angles are used. Figure 9.10(a) illustrates the heel effect in mammography. The beam intensity decreases quite rapidly toward the anode end of the tube. The focal spot dimensions also vary across the field of view giving poorer resolution at the chest wall. The magnitude of the heel effect is plotted in Fig.9.10(b). At the nipple region of the breast the beam intensity has dropped to 60% of maximum but the focal spot dimensions still enable optimum resolution

In order to reduce the heel effect on the image the tube itself is angled placing the cathode over the chest wall (nearest patient) where greater intensity is needed; the anode is further from the patient.

9.1.4 Patient radiation dose

The high proportion of photoelectric absorption is responsible for potential high patient radiation dose. Absorption of low energy scatter within the tissue also increases dose. This is a problem with low kV imaging. In order to reduce it to optimum levels (lowest dose versus diagnostic quality image) the major

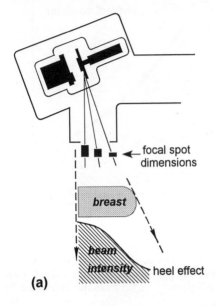
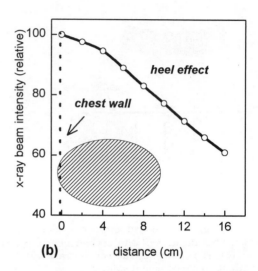

(a)
(b)   distance (cm)

Figure 9.10   **(a)** The combined alteration in focal spot dimension and heel effect from the edge of the support plate. The focal spot is larger at the cathode end and decreases toward the anode. **(b)** The heel effect for a typical mammography machine operating with a 0.4mm focal spot.

factors influencing patient dose must be carefully controlled:

- Tissue thickness (breast compression)
- X-ray beam quality
- Detector sensitivity

Breast compression   A plastic paddle parallel with the support surface compresses the breast and maintains uniform tissue thickness. This improves image resolution throughout the breast volume by reducing object-to-film distance (OFD) and reducing geometrical unsharpness. Subject contrast is also improved due to scatter reduction within the breast volume.

Tissue compression also significantly lowers patient radiation dose by minimizing photon scatter since is low energy and would be absorbed. The high fraction of photoelectric absorption by the primary beam is responsible for potential high patient radiation dose in mammography, so photon density must be reduced for minimum radiation dose therefore mammography uses the most sensitive film-screen units for maximum efficiency. Patient dose is also influenced by anode material and filters.

Patient radiation dose is strongly influenced by the choice of grid, cassette, screen and film so that there is efficient capture of all emerging x-ray photons for image formation. Grid septa thickness has already been discussed and efficiency can be further increased by using carbon fiber for all non-metal construction grid and cassette. Film sensitivity can be improved by using longer film processor times and an elevated developer temperature.

Entrance dose   The dose at the surface of the patient can be measured directly with a dosimeter. Measurements of surface dose usually assume soft tissue or a soft tissue equivalent material (plastic or water).

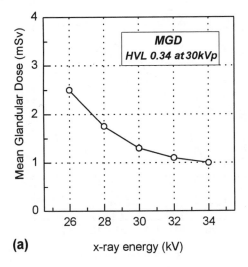

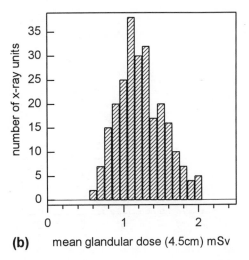

(a)   x-ray energy (kV)   **(b)**   mean glandular dose (4.5cm) mSv

Figure 9.11   **(a)** The Mean Glandular Dose decreasing with increasing beam energy (kV) **(b)** a histogram of the MGD obtained for a group of breast screening centers showing a mean value of about 1.3mGy.

The beam energy (effective or peak) and the beam's half-value-layer (HVL) must be known since low energy photons will be preferentially absorbed in the surface layers. Any dose measured at the surface of the patient will include a fraction from photons back-scattered from deeper tissue layers. This is the Back Scatter Fraction (BSF). This contribution to the entrance dose is not present when simple air readings are taken without a patient or suitable phantom being present in the beam. The terms entrance exposure and entrance surface dose are sometimes used to distinguish measurements made with and without BSF correction respectively.

Mean Glandular Dose Glandular tissues receive varying doses depending on:

- Depth from the skin entrance site
- Beam quality (kV and filtration)
- Breast thickness
- Breast consistency
- Optical density of the mammogram

The mean glandular dose (MGD) to the standard breast for a standard optical film density allows direct comparison between different mammography systems. It also allows a better estimation of risk to the patient. The standard breast which is used for these measurements comprises a 50:50 mixture of adipose and glandular equivalent material with a superficial adipose layer of 0.5cm giving an overall thickness of 5cm which represents the average compressed breast. The mean glandular dose is energy dependent as shown in Fig.9.11(a) which is a plot of MGD for effective beam energies from 26 to 34keV at the stated HVL.

Factors used in the MGD calculation which relate entrance exposure values to the average MGD have been measured by several workers. The breast phantom is exposed for optimum image quality having a mean background optical density of 1.5. The incident air kerma K is obtained in Grays. These factors depend on the x-ray tube target material and the beam HVL. The glandular dose is then obtained for the air kerma value K as:

$$MGD = K \times p \times g \qquad (9.3)$$

Factors p and g are conversion values obtained from tables for the HVL as measured an example is given in Tab.9.3.

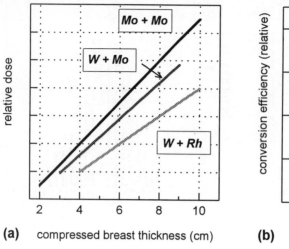

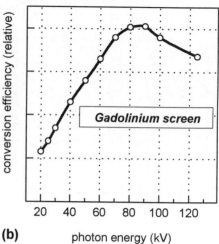

(a) compressed breast thickness (cm)   (b)   photon energy (kV)

Figure 9.12   **(a)** Breast surface dose increase with tissue thickness for different anode and K-filter combinations. **(b)**   Intensifying screen conversion efficiency variation with photon energy.

The MGD to the standard breast should not exceed 5mGy and more recent reports suggest 3mGy. Surveys of MGD values using current equipment now give recommendations that values should not exceed 1.3mGy for the standard breast.

Figure 9.11(b) indicates the range of MGD values published by a number of breast screening centers confirming the new recommended limit of 1.3mGy

Table 9.3 Conversion values for MGD

HVL	p	g (mGy Gy^{-1})
0.30	1.10	183
0.35	1.10	208
0.40	1.09	232
0.45	1.09	258
0.50	1.09	285

The anode target material also has a significant effect on overall dose to the tissue and Fig. 9.12(a) shows the level of dose reduction given by various combinations of molybdenum and tungsten targets with K-edge filtration.

Film-screen type The single screen/single emulsion design gives a very high efficiency and superior resolution. Figure 9.7(b) has shown the potential resolution using 0.4 and 0.1mm focal spots can exceed 20Lp mm^{-1}. Mammography film/screens can almost match this giving approximately 20Lp mm^{-1} as against 5-10Lp mm^{-1} for high detail conventional radiography. Screen materials are almost always rare earth, although these show a reduced sensitivity for low kV photons Fig. 9.12(b).

9.1.5 Automatic Exposure Control (AEC)

The conventional AEC (photo-timer) would use an ionization chamber placed in the primary beam. If used at low kV's it would absorb a significant proportion of x-ray photons so a different procedure is used. A very sensitive balanced detector is placed behind the film cassette; the arrangement is shown in Fig.9.13(a).   These are twin detectors in a sandwich design comprising 2 detectors (D1 and D2) separated by a metal filter. The output signals from D1 and D2 are

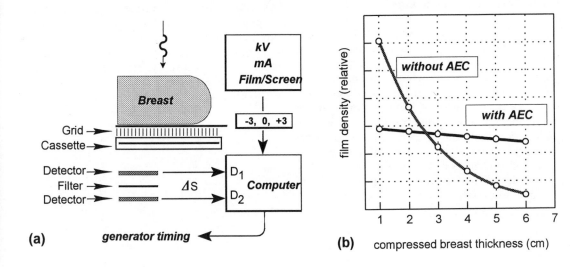

Figure 9.13 **(a)** Typical AEC design for mammography showing balanced detectors placed beneath the film cassette. **(b)** Graph showing constant image density for increasing breast thicknesses. The image density would sharply decrease without automatic exposure control.

electrically balanced; detector D2 behind its beam hardening filter acts as a reference. Any small change in low kV photon flux caused by a change in breast density influences D1 more than D2 and a signal difference will be given. The magnitude of this difference signal controls the film exposure (mAs value). Information concerning screen and film sensitivity, kilovoltage and tube current influence this difference signal to give an optimum exposure value for all variables.

The film density is kept quite constant for a wide range of breast thicknesses. Fig. 9.13(b) shows the difference between exposure levels with and without this automatic exposure device (photo-timer). The controlled range (black line) shows very little variation in film density for a 1-6cm variation in breast thickness. The film density can be varied by the operator; this is the +3,0,–3 density control in the illustration.

Table 9.4 lists the minimum requirements for a mammography unit that would be used for a screening program.

Table 9.4 Specification for mammography unit.

X-ray Tube:	Current rated >200mA for short exposure times
Focal Spot:	0.4 and 0.1mm
Generator:	High frequency with feedback control for kV, mA and time.
FFD:	60cm
Filters:	Automatic K-edge filter change with kV (Mo Rh Al).
AEC:	Compensation for kV film screen and breast thickness
Compression	Motor driven (150N max.)
Grid:	5:1 to 4:1 27 - 40 lines cm^{-1}

9.1.6 Basic machine design

Figure 9.14 shows the essential features of a modern mammography machine itemized in Tab.9.4. The x-ray tube is commonly tilted to angle the x-ray beam which minimizes heel effect problems which are encountered with small focal spot sizes. Tissue compression is obtained by using a thin plastic compression paddle so that the breast has a uniform thickness. This significantly reduces patient dose and improves image quality by reducing geometrical unsharpness (object to film distance minimal).

Automatic exposure control (AEC) is obtained by placing the detector under the support plate, grid and film cassette, in this way there is no added absorber between the cassette and the x-ray beam. At low kilo-voltages even the thin walls of the AEC ionization chamber would offer significant absorption.

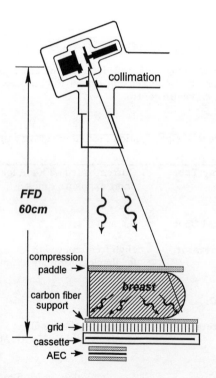

Figure 9.14 Overall design for a mammography x-ray set showing angled x-ray tube positioned 60-65cm from the image plane, the compression paddle of thin plastic and the automatic exposure device under the cassette

9.2   HIGH KILOVOLTAGE IMAGING

The use of x-ray photons with energies in excess of 100kVp presents several important advantages in diagnostic imaging. High kV is widely used where different tissue types are being imaged (bone, soft tissue or iodine/ barium contrast materials). High kV techniques give fast exposure times which freeze motion (movement unsharpness) due to either patient movement (during breath hold) or cardiac motion. The common applications are found in:

- Chest radiography,
- Fluoroscopy (gastro-intestinal tract)
- Obstetric pelvis
- Lumbar and dorsal spine investigations.
- Computed tomography (CT)
- Digital subtraction angiography (DSA)

9.2.1 Subject contrast

Above 70kV tissue interactions are predominantly Compton and image formation relies on the primary beam being scattered away from the image plane in its passage through the body. A high ratio grid is necessary to block this radiation from reaching the film since unlike low kV imaging it travels in a forward direction.

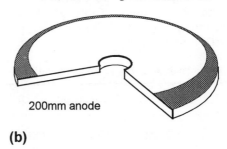

dual target 100mm anode

target 1.
target 2.
← Graphite

(a)

double bearing all metal anode

200mm anode

(b)

Figure 9.15 **(a)** Anode design for high voltage uses a dual focus anode between 100-200mm diameter. Graphite increases the radiation surface. **(b)** A large diameter anode used in dual bearing tubes with sleeve bearings where the majority heat loss is by conduction.

Since image formation is dependent on Compton scatter the subject contrast depends on electron density and not atomic number and bone appears more transparent. This property is exploited in chest radiography where the rib cage is rendered more transparent.

X-ray intensity and FFD It has been seen in Chapter 3 that increasing the tube kilovoltage increases the intensity of bremsstrahlung production as kV^2. The overall effect on film blackening is further influenced since the proportion of radiation transmitted by the patient (and so reaching the film) is increased and the intensifying screen response to higher energy photons is greater. At higher kVs (above 80kV) film density doubles for every 15kV. The increased x-ray intensity at high kilovoltages has a valuable practical application: to maintain the same mAs value the exposure time can be greatly reduced - typically 20mS for chest radiography; movement unsharpness is therefore not a problem. Table 9.5 demonstrates how, by increasing kilovoltage but keeping the tube

current the same, the required mAs can be achieved by shortening exposure times. This produces anode rating problems, however, since only a part of the available target length will be used for these very fast exposure times unless fast anode rotational speeds are used.

Table 9.5 X-ray intensity increases as kV^2

kV	Current (mA)	mAs	time (s)
60	200	20	0.1
80	200	11	0.055
100	200	7	0.035
120	200	5	0.025

9.2.2 High kilovoltage machine design

X-ray tube The two anode designs shown in Fig.9.15(a),(b) are for heavy duty use (high loadability). The first has a diameter of 100mm and graphite backing where heat dissipation is predominantly by radiation. The second anode has a 200mm diameter designed for a double sleeve bearing where heat loss is by conduction through the bearing itself. These two factors enable the anode to have a very high thermal rating since both these tubes are operated at near maximum specification. Table 9.6 lists the specifications for 3 tube types: chest, fluoro/DSA and CT.

Table 9.6   High kV x-ray tube specifications

	Chest	Fluoro.-DSA	CT
Heat	600kHU	1.35kHU	3.5MHU
Focus	1.2	0.6/1.0	1.6
Power	450W	2kW	30kW

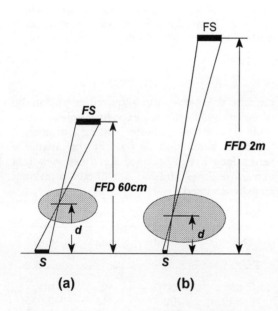

Figure 9.16 (a) Image unsharpness (S) is a major problem at short FFD's **(b)** Increasing the FFD decreases the unsharpness for the same focal spot size (FS).

Focal spot size   The size of the focal spot can be larger than those in low-kV imaging since the FFD can be 70 to 200cm. Chest radiography is the least limited since at an FFD of 200cm a 2mm focal spot will give an unsharpness of only 0.2mm using eqn. 9.2

from Box 9.1 and recalculating image unsharpness for an FFD of 2m. Box 9.2 demonstrates that small detail is not lost even with focal spot sizes of 2mm. Figure 9.16(a) and (b) indicates the degree of unsharpness S for short and long FFD's and how, in the case of mammography, deep lesion (large values of d) resolution can be lost. At an FFD of 200cm the anode angle should be at least 11° for full coverage of the thorax.

Grids   Low energy oblique scatter in mammography can be stopped by employing a low ratio grid (Pb 3.5/77 or Pb 5/44) as illustrated in Fig.9.17(a). High ratio grids are necessary to reduce the amount of forward high energy scatter reaching the film in the chest radiograph (Pb 16/44). These are usually parallel grids since high ratio focused grids are difficult to align. High voltage fluoroscopy uses lower ratio focused grids (Pb 8 or 12/44) which can produce problems with high resolution (1000×1000) digital matrices.

A 125-133kV chest radiograph exposure time is about 20ms using a large FFD. A valuable diagnostic property of high kV chest imaging is the easy penetration of the mediastinal regions.

Box 9.2

Chest radiography at 2 meters FFD
(from Fig.9.16)

FFD	= 200cm
d (OFD)	= 12cm
FS	= 2mm

From eqn. 9.2 (Box 9.1)

$$s = 2 \times 120/2000 - 120 = 0.12\text{mm}$$

A focal spot of 2mm will give adequate resolution. In practice the focal spot is typically 1.6mm.

Tube rating   For the short exposure times given in Tab.9.4 an anode revolving at 300rpm will make one revolution in 20ms; at shorter exposure times only a fraction of the target will be used so the entire electrical

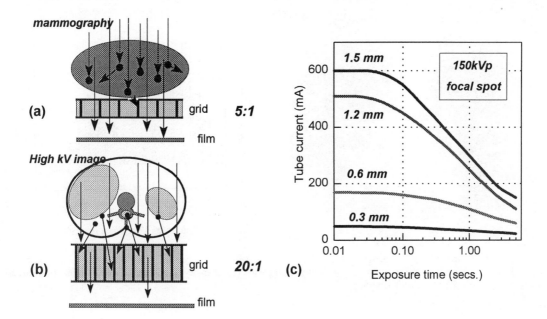

Figure 9.17 **(a)** Grids used for low kilovoltages have a low ratio of 5:1 since scatter is oblique. **(b)** high kV radiography requires high ratio grids 20:1 to stop the forward scatter. **(c)** The electrical rating for an x-ray tube operating at high kV decreases with focal spot size.

energy is dissipated only over a small area. For this reason increasing anode diameter can improve the tube's rating. Since these x-ray tubes are operating at near their maximum rating heat dissipation is of prime importance. The focal spot size influences the tube loadability as shown by the family of electrical rating curves in Fig.9.17(b). Increasing anode loadability can be achieved by:

- Large diameter anodes
- Fast rotation speeds
- Ceramic metal housing
- Sleeve bearing instead of ball-bearings

Automatic exposure control This is provided by an ionization chamber positioned in front of the cassette. This is transparent to the x-ray beam at higher kilovoltages. More than one ion chamber can be used as already seen in Chapter 6. Because of the greater penetration, less absorbed and shorter exposure times the patient dose is low in high kV work, typically 20-100µGy for a chest radiograph.

9.2.3 Image quality

Resolution Since image formation is dependent on scatter the image resolution is poorer than mammography. Fig 9.18(a) shows a high kV chest radiograph whose resolution is approximately 2Lp mm^{-1}, the limit for high kV imaging without contrast media.

Subject contrast At high kilovoltage this depends on differing electron densities between tissues. It has already been seen in Chapter 8 that for photoelectric reactions there is a wide contrast between the different tissues (muscle, fat and bone) however subject contrast due to Compton scatter

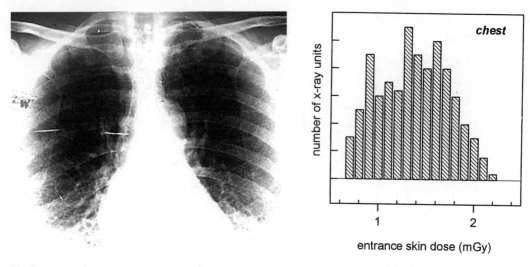

Figure 9.18 (a) Chest radiograph (CXR) using 125kVp at 5mAs. The rib cage is relatively transparent allowing a clear view of the lung fields. (b) The range of entrance skin doses measured from a large number of chest units.

obeys the approximate rule:

$$\rho \times \frac{electron\ density}{kV} \qquad (9.4)$$

where ρ is tissue density; it is independent of the atomic number Z. Soft tissue differences are reduced and also bone will be more transparent allowing features behind to be observed. Air (as with the photoelectric effect) is virtually transparent and would give a dense black shadow. These points are particularly valuable in high kV chest radiographs where the rib cage is more transparent allowing visibility of the full lung fields. Pneumo-thorax would be a black shadow.

High kV fluoroscopy using dense iodine or barium contrast materials depend on photoelectric reaction in these high Z materials to give fine details. Very fast exposure times of 10 to 20ms freeze all involuntary movement; movement unsharpness is almost zero. CT images depend almost entirely on Compton interactions for image formation; very sensitive electronic detectors replace film. These are tightly collimated to remove scatter events in the same way as high ratio grids. Comparisons between low and high kV imaging techniques are summarized in Table 9.7. Photoelectric reactions preferentially occur at low kilovoltages and the primary beam photon is removed entirely. Their probability increases with the atomic number Z of the absorber. Total photon absorption is very effective in producing a high contrast image.

Compton reactions decrease slightly with energy (eqn. 9.4) and they are not influenced by absorber Z. Scatter photons are produced that travel at narrow angles to the primary beam and are removed by high ratio anti-scatter grids. Compton reactions depend on the electron density in the absorber and are less dependent on photon energy above a certain threshold (~80kV).

Patient dose When comparing entrance surface doses there is a very wide range between analog and digital radiography. The fastest film/screens used in conjuction with high-kilovoltage systems (140-160kVp) give about 700µGy and image phosphor plates return approximately the same value.

Large field of view image intensifier units using either digital output or 100mm cut film cameras give an entrance dose of about 100μGy. Figure 9.18(b) indicates typical surface doses from a wide range of chest x-ray units usinng a mixture of film/screen combinations and using kilovoltages ranging from 110 to 140kVp. There is a considerable spread of values over the 1-2mGY range but a fair number of units are capable of doses below 1mGy

Table 9.7 Overall properties of low and high kV techniques.

	LOW kilovoltage (25-30kV)	*HIGH kilovoltage (100-150kV)*
X-ray Tube		
Focal spot	small 0.4 and 0.1mm	medium 0.6mm/large 1.6mm
Anode material	molybdenum or tungsten	tungsten with graphite or large diameter.
Filament	double	single
Tube Current	limited (space charge effect)	large
Exposure Time	long	very short
Unsharpness		
Geometrical	FFD 60cm. FS critical	FFD to 200cm. FS not critical
Movement	Present. Long exposure times	Not present. Very short times
Grid		
Ratio	4	12 to 15
Factor	<2	<4
Film		
Emulsion	single	double
Contrast	high	variable
Intensifying Screens		
Number	single	double
Thickness	thin	thin and thick
Sensitivity	low	high
Film processor		
Developer	35°C	34-37°C
Time	3 minutes	choice
Film image		
Contrast	high	low-medium
Resolution (Lp mm^{-1})	20	2 to 5
Noise/Mottle	low	fair-poor
Patient dose		
Organ	high	low
Whole body	low	low

10

Fluoroscopy

10.1 Fluoroscopic image

10.2 Performance parameters

10.3 The fluoroscopy system

10.4 Feedback controls

10.5 Specific system designs

10.1   FLUOROSCOPIC IMAGE

Conventional film radiography is restricted to static patient investigations. If dynamic events need to be studied i.e. movement of contrast material through blood vessels or the gut, the image must be viewed directly using fluoroscopic methods.

The earliest fluoroscopic systems used phosphor screens when the transmitted x-rays caused scintillations that were viewed directly by the radiologist. The fluorescent screen was backed by lead glass so reducing radiation dose to the eyes. The images were of very poor quality for a number of reasons.

- Poor light output by the fluorescent screen for safe exposure rates
- Low efficiency of the light conversion mechanism of the screen
- Poor spatial resolution.

Only a small percentage of the light from the screen was available to the eye owing to a very narrow viewing angle (about 6°) to the light photons Fluorescent screens also give poor image quality because the visual acuity of the eye is ×10 less at low light levels (see Chapter 8).

Fluorescent screens are no longer used since they gave high radiation dose to the operator and the sensitivity of fluoroscopy is greatly improved by electronic intensification of the x-ray signal using an image intensifier.

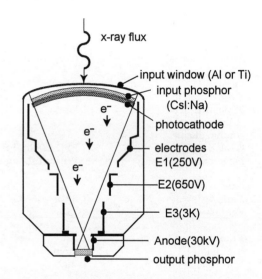

Figure 10.1 Image intensifier design. A metal window encloses the input phosphor (CsI:Na) and photocathode. Electrons ejected from the photocathode are accelerated by the electrodes E1, E2 and E3 towards the anode (+30kV) and onto the output screen.

10.1.1 The image intensifier

The general design is shown in Fig.10.1. Electronic intensification of the incident x-ray beam is achieved by first converting it to light using a fluorescent input phosphor CsI:Na. The light photons are then converted to photoelectrons using a photocathode. The electrons are accelerated by high voltage electrodes which focus them onto a much smaller fluorescent screen.

The following basic features can be identified in the figure:

- a thin glass or metal (aluminum or titanium) input window,
- an input fluorescent screen (CsI:Na)
- a photocathode.
- high voltage focusing electrodes E_1,
- E_2 and E_3 electrodes leading to the anode.
- output fluorescent screen coupled to a video camera and/or film cameras

The casing or **housing** of the image intensifier is mu-metal and (except for the input and output windows) is enclosed by a protective steel/lead cover which improves radiation safety for the operator. Mu-metal is an alloy which is highly permeable to magnetic fields so strongly reducing magnetic interference from the earth's magnetic field and other equipment (MRI machines) which would seriously distort the electronic focusing.

10.1.2 Image intensifier input

The face of the image intensifier is drawn in Fig.10.2(a). The entrance window is thin metal through which the x-ray beam passes onto a scintillator (CsI:Na); this converts the x-ray energy into light photons. The light photons interact with an antimony/cesium photocathode material which produces photo-electrons, these are then accelerated by a large potential difference (30kV) onto a small display screen.

The input window This was originally glass in early designs but is now commonly aluminum or titanium which allows approximately 95% transmission for 60kV x-rays (effective energy); glass provided only 80% transmission. Figure 10.1 shows that the input window of the intensifier has a convex shape; this is the origin of slight pincushion distortion in all image intensifiers.

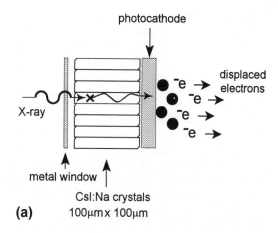

(a)

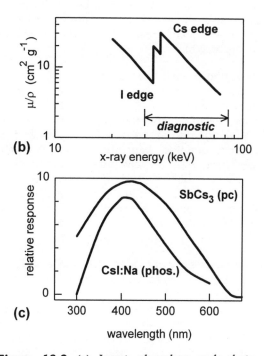

(b)

(c)

Figure 10.2 (a) Input phosphor and photo-cathode. The x-rays penetrate the input window, undergo photoelectric absorption by the CsI:Na phosphor and the resulting light photons eject a cloud of electrons from the photocathode. **(b)** Absorption of x-radiation for cesium iodide showing the K-edges for iodine and cesium giving optimum absorption over diagnostic photon energies from 30-80keV. **(c)** The peak sensitivity of the photocathode matches the peak wavelength of light from the cesium iodide phosphor at about 400-500nm.

The input phosphor Directly behind the window is a phosphor or scintillator which converts the incident x-radiation into visible light. Modern intensifiers use cesium iodide doped with sodium (CsI:Na), deposited as monoclinic columnar crystals on the input window itself.

These crystals form an array of tiny needle elements which collimate the light photons produced by photoelectric interactions within the scintillator crystals. **Light collimation** improves spatial resolution by reducing dispersion or **flare** at the phosphor surface.

Overall image quality depends on efficient x-ray absorption by the input phosphor. The CsI:Na phosphor absorbs about 60% of the incident x-ray beam assisted by the favorable position of the K-edges of cesium and iodine at 36 and 33keV respectively which is shown in Fig.10.2(b).

The photo cathode This is a layer of complex cesium antimony compound ($CsSb_3$) directly applied to the surface of the input phosphor and converts light photons from the scintillator into an electron cloud whose flux is proportional to light photon flux. The light spectrum from the cesium iodide phosphor and the photocathode is matched for wavelength as shown in Fig.10.2(c). There is a linear relationship between x-ray intensity at the intensifier face, light production and electron density from the photocathode.

The focusing electrodes The electrons produced by the photocathode are accelerated by a high voltage applied to the internal electrodes identified in Fig.10.1. as E_1, E_2, E_3 with the anode which carry an increasing voltage level. The electrons, produced by the photocathode, are accelerated towards a cylindrical anode, and focused onto the **output phosphor**. The focusing electrodes act as electrical lenses by modifying the electrostatic field between the photocathode (at earth potential) and the anode which is set at a very high potential, typically 25-35 kV.

Altering the voltage levels on the electrodes (electronic switching) controls the **area** of the input screen used by the image intensifier. This provides a **zoom** or **multi-field** facility.

A single image intensifier can be electronically switched to give up to 3 fields of view: e.g. 33cm (13″), 23cm (9″) and 17cm (7″); image resolution improves with decreasing field size.

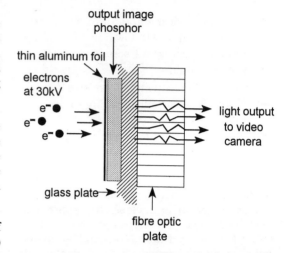

Figure 10.3 The output screen of an image intensifier designed for a dedicated video output showing the fiber optic plate which is in contact with the screen and video camera face.

10.1.3 The image intensifier output

The output screen scintillation phosphor is a few microns thick deposited on a glass base which serves as the output window of the intensifier. Fig.10.3 shows a general design for an image intensifier output screen. A complex silver-zinc-cadmium sulfide is frequently used as the scintillator (type P20) although several other compounds are available. Typical output diameters range between 20-25mm, the area being about one hundredth of the input area.

The accelerated electrons, from the photocathode, acquire enough kinetic energy to produce multiple light photons when they bombard the output phosphor. The image produced is an inverted, reversed and minified version of the light pattern from the input phosphor.

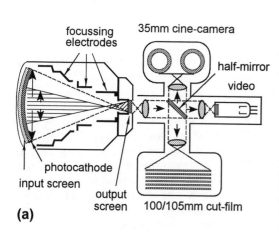

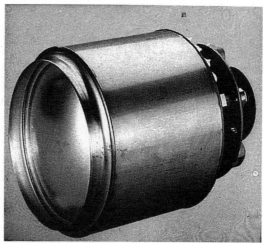

Figure 10.4 **(a)** Image intensifier output shared by a 100mm cut-film camera, a cine camera and a video camera. The input can be switched between two fields of view. **(b)** An image intensifier showing metal construction (courtesy Philips Inc.)

The inner surface of the output phosphor is coated by a layer of very thin aluminum foil which allows electron transmission but prevents the light produced by the phosphor returning to the photo cathode where it might release secondary electrons not associated with x-ray transmission causing **veiling glare**.

Output coupling Some designs of output screen for dedicated video camera output have a fiber optic plate which acts as an interface between output screen and video camera tube. This design is shown in Fig.10.3 and significantly reduces light dispersion at the camera face, however it restricts output to a single video camera.

Image intensifiers which share output devices (cine-camera, 100mm cut-film camera and video camera) use a system of lenses and a split mirror to share the light signal from the output screen. This arrangement is shown in Fig.10.4(a) where the output screen is shared between a cine-camera, a 100mm cut-film camera and video tube.

In most fluoroscopic systems the output from the image intensifier passes through a two lens system serving a film recording device and video-camera. The first and second lenses transmit the image as a parallel beam to the video camera. A rotating split mirror intersects the parallel beam directing light to either a cut film- or cine-camera for a permanent record. The lens system reduces the light output from the image intensifier and the light intensity is reduced for each imaging device added to the output. In practice only one film camera would be used and this would receive about 70% of the available light.

A dedicated video output for digital systems (digital fluorography: DF) uses a direct fiber optic link between the image intensifier and camera. This would capture 100% of the available light and film records would be taken as video or digital images. A commercially available image intensifier employing metal construction is shown in Fig.10.4(b); the diameters vary between 15 to 40cm (6 to 16 inches).

10.2 PERFORMANCE PARAMETERS

The magnitude of signal amplification given by an image intensifier depends on the transparency of the input window (glass or metal) and the conversion efficiency of the input phosphor, photocathode and output phosphor. Figure 10.5 identifies the losses incurred by converting x-ray information into a visible image using a *phosphor → photocathode → phosphor system.*

The metal window has an absorption loss of about 5-8% and following this the x-ray absorption by the CsI phosphor is about 50-60%. The calculation in Box 10.1 explains the bar-graph presented in Fig. 10.5; for an image intensifier having a 23cm diameter field of view and 2.5cm output screen the incident dose is $0.2\mu Gy\ s^{-1}$ which would represent a $5\times10^5\ cm^{-2}\ s^{-1}$ photon flux.

The lowest efficiency in the chain is the x-ray absorption by the input phosphor, which depends on two major factors: the phosphor's composition (K-edge energy), phosphor thickness and x-ray to light conversion efficiency; this is the area of most statistical uncertainty termed the **quantum sink** which sets a limit to image quality. All subsequent stages will only amplify the fractional difference (contrast) between any two points on the input phosphor. The intensification factor is a measure of the electronic gain or increase in the light intensity at the output compared with the input phosphor. There are two parameters for measuring intensification factor:

- Image minification
- Flux or electronic gain.

10.2.1 Minification gain

This is derived simply from the area ratio between the input and output screens of the intensifier which produces an increase in gain in proportion to the relative radius of the input and output phosphors. The image is brighter when minified since the number of photons will be squeezed onto a smaller area, giving a minification gain in brightness, so:

$$\frac{\pi r_{in}^2}{\pi r_{out}^2} \qquad (10.1)$$

The output phosphor diameter is typically 2.5cm. Since area also varies with the square of the diameter $(\pi r^2 \equiv \pi/4 \times d^2)$ a 40cm diameter image intensifier will give a minification gain of $40^2/2.5^2 = 256$. The minification gain varies with input field size and has typical values between 50 and 250.

Radiation exposure increases with decrease in field size (zooming) since the minification gain is smaller. The increase in exposure rate is obtained by simply squaring the diameters i.e. zooming from 36 to 17cm produces a $36^2/17^2$ or 4 fold increase in dose maintaining the same noise figure.

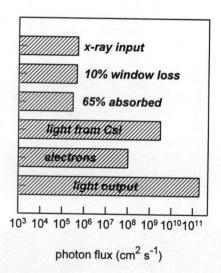

Figure 10.5 Gains and losses from the input of the image intensifier to the output. Calculations are given in Box.10.1

10.2.2 Flux gain

As the high voltage electrons are accelerated from the photocathode onto the output phosphor they gain kinetic energy. The amount of light produced at the output phosphor depends on the kinetic energy deposited by the electrons on the phosphor. The number of light quanta emitted by the output screen for every light quanta emitted by the input phosphor is the lumen, electronic or flux gain:

$$\frac{\text{Light photons from output phosphor}}{\text{light photons at photocathode}} \quad (10.2)$$

This depends on the operating potential of the image intensifier; typically 25 to 30kV. Box 10.1 calculates flux gain by comparing input light to output light ratio.

Box 10.1

The flux gain of an image intensifier

Using the reference values for exposure stated at the beginning of this section. For a useful x-ray flux of 3×10^5 (after window and absorption loss):

Light conversion: The input phosphor CsI:Na has 50% conversion efficiency to light. X-ray effective energy 60keV and the mean photon energy of the light produced is 3eV so:

$$\frac{(3 \times 10^5) \times (60 \times 10^3) \times 0.5}{3} = 3.0 \times 10^9$$

so there are approximately 7000 light quanta produced for each x-ray photon

Photocathode electrons: Only a fraction (~3%) of the above light photons produce useful photoelectrons. So the above light flux would give approximately 10^8 photoelectrons; these are accelerated by the high voltage onto the output phosphor, each absorbed x-ray photon producing about 300 electrons.

Output phosphor: The kinetic energy of the accelerated electrons is converted into visible light at the output phosphor. Depending on the output phosphor type approximately 0.063 light photons are produced for each electron of energy 1eV. For an electron stream having an effective energy of 30kV this would give

$$10^8 \times (30 \times 10^3) \times 0.063 = 2 \times 10^{11} \text{ photons}$$

producing approximately 2000 light photons per photoelectron.

Flux gain: The total light produced at the output screen by the electrons is $10^8 \times 2000 = 2 \times 10^{11}$. The available x-ray flux produces 3×10^9 light photons at the input so the flux gain is $2 \times 10^{11}/3 \times 10^9 \simeq 60$.

These are the gains and losses plotted in Fig. 10.5

The differing luminescent spectra from input and output screen make this a somewhat dubious measurement. The luminance (candela m^{-2}) is increased also by the minification gain by up to 200 so a **total gain** (luminance, brightness or intensification gain) of 10000 is available; this increases to 15000 for large field (40cm) intensifiers.

A more useful measure of image intensifier performance is given by the conversion factor, which directly compares the light output with x-ray exposure.

10.2.3 Conversion factor (CF)

This is a measure of the efficiency of image intensifier converting ionizing radiation (x-rays) measured in µGy s^{-1} to light output whose luminance is measured in candela (cd) as cd m^{-2} So the conversion factor is:

$$\frac{\text{output phosphor luminance} \, (\text{cd m}^{-2})}{\text{input phosphor dose} \, (\mu\text{Gy s}^{-1})} \quad (10.3)$$

The output phosphor luminance is measured with a photometer; the incident radiation with a calibrated dosimeter. The x-ray beam quality must be defined and is usually taken as 2mm Al pre-filtration giving 7mm HVL. If a 0.5µGy s^{-1} input phosphor dose gives 400cd m^{-2} output luminance the CF would be 200. Typical values of conversion factor range from 100 to 1000 cd m^{-2} per µGy s^{-1} depending on intensifier input area.

The conversion factor varies with the area of the input field, since although the radiation dose per unit area does not change minification gain will alter, so the CF value for the same dose rate increases with intensifier input area since the intensification factor (light output) increases.

If the amount of light seen at the output is kept constant then as conversion performance decreases (as the image intensifier gets older) more radiation will be required at the input.

Units for the conversion factor The conversion factor for an image intensifier can be expressed in:

- milliRads (cd m^{-2} mR^{-1} s^{-1})
- microGrays (cd m^{-2} μGy^{-1} s^{-1})
- microCoulombs (cd m^{-2} μC kg^{-1} s^{-1})

The approximate multipliers for these are given in Tab.10.1

Table 10.1 Conversion factor multipliers

Given	Required		
	mR^{-1}·s	μGy^{-1}·s	μC kg^{-1}·s
mR^{-1} · s	1	0.115	3.9
μGy^{-1} · s	8.7	1	34
μC kg^{-1} · s	0.256	.03	1

10.2.4 Detective quantum efficiency (DQE)

Quantum noise The image intensifier image is inherently noisy owing to the low x-ray photon density used during fluoroscopy investigations (screening). A typical noise figure can be calculated for an incident exposure of 0.2μGy s^{-1} photon density to estimate the quantum noise figure for a real time fluoroscopy images calculated in Box.10.2.

In order to obtain diagnostic quality images from an image intensifier with minimum noise level a certain density of x-ray photons are required. The detection quantum efficiency (DQE) relates the intensifier's input screen absorption efficiency and its x-ray-to-light conversion efficiency as an SNR figure. This then describes the signal to noise ratio (input SNR) at the input phosphor, for total absorption, compared to the output SNR of the image:

$$DQE = \left[\frac{output\ SNR}{input\ SNR} \right]^2 \qquad (10.4)$$

An ideal system would convert 100% of the photons into useful information but in practice losses occur at both the input and output window of the image intensifier, as already shown. The DQE measurement therefore takes into account:

- The percentage of x-ray photons penetrating the input window
- The percentage of x-ray photons absorbed by the input screen
- The percentage of absorbed quanta forming the image.

Typical DQE values from modern equipment vary between 50 and 70%. It is a critical measure since the difference between a 40% DQE and a 50% DQE would give a relative contrast improvement of approximately 25% with a 20% lower radiation dose. In order to obtain maximum DQE:

- The input metal window must give maximum transmission.
- The input phosphor must offer maximum absorption to x-rays.
- Maximum light conversion.
- Increase detector size
- Highest SNR for imaging chain

Box 10.2

Image noise

Overall resolving power: 2.5Lp mm^{-1} giving 5 resolvable elements per mm (2500 resolvable elements per cm)

Integration time of image chain: 0.2s including the eye.

Fluence at face: 0.2μGy s^{-1} input dose is about 5×10^5 x-ray photons per second.

Overall absorption/conversion efficiency: 40% so useful photons equals 2×10^5

Image frame rate: 5 fps (0.2s per frame) giving (2×10^5) /5 = 40000 photons cm^{-2} per image.

The x-ray photons available for each resolvable element are then: 40,000/2500 = 16

The **quantum noise** associated with each resolvable element is therefore √16 or 4 giving a quantum noise figure of 25%. A slower picture integration time of 0.5s will decrease quantum noise to 15%.

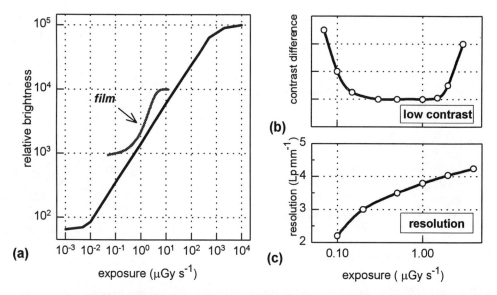

Figure 10.6 **(a)** The dynamic range of an image intensifier covers several orders of magnitude. The lower limit is given by the dark current noise of the photocathode; the upper limit is due to the x-ray exposure on the conductivity between photocathode and output phosphor. **(b)** low contrast visibility (plateau region) is optimum between 0.15 and 1.0µGy s-1 and resolution **(c)** is approaching maximum.

The electronic noise in a video camera determines the dynamic range of the image intensifier/video image chain; a common SNR value is 1000:1 with current systems approaching 2000:1.

The DQE is commonly measured using a ^{241}Americium source, which gives a gamma-ray with a single 60keV energy; this corresponds to a filtered x-ray beam with a peak energy of 120kVp. The output signal is measured using a photometer with a time constant (integration time) which closely matches the eye. There is a great deal of variation in methods chosen for measuring the DQE and manufacturers' figures should only be taken as a very rough guide.

10.2.5 Dose response

Dynamic range The linear transfer curve in Fig.10.6(a) shows the dynamic range of an image intensifier as output luminance for an input dose rate; this range covers several orders of magnitude. The limiting factors are:

- The **lower limit** is due to the image intensifier dark current which is inherent electronic noise in the system equivalent to a dose of 0.001µGy s^{-1}.
- The **higher limit** is imposed by the high x-ray photon flux which induces a separate current within the photocathode which reduces electron velocity and produces a decreased light output.

Image contrast The minimum detectable difference between two low contrast objects depends on the dose rate to the surface of the image intensifier. The optimum level is therefore set by the manufacturer and automatic dose control devices aim to keep this reference level so that high quality images are displayed. The 'bath-tub' graph shown in Fig.10.6(b) demonstrates that there is an optimal dose rate below which quantum noise degrades low contrast visibility and above which saturation effects influence display

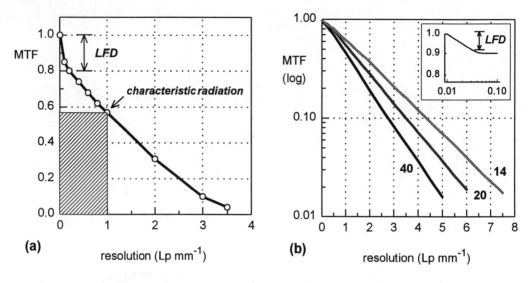

Figure 10.7   **(a)** MTF of an image intensifier (linear plot) showing the low frequency drop influencing the entire MTF curve.   Characteristic modulation is the MTF value for 1Lp mm^{-1} which is 0.57 in this case. **(b)** MTF curves (log-linear scale) for three sizes of input field showing an increased resolution with decreasing field (zoom) size.

quality. The dose rate for modern image intensifiers is typically kept within the 0.15 and 0.2μGy s^{-1} band; this limit allows an optimum patient dose: image quality ratio.

Image resolution   The spatial resolution is often conveniently measured in terms of line pairs per millimeter (Lp mm^{-1}) by using a line pair test pattern consisting of an etched tungsten or tantalum grating. This is a measure of fine object detail in the output image.   Overall resolution of the image intensifier improves with increased dose rate at the image intensifier face but low contrast visibility is the limiting factor which again restricts the dose rate to within 0.15 to 0.2μGy s^{-1} as shown by the resolution curve in Fig.10.6(c) where 3.5 to 4.0Lp mm^{-1} is currently the best performance value.

Low frequency drop   A typical MTF for an image intensifier is shown in Fig.10.7(a) using linear axes in order to emphasize the low frequency fall off, common to all image intensifiers. The MTF response quickly drops

from an initial value of 1.0 to about 0.8; the percentage drop is called the low frequency drop (LFD) and represents a fall of 8 to 10% in resolution value and is responsible for the degradation of all spatial frequencies.

There are two main reasons for this rapid fall in resolution:

• X-radiation scatter in the input window and phosphor
• Light diffusion at the output window.

The first can be reduced by using a thin metal window (aluminum or titanium) and a CsI:Na crystalline input phosphor. Light diffusion at the output screen can be reduced by using a fiber optic plate as an interface. The contrast improvement for larger objects is significantly improved as the LFD is reduced to about 6 or 8%. The **characteristic modulation** of an image intensifier is measured as the MTF value for 1Lp mm^{-1} (typically 0.57); this is sometimes used as a measure of overall resolution.

The spatial resolution is increased by decreasing the input field of view. The MTF's

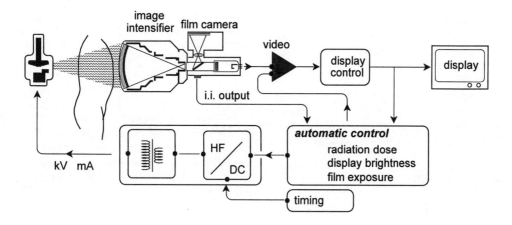

Figure 10.8   General design of a fluoroscopic system with an image intensifier. Fluoroscopy imaging chain showing the image intensifier feeding a cut film camera for hardcopy. A video camera gives real time monitoring. A conventional film cassette can be moved in front of the intensifier face; this would carry its own ionization chamber for exposure control

in Fig.10.7(b) show a 40cm image intensifier zoomed to decrease the field size through 20 to 14cm so improving resolution.

10.2.6 Contrast ratio

The ability to register low contrast differ-eneces also depends on the SNR. Image noise can be introduced by a variety of factors:

- x-ray scattering at the input window.
- x-ray scattering at the input phosphor.
- light scattering within the phosphor itself.
- visible light not absorbed by the photocathode.
- back-scattering of light from the output phosphor toward the photocathode.
- scattering of light at the output window (reduced by fiber optic plate).

The overall effect of these scattering events is to reduce image contrast by causing **veiling glare**. This can be measured as a **contrast ratio** C_v by measuring output light intensity at the display before and after placing a lead-

disc in front of the image intensifier face so:

$$C_v = \frac{L_c}{L_d} \qquad (10.5)$$

Where L_c is the light intensity at center of image and L_d the light intensity at the same point when a lead disk blocks 10% of the central input area.   For a perfect image intensifier L_d would be zero and C_v would be infinite but due to scattering the contrast ratio can vary from 17:1 to 40:1 depending on the condition of the unit.

10.3   THE FLUOROSCOPY SYSTEM

The basic electronic fluoroscopy imaging chain is shown in Fig.10.8. It includes:

- X-ray tube
- High frequency generator
- Image intensifier
- A video camera
- A hard copy film camera
- A video display for real-time viewing

10.3.1 The x-ray tube and generator

Table.10.2 lists the specifications for a typical x-ray tube suitable for fluoroscopy. X-ray tubes have maximum thermal capacity and heat dissipation. These permit high patient throughput and are usually synchronized with imaging systems (e.g. cine-camera) using pulse mode.

The influence of focal spot size on resolution is critical, as the curve in Fig.10.9 demonstrates. The influence of focal spot size on image resolution follows a general formula:

$$R = \frac{m}{F(m-1)} \qquad (10.6)$$

where m is the image magnification and F the focal spot size of the x-ray tube.

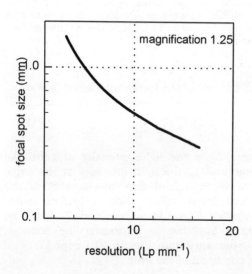

Figure 10.9 The change of potential resolution with x-ray tube focal spot size.

Patient separation from the image intensifier face usually gives a magnification of about 1.25 yielding a resolution of 6.25Lp mm^{-1} for a focal spot of 0.8mm and 4Lp mm^{-1} for a 1.2 mm focal spot. However the focal spot size is not a limiting factor for image resolution since the image intensifier has an upper limit of about 4Lp mm^{-1}. However if magnification

views of ×2.5 are chosen large focal spot sizes will significantly influence image unsharpness. Fluoroscopic x-ray tubes typically have dual focal spot sizes 0.3 and 1.0mm which allow magnification views with minimum unsharpness and optimum thermal rating.

High frequency power supplies are used almost exclusively with power ranges from 15 to 80kW depending on application (small mobile or large fixed installation). The larger generator should permit continuous operation at 2000W and allow an acquisition rate of up to 8 frames per second (fps). Since the K-edge of iodine is 33keV an effective x-ray energy of ×2 or 70keV is chosen which translates as a 100kVp.

Table 10.2 X-ray tube specifications

	Medium Duty	*Heavy Duty*
Construction	glass	metal/ceramic
Focal spot (mm)	0.6/1.2	0.4/0.8
Target	12°	8°
Heat storage	0.4MJ (0.6MHU)	1MJ (1.35MHU)
Maximum power	450W	2000W

10.3.2 Image intensifier performance

The general specification for a large field image intensifier having three zoom settings is summarized in Tab.10.3. Both conversion factor and image pincushion distortion **increase** with **increasing field size**. Resolution and contrast ratio both improve with **decrease** in field size and relative patient dose also increases.

Image intensifiers have undergone major improvements owing to the stringent requirements for digital fluorography. A typical signal to noise ratio exceeds 1000:1 and low frequency drop would be less than

8% due to aluminum or titanium input windows having a transmission factor of >95% at 60keV.

A 100mm film cassette for hard copy is shown in Fig.10.8 but various hard copy devices are used. Automatic exposure and display brightness controls are incorporated into all fluoroscopy systems. These alter the generator kV and mA to give a constant input dose rate to the image intensifier.

Table 10.3 Image intensifier specifications

Field diameter	40cm 16"	32cm 12.5"	20cm 8"	15cm 6"
Resolution (Lp mm^{-1})	4.0	4.2	5.5	6.0
Contrast ratio	20:1	25:1	30:1	30:1
Dose (relative)	0.25	0.5	0.75	1.0
Pincushion (%)	9	4.5	1.4	1.0
CF (cd m^{-2}mR^{-1}s^{-1})	166	100	60	50

DQE 52%
LFD 6%

10.3.3 The video image

The basic domestic video display has been described in Chapter 8. Fluoroscopy uses a high definition video display (1023/2046 lines at 60Hz or 1249/2498 lines at 50Hz supply frequency) to give real-time images of iodine or barium contrast enhanced radiographs. The high definition video images are digitized for subsequent storage or laser imager film recording.

The video camera shown in Fig.10.10(a) converts light images on the output phosphor of the image intensifier into a video image signal for transmission to display devices. Light enters the camera tube and strikes a light-sensitive double layer of a photo-conductive material, usually Sb_2S_3 embedded in a substrate of insulating mica on the glass window. The type of photo conductive material distinguishes the camera tube:

- Vidicon: photoconductive layer is antimony based

- Plumbicon: photoconductive layer constructed from lead oxide

Photoelectrons are released from this photoconductive layer by the light photons, but leave behind fixed positive charges on the image plate which faithfully reproduce image detail and light intensity. A focused beam of electrons accelerated from the camera cathode scans across the image plate in a raster pattern. The negative electron beam current is influenced by the positive charges on the image plate and a signal current is set up proportional to the amount of stored charge. This signal current is amplified and timing pulses added forming the video waveform.

Charge Coupled Device (C.C.D.) This is a solid-state imaging sensor commonly found in domestic 'Cam-Recorders'. The device needs no electron gun, deflection system or evacuated tube seen in video camera tubes. Its simple design is shown in Fig.10.10(b) where a semiconductor photosensitive surface (8×6mm being typical) is divided into many thousands of separate islands of photodiodes arranged in rows and columns. Present CCDs can offer resolution of 2048 × 2048 pixals. Electrons liberated by light photons are captured in the charge coupled layer of the semiconductor, the electron number is in proportion to light intensity.

Readout of this stored information is different from other camera technology. An electron beam is not used, but each line of information (stored electrons) is shifted electronically and read out as a video waveform. The camera operates on a voltage of about 12 volts, compared with 200-300 volts for a video tube. A lens system focuses the image onto the semi-conductor surface. The photosensitive sur-face releases electrons in proportion to the amount of incident light and these electrons

Spatial resolution is not quite as high as conventional cameras but since the output is more amenable to digitization higher quality CCD cameras being developed should slowly replace the tube cameras; however at present the resolution for video camera tubes is not a

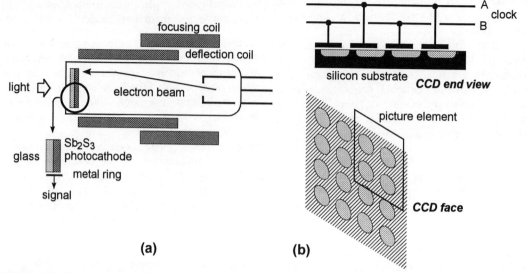

(a)   **(b)**

Figure 10.10   **(a)** A vacuum tube video camera which uses an electron beam to scan a photocathode which holds the image data. The scanning pattern depends on the video standard (typically 1023 or 1249 lines) **(b)** a CCD semiconductor camera uses an array of photosensitive diodes which are read out by clock pulses to give a video signal. A group of four diodes contributes to a picture element.

limiting factor in radiology. Table 10.4 compares the performance of a vidicon, plumbicon and CCD camera.

Table 10.4 Properties of video cameras

	Vidicon	Plumb.	CCD
Target	Sb_2S_3	PbO	Si
Sensitivity (µA/lumen)	Varies	400	700
Resolution (relative)	0.55	0.65	0.4
Lag (relative)	10	1	0.1
Dark Current (nA)	20	<1	5
Life (hours)	4500	4500	>500k

Video resolution and bandwidth (bandpass):   The total range of frequencies in a mixed signal (sound, radio-frequency, video) is called the bandwidth or bandpass.

Vertical resolution V uses a Kell factor K which represents the useful fraction of the scan line which takes part in image registration. This is usually a fraction of about 0.7, so:

$$V = KN \qquad (10.7)$$

The vertical resolution for 525 and 625 line video display would be 367 and 437.

The bandwidth B necessary to transmit the video display is calculated as:

$$B = Lp \times V \times fps \qquad (10.8)$$

Where Lp are the number of line pairs and fps the number of frames per second. The vertical resolution V equals Lp for an aspect ratio of 1:1 so for V equals 367 and 437 the necessary bandwidth is 4.0MHz and 4.7MHz and for 1023 lines and 1249 lines a bandwidth of 19 and 25MHz is required. A bandwidth of over 100MHz is needed for a non-interlaced (progressive scan) high resolution display having 2000 lines which is becoming the preferred display for radiology. The horizontal resolution H is calculated as:

$$\frac{2 \times (bandwidth)}{fps \times scan\ lines} \qquad (10.9)$$

A 525 line display would have a horizontal resolution of 507 picture elements and 625 a resolution of 601 picture elements, the horizontal resolution depending on the system bandwidth. The image detail in conventional radiology video systems requires at least twice the bandwidth of domestic television signals and in the case of high definition 1249 line displays (50Hz supply) the bandwidth is five times larger and requires a range from a few hertz up to 25MHz.

Combining image intensifier size with the available video resolution gives the final display resolution of the entire imaging chain. For a 40cm image intensifier and a 1023 line display the resolution would be:

$$\frac{400}{1023 \times 0.7} = 0.55mm \text{ or } 1.8Lp \text{ mm}^{-1}$$

a 2000 line display would increase this to 3.5Lp mm^{-1} and a 3000 line display to 5.25Lp mm^{-1}; this definition compares very favorably with the best film image. The expected resolution figures for various output devices are given in Table 10.5

Table 10.5 Overall resolution Lp mm^{-1}

Image intensifier	Output	100mm film	Cine	Video 1023	1249
15cm	6.0	5.2	3.0	4.7	5.8
20cm	5.5	4.8	2.7	3.5	4.3
40cm	4.0	3.5	2.0	1.8	2.2

10.3.4   Video recording

This is used to capture the video image for subsequent display or hard copy film recording. Multiple film copies using a film formatter can be readily achieved. Rapid video recording is obtained by using a solid-state image memory. It provides limited storage (4-5 frames) but offers instant playback and reduces patient's radiation dose.

Video tape recorder   Although the economics of a video recorder are very favorable (maximum number of images on a video tape cassette), the quality of the images commonly recorded is much poorer than those obtained by cine-fluorography since the images are obtained from a relatively low resolution television system.   High definition video recorders matching HD-video standards are becoming available. Major disadvantages are:

- Access times to individual images stored on magnetic tape may be long.
- Direct or random access is not available.
- Contact between the heads and the tape causes wear and leads to image degradation.
- Video tape deteriorates in storage and images become noisier.

Video disc   An alternative video image storage device which has a limited storage capacity but allows instant playback of any stored image uses a video magnetic disc. Images can be selected after a patient investigation for film recording before the disc is erased and re-used.

Digital recording   The output from the video camera is digitized and the image is stored as a matrix (512×512, 1024×1024 or larger matrices). Many such digital images can be stored during a patient study and then selected for film hardcopy on a laser film formatter. Dynamic frames can be collected at up to 30 fps.

10.3.5 Hard copy film recording.

Real-time events can be viewed on the video monitor but it is sometimes important to obtain permanent records during patient investigations. There are four common methods for obtaining permanent film images:

- Spot film cassette,
- Rapid sequence 100 or 105mm cut film
- Serial film changer (film cassette)
- Cine-fluoroscopy
- Digital recording

The video camera monitoring an image intensifier input can also be used for providing a video or digital image for storage and retrieval.

Spot film cassette This is the traditional method of film recording. Fluoroscopy is interrupted and the cassette moved sideways from its protective shelter to be in front of the image intensifier face. The tube current is then increased from 1-3 mA used for fluoroscopy to 300-400 mA for film exposure. The area for film recording can be selected thus allowing for multiple exposures on the one film-cassette combination. The major disadvantage of this technique is the time required for the cassette to move into place and for the x-ray tube to deliver the increased current (filament heating). The overall delay time is about 0.75 seconds and the image cannot be viewed on the video monitor while the cassette is in place. Modern systems allow up to two exposures per second for a range of format sizes.

The spatial resolution is the highest of the hard copy devices, about 5-6 Lp mm^{-1}, which is limited by the size of the focal spot (Fig.10.9). The radiation dose to the patient is the highest of any of the hard copy devices per image obtained.

Rapid sequence cut film camera (100 and 105mm). These devices can acquire permanent images on small format, 100mm cut film or 105mm roll film, at a rate of up to 10 images per second. A typical design is shown in the photograph of Fig.10.11

The camera views the light output of the image intensifier deflected from the semitransparent mirror between the tandem lens system (see Fig.10.4(a)). When the mirror is in place about 85% of the light is directed onto the cut-film camera.

The main advantage of this recording system is the reduction in patient and staff radiation dose, about one third of that from a spot film cassette, however the spatial resolution of the 100mm camera is inferior to the film cassette. An advantage however is the reduction of unsharpness (caused by organ movement) by the short exposure times. Cut film typically requires 1.5μGy per

frame. Frame rates are usually 1 to 6fps and the film resolution 3 to 4.5Lp mm^{-1} depending on image intensifier field size.

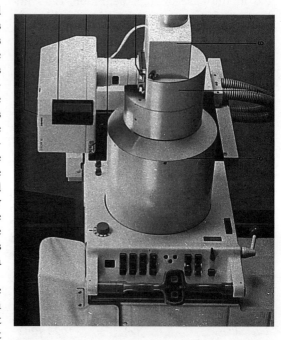

Figure 10.11 A 100mm cut film camera at right angles to the intensifier sharing its output with an 'in-line' video camera (courtesy Siemens Inc.)

Serial film changers Serial film changers acquire rapid full size radiographic images. The image intensifier video display provides positioning information. Typical exposure rates are about eight to ten exposures per second for about five seconds. The x-ray tube is pulsed during film changing. The spatial resolution is higher when using the serial changer and the images do not require projection when viewed. The disadvantages of using serial film changers are mechanical difficulties associated with the transport system which may lead to jamming and curling of the films.

Cine-fluorography this records the moving image, in real-time, on 35mm cinematographic film. After the reel of film is processed the images are projected viewing in cine mode.

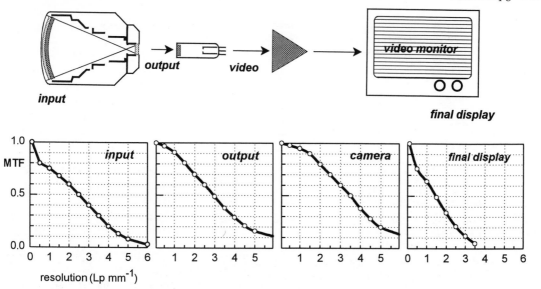

Figure 10.12 MTF's for the fluoroscopy chain showing the input face, the output screen and the video output. The MTF product shows a final resolution of about 2Lp mm^{-1}, this can be improved with increased scan lines.

A variety of framing rates are available in Europe: 12.5, 25, 50, 100, 150 frames s^{-1} and in the USA: 15, 30, 45, 60, 90 and 120 frames s^{-1}. Rapid heart rate in pediatric cardiology can be followed at 120 to 150 frames s^{-1} (90 to 120 fps USA) and typically adult cardiology at 50 to 60 frames s^{-1} (30 to 60 fps). Cine-fluorography normally employs a double imaging system involving both anterior and lateral planes of the heart where pulsed radiation exposures are synchronized with the film transport mechanism; this will be described in more detail later.

10.3.6 The image chain

The overall image resolution, contrast and noise is the product of the image intensifier, video camera and display type. Of this image chain the image intensifier is the major weakness due mostly to the quantum sink effect described earlier so significant improvements in image quality will depend on image intensifier improvements.

The image intensifier is capable of about 6 Lp mm^{-1} for a 17cm (6.5″) diameter field-of-view. Resolution decreases with increasing input diameter as shown previously in Table 10.3. A 36cm (14″) image intensifier is chosen for imaging the full body width. It has a DQE of 52%; a low-frequency-drop of 6%; a conversion efficiency (G_x) of 150 cd m^{-2} mR^{-1} sec^{-1}. The final resolution of the fluoroscopy display is the product of all the components of the system. Fig.10.12 shows 3 MTF's from regions of the image intensifier/input/output and the camera. The overall MTF is seen by the display.

Improved input face materials (thin metal window and CsI:Na phosphors) have produced significant improvements in resolution. A 20cm image intensifier has a resolution of 5Lp mm^{-1} when using cut film, almost matching spot film, and the cut film fluoroscopy investigation has a much lower radiation dose. High definition video displays (1049/1249 lines) approach the resolution of modern image intensifiers and this is not a limiting factor particularly with the current 2046 and 2498 line video displays.

The resolution of the image-intensifier and video display combined can be estimated from the resolvable video line-pairs derived from eqn.10.8 where V is the vertical resolution:

$$R_S = \frac{image\ intensifier\ size}{V} \qquad (10.10)$$

This is used for calculating the system resolution already given in Table 10.5.

Sensitivity   This is the ratio of the camera signal strength to the input illumination and is analogous to the film/screen characteristic curve.   The gamma for plumbicons is 1.0 and for vidicons 0.7 so the image contrast is preserved at the output of a plumbicon but slightly reduced for a vidicon. The sensitivity, signal strength for the same illumination, is higher in plumbicons than in vidicons. The dark current that flows when no illumination is present is equivalent to film fog and ideally should be zero. The dark current in plumbicons is about 25 times less than that of a vidicons. CCD gamma value is also 1.0 and the dark current is very low (see Tab.10.4).

Image lag or persistence   Theoretically the electron beam of the video camera neutralizes the charge on the photoconductive layer during subsequent raster scans and therefore the image data at that location is removed. In practice neutralization is not complete, which results in persistent remnant image data called after-image or image lag.

Only 60-70 % is neutralized in the vidicon and 90-95% in the plumbicon. Since the vidicon exhibits a considerable amount of image lag or persistence it will not be suitable for certain applications, such as cardio-vascular work, where rapid movements are being recorded.

Plumbicon cameras exhibit very little lag but produce images that are more mottled or noisy than those produced by the vidicon since the relatively high lag in the vidicon smoothes or integrates the statistical variation of light in the image. CCD cameras have a very quick response and minimum lag.

10.4 FEEDBACK CONTROLS

The absorption of x-rays depends on the transparency of the object and for different thicknesses of patient the image intensifier output will vary greatly in brightness producing a changing image quality. In order to stabilize the image signal two methods are used:

- Automatic Brightness (or Dose) Control (ABC), maintains a constant dose rate at the intensifier face.
- Automatic Gain Control (AGC) maintains a constant video display brightness

Both types of regulation are used in modern fluoroscopy equipment.

The image intensifier-video image chain is calibrated at the time of manufacture so that a certain dose at the image intensifier face produces optimum image quality at the output. The dose rate which provides optimum image brightness is pre-set by the manufacturer and is typically 0.15 to 0.2 µGy s^{-1}.

10.4.1 Automatic controls

Several feedback signals are used to maintain consistent optimum display quality. The automatic brightness control (ABC) maintains a constant average dose rate at the input window of the image intensifier so giving a constant displayed image brightness independent of x-ray absorption by the patient. Manufacturers use various techniques for measuring this input dose, two of which are:

- The image intensifier light output monitored by a small photomultiplier or photodiode
- For a dedicated video camera where the output screen and camera face is connected by a fiber optic plate, the video signal from a central (dominant) area of the image is monitored.

The first method is preferred since it provides a direct measure of image intensifier performance prior to the video chain.

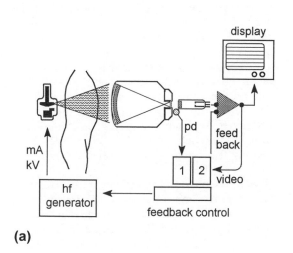

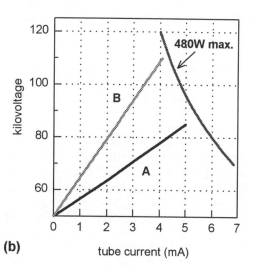

(a)

(b)

Figure 10.13 **(a)** Automatic brightness (dose) control using signals from [1] a photo-detector (pd) and [2] the display video signal controlling the x-ray generator to provide a consistent image quality at the display. **(b)** Two plots A and B of an Automatic Brightness Control program which alters kV and mA for increasing thicknesses of patient, so that the same input dose rate is maintained at the intensifier face.

Slight signal loss is inevitable since the optical coupling is modified and is not as efficient as the fiber optic plate. Signal sensors which provide feedback control are shown in Fig.10.13(a):

- A photo-detector which monitors image intensifier output controlling kV and mA.
- The display video signal whose amplitude alters video amplifier gain

The photo-detector system monitoring the image intensifier output (pd in the diagram) also adjusts the luminance levels for film exposure when using 100mm cut film or cine-camera.

Dominant region If the object is moving within the region of interest this can lead to large changes in brightness levels. In order to minimize this the feedback controls can:

- Monitor the peak video value
- Monitor the minimum value
- Use the mean value of these extremes

Monitoring the peak value does prevent the display from being overdriven, however other parts of the image can become too dark and for this reason the minimum value should also play a part. Control taken from a photo-detector (photomultiplier) sampling the image intensifier light output can only give a mean value. A better method selects regions of the image (usually splitting the display into three rectangles).

The particular display region which covers the anatomy of interest is operator selected and this is then the dominant region which supplies luminance information to the ABC circuit.

Exposure level Fluoroscopy uses a low input dose rate of about $0.2\mu Gy\ s^{-1}$ but during cut-film or cine this dose must be increased to about $0.9\mu Gy$ per frame for correct film exposure. Cine film exposure depends on frame rate which can vary between 30 and 150 frames per second. Increasing frame rate increases radiation dose

proportionally since each cine-film frame requires the same exposure level per frame.

10.4.2 Automatic Brightness Control

The Automatic Brightness Control (ABC)
(Fig.10.13(a)) ensures consistent dose rate at
the image intensifier face which maintains
image quality at the display monitor.

Feedback control of the tube current is a
simple operation but the response may be
slow since it takes time for the filament to
heat up; this type of exposure control is not
suitable for cine applications. Current control
of the x-ray tube can lead to difficulties when
imaging very thin patients, since these patients are relatively radio-transparent leading
to high transmission values at the image
intensifier. If feedback is obtained using current control only the current reduction may
be too great and lead to noisy images.

Automatic brightness control is therefore
achieved by adjusting both current and kilovoltage levels. The radiation dose at the image
intensifier input can be maintained in one of
three ways:

- A change in kVp at fixed mA
- A change in mA at fixed kVp
- Both kVp and mA changed

Current control usually dominates, but a
kilovoltage over-ride exists when preset values
of current might be reached which would
exceed rating levels. Figure 10.13(b) plots
kilovoltage against tube current control and
shows the maximum permitted level (480W in
this case) which forms the 'isowatt' limit for
the particular x-ray tube.

In some x-ray tube designs this can
approach 2000W. A function similar to the
ones shown plotted here is used by the
fluoroscopy system to calculate the kVp, mA
and dose rate so maintaining a constant
object transparency. The linear functions
plotted in Fig.10.13(b) differ according to the
emphasis placed on mA or kV; slope (A)
predominantly alters mA while (B) alters mA
and kV with equal measure.

In addition the video signal itself can be
maintained by applying an Automatic Gain
Control or AGC; both types of regulation are
used in modern fluoroscopy equipment as
shown in Fig. 10.13(a). Choosing a 'worst
case' condition of an extra large patient acting
as an effective x-ray absorber the ABC first
adjusts the tube current in order to maintain
the set input dose figure for the image
intensifier (typically 0.2 µGy s^{-1}). If a current
limit is reached the kV is then increased
keeping the overall power within the rating of
the x-ray tube.

When investigating thick body parts the ABC
will increase mA and then kV in order to
maintain video signal strength (display brightness). This may not be sufficient to maintain
image brightness and if exposure limits are
operating the machine will change the iris
aperture or increase video amplifier gain
(automatic gain control AGC); both these
adjustments will increase image noise. In
special cases high level control (HLC)
increases mA still further in order to
overcome limitations but this results in a
much increased patient dose, exceeding the
upper limit of 100mGy min^{-1} (10R min^{-1}) at
the patient surface. In most fluoroscopic
machines the ABC uses a reference central
area of the image intensifier; this is the
dominant area so the anatomical area of
interest should always be central in the field
of view. Fluoroscopic equipment with automatic brightness control commonly give a
range of exposure rates for particular studies.

10.4.3 Automatic Exposure Control

When radiography (spot film) is being performed by placing a film cassette in front of
the image intensifier a thin walled ionization
chamber, located in front of the film cassette,
controls exposure cut-off by comparing to a
reference signal.

Both cine and 100mm/105mm photospot
cameras require higher light intensities from
the image intensifier when recording an image
and the exposure signal for these cameras is
obtained from the photo-detector feedback.

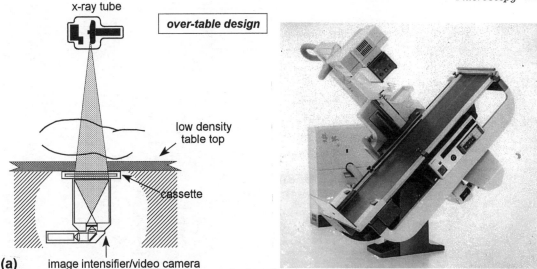

x-ray tube

over-table design

low density table top

cassette

(a) image intensifier/video camera

Figure 10.14 **(a)** An over-table fluoroscopy system. The table top can be moved at set angles for various patient investigations. The operator usually controls the exposures behind a protective screen consequently this design is more commonly called a remote control fluoroscopy system. **(b)** A standard design remote fluoroscopy system (courtesy Siemens plc).

Other methods of automatic exposure controls are used where the exposure can be timed (pulsed) by a grid controlled x-ray tube when switching is instantaneous. This technique is useful for bi-planar cine-angiography.

There is an optimum exposure level that will give the best contrast with good resolution Fig.10.6(b),(c). Any increase in dose rate would improve resolution but at the expense of contrast. This may be acceptable in vascular contrast studies.

10.5 SPECIFIC SYSTEM DESIGNS.

Three major radiography/fluoroscopy (R/F) designs are commonly used:

- An 'over-table' model where the x-ray tube is placed above the table top, irradiating downwards onto the image intensifier under the table surface.
- An 'under-table' model where the x-ray tube is under the table surface shielded by the table side panels irradiating upwards onto the image intensifier

- Single or bi-planar cine-fluoroscopy where x-ray tube and image intensifier are fixed to C-arms.

All three models allow the source-to-image-distance (SID) to be altered but this is more limited in the under-table design.

10.5.1 Over-table (OT) x-ray tube

This is a very versatile design allowing a great number of patient investigations and incorporating a variety of imaging devices. This is a remote control fluoroscopy system, a general design shown in Fig.10.14(a). The x-ray tube is placed above the table or couch and the image intensifier below. Exposures are controlled remotely from a shielded control station. This design allows:

- Image intensifier fluorography
- Spot filming using an under-table cassette
- Serial film exposure using a film changer
- Cut film using a 2-channel light distributor (lens and mirror between output phosphor and video camera)

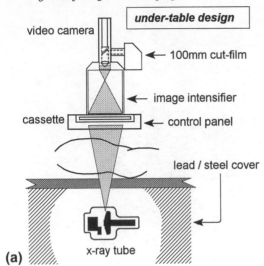

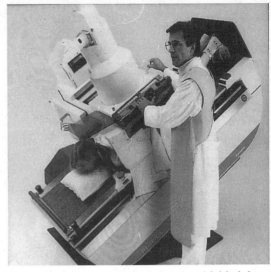

Figure 10.15   **(a)** An under-table fluoroscopy system where the x-ray housing is shielded by a lead/steel cover on the side of the table. The operator can be near the patient during investigations and operate the table and exposure controls locally. **(b)** This is shown in the photograph where a lead-lined curtain enclosing the patient provides added protection (courtesy Siemens plc.)

- Tomography, since the x-ray tube support can be angled.

The table itself can be tilted (shown in Fig.10.14(b)) and the focal spot (source) to image distance (SID) is large, from 115 to 150cm which minimizes geometrical unsharpness and reduces patient radiation dose. Anti-scatter grids are fitted but can be removed for low dose but lower quality imaging.

10.5.2 Under-table (UT) x-ray tube

The x-ray tube is placed beneath the table whose side-panels provides additional radiation shielding for the operator standing at the side of the table; the general design is shown in Fig.10.15. There is a control panel for local operation attached to the image intensifier housing. Most of the facilities offered by the over-table design are available but tomography requires separate ceiling mounted x-ray tubes.

The limited SID is 68 to 98cm which requires an x-ray tube with a larger anode-angle which can cover the necessary field of view at this low source to image distance. This can limit resolution by increasing geometrical unsharpness. The table material in both designs must have a high transparency to x-rays and consequently is almost always carbon fiber. The over/under table design is combined in a universal cantilevered C-arm which uses a large field (40cm) image intensifier. This design has been developed from specialized C-arm bi-planar machines but uses digital imaging techniques ex-clusively.

10.5.3 Mobile C-arm

Small mobile C-arm machines with image intensifier and x-ray tube fixed as an integral unit (Fig.10.16) find a ready application in surgery including orthopedics, bone fracture inspection, foreign body localization, and pacemaker implantation. Both fluoroscopy and radiography can be employed since film cassettes can be clipped to the image intensifier housing.

The image intensifier is linked via a fiber optic plate directly to a video camera tube or CCD device. The video signal provides a measure of light intensity which is related to x-ray exposure input. This forms the ABC feedback maintaining a constant dose rate at the image intensifier face. Table10.6 lists a typical specification for a small mobile image intensifier unit.

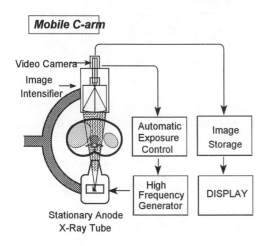

Figure 10.16 A small mobile C-arm complete with image storage facilities and automatic exposure control operated by video signal feedback.

Table 10.6 A mobile C-arm unit.

	Specification
X-ray tube	dual focus stationary anode Focal spot 0.6mm fluoroscopy 1.8mm radiography
Image intensifier	15cm 560 cd m^{-2} μC kg s^{-1}
SID	90cm
Grid	circular Pb8/40
Video display	1249/1023 lines 50/60Hz

The images can be stored on a video disc or on a digital storage device. Patient radiation exposure can be reduced considerably by using last-image-hold storage (LIH) on the video disc or digital image capture.

10.5.4 C-arm bi-planar cine-fluoroscopy

Cine-fluoroscopy is used for investigating rapidly moving organs as seen in angiography or more specifically cardiology. The images are typically recorded from two opposed image intensifiers covering lateral (horizontal) and AP (vertical) views as shown in Fig.10.17(a); a 35mm cine-camera views the output screens. Each frame of the cine-film receives the same exposure dose so slow frame rates require less photon fluence (exposure rate) than fast frame rates. The fastest frame rates (pediatric cardiac studies) are between 90-120 fps.

The drive control is connected to the x-ray generator so that frame rate and exposure levels can be synchronized along with exposure and camera shutter timing. Opposed C-arm biplanar cine-acquisition must be switched on and off alternately to prevent scatter from one plane interfering with the other. An alternating pulse switches each x-ray tube on and off sequentially shown in Fig.10.17(b) where a simple pulse sequence which enables film transport and shutter to be synchronized with the two pulsed x-ray sources. Instead of a pre-set pulse width an ideal system uses a photo-multiplier light sensor which tailors the pulse width according to radiation exposure and the x-ray tube is controlled by an automatic exposure control. A special grid-controlled x-ray tube is commonly employed for the fast frame rate switching that is required in cine-angiography. A high frequency generator with a very low ripple component allows a high degree of dose reproducibility. Owing to high frame rates required cine-angiography remains the recording method of choice since digitized frame rates offering the same resolution only achieve 30 fps at present digitization rates.

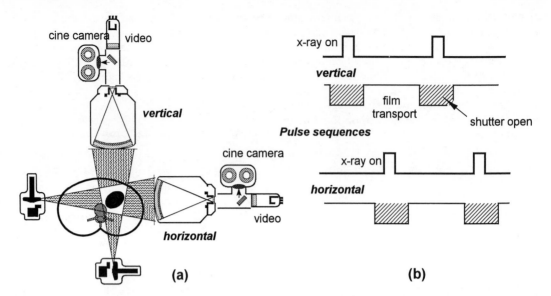

Figure 10.17 **(a)** A double C-arm cine-fluoroscopy system allowing simultaneous viewing in 2 opposing planes (bi-planar unit). Cine film recording is used for capturing heart movement at up to 150 fps. **(b)** Both image intensifier and x-ray tube are switched during acquisition to prevent scatter radiation interference from the opposing plane. The shaded pulse indicates when the image intensifier is switched on.

10.5.5 Staff dose exposure

The staff dose for both over and under-table x-ray tube fluoroscopy units is influenced by:

- The size of the patient
- The tissue being investigated (soft tissue or bone)
- The tube current and kilovoltage

The remotely controlled over-table design shown in Fig.10.18(a) gives a high dose rate in the vicinity of the table but this can be reduced by fixing lead-fabric curtains below the x-ray tube. This design tends to give lower patient doses due to a larger FFD.

The use of an under-table x-ray tube reduces the amount of scattered radiation reaching the radiologist in the vicinity of the table since substantial lead shielding is incorporated into the table side panel reducing staff exposure to about $1\mu Gy\ min^{-1}$. (Fig.10.18(b)). There is an in-built timing mechanism for all fluoroscopy machines which automatically switches off the x-ray tube supply after a fixed period of 'screening'; this is typically 3 minutes.

Cine-angiography can be responsible for high staff radiation exposures since the bi-planar design allows horizontal C-arm positioning and a high level of radiation scatter can reach the cardiologist. Ceiling mounted swivel arms carrying transparent lead-acrylic panels placed between the machine and its operator can reduce this scatter significantly.

Image storage High definition video or digital image storage devices can dramatically reduce patient (and staff) radiation dose since the x-ray tube is only switched on for a brief time, the picture is captured by the storage device and can then be viewed without continuous patient exposure. Figure 10.19 shows the dose reduction that can be obtained by using a video disc store which allows last-image-hold (LIH). Faster digital image capture uses smaller exposure levels and further patient dose reduction can be achieved.

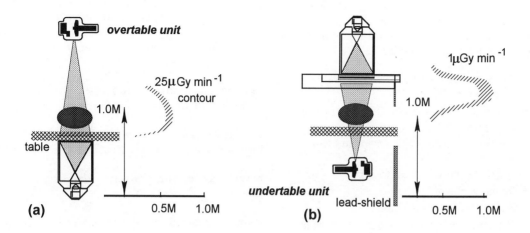

Figure 10.18 (a) Staff dose contours at 1 meter height from a remote control over-table design showing 25µGy contours and (b) an under-table design showing 1µGy contours. The considerable reduction in dose rate is due to table shielding .

If the irradiation time to the patient during fluoroscopy is reduced then the dose to the operator will likewise be reduced particularly when they must remain close to the patient during investigations.

Fluoroscopic procedures account for the greatest contribution to the total dose received by workers in diagnostic radiology. Particular attention should therefore be paid to the efficiency of x-ray image intensifier performance so that high exposure rates are not necessary in order to compensate for poor image quality. In general patient and staff radiation dose can be reduced by:

• Use of pulsed systems
• use of image storage
• maintaining short screening periods
• installation of low absorption material in the table and cassette (carbon fiber)
• prominent display of fluoroscopic timing on the monitor
• installation of dose-area product meter (Diamentor)
• in some instances removal of the anti-scatter grid
• cine-cardiology frame rates below 30fps and short cine runs (3-5s) although this is not always practical in pediatric studies.

The maximum output from the x-ray tube is limited to a patient entrance dose of 100mGy min^{-1} (10R min^{-1}). This is an upper limit and a more acceptable limit would be 50mGy min^{-1} for modern sensitive image intensifiers and in practice should be well below this figure. Using a properly operating modern image intensifier factors of about 90kV and 0.5mA should give adequate image quality with a patient absorbed dose rate of 10mGy min^{-1}. The minimum focal spot to skin distance should be 30cm and preferably not less than 45cm.

Since the application of digital imaging techniques has considerable advantages it is seen as a direct benefit to patient and workers to upgrade and retrofit a digital imaging system in the form of a high efficiency large field image intensifier and high definition video chain either in the form of a plumbicon tube or CCD camera (1024×1024 or 2048×2048 array) with a low dark current. A minimum resolution of 2Lp mm^{-1} should be obtained for a 33cm field size. A digital imaging system offers the following benefits:

- Patient dose reduction due to image storage (see Fig.10.19)
- A wide exposure range through image post processing.
- Time saving due to unnecessary film processing.
- Exposure series of up to 8fps
- Image archival
- Image data transmission
- Multiple images on a single sheet of laser imager film

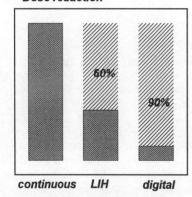

Dose reduction

60%

90%

continuous   LIH   digital

Figure 10.19 An indication of patient dose reduction comparing non-image store fluoroscopy with video and digital image storage.

Further reading

The Physics of Medical X-ray Imaging
Hasegawa
Medical Physics Publishing 2nd Edition.

Imaging Systems for Medical Diagnostics
Krestel
Siemens Aktiengesellshaft

KEYWORDS

automatic brightness control (ABC): adjusts generator output to give constant dose rate at image intensifier face for different patient thicknesses

automatic exposure control: adjusts image intensifier light output for film recording.

automatic gain control: adjusts video signal for constant display brightness.

barrel distortion: display distortion (also pincushion distortion).

C-arm: cantilevered connected image intensifier and x-ray tube.

charge coupled device (CCD): semiconductor position sensitive detector (camera)

cine-film: 35mm panchromatic film.

contrast ratio: a low contrast measure. Output light intensity before and after a 10% central region is shielded. (see veiling glare).

conversion factor: ratio of output phosphor luminance (cd m^{-2}) to input dose (μGy s^{-1}) typical values 100-1000 cd m^{-2} μGy s^{-1}.

cut-film: 100mm or 105mm square film stock.

dark current: background current during no input conditions.

field size: area seen by image intensifier input

flare: light dispersion at the input phosphor surface.

flux gain: gain in light intensity between input and output phosphors (electronic gain).

focusing electrodes: high voltage electrodes accelerating electrons

image lag: temporal response time

intensification factor: product of minification gain and electronic gain.

low frequency drop: drop in MTF value which influences entire resolution range.

minification gain: ratio of input to output screen area.

photocathode: placed immediately behind the input phosphor converting light to electrons.

pincushion distortion: display distortion

quantum efficiency: efficiency of converting photons to electrons or vice versa.

quantum sink: point loss of signal data.

veiling glare: ratio of light intensity at center of image with and without lead disk.

vignette: loss of peripheral display detail.

zooming: changing input field size.

11

Computers

11.1 Computer architecture

11.2 Central processing unit (CPU)

11.3 Bulk storage

11.4 Data input/output

11.5 Software

11.6 Networking

11.1 COMPUTER ARCHITECTURE

Computers form as essential part of our personal lives and of course the workplace which includes radiology.

The concept of computer design starts with Charles Babbage (1792-1871, British mathematician) who in 1822 described an analytical engine to the Royal Astronomical Society. Countess Augusta Lovelace (daughter of Lord Byron) was his assistant and could be identified as the first computer programmer. Important foundation work was started by George Boole (1815-1864, British/Irish mathematician) who developed a analysis of logic in 1847 and Boolean algebra later became the cornerstone of modern computer design. Herman Hollerith (1860-1929, American inventor) meanwhile devised a method in 1880 for automating the process of data handling into an electro-mechanical counter using a series of cards with punched holes. A similar method was already being used by the weaving industry for controlling their machines. In 1911 Hollerith merged with three other companies to form the Computing Tabulating Recording Company later to become part of IBM.

Alan Turing (1912-1954 British mathematician) published an article in 1936 on 'computable numbers' which gave a precise mathematical concept of computers and he was instrumental in the construction of an automatic computing engine (ACE) in 1948.

Meanwhile in 1938 an independent development in Berlin by Konrad Zuse (1910-1995, German engineer) resulted in a mechanical computing machine the Z1 which was later developed in 1941 into the first automatic digital programmable calculator (Z3) using 2,600 electromechanical relays. He later constructed a Z4 model weighing more than one ton.

John von Neumann (1903-1957, Hungarian/American mathematician) studied the art of numerical computation and designed some of the earlier electronic computers. His theoretical treatise on computer architecture governed their design until quite recently.

The parallel development of semiconductor micro-electronics: the transistor by Bardeen, Brattain and Shockley in 1947 (American physicists) and the first integrated circuits by Noyce and Kilby in 1957 (American physicist and engineer) gave the much needed reliability which heralded the practical everyday computer. Noyce also co-founded Intel the microprocessor manufacturer. Modern computers now encroach on all aspects of business, entertainment, education, science and medicine. Diagnostic radiology relies on them for:

- CT, MRI, ultra-sound, nuclear medicine machines as well as microprocessor controlled x-ray generators.
- Radiology information systems (RIS), as a computer network for digital image storage and transmission, handling text as well as image data.

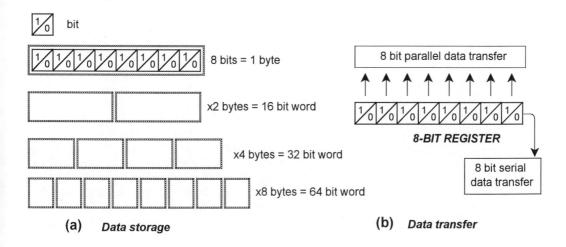

Figure 11.1 (**a**) The single bit forming an 8-bit byte which is then used to form a 16-bit or 2-byte word. Other word lengths are 32-bit and 64-bits which use 4 and 8 bytes consecutively (**b**) a single byte shift register which can move data in serial or parallel fashion.

- Quality control systems where measurements are taken, stored and compared to reference values. A report is then generated.
- Nuclear medicine and radiopharmacy inventory and monitoring
- General office word processing, spreadsheet, database and graphics.

Before outline descriptions of these computer systems can be given a basic knowledge of computer science is useful starting with their arithmetic fundamentals.

11.1.1   Computer code

Binary   The computer uses the binary system as the numerical base for all its internal working. All input signals from radiology equipment or otherwise must first be converted into binary format.

Since the Base$_2$ number system is awkward to describe two common formats are used for describing it: octal, using a modulo of 8 and

hexadecimal using a modulo of 16. Table 11.1 compares decimal, binary, octal and hexa-decimal numbering and demonstrates the convenience of octal and hexadecimal when tackling computer programming or problems involving binary notation.

The fundamental unit is the **bit** (short for binary integer) which can either be on or off: this is binary or 2 state logic 0 or 1. Figure 11.1(a) shows this basic building block and the way it is used to construct larger units. Bits can be put together in groups of 8 to form **bytes** which hold a maximum decimal count of 256 the 8 bits giving 2^8 or 256 decimal possible variations. Bytes can be further grouped into words of 2 bytes forming a 16 bit **word** giving $2^{16} \approx 65,000$ decimal, which was the basic word size used in earlier computers, and 4 bytes forming a 32 bit word $2^{32} \approx 4.3 \times 10^9$ decimal, which has now become the standard word length.

Larger word sizes of 64 bits are also available in very fast computer systems. These words form the computer memory. Bulk storage devices such as disks have sizes measured in mega-bytes (M-bytes).

Table 11.1   Four numbering systems

Decimal	Binary	Octal	Hexadecimal
00	00000	0000	0000
01	00001	0001	0001
02	00010	0002	0002
03	00011	0003	0003
04	00100	0004	0004
05	00101	0005	0005
06	00110	0006	0006
07	00111	0007	0007
08	01000	0010	0008
09	01001	0011	0009
10	01010	0012	000A
11	01011	0013	000B
12	01100	0014	000C
13	01101	0015	000D
14	01110	0016	000E
15	01111	0017	000F
16	10000	0020	0010

11.1.2 Data transfer and storage

Data transfer can be achieved by either **parallel** or **serial** methods, both are shown in Fig.11.1(b). Parallel connection is much faster than serial but sometimes the device can only handle data at a slow rate, a modem serial connection is an example. Some printers and film formatters are serial devices where slow mechanical speed cannot match the fast data transfer. Fast devices such as memory or VDU displays are always parallel.

The terms kilo- and mega- do not strictly work out to 1000 and 1 million in binary arithmetic:

$$2^{10} = 1024 \text{ bytes} \quad = 1\text{k-byte}$$
$$2^{20} = 1048 \text{ k-bytes} = 1\text{M-byte}$$
$$2^{30} = 1073 \text{ M-bytes} = 1\text{G-byte}$$

Accurate determination of storage requirements converting bits to bytes uses these values. An image matrix having x and y dimensions 512×512 and 10 bit deep (z axis) would have a total of 2621440 bits:

$$\frac{2621440}{8 \times 1024} = 320\text{k-bytes}$$

Using a similar conversion factor, a high resolution image of 1024×1024×10 bits is equivalent to 1.25M-bytes and a computed radiography image plate of 2176×2640×12 bits would require 8.2M-bytes of disk storage.

ASCII (American Standard Code for Information Exchange). This is a second computer coding system that uses binary numbers in groups of 8 digits (bytes). These represent display characters and are commonly met when representing alphanumeric characters. The byte values range from 00000000 to 01111111 which will define 128 separate characters, including upper and lower case alphanumeric. For example 'A' is represented by 01000001 (65 decimal, 101 octal) and 'B' by 01000010 (66 decimal, 102 octal), etc.

11.2   CENTRAL PROCESSING UNIT (CPU)

A block diagram of a basic computing system, based on a common PC, is shown in Fig.11.2. The central processing unit (CPU) is a microprocessor semiconductor chip (486 or Pentium series etc.). The external devices (disks etc.) connected to a CPU make up a practical computer. Some of these devices only accept information as output devices such as the video display unit (VDU), various printers and film formatters. Others are exclusively input devices such as the keyboard and boot-up ROM. Most of the other peripherals are both input and output devices.

The local bus is a pathway directly linking peripheral components such as the visual display unit (VDU) and hard disk. An Expansion Bus allows a wider range of peripherals (including other computers) to be connected. An Industry Standard Architecture **ISA** is an expansion bus that is either 8 or 16 bits wide whereas an Enhanced Industry Standard Architecture **EISA** uses 32 bit transfer.

Hard disk interfaces have a bus standard that allows efficient data transfer.

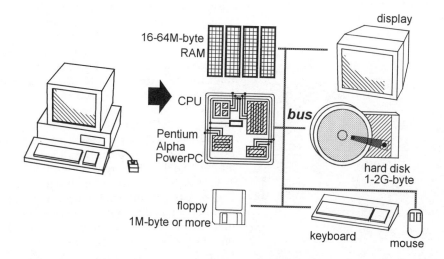

Figure 11.2 The basic personal computer (PC) broken down into its building blocks of central processing unit (CPU), random access memory (RAM), floppy and hard disks, keyboard, pointing device (mouse) and high resolution display (VDU). These are connected by a data bus for information transfer between the devices.

The Integrated Drive Electronics **IDE** is a part of the computer motherboard. An expanded version of this is the Small Computer System Interface **SCSI**, pronounced 'scuzzi', which accepts a far wider range of devices including disks and printers.

The CPU is the main organizing center of the computer and handles program instructions. Within it are electronic circuits:

- The arithmetic unit which carries out arithmetic operations on binary numbers.
- Instruction decoders which examine program instructions
- Logic gates which are the pathway for these programmed instructions.

The CPU also has registers which temporarily store words as the CPU is carrying out the various operations. The entire CPU is under a master clock control which provides synchronizing pulses and dictates to some extent the speed at which the CPU can run. Most radiology computer CPU's have the common micro-processor families manufactured by IBM/Intel, Macintosh or Sun.

11.2.1 Processor families

A microprocessor chip is shown in Fig.11.3 as part of a computer mother board which includes other integrated circuits such as memory and control circuitry. The mother board represents the complete working computer to which peripheral devices (e.g. disk storage units) are connected.

Design specifications Within many microprocessor chips there are additional components that let the microprocessor handle complex mathematical calculations and graphical functions more quickly. The Pentium chip, for example, has a special characteristic called 'superscalar technology' which gives this chip-set more than one pipeline to execute instructions making it much quicker than those that use just one.

Older design chips used Complex Instruction Set Computing **CISC** which gave a slower performance than the Reduced Instruction Set Computing **RISC** found in PowerPC and Alpha microprocessors. RISC is based on the concept that most computers use only a few simple instructions most of the time thus RISC chips execute those fewer instructions faster in a single clock cycle.

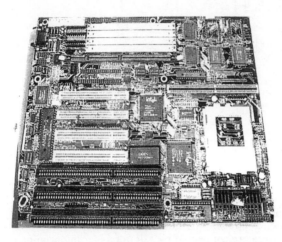

Figure 11.3 A microprocessor chip attached to its holder on a motherboard.

486 family   This has a 32-bit addressing, 32-bit data bus and can address 64 giga-bytes of main memory. Its has additional features such as an on-board buffer or cache memory and a built-in math co-processor (except 486SX). The original DX versions would run at clock speeds of 25,33 or 50MHz. Later additions to this range included DX2, designed to execute code twice as fast as the earlier 486DX. The DX2 is faster because clock doubling gives speeds of 50 and 66MHz. Another advance was the DX4 processor which tripled the internal clock speed to 75 and 100MHz.

The 486 chips were the first to have a cache memory which stores frequently used data. This is usually 8k-bytes but the DX4 models used 16k-bytes. An extra processing capability is give by the math co-processor which executed floating point calculations, significantly increasing mathematical and graphical functions. The 486 chips were also the first to include a RISC-like core; previously Intel used a CISC core.

Pentium   This is the next in the Intel series, the successor to the 486. The 486 design evolved into a more advanced processor the 586 or Pentium. Although the size of the Pentium's data bus was not changed from 32-bits the amount of information the Pentium can process internally through the chip itself is increased to 64-bits so it can operate much faster internally. Originally the Pentium was introduced with two clock speeds 60 and 66MHz but these were upgraded to 90, 100 and 120MHz; they now extend to 133 and 150MHz. The Pentium includes a 16k-byte cache, an 8k internal cache for data and another for instructions. The Pentium has an instruction set double that of the 486DX2 and has become more RISC-like than the 486. Multiple data pipelines allow multi-tasking (more than one instruction at a time). The Pentium has a better math co-processor than the 486 and will execute floating-point instructions 10 times faster than a 486DX processor running at 33MHz.

Pentium Pro (P6) The next generation Pentium processor is still faster. This sub-family consists of micro-processors running at 150 to 200MHz. With 32bit software the 150MHz Pentium Pro is over twice as fast as the 100MHz Pentium executing about 300 MIPS in contrast to the 100MIPS of the Pentium.   It is well suited to file-server applications. It has 5.5 million transistors compared to the Pentium's 3.1 million. The Pentium Pro competes with the Sun SPARC-stations and Digital Equipment's Alpha-Servers.

Macintosh PC   The Apple Macintosh computer uses a different microprocessor family produced by Motorola.   It is not compatible with the Intel family described above. Apple Computer, IBM and Motorola combined forces to produce the PowerPC microprocessor. The 601 chip runs at 100-132MHz and can execute 3 instructions per cycle and has 32k-Byte of on-chip cache. Models 603 and 604 are faster and process six independent instruction pathways and an increased cache size. All PowerPC microprocessors use a 64-bit RISC architecture and multiple pipelines.

Alpha   Digital Equipment produced this chip design in 1992 as two basic designs 21064 and 21164. The 21064 and 21064A have a range of clock speeds up to 275MHz. Both microprocessors have a 128-bit data bus and up to 32k-bytes of on chip cache memory. The 21164 has a 300MHz clock speed and delivers 1000MIPS. Alpha processors use RISC architecture and would be found in network servers or mainframe computers.

Sun workstations   These are designed specifically to handle high resolution graphics and use their own SPARC processor whose speed typically exceeds 100 MIPS. Their memory can be expanded from 8M-bytes to more than 100M-bytes and their hard disks can hold 2.3G-bytes of data. This large memory is necessary since complex graphics, drawings and images occupy a lot of space.

Clock speeds   Although there are numerous types and standards for microprocessors they all have one measurement in common: the system clock speed measured in MHz or millions of clock cycles per second.
 Clock speed helps to distinguish chip types although they should not be used for judging processing speed since a 486DX4 microprocessor and the Pentium have similar clock speeds but the Pentium, due to its internal design, has the greater processing power.
 Computer speed is often quoted as millions of instructions per second or MIPS and millions of floating point operations (mega-flops or MFLOPS). A speed of one MIP is equivalent to an integer calculation performed on a 1024×1024×8 bit matrix (1M-byte). Typical speeds given by modern computers are given in Tab.11.2., the fastest exceed 200MIPS.
A MFLOP would involve a floating point operation on the above matrix; an example would be a count density normalization. A typical range would be 4 to 100 MFLOPS for most radiology computers.

11.2.2 Memory

The microprocessor has three types of memory:

- Read and Write (RAM)
- Read Only Memory (ROM).
- Cache memory

Read and Write Memory (RAM)   The computer memory uses semiconductor capacitors and transistors for storing information as bits. The most common type of memory is the RAM (random access memory) or DRAM (Dynamic RAM) which uses electric charges held by etched capacitors on a silicon chip. This memory is **volatile**; it only holds information when the power is on. The electric charge representing the stored information drains away so these chips must be constantly refreshed in order to prevent data loss. This makes this type of memory slower than Static RAM or SRAM which uses thousands of transistors to store information. Although SRAM is still volatile it does not need refreshing so is many times faster than RAM however it is more expensive and less compact. If power is removed from either kind of RAM chip all data is lost.
The RAM is where programs and data are stored and constitutes the main computer memory. This can be several mega-bytes in size, using either 16 or 32 bit words according to CPU type. Figure 11.4(a) represents a block of computer memory having x, y dimensions. Each x and y location is an address which can be 8,16 or 32 bits deep. Program instructions or data in the form of images are stored here. In radiology systems working memory is typically 50 to 64M-bytes. This size of memory will typically hold several 512×512 images with a gray-scale depth of 10 bits; memories up to 128M-bytes have definite advantages if large image matrices are being handled.

Cache memory   Although RAM composes the largest amount of memory in a computer other forms of memory exist. CPU chips have built in memory space called cache memory. Several types of cache memory exist but their common purpose is to serve as transitional storage between conventional RAM and storage devices such as disk. The cache acts as an intermediate store allowing the CPU to

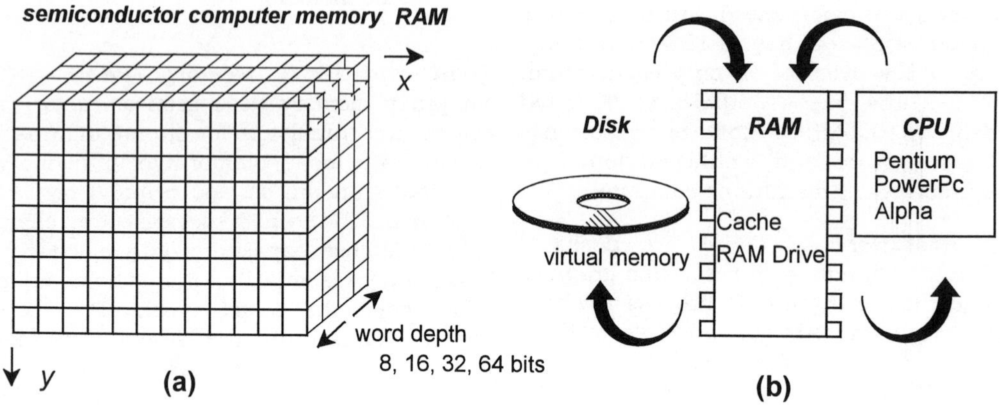

Figure 11.4 **(a)** Basic memory structure showing x and y dimensions as well as depth which is measured in bytes. **(b)** Memory organized as CPU semiconductor RAM or virtual memory residing on hard disk or RAM Disk residing in memory.

complete some other task; this greatly increases computational speed.   Most video display adapter cards which drive video monitors also have dedicated cache memory for image display.

ROM   A specific Read Only Memory ROM contains a permanent pre-programmed instruction set that users cannot alter. These instructions form part of the boot-up sequence when the computer is first switched on by loading input/output instructions into RAM.

Virtual memory   This is commonly supplied by the hard disk as swap files. When the RAM gets full some data can be written to disk which frees up RAM for more immediate work. RAM and the hard disk then swap data back and forth.

Virtual drive or a RAM disk can be supplied by sections of RAM being treated as a disk. This speeds up the CPU by supplying frequently used programs, that would be stored on the hard disk, from the RAM disk which has a much faster access and data transfer time.   A general scheme using the

different memory types is illustrated in Fig.11.4(b).

Table 11.2   Estimated speed of some microprocessors in MIPS

CPU	MIPS
Intel 486	20
Pentium	100
Pentium-Pro	200
Motorola 68040	15
PowerPC 603e	100
IBM RISC/6000	55
Sun SPARC	75-100
Alpha	1000

11.3 BULK STORAGE

In most situations in which digital images are acquired in radiological examinations the diagnosis will not be made immediately. Some means must be available to store the examinations images, perhaps on a semi-permanent basis, for viewing and for making hard-copy images of, later.

Also the digital imaging system must be capable of performing many digital examinations and so information from one examination must be set aside safely while data from the next examination is being acquired. There are many devices used to store images in a digital format:

- magnetic disks,
- magnetic tape,
- optical disks.

The important features to be considered when choosing and specifying a digital auxiliary storage device are:

- **storage capacity**, the number of bytes that can be stored,
- **transfer time**, the rate (M-bits s^{-1}) at which the information can be moved from main memory to storage device and vice-versa,
- **access time**, the time required to retrieve a stored piece of information.

Typical values for these characteristics are shown in Tab.11.3. Other factors which must be taken into account are the relative cost of storage per image, ease of operation and avoidance of any errors which might occur during image transfer.

Table 11.3 Storage devices compared to RAM

Storage	Capacity (M-bytes)	Access time	Data transfer (M-b s^{-1})
HD floppy	1.4	300ms	30k-byte
MiniDisc	140	~200ms	150k-byte
Hard disk	500-2000	10-20ms	2-4
Optical	400-650	150ms	v. slow
DAT	4000	slowest	slowest
RAM	64-120	15-100ns	10-250

There are four main options for storing the high number of images produced during digital imaging procedures. Fast access short

term storage is always the realm of semiconductor solid state memory but this is expensive and is normally restricted to a few tens of megabytes. Slow access, long term storage which can hold up to 3G-bytes per disc includes magnetic and optical disks as well as magnetic storage tape.

11.3.1 Magnetic disk

The stored data are recorded magnetically on the disc surface and organized in tracks and sectors as shown in Fig.11.5(a).

Floppy discs Also known as diskettes; these are removable 3½ inch diameter discs. The disk material is coated magnetic plastic and is vulnerable to damage.

The standard disk density is 1.4M-bytes but high density disks based on MiniDisk audio disks launched by Sony in 1992 promise to give a capacity of 140M-bytes with a data transfer rate of 150k-bytes per second.

Hard disks Sometimes known as a Winchester disk this consists of one or more magnetic disks arranged on top of the other and rotating at high speed. These bulk storage devices are fixed and not removable. The disk is aluminum coated with magnetic material. The Winchester design is hermetically sealed against environmental contamination. It spins at 3600 rpm as compared to the floppy 300 rpm so data transfer is very much faster. An example of this design is shown in Fig.11.5(b).

The sizes of early hard disks ranged from 20 to over 100M-bytes but most recent models are typically more than 500M-bytes and even 8-10G-bytes is possible. They are the main medium for short term image storage in a radiology computer.

Essentially the surface of the disk is treated as an array of data points, 1 or 0. The position of each point is decided by the disk format so the disks need to be formatted before they can be used. Accessing the data in any reasonable time requires the disk to spin

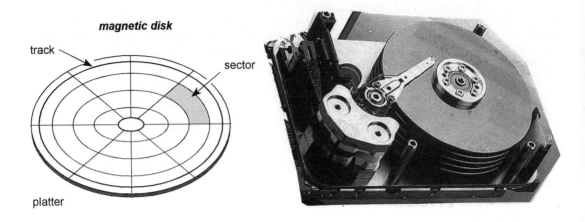

Figure 11.5 **(a)** The computer floppy and hard disc is organized as tracks and sectors which are addressable. **(b)** a Winchester disc used for storing up to 2G-byte of information (Courtesy Seagate)

very fast. Floppy disks spin at 300rpm and it takes about a fifth of a second for any given part to be identified. Hard disks spin much faster at about 5400rpm and this speed is being superseded with new designs.

Data retrieval. The performance of a hard disk is crucial to the speed of a computer system. Slow data retrieval will hinder a fast processor performance. The disk average **access time** is the time taken by the drive to locate the right track on which data are stored and the specific place on the track were the data starts. This is quoted in milliseconds and ranges from 65 to 80ms for slow disks to 10 to 12ms for the large fast disks. The **transfer rate** is the speed of data transfer and is measured in M-bytes s^{-1}. In order to get an accurate view of a hard disk performance both access time and transfer rate should be looked at together. A high access rate with a slow transfer rate produces a slow drive. A less important measure is the **seek time** which defines the amount of time it takes the hard drive's read/write head to find the data location point

The main purpose of a hard disk in radiology is to store images. High image transfers of up to 25 images per second are typical for some systems. Magnetic disks with capacities up to about 1G-byte are available. Such a store would be capable of holding up to about 4000 512×512 images having a 10 bit gray scale. The access time is typically about 10 ms.

11.3.2 Magnetic tape

Magnetic tape systems are available for archival purposes which have capacities up to about 4G-bytes and transfer rates of typically 500 to 800k-bytes s^{-1} and so have slow data retrieval times. However it is relatively cheap storage medium and its portability has made it a popular medium of image data transfer. There are two types of technology used for tape streamers: helical scan recording and linear (or longitudinal) recording. The linear type offers a better performance over the helical but has lower capacities

Helical scan This includes the 4mm and

8mm DAT (digital-audio) tape. Helical scan recording uses the same principle as video tape recorders and is inherently slower than the linear type. For this reason it is usually found as a back-up medium. The read/write heads are attached to a helical scanning drum and data are recorded in a stripped pattern. The tape moves at less than 1 inch per second. A typical DAT tape can store 4G-bytes of data.

Linear This includes QIC (pronounced quick) tapes. QIC-WIDE tapes offering higher capacities cost appreciably more than the equivalent DAT tape. When data is recorded onto linear tape the tape heads are stationary and the tape moves past at about 100 to 125 inches per second. The data is recorded in straight lines. Extra heads can be added to improve data transfer. The 800 k-bytes s^{-1} can be increased to 1.6M-bytes s^{-1}. A linear tape stores typically 2 to 4G-bytes of data.

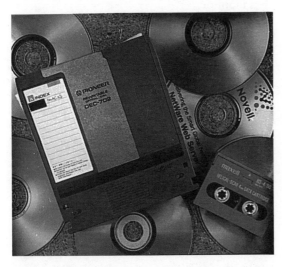

Figure 11.6 A collection of large volume storage media showing (from the left) a DAT tape cartridge, a CD ROM or WORM and a magneto-optical disc.

11.3.3 Digital optical disk

Optical drives include WORM (write once/read many), magneto-optical (MO) and re-writeable optical. These devices are well suited as an archival medium because of their very large storage capacities, typically in the giga-byte range, and slow transfer rate which is much slower than that of digital magnetic disk. A collection of magnetic and optical storage media are shown in Fig.11.6.

WORM The information is physically stored in memory by burning a tiny indentation, using a laser, in the glass substrate. Because of this most optical disk system can only be written to once, but read from many times, hence their name. This is very different to the digital magnetic disks which can written to many times, i.e. data stored on the disk can be erased and over-written by new data. So while it is not possible to overwrite information, once written the data cannot be replaced. Radiology archives are particularly keen on this type of media for storage since it provides sufficient security for patient data. Typical storage densities are 2 G-bytes which can hold up to 450 CT images of 512×512×16 bits deep. Banks of disks can be held in 'juke-boxes' where many of these optical disks can be kept on-line holding thousands of images representing weeks and perhaps months of patient image data.

Re-writeable optical disks Re-writeable or erasable optical disks provide the same high capacities as those given by WORM or CD-ROM but the data can be erased. Most users who store large amounts of data (hundreds of megabytes) very seldom erase so the application for erasable disk drives is for large files that are being continually altered. The average access time for a 5¼" erasable optical drive is about 40 to 60 ms with smaller 3½" optical drives producing times of 30 to 40ms; about three times slower than a magnetic disk.

Magneto-optical (MO) Discs These use a combination of laser and a small electromagnet to store data. To change the magnetic information on part of the disk a tiny area on the magnetic surface is heated by the laser. This brings the magnetic layer to its Curie point when new magnetic information can then be written. Once cool the magnetic state is fixed. The process is fast but the extra heating step takes time and consequently slows the writing speed.

Data access is as fast as the optical disk and relies on the polarization of laser light by the magnetic polarity of the data area. The main drawback of magneto-optic disks is the extra time to write information. They have a smaller storage capability than optical disks: typically 128 to 512M-bytes.

11.4 DATA INPUT/OUTPUT

The central processing unit communicates with the outside world by exchanging information very much as human beings do. There are input 'sensory' signals in the form of image data or keyboard instructions and output 'motor' signals driving disks and printers. Each input and output connection must first go through an interface with the computer which is a simple logic device packaging the digital information in coded words or blocks recognizable by either the computer or device. Some devices need confirmation or 'handshakes' after each data transfer so that synchronization can be maintained

11.4.1 Interfaces

An interface is the connection between hardware either within the computer (disk interface, display interface etc.) or between the computer system and an application device (gamma camera etc.). Interfaces are of two types: serial and parallel depending on the transfer of data; parallel interfaces are obviously much faster than serial interfaces but some data lends itself more readily to serial transmission such as optical data transmission. There are common standards that define interface performance:

- SCSI: Small Computer Systems Interface 'scuzzi' is a general purpose high-speed multi-tasking interface used to connect a computer peripheral device such as printers and disk drives.

- EISA: Extended Industry Standard Architecture competitor of IBM's Microchannel Architecture (MCA) which is a PC design.
- IDE: Integrated Drive Electronics refers to the hard disk drive interface

Ports These are serial (RS232) which connect the mouse, keyboard, modem or pen plotter. Data is fed out in serial mode. The parallel (Centronics) port is usually used by printers and imagers. The mouse is the most common form of pointing device. There are two basic designs for pointing devices. Those based on a roller ball include the mouse and tracker ball devices; the latter is more accurate in placing an exact location on screen and is seen in radiology imaging systems. Joysticks, which use wheels instead of a ball, are rarely seen in radiology equipment. The second type of pointing device is a light pen which is useful for identifying text locations and instructions on a monitor.

The keyboard is the standard item on almost all computers. It is used to enter information and instructions. The computer keyboard has special keys which are not found on a typewriter keyboard. Modifier keys are used in combination with other keys to change commands, the most useful key being the control key or 'Ctrl'. Other keys are the function keys F1 through to F12 which represent **macro functions** (small programs) or specific commands that launch an application that would otherwise require a set of commands, sequences or multiple keystrokes.

Displays These can show gray-scale or color images. The video interface or video card allows the monitor to decipher DAC instructions and defines display resolution. Gray-scale monitors are able to display a wide range of grays. The common monitor has 8-bit pixel depth so can display 256 gray levels but high brightness monitors are capable of handling up to 2000 gray levels. These are most valuable for diagnostic radiology displays. Color displays exist as 24 and 32-bit monitors. The 24-bit monitor can display 2^{24} colors or 16,777,216 and gives a true color representation. A 32-bit monitor displays the same number; the extra bits are used for display manipulation which is used for photo-retouching or video production.

11.4.2 Communications

The common computer communication uses cables to connect peripheral equipment such as displays, printers and keyboards. The communication with other equipment, including other computers, is more complex since the speed of communication is most important. This is measured in bits per second or **baud**. The baud rate is roughly equivalent to characters per second: 1200 baud $\cong$120 characters per second. Common baud rates for data transmission are 1200, 2400, 4800 and 9600. The transmission speed between two devices is restricted to the lowest baud rate that they have in common.

Modems These allow computers to communicate over telephone lines. They require special application programs that set the baud rate and transmission characteristics. A FAX-modem has software and hardware that enables the computer to act as a FAX machine however hardcopy can only be produced if the computer is connected to a printer.

11.5 SOFTWARE

The computer is quite dumb unless it is given some form of instruction for the task in hand. All the previous sections have concerned themselves with the mechanisms or 'hardware' that go together to make a working computer but this will only 'come alive' and do useful work when the appropriate 'software' is loaded into memory instructing the computer to carry out a logical sequence of events such as a simple addition of two numbers received from the keyboard which is then displayed on the monitor or (at the other end of the complexity spectrum) reconstruction of x-ray signal data from CT detectors and forming these into an axial-section gray-scale image. The software consists of programmed instructions carefully written in a logical sequence. Programs can be quite simple (macro-functions mentioned in 11.4.1) using a simple English instruction set; these are not very efficient with computing power so can be rather slow. Longer more complex programs which must be very fast and efficient use special coded instructions.

11.5.1 Languages

Both the computer instructions or program and image data are stored in memory and also on disk, in binary format. A computer program consists of a series of binary numbers which when processed identify a unique coded instruction e.g. add, subtract, fetch data, etc.

Early programs consisted of strings of these numbers and consequently programs were very difficult to write. Programs now exist in various languages which simplify program composition. Assembly language is the most primitive but enables precise control of the computer and the way it handles data. Assembly languages are extremely efficient and offer the greatest speed of computation. They are mostly used for fast data handling.

More complex program languages, i.e. C or C++, Pascal, FORTRAN, are more understandable having short English-like instruction set. Both types of programs must be translated into the binary coded instructions. This is achieved by using a compiler. The easiest language is BASIC which is a high-level language which is usually compiled as the program is run. It is therefore much slower than the low and medium-level languages but this is not a limitation if the data itself is keyboard limited. A BASIC program can be rapidly tailored to suit the particular task in hand.

11.5.2 Operating systems

This is a master control program that manages the internal functions of a computer and essentially makes it work as a computer moving data in and out of the RAM and finding room for new data by freeing up or swapping memory or copying it onto disk.

Multi-tasking   This describes the ability of the operating system to run more than one application in memory simultaneously. Since CPU's and operating systems are extremely fast and memory management is very efficient, the computer can seem to be handling more than one operation at once, using pauses in one application to implement instructions in another program.

One type of multi-tasking is **time-sharing** where the processor works with several users on a cyclical basis. Users do not notice this unless there are many users requiring fast response. Some operating systems allow multi-tasking either on a local scale where different jobs are carried out simultaneously (keyboard input, saving to disk and printing) or between machines on a **network**.

Common operating systems that have been designed for single or multi-user personal computers are:

- MS-DOS
- MS-Windows
- OS/2
- Macintosh System
- UNIX

MS-DOS is the primary single user operating system for IBM compatible computers. It was introduced in 1981. It is a command line operating system that issues prompts of the form C:> requiring the operator to respond with a properly coded reply. MS-DOS has a severe limitation since it imposes a 640k memory barrier and has no memory management capabilities.

MS-Windows   This is a windowing environment or graphical users interface (GUI) similar to Macintosh. MS-Windows is an operating system that utilizes MS-DOS but introduces multitasking and memory management. The latter increases the apparent size of RAM by allowing expanded memory, extended memory or virtual memory situated on disk.

Both MS-Windows 95 and MS-Windows NT have no DOS background and run 32-bit applications.   Freed from this restriction it allows the full 32-bit code capability of 32-bit processors such as the 486 and Pentium and treats memory as one long segment rather than splitting it up into sections as previously. Each 32-bit program runs in its own protected memory space. While 16-bit programs are more likely to cause trouble they are more stable in a Windows 95 environment. Both 95 and NT require much larger memory ($\geq$16M-bytes) and large hard-disk storage.

OS/2   (Operating System/2) is a multitasking operating system designed for IBM PC's. Windows was originally developed as a temporary measure while OS/2 was undergoing preparation. OS/2 is not limited by the 640k memory barrier and provides a degree of protection for parallel program operation, allowing exchange of data between applications. Version 2 runs MS-DOS and Windows applications.

Macintosh   An operating system specifically developed for Macintosh computers; this is Mac7 which has all the virtues of Windows, that is pseudo-multitasking, virtual memory, a graphics toolbox and has the same memory limitations. It is designed to support Claris application software.

UNIX   This is used on a large variety of computers from PCs to large mainframes. It is designed to support multi-user and multi-tasking. It is a common operating system for radiology. It still has its limitations since it is not very user friendly having more than 200 commands and somewhat restricted error messages. UNIX is able to link computers of different families together (i.e. PCs and main-frames).

NetWare   This is a network operating system manufactured by Novell for LAN's. It is a major operating system designed for PC network file-servers. It is also available on OS/2.

11.5.3 Application software

These are the common programs that make the PC an invaluable tool for clinic, laboratory and office. They include:

- Word processing
- Spreadsheets
- Databases
- Graphics
- Technical drawing
- Computer aided design and drafting (CAD and CADD)
- Desktop publishing

All applications are specific to the computer operating system but most software publishers have versions of their applications that will run on MS-DOS, Windows, OS/2 or UNIX. Macintosh applications are mostly unique to that computer type (Claris).

Scientific applications Software is available for more specialist applications. Radiology applications would be:

- Laboratory / radiopharmacy management
- Spectrum analyzers
- Equipment quality control
- Image communication and management
- Patient management.

11.6 NETWORKING

This is a way of linking several PCs and larger main-frame computers so that they can swap data and share resources such as printers and hard disks. Network servers commonly form the nucleus of a networked computer system where many separate PC type work-stations use a common database and program set. In theory any computer on the network can be a server but in practice this is a specialized unit consisting of a fast micro-processor (Intel Pentium) with 64M-bytes of RAM and CD-ROM with a very large hard disk (1-2G-bytes) which have typical transfer rates of 10M-bytes s^{-1}.

Cabling Connections between computers can rely on single twisted pair wires commonly seen used with telephones which will handle a restricted data flow to co-axial cables which will handle much faster data rates. Fiber optic cables are becoming the connector of choice however since these can handle extremely fast data rates and are not prone to electrical interference. Cable-less or wireless interconnections that use infra-red or GHz radio-frequencies are available for local area networks.

- **Twisted pair** connections connect low speed peripherals handling 300-9,600 baud (bits per second). The cable may be unshielded (unshielded twisted pair UTP) or shielded to reduce electro-magnetic interference (EM). Shielded twisted pairs can handle up to 16M-baud in token ring networks.
- **Coaxial cable** dramatically reduces EM interference and provides a high bandwidth of up to 250M-baud. The transmission speed does not decrease at such a fast rate as the twisted pair.
- **Fiber optic cable** gives a very large bandwidth of up to 2G-baud and greatest immunity to EM interference. This is fast becoming the standard communication medium.
- **Wireless** connections or Radio-LAN is simply radio communications on an allocated frequency between 2 and 3GHz. Transmission is coded for security and it can quickly link computers in the same building. It has distance limitations.

11.6.1 LAN/WAN

This is a method for connecting a group of computers, usually near to one another so it is called **Local Area Network (LAN)** as distinct from a **Wide Area Network (WAN)** which uses remote communication devices. LAN enables resources to be shared within a department. The computers and peripherals (laser film formatters, large disk storage etc.)

are connected by a simple cable or optical fiber link. Points or **nodes** on the network provide connections which can transmit, receive or repeat a message. The node is normally synonymous with a **work-station**. Networking is commonly met in radiology in management systems or when similar digital imaging machines are linked: CT, MRI, and DSA to diagnostic work stations. The advantages of networking radiology machines are:

- Images can be accessed from different machines and reported from a single point
- Single film output devices can be used for department hardcopy
- Uniformity of program format in the department.

There is usually a fast machine controlling a large disk store transmitting or **down-loading** information and programs as well as sending it back or **up-loading**. The central archive storage medium of the LAN (large disk) is itself part of a dedicated fast computer and holds all the department's image and program data; this is the **file-server** supplying other machines in the network that are called **work-stations**.

File servers The basic design of a network often contains a central file server that is the central mass storage. The file server is commonly a very fast PC with a large disk store which holds the applications programs and data files or image files for all the workstations in the network. In a peer-to-peer network all the workstations act as file servers. In a more common client/server network a single large PC with a very large disk store is the central file server for all the work stations or clients. Most network servers run 24 hours a day seven days a week so reliability is essential. A network serving a small number of users (15-20) is called a **work-group server** and typically has 16M-byte RAM and a 1G-byte disk as a starting size which can be expanded as necessary.

A local area network can form the basis of a Picture Archiving and Communications System (PACS) that communicates with other departments, clinical centers and hospitals so that patient diagnostic images can be dispatched more effectively.

11.6.2 Network design

Computers connected together allowing data exchange and communication uses a local area network (LAN) or a wide area network (WAN). The most basic form of computer connection use cables and the data is quantized as information packets which travel at various speeds depending on transmission technique. The speed of transmission is measured in bauds or bits per second. The baud rate approximately equals characters per second 1200 baud is 120 characters per second. Transmission speed is limited to the highest baud rate that connected devices have in common.

PC networks range from LAN's connecting just two or three computers to common output devices (laser printers) but may include 50 to 80 computers. WAN's use telephone or fiber optic lines to link computers at a distance.

Tree or Bus topology The extension of the computer bus is only suitable for very limited distances. Bus topology is a method of extending this communication using nodes to connect various computer systems or input output devices. Bus topology is a special case of tree topology which has a single trunk shown in Fig.11.7(a).

Using this design the bus can be extended by up to 300m (1000ft) without a repeater, which is a data amplifier used for extending the length of a network. Each branch of a tree network can act at full bandwidth since many messages may be sent along the bus at the same time. It is possible for messages to collide with each other and need to be retransmitted. Tree topology is a decentralized LAN used by EtherNet and AppleTalk where a single connecting line or bus is shared by a number of nodes including shared peripherals and file server. AppleTalk used by Macintosh, is a low bandwidth network design suitable for small network system. The advantage of a tree topology is that failure of a node does not disrupt the network.

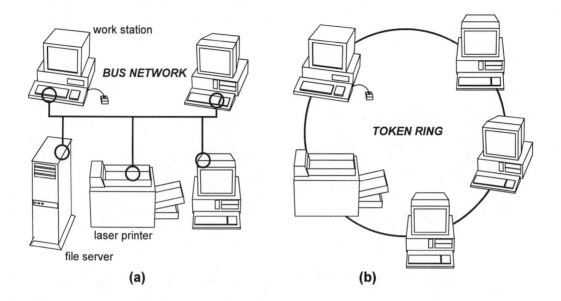

Figure 11.7 **(a)** A Bus is basically a backbone that each workstation or terminal is attached. **(b)** a token ring network has each workstation attached in a chain.

Ethernet This was developed at Xerox PARC and uses a special protocol (plan) for sending data. Ethernet tends to be faster and more efficient than many other network designs and is capable of handling a great deal of information data and allows work-stations to send data virtually simultaneously. Data collisions are detected and retransmitted.

Token Ring topology This is typified by point to point connections forming a closed loop shown in Fig.11.7(b). Each node acts as an active repeater to the next so ring networks can extend a greater distance than bus networks. Computers and other equipment on a token-ring communicate by means of a piece of software called a token which is passed between the devices. The token is a "pass" that gives priority to the machine that possesses it at any time. The token is passed from machine to machine. A machine can only send a message (image or data) on the network if it has the token. The drawback is that only one computer can use the network

at any one time slowing down the system. Other disadvantages of the ring system include the need for active repeaters at each node and the lengthening of the communication path as the ring expands. Failure of a node can disrupt the network. Fiber optic distributed data interfaces (FDDI) use ring topology.

Star topology In this design all nodes are connected to a single central exchange. At the center is the **router** or star controller which can be seen as a file server in Fig.11.8. Wiring costs are high since each workstation connects to the central router. Timing can be controlled more easily preventing messages from colliding.

Multiple interconnected star topologies exist where two or more hubs are connected to form an extended network. The main disadvantage is that the hub can be a single point of failure. The UltraNet design network is an example of the star topology. **Gateways and bridges** allow separate networks to be connected so that local traffic within a network does not add to the overall traffic of the combined network. When users need to communicate with others in different zones they send information through the gateway.

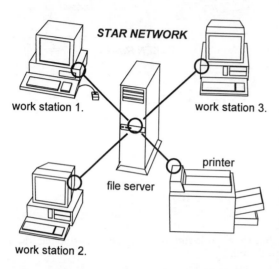

Figure 11.8 A star network with file-server supplying data and programs to all terminals.

Internet This was set up in the early 1970's for the United States military as a computer network able to survive nuclear war-fare. Four university computers were linked to form a high speed network. Eventually the backbone network accepted non-commercial from any location and in 1988 the administration of the network passed to the science foundation. Other independent networks around the world found it easier to route their traffic through this common backbone than link directly to each other.

The Internet is a Wide Area Network (WAN) connecting millions of PCs, mainframes by cable and radio links across the world using common communication protocols, the major one being TCP/IP (Transfer Control Protocol/ Internet Protocol). This allows very different types of computers to communicate with each other. Communication can be via a **modem** which allows digital data to be transmitted down a telephone line. Modem speed should be at least 14,400 baud. Modems are commonly classified by a series letter V.32 and V.34 being typical. These refer to 14.4 and 28.8k-baud respectively. An Internet **provider** connects the user to the on-line community. An account is provided on the central computer service provider enabling the user to log onto the server via a modem. The user's PC then acts as a terminal for the central **server**.

Computers on the Internet are divided into **clients** and servers. Clients are the desktop units that access the Net. Servers are the 'workhorses' many of them mainframes which use UNIX as their primary operating system. TCP/IP allows users to operate their normal operating systems (Windows, OS/2, etc.) and translates this information into a version that can be understood by the internet UNIX servers. Lines of communication are controlled by routers.

Medical interests on the internet are handled by various servers around the world having archives containing, for instance, radiology teaching files belonging to various university medical schools; these can be downloaded by the internet user. There are now 168 countries linked to the net and in May 1995 responsibility for the internet's backbone was handed over to private companies.

11.6.3 Radiology computer

A typical computer used for image data capture is shown in Fig.11.9 and serves as a simple demonstration. This can be part of the CT, MRI etc. The signal is first digitized by an ADC then the system processor steers the digitized signal into an **array processor** which is a dedicated computer designed for image reconstruction and handling. From here it can be simply displayed, undergo image processing (smoothed, edge enhanced etc.) or recorded on hardcopy (film). A local disc storage device can accept this image for further processing by work-stations on the network or it can be archived by the file-server which may be part of the departments radiology information system (RIS).

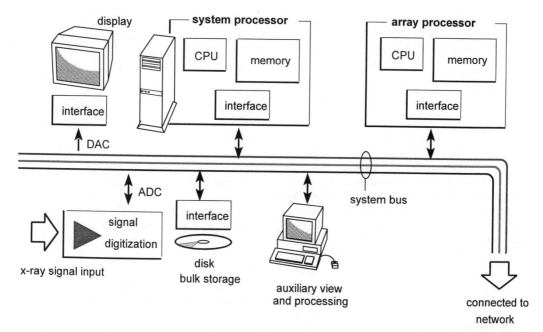

Figure 11.9 A basic design for a radiology computer accepting image signals from a piece of equipment and storing these as an image matrix on an array processor. The system is controlled by a central processor. The system bus is connected into a network.

The DICOM standard This is the standard data transmission protocol for clinical data and images set up by the American College of Radiology (ACR) with members of the National Electrical Manufacturer's Association (NEMA) in 1984. The ACR-NEMA Digital Imaging and Communications in Medicine (DICOM) standard has now been adopted by the majority of medical product manufacturers inside and outside radiology. The DICOM standard is a means for getting image data and associated information into and out of imaging equipment, whether it be an acquisition, archiving, display or hardcopy device.

In a radiology department operating different makes of equipment specific inter-facing is necessary to get the machines to talk to one another (if at all). If each piece of equipment, regardless of manufacturer, has a DICOM interface then interconnection between these machines is straightforward. The DICOM interface uses its own software operating system and executes the DICOM protocol so that the image data are formatted for transmission and provides network connection with other devices. Intra-hospital and tele-radiology applications are accommodated into this protocol. The key features of the DICOM standard include:

1. An effective framework necessary for claiming conformance to DICOM, requiring product manufacturers to complete a DICOM conformance statement.
2. Communication of patient and scheduling information thus integrating equipment with hospital and departmental information systems.
3. A means for querying patient studies and retrieve images as selected by the user.
4. The management of hardcopy devices connected to the network with basic film layout and remote hardcopy tracking.

5. The transfer of imaging studies from computer radiography, computed tomography, magnetic resonance, nuclear medicine and ultrasound.
6. The interchange of images on storage media such as optical or magnetic discs.

The European standards body (Comite European de Normalisation: CET TC 251) has adopted DICOM for the European Standard MEDICOM and the Japanese Industrial Association of Radiation Apparatus (JIRA) has incorporated DICOM into its standards.

The direct connection of medical equipment to standard TCP/IP network environments is also specified by DICOM bringing flexible network solutions using a variety of network standards.

Further reading

A special course in Computers for Clinical Practice and Education in Radiology.
Ed. Honeyman and Staab
RSNA Publications 1992

KEYWORDS

ASCII American Standard Code for Information Exchange. Each Character of text is represented in byte mode. Capital A is 65 decimal; B is 66 and so on.

assembly language: a type of computer language which is complex but enables the most efficient way of programming the computer, particularly for speed.
back up: copying data from one storage medium to another i.e. from Hard Disc to Floppy disk. Protection against data destruction.

BASIC Beginners All purpose Symbolic Instruction Code. A very user friendly programming language (unlike assembler). Versions are GW Basic, Quick Basic.

binary: numbers written in base 2, the fundamental counting system used by computers (see bit and byte)

BIOS (basic input/output system) A set of programs encoded on a ROM chip. It enables the computer to perform basic input/output instructions during boot-up.

bit: each bit in a computer memory can represent 1 or 0.

boot: the process a computer goes through when it starts up. BIOS loads the operating system from the disk (hard or floppy)

bus: A multi-wire connection that carries data between different parts of the computer or between computers.

byte: a unit of storage capacity made up from 8 bits. This will hold any number from 0 to 256. The byte is the composite building block common to all computers. Several bytes make up a Word. Memory and disk sizes are usually quoted in bytes: kilobytes (1000 bytes), megabytes (1 million bytes), giga-bytes (10^9 bytes)

C: A fast and widely used programming language.

cache: an area of memory used to store a copy of information recently read from or written to a hard disk. This greatly speeds up program operation. Cache sizes can vary; the bigger the better.

CD-ROM Compact Disc read only memory. Used as a storage medium for programs and data. Very high capacity (2 giga-bytes) can store images but quite slow to read them out.

CPU Central Processing Unit. The central microprocessor chip e.g. i486, Pentium.
database: a program that stores information so that it can be easily retrieved by searching and sorting facilities.

default: when a program requests an

answer and gives you the most common answer which is accepted as a default when the Enter or return key is pressed.

expanded/extended memory: methods of adding extra memory beyond the basic 640k-bytes. Expanded Memory can be fitted to all PC computers. Extended memory can be added and simply extends the existing main memory from 1M-byte up to 8 or sometimes 16 or 64M-bytes.

file: a section of information stored on disk and given a name.

floppy disk: a small disc either 5¼ or 3½ inches, which can be removed and used on other machines.

hard disk: a fixed disk drive and rigid disk used as the main bulk storage device on a computer usual sizes are 200, 500 and 2000M-bytes (1-2G-bytes).

interface: hardware or programs that sit between two or more pieces of hardware and acts as an intermediate data exchange mechanism or translator for dissimilar machine types.

macro: a stored sequence of instructions (usually keystrokes) that can be implemented by pressing just one key.

math co-processor: a companion chip to the CPU that carries out arithmetic functions. Program speeds increase by up to 6 times when using image processing or graphics.

modem: modulator/demodulator. A piece of hardware that connects the computer to a telephone line for communication.

multi-tasking: running more than one program or doing more than one job simultaneously on the same computer or connected group of computers.

network: several computers linked together with their output devices shared (printers, film-formatters etc.)

operating system: a program that is automatically loaded into the machine at start up (boot-up), and performs all the basic or housekeeping instructions i.e. disk transfer of program material, erasing or relocating data etc.

parallel port: input/output connection connecting the PC with usually display devices (printer or film formatter). The fastest method of data output.

pixel: picture element, represented by dots on the display screen. Images can be from 512×512 to over 2048×2048 pixels.

RAM: Random Access Memory where data can be written to and read from. Stored data is lost when power is removed (computer switched off).

ROM: Read Only memory. Contains the start-up programs of the computer. This data is obviously not lost when the computer is switched off.

serial port: connection between input/output devices where data queues up 'in line'. This is much slower than the Parallel Port but is more universal between computer types (RS232 interface line)

The digital image

12.1 Signal input
12.2 The image matrix
12.3 Digital image quality

12.4 Digital image processing
12.5 Picture Archiving and
      Communication Systems (PACS)

12.1 SIGNAL INPUT

Essential devices connected to radiology computers are the keyboard, a pointing device such as a mouse, disk drives (floppy or hard disk) and a source of signal data from machines such as ultrasound, gamma camera, CT or MRI as well as digital or video image data from radiographic equipment: DSA and image plate.

12.1.1 Analog to digital conversion

The input data is first converted to binary format using an Analog to Digital Converter (ADC); the principle is shown graphically in Fig.12.1 where the varying voltage levels are converted to their binary equivalent numbers. Conversion accuracy depends on the number of bits used which influences the step size.

An ADC with $2N$ steps can more accurately handle the analog voltage but takes a longer time for its conversion than an N step converter.

Most signals from radiology equipment start as varying analog voltages seen in Chapter 8 as film density changes or video signals. These varying signal voltages must be represented as a digital value before being accepted by the computer for signal processing and displayed as a digital image.

This is represented as a stepped graph in Fig.12.1 where a varying voltage is sampled and the voltage level converted into a binary number which represents voltage amplitude or height.

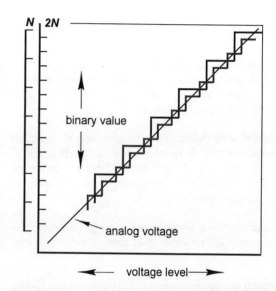

Figure 12.1 The conversion of analog voltage signals (*x*-axis) into digitized values (*y*-axis), showing step digitization using a low and high bit number ADC.

12.1.2 Data sampling

If the analog signal is represented by a moving voltage waveform then how often should it be sampled? Too slow sampling will fail to pick out rapid fluctuations and too many samples would require excessive data points and create storage problems.

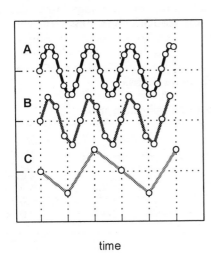

time

Figure 12.2 The sinusoidal waveform (A) is being over sampled. The waveform (B) is sampled at the Nyquist frequency which achieves accurate signal digitization. Fewer sampling points (C) misrepresent the original data which now has a lower frequency; this signal has undergone aliasing.

Aliasing The example in Fig.12.2 shows the same signal (A) being sampled prior to AD conversion. The number of samples taken faithfully represents the sinusoidal waveform but is the signal being over-sampled? Since the fastest fluctuation of the waveform corresponds to the highest frequencies this information will be lost if the sampling is reduced. It is important to digitize or sample the signal at a rate which faithfully reproduces the original detail (resolution or signal frequency).

If the original signal (A) is considered as a simple frequency f then this can be digitized accurately if the sampling frequency is at least $2f$. This is represented by waveform B in the diagram. The critical sampling frequency of $2f$ is the **Nyquist frequency** (H. Nyquist USA mathematician 1889-1976). Sampling rates below this frequency would lose high frequency information (example C in Fig.12.2) causing aliasing artifacts in the image. This can be seen in the common 'wagon wheel effect' in western movies, where the film transport rate is slower than the revolutions of the spoked wheel, which then seems to be rotating backwards.

Shannon sampling theorem (C.E. Shannon US mathematician, 1916-) The sampling theorem by Shannon states:

"An analog signal containing components up to a maximum frequency f-Hz may be completely represented by regularly spaced samples of $2f$ or twice the signal frequency".

The sampling rate T is:

$$T = \frac{1}{2f} \tag{12.1}$$

The minimum sampling frequency $2f$ is the Nyquist frequency.

For example an audio waveform with frequency components of 20kHz must be sampled at least 40kHz intervals. A frequency of 1MHz should be sampled at 2MHz. The sampling interval would be $\frac{1}{2}f$ or $\frac{1}{2}(2 \times 10^{-6})$ which is a sampling period of 5×10^{-6} seconds. This sampling frequency implies that we can recover the complete analog signal avoiding spectral overlap or **aliasing**. In practice a slightly higher rate is chosen to capture all the fast frequencies. Aliasing is a serious artifact in high resolution digital images (CT) where fine detail is smoothed out (bony structure) because high frequency information has been lost through data sampling error.

Quantization error (q) Since analog signals are constantly varying the action of sampling and converting to a binary value introduces errors. Digitization accuracy depends on the bit number n of the ADC. The maximum error q_{max} when digitizing an analog signal with an amplitude range of A and increment size N where $N = 2^n$ is:

$$q_{max} = \frac{A}{N} \tag{12.2}$$

For a range of 10 volts and a 3-bit ADC the q_{max} value is 1.25V.

The average error q_{av} is half this at 0.625V so:

$$q_{av} = \frac{A}{2^{n+1}} \qquad (12.3)$$

The average digitization error for a range of bit sizes is listed in Tab.12.1. Quantization error in a digital image is illustrated in Fig.12.3 where a single digitized step value can represent a range of analog voltages. A video signal of 1 volt with a noise of 1mV (dynamic range or SNR of 1000:1) will require at least a 10 bit conversion since the least significant bit would represent 1mV.

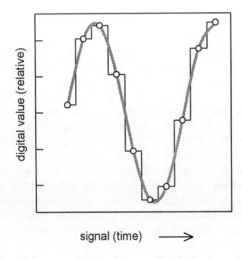

Figure 12.3   The stepped conversion by the ADC produces varying heights which translate as varying degrees of accuracy in digitization. This is the quantization error.

The original signal from the video camera (attached to an image intensifier) is a varying analog voltage   i.e. a moving video voltage level, that describes the light intensity on the camera face which in turn is directly related to the x-ray intensity at the image intensifier input face. The video voltage is transformed into a digital signal using an analog to digital converter (ADC) as previously described. The ADC must have a linear response over the full dynamic range of the image intensifier otherwise **differential non-linearity** will cause stretching or compression of values during conversion leading to image distortion.

The binary output from the ADC forms the digital image matrix.

Table 12.1 Digitization error

Bits	Range	q_{av} (%)
4	16	3.125
8	256	0.2
10	1024	0.05
12	2048	0.012

12.2   THE IMAGE MATRIX

While they are being acquired digital images are held in a block of semiconductor memory either in the main central processor memory or in a special image computer called an **array processor**. The array processor is a dedicated computer with some functions 'hardwired' to give extra speed. These functions would include data steering into the image memory independent of software program control.

A variety of matrix sizes are used in radiology depending on the degree of resolution required. Common matrix sizes are 512×512, 1024×1024 and 2048×2048 although smaller matrices are used in ultrasound and nuclear medicine.

12.2.1 Forming the image matrix

Separate elements of the matrix are **pixels** and carry intensity information represented on the video display as a gray-scale. The analog signal in this case is a video scan line, from a fluoroscopy system image intensifier, which is digitized prior to storage in the image matrix.   Figure 12.4 shows how a single scan line is sampled and digitized and each binary value stored in an x and y-matrix to form the digitized image.   The video waveform is measured in decimal millivolt levels (64, 82 etc.) and then converted into a binary value,

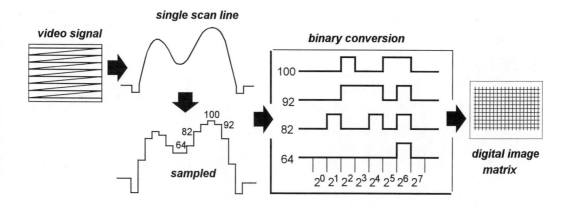

Figure 12.4 The digitization of a video scan line showing the continuous waveform broken down into discrete values at regular intervals. In this example the intermediate decimal figures are converted to binary format.

for instance 92 would be 00111010 and 100 would be 00100110 etc. These values represent signal intensity (gray scale) and are stored in the individual addresses of the image matrix. The signal first undergoes some filtration to remove noise which would interfere with the subsequent analog to digital process in the analog to digital converter (ADC). Each voltage level is represented by a digital binary value as shown by the pulse sequences in Fig.12.4. The stream of binary digits is accepted and stored by the computer processing unit (CPU) as the digital image.

The positional information (x and y) is obtained from the video raster timing and scan speed. Pixel positions within the matrix is governed by spatial information (position along the scan-line) and timing (end-of-line and sync. pulses) of the scanning beam; the video time-base of the camera or display supplies these signals from stable clock pulses. The video voltage level, which is proportional to image-intensifier light intensity, is digitized giving the gray scale information which is stored in each pixel.

Digitizing a video frame acquired in $\frac{1}{30}$th second for a 512×512 matrix requires that 512^2 samples are digitized in:

$$\frac{0.0333}{512^2} = 127 \times 10^{-9} \text{ s}$$

or 127ns or 8MHz. This sampling frequency would limit the bandwidth to 4MHz for faithful digitization (½ Nyquist rate). Specific signal handling for imaging devices used in nuclear medicine, ultrasound, CT and MRI are described in their relevant chapters.

12.2.2 Matrix size

Image matrices used for capturing radiology picture data range from a very low definition 32×32 pixels to extremely high definition 2048×2048. Some image plate digital images exceed even this high figure. Table 12.2 lists typical applications seen in Radiology.

As already discussed in Chapter 9 the image matrix is stored in computer memory as a 2-dimensional array (x and y axes). Each pixel address is from 8 bits to 16 bits deep which is

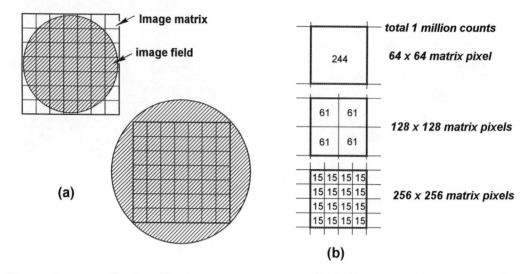

Figure 12.5 **(a)** A nuclear medicine gamma camera field within a rectangular image matrix showing exact and over framing **(b)** the individual pixel values N for three matrix sizes 64×64, 128×128 and 256×256. Image noise is related to $\sqrt{N}$.

displayed as a gray-scale describing signal intensity (nuclear medicine, DSA, MRI), attenuation (CT). Figure 12.5(a) shows alternative methods for framing the circular field of view offered by many radiology machines (e.g. fluoroscopy, CT, gamma camera, etc.). **Exact framing** encloses the total area within the matrix but is wasteful of matrix area. The alternative is **over framing** where the whole matrix is within the field of view. This closely represents the collimated field of view or the area of patient being examined and gives a larger working image than the exact framing method.

Figure 12.5(b) shows the decrease in count density for a fixed total count (1 million) as the image matrix increases in size from 64×64 to 256×256; the individual pixel count N decreases by a factor of 4 from 64^2, 128^2 to 256^2. Since noise content is related to $\sqrt{N}$ the noise component increases with matrix size (for the same total count). Resolution may be improved with larger matrix sizes but low contrast definition will be lost due to increasing noise.

Table 12.2   Matrix sizes common in radiology

Recording Medium	Matrix Size	Pixels	Pixels mm^{-1}
Film			
(14″×17″)	3500×4000	14 M	10
Image Plate	2048×2048	4 M	4
Video			
625 line TV	512×512	262 k	1
1249line TV	1024×1024	1 M	2

12.2.3   Image storage

Image memories are specified by:

- Storage capacity
- Transfer rate
- Access time

Storage can be located in the computer RAM memory which has very fast transfer rates and data access time but has limited storage capacity or disk storage (Winchester disk) which has a transfer rate of 1MByte s^{-1}

corresponding to an image transfer rate of 4fps at 512^2 as shown in Table 12.3; disk retrieval or access is about 10ms. Optical or magneto-optical disks are suitable for long term (archival) image storage since their access times are much longer

Table 12.3 Data storage for two image sizes.

	$512^2 \times 8$	$1024^2 \times 10$
Total Memory	256kByte	1.25MByte
Transfer Rate		
4 fps	1MByte s^{-1}	5MBytes^{-1}
15fps		18MByte s^{-1}
60fps	15MByte s^{-1}	
Storage		
5 s duration	75MByte	90MByte

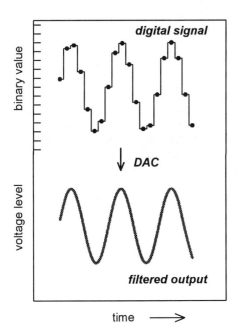

Figure 12.6 A simple DAC example showing conversion of digital values to voltage levels and filtering the step waveform to get a smooth analog signal for display.

12.2.4 Image display

Digital to Analog Conversion (DAC) Data output from the computer most commonly appears as images on a color or black and white monitor; other output devices would be film-formatters and printers. Digital data for display is converted to voltage levels by a Digital to Analog Converter (DAC), the converse of the Analogue to Digital Converter.

The action of a DAC is shown in Fig.12.6 where each digital value (represented by a different height column) gives a 'staircase' waveform which is then filtered giving a smooth output waveform which is mixed with video sync pulses to give a complete video scan line for the display.

12.3 DIGITAL IMAGE QUALITY

Quality of digital images depends primarily on the image matrix size. Smaller matrices have poor resolution but better noise characteristic and therefore better low contrast discrimination. As the matrix size is increased resolution improves but the count or photon density in each pixel must be increased in order to maintain a certain minimum noise level. This factor is crucial to digital image quality so the size of the image matrix should be chosen with care and should not be unnecessarily large.

12.3.1 Noise

Since the number of photons available for image formation is related to patient dose image quantum noise increases as patient dose is decreased (all other parameters being unchanged, i.e. detector efficiency, matrix size).

The interaction between a position sensitive detector (gamma camera, image intensifier etc.) with a uniform flux of radiation (γ- or x-ray) obeys the random processes covered by statistical laws i.e. Poisson and Gaussian distributions described in Chapter 1. Thus if such a detector was represented by an image matrix each matrix pixel would contain a mean number x counts with a standard deviation of approximately $\sqrt{x}$. The statistical error or noise can be expressed as:

$$\frac{\sqrt{x}}{x} \qquad (12.4)$$

For a pixel count of 100 the estimated noise figure would be 10% and the standard error 0.1. For a pixel count of 10,000 the values would be 100 and 0.01 respectively. Box 12.1 gives other examples involving low contrast detection demonstrating that noise content influences the level of low contrast differences that can be visualized in a digital image.

Box 12.1

Low contrast and noise

Fluoroscopy
3×10^5 photons mm^{-2} gives an approximate skin dose of 10mGy. The quantum noise is:

$$\sqrt{3 \times 10^5} = 547 = 0.18\%$$

so low contrast differences of 1% will be visible even at reduced patient radiation dose.

Nuclear Medicine
An Image having a total count of 10^6 on a 128×128 matrix has an individual pixel density of:

$$\frac{10^6}{128^2} = 61$$

so the quantum noise per pixel is $\sqrt{61} = 12\%$. Increasing the total counts to 2 million reduces this to 9%

Tomographic imaging (SPECT) requires an accurate uniformity measurement with a variation of only 1%. A 30 million flood field collected by a 64×64 matrix would give 7324 counts per pixel and a quantum noise figure of approximately 1%. A 128×128 matrix would require 4 times the number of counts.

Digital image matrices can contain multiple noise sources including:

- **The detector.** This is responsible for quantum noise or the interaction of the photon flux with the phosphor. The number of quanta making up the image determines the image noise content. This is seen in low radiation dose investigations using image intensifiers, image plates and low count density scintigraphs.
- **Digitization accuracy**. Conversion of the analog event into a binary coded precision gives error to the image (Fig.12.3).
- **Magnification**. Decreasing the field of view can decrease photon density and so increase noise.
- **Image subtraction**. Digital subtraction of one image from the other leaves behind the sum of the noise content of both images (e.g. digital subtraction angiography or DSA).

12.3.2 Resolution and contrast

Image resolution for a digital matrix cannot be better than the dimension of an individual pixel. The real dimensions of a pixel as mm^2 or cm^2 depend on the size of the field of view.

From Chapter 8, image resolution is measured in line pairs per mm (Lp mm^{-1}); if two lines are x mm apart then $1/x$ mm represents x Lp mm^{-1}. If two lines separated by 0.5mm can just be resolved then the image resolution is 2Lp mm^{-1}. The resolution of a digital image held in matrix form depends on pixel size p so line pair resolution is:

$$\frac{1}{2p} \qquad (12.5)$$

Pixel size is determined by the field of view (for instance film size or image intensifier size) and matrix size m so that pixel size is FOV/m. A 43×43cm film (14″×14″) digitized on a 1024 matrix would have a pixel size of 0.4mm giving a resolution of 1.25Lp mm^{-1}; hardly acceptable considering the original film data may have yielded 3Lp mm^{-1}. Table 12.4 lists some common digital images used in radiology and the area occupied by the individual pixels

The resolution of a digital matrix usually matches the machine resolution. Information cannot be gained by using a 1024×1024 matrix having resolution of 1.25Lp mm^{-1} if the machine is only capable of 0.5 Lp mm^{-1} resolution.

This point is clearly seen in nuclear medicine where digital images of 256×256 represent the maximum resolvable detail that the gamma camera is capable. Employing larger image matrix sizes degrades image quality by introducing more noise into each pixel. For a fixed total count density each pixel n would reduce in magnitude so increasing noise as $\sqrt{n}$.

Table 12.4   Pixel sizes for radiology matrices.

System	Matrix Size	Pixel size (mm^2)
Nuclear Medicine		
38cm Camera	256×256	1.5
CT		
28cm (Head)	512×512	0.55
45cm (Body)	512×512	0.87
DSA		
20cm II	512×512	0.4
	1024×1024	0.2
Image Plate		
8″×10″	1760×2140	0.01
Laser Imager		
14″×17″	4260×5182	0.008

Line-pair value   A resolution of 1Lp mm^{-1} would require 2 pixels mm^{-1} and 5Lp mm^{-1} would require 10 pixels mm^{-1}. An image intensifier having an input face of 250mm would give a resolution of 1mm on a 512×512 matrix. Mammography using a field size of 7″×9½″ (18×24cm) would need a matrix of 2048×2048 to resolve detail approaching 0.1mm.

Matrix size is sometimes increased for display purposes. Some CT machines reconstruct their images using a 512×512 matrix but display them as a 1024×1024 matrix by **interpolation**. This does not increase system resolution, merely improves the cosmetic appearance of the image.

Contrast   This is dependent on count density in a digital image matrix. It was shown in 12.3.1 that noise plays an important role if small density differences are to be seen. Contrast is therefore a question of signal to noise which is demonstrated in Box 12.1. The low contrast visibility depends on noise fluctuations.

12.4 DIGITAL IMAGE PROCESSING

The great advantage of digital image matrices is the ability to manipulate the raw image data using computer techniques. Real improvement and feature enhancement can be achieved that contributes significantly to diagnosis.

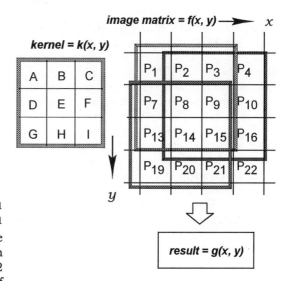

Figure 12.7   Action of matrix filtering using a small mask (kernel) which is moved over the image matrix. The center pixel in the image matrix is modified for each mask position.

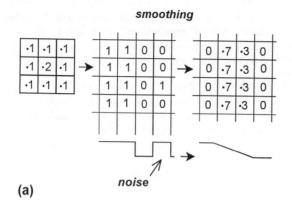

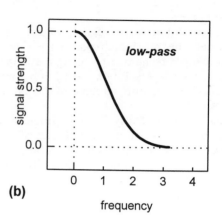

smoothing

(a)   *noise*

(b)

Figure 12.8   **(a)** Smoothing a section of a digital image using a 9-point kernel to remove a noisy pixel (last in the 3rd row); The profile for this row is shown below the matrix. After filtering the sharp edge (between the 1's and 0's) is smoother but the noise component has vanished. **(b)** the shape of a low pass filter which will reject higher frequencies.

12.4.1 Spatial filtering

Contrast occurs at different scales in an image; fine structure occurs on a small scale while slow changes in gray level occur over a large scale. Spatial filtering techniques can be used to emphasize features of different sizes. Sharp edges, fine detail and image noise or mottle all occur over a small scale. Spatial filtering techniques can be used to enhance these edges and fine structure and reduce the effects of noise. There are two types of digital spatial filter: a **low pass**, smoothing filter used to reduce noise and a **high pass** edge or contrast enhancing filter.

The general application of a small filter mask or kernel to an image matrix is shown in Fig. 12.7. Using the labels from this diagram the mathematical expression for the 3×3 filter (9-point) can be described, either as:

$$P_8 = (A \times P_1) + (B \times P_2) + (C \times P_3) + (D \times P_7) + (E \times P_8) + (F \times P_9) + (G \times P_{13}) + (H \times P_{14}) + (I \times P_{15})$$

$$P_8 = \sum_{x,y}^{3} k(x,y) \cdot f(x,y)$$

$$g(x, y) = \sum_{x}^{3} \sum_{y}^{3} k(x,y) \cdot f(x,y)$$

or $$g(x, y) = k(x, y) \otimes f(x, y) \qquad (12.6)$$

These same equations describe placing the kernel $k(x, y)$ over the image matrix $f(x, y)$ and storing the product of the entire matrix multiplication $\otimes$ as the output filtered matrix $g(x, y)$.

Low pass filter (smoothing) Low pass filters are used to reduce noise or mottle. The process is often called image smoothing, i.e. removing the apparent 'graininess' due to image noise. Figure 12.8 shows that for each pixel in an image the gray level value is added to the sum of the gray levels in the eight surrounding pixels.

The example in Fig. 12.8(a) shows a single profile through a section of an image having a uniform pattern interrupted by a noise spike. The average of each pixel is obtained by addition of the gray levels of the adjacent pixels.

edge enhancement

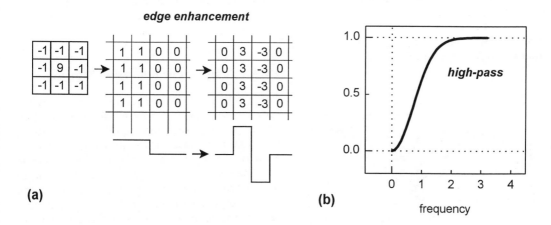

Figure 12.9 **(a)** Edge enhancement produces an exaggerated differential profile. **(b)** the shape of a high pass filter which will reject low frequencies while accentuating high frequencies.

This new averaged or smoothed data is shown after filtering with this smoothing kernel. The effect of the noise spike has been reduced with a loss however in spatial resolution or detail. The original pixel gray level is replaced by the average of these nine pixels. This process is repeated for all the pixels in the image. Figure 12.8(b) shows the frequency shape for this low pass filter. The smoothing action given by this filter when applied to a noisy image is shown in Fig.12.17 at the end of this chapter.

High pass filter (edge detection) These are used to enhance of an edge or contrast in an image. An edge is defined as a change in gray level and contrast is defined as a change in optical density in an image. Figure 12.9(a) shows a pattern of numbers representing a step change in an image matrix and the kernel used to modify the values in the matrix. This 3×3 filter now has negative values. Each of the original values is multiplied by the central kernel value, 9, while the neighboring values are multiplied by the outer −1 kernel values. The original data is replaced by the sum of these three operations, giving the filtered matrix. The effect of this

operation is to emphasize the location of edge structures in an image.

The image data in a matrix can be enhanced by using low pass or high pass filters. Since noise contains a great deal of high frequencies it can be greatly reduced by passing the data through a low pass filter removing scattered noise peaks in an image or reducing them in height. If edges are an important feature in the radiograph then an edge enhancement can be applied. This can be seen in Fig.12.18 at the end of this chapter. Digital filters can be used to enhance detail in an image and help to reduce noise but they are computationally expensive. For example each pixel in a 1024×1024 image (about a million pixels) require nine multiplication and one addition.

Specific filters Two commonly used filter types are Hanning and Butterworth. The filter amplitude at any particular frequency depends on the cut-off frequency F and the 'roll-off' value Q decides the filters shape. If F or Q is high then the filter is high-pass: accentuating edges in the image. Low values of F and Q give a smoothing action. These filters can be designed so that even though a general smoothing is carried out the tail of the filter characteristic passes sufficient high frequency information to preserve edge detail.

Figure 12.10 shows three filter shapes (A) a simple linear ramp and two varieties of Butterworth filter (B and C).

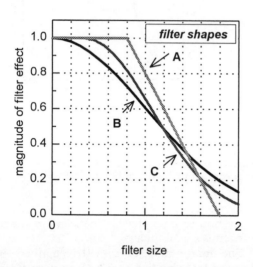

Figure 12.10 A linear filter (A) and two types of Butterworth filter (B and C). The *x*-axis is a measure of the filter matrix size.

Unsharp masking   Many techniques are available for edge detection and enhancement and certain manufacturers (Kodak) have produced Adaptive Unsharp Masking (AUSM) for effective and rapid edge enhancing of their computed radiography image plates. Unsharp masking follows a common principle which is the formation of the initial mask by over smoothing the clinical image. This is then subtracted from the initial image and the resulting matrix added to the original image. This action reduces noise and emphasizes any detail that may be present.

The AUSM is thus not a linear process. The general equation describing it would be:

$$O(j,k) = I_i(j,k) + \beta \left[I_i(j,k) - I_b(j,k) \right] \quad (12.7)$$

Where $I_i(j,k)$ is the input image $I_b(j,k)$ is the

unsharp mask formed by blurring or over-smoothing the initial image and β is a boost function which depends on the application. $O(j,k)$ is the output image.

12.4.2 Temporal or Recursive filtering

Noise reduction is particularly important in radiological imaging where patient radiation protection requires that the minimum amount of radiation is used for the imaging procedure. As a result the noise component in an image can be significant, e.g. fluoroscopy or in nuclear medicine examinations. When dealing with a sequence of similar digital images such as a dynamic acquisition, noise reduction can be obtained by averaging a number of images in the sequence. The signal to noise ratio obtained by averaging any number of images N, will be improved by a factor $\sqrt{N}$ as plotted in Fig.12.11(a).   When several images are added together any image signal (feature) remains relatively constant, however the noise due to its random nature is uncorrelated and the fluctuating values will tend to average or cancel out. This is described more fully in Chapter 13. It has already been seen that image noise decreases as the pixel count increases. Increasing the pixel count can either be achieved by increasing radiation dose or time per study in the case of nuclear medicine and MRI; an alternative procedure is to add successive images.

12.4.3 Look up tables (LUT)

Signal pre-processing is achieved by both analog and digital means where non-linear outputs are desirable. The analog method relies on fixed circuits whereas digital methods use a 'look-up-table' (LUT) which holds stored values of the desired non-linear conversion (i.e. logarithmic numbers).   An LUT is stored in ROM or RAM depending on whether the signal conditioning is fixed or variable. A display look-up table (Figure 12.11(b)) relates the brightness produced on the screen to the number stored in memory.

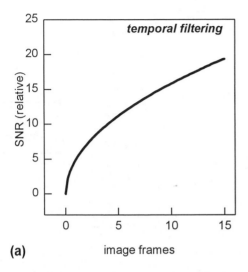

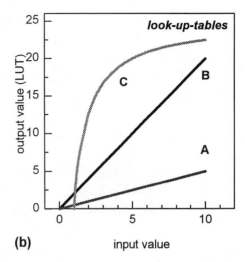

(a) image frames   **(b)** input value

Figure 12.11 **(a)** Temporal filtering reduces image noise as a square root function of the image frames that are summed. In practice five images are usually averaged. **(b)** Three LUT examples linear (A and B) and non-linear (C) that can be used for input signal modification. The input values are represented by the *x*-axis while the output values derived from the stored LUT are given by the *y*-axis.

Usually a linear look-up table is used (curves A and B) which produces a steep or shallow linear change in monitor brightness for a given linear change in the input digital data. However it is possible to vary the shape of the look-up table so as to enhance dark or bright sections of the image (curve C). Table 12.5 gives an example where a linear input can be converted into a clipped-linear function or a logarithmic function.

Table 12.5 Values for a LUT which gives a clipped or logarithmic output.

	LUT	value
Table Entry	*Clipped Linear*	*Logarithmic*
20	20	3
40	40	7
60	60	20
80	80	55
100	80	148
120	80	–

Translation tables A common application for look-up tables involves the alteration of display characteristics. When a video signal is acquired and digitized it is converted to a sequence of numbers. Each number represents the amount of radiation detected in different parts of the field of view. The image may be displayed on a viewing monitor in its raw state but some form of data processing is usually required. Figure 12.12(a) shows an input video signal that can be shaped in order to correct for detector response non-linearity before conversion to an analog display signal.

The common linear gray scale can be transcribed into other formats including color scales, both linear and non-linear. This is achieved by digitally changing the original linear gray-scale into three non-linear signals and feeding these into the RGB amplifiers of the color display. Figure 12.12(b) shows the generation of a red, orange, yellow, white thermal scale from the original linear gray scale.

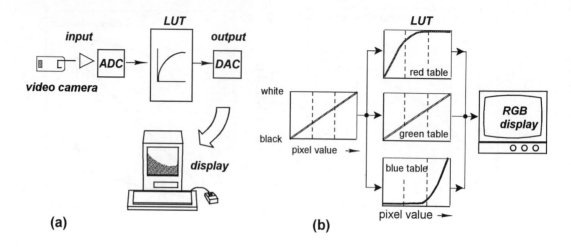

Figure 12.12   **(a)** The position of a look-up-table after the ADC in an imaging system (digitized video signal) which alters the detector characteristic before display. **(b)** Three LUTs used for driving the red-blue-green guns of a color display to give a thermal color scale (red, orange, yellow, white).

The gray scale pixel values are sampled by the RGB amplifiers. The green LUT has values linearly following the gray scale value. The Red LUT saturates rapidly with the gray scale so is only evidently changing at low values. The blue LUT only responds to high pixel values giving white saturation.

12.4.4 Histogram equalization

If the total image gray scale is represented as a histogram by plotting image densities against frequency of occurrence as shown in Fig.12.13 it can be seen that a considerable number of pixels are either entirely white or entirely black and contribute nothing to the image content. If these pixels are removed from the displayed image then the pixels holding gray-scale information in the middle of the histogram can be displayed utilizing the full gray scale range. This enhances the contrast differences. The image in Fig.12.13 shows an example where extreme pixel values are ignored leaving the entire gray scale to represent the pixel values which contain useful diagnostic information.

12.4.5 Windowing

Histogram equalization and LUT's are effective methods for improving the image contrast. The contrast resolution of modern digital imaging systems is 10 to 12 bits, i.e. the range of contrast presented to the digitizers can be divided into 2048 and 4096 gray levels respectively. However the eye is only capable of distinguishing about 35 gray levels, a fraction of the information provided. Windowing a section of the stored data allows a selected anatomy to be viewed with improved contrast. This is a common method for improving low-contrast visibility in CT.

Windowing can be used to display only a small range of contrast in which low contrast variations will be enhanced. Figure 12.14(a) shows windowing of a large digital scale 0–4095. Most display systems have a resolution of eight bits i.e. only a maximum of 256 gray levels can be displayed simultaneously.

A window permits a small section of these stored values to be displayed using the full 8-bits or a reduced bit number if greater contrast between structures is required.

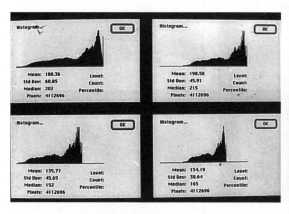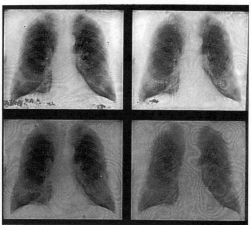

Figure 12.13 Histogram equalization of an image showing the full gray scale applied to a selected group of pixel values. (Courtesy Philips)

By varying the position and width of the window it is possible to display a section of the total range on a black to white scale.

The center and width of the window may be chosen independently. It is therefore possible to represent any gray level range of the digitized signal with maximum contrast resolution on the viewing monitor. The maximum window possible is all 4096 gray levels displayed simultaneously as black to white. The minimum range occurs when one level is set to black and the next level up is set to white. Thus the maximum contrast between adjacent levels is obtained.

12.4.6 Interpolation

A degree of image improvement can be obtained by pixel doubling or interpolation. Interpolation is commonly found in CT displays where 512×512 images are interpolated as 1024×1024. The distribution of pixel densities shown in Fig. 12.14(b) shows a coarse bell shaped profile. If the number of pixels of this data-set is increased by inserting pixels which have an average value of their neighbors then a much smoother image results as seen in the example by the curve outline. The appearance of the image improves but the resolution remains the same.

12.5 PICTURE ARCHIVING AND COMMUNICATION SYSTEMS (PACS)

Picture archiving and communication systems is a method for storage and transmission of radiology images so that once a clinical study is acquired from one modality (CT, MRI etc.) they can be first stored on a fast access medium for reporting (semiconductor memory) and then held by an intermediate storage device (magnetic disk) and eventually archived on a large capacity optical disk.

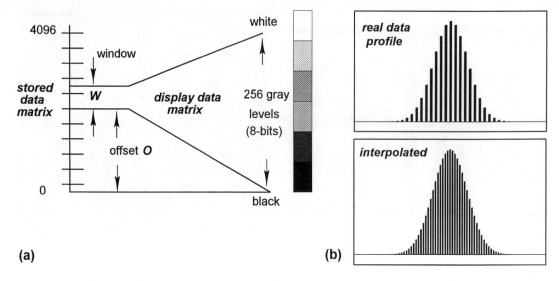

Figure 12.14   (a) Windowing a selected group of values stored in image memory for display using 256 gray levels. The full range of stored values covers 0 to 4096. Window width W and off-set O is indicated. (b) Interpolation showing how the real data in a coarse matrix ($n{\times}n$) can be interpolated to give a larger matrix ($2n{\times}2n$). This is commonly performed with CT images where 512 acquisition matrices are interpolated as 1024 display matrices.

A PACS is only effective in radiology if it can produce images of diagnostic quality that are easily accessible and of high quality. PACS connects imaging devices as a network and allows connections to other networks in wider localities so that images can be transported from place to place.

It also catalogs and stores each picture on electronic media (optical or magnetic disks). The clinician reporting the patient's various imaging studies can call-up these images from various centers and view them in his office. The pictures do not need to be on film; all viewing takes place on a high-resolution video terminal. Amongst the various advantages:

- PACS eliminates the need to generate film so cutting costs and loss of data.
- Images can be transmitted over long distances (satellite link) to other clinicians for consultation.
- Various data handling techniques can be employed: zooming, image enhancement etc. not available with film images.

The American College of Radiology (ACR) and the National Electrical Manufacturer's Association (NEMA) representing the equipment manufacturers, produced an interface standard intended to make digital image data available from all devices that produce digital images (CT, MRI, DSA, computed radiography, nuclear medicine and ultrasound). The standard interface is called ACR/NEMA which now has a digital image communication standard (DICOM). While DICOM is an advance there are still many problems with the acceptance of PACS in general.

It must be justified on the basis of cost savings which has yet to be realized. Digital displays are still technically inferior to back-lighted film as seen in common procedures such as chest radiographs. For this reason only PAC subsystems have proved practical for nuclear medicine, ultrasound, CT or MRI.

12.5.1   Image archiving

The capacity of a PACS facility can be measured by the number of images accessed.

Storing 1024×1024×10 bits requires 1.3M-bytes. Table 12.6 lists bulk storage devices available for PACS systems and their capacity.

A standard imaging system (fluoroscopy) has a basic image memory of 64M-bytes so can store approximately 40 such images for immediate display. Further images must then be stored on fast bulk storage such as 1 to 3G-byte magnetic disks which has a slower retrieval time.

Optical discs can be arranged in a 'juke-box' configuration holding tens of giga-bytes but retrieval time can be very slow indeed. Critical design problems now emerge. In order to increase storage capacity and access time some form of **data compression** must be introduced, preferably without image data loss.

Table 12.6 Image size and storage requirements.

Study	Image size	Bytes	1G-byte
CT	512×512×12	390k	2564
Fluoro.	1024×1024×10	1.3M	800
Image plate	1760×2140×10	4.5M	220
Selenium	2000×2000×12	5.7M	175
Mammo.	2048×2048×12	6.0M	166

12.5.2 Image compression

Image data from large matrices occupies a great deal of room in the computer memory and disc store. A radiographic image contains a great deal of redundant information. If this is removed before storage then simple image compression can be achieved without information loss. Other more complex forms of image data compression alter the pixel depth from 8 to 3 or 4 bits.

Difference value Instead of storing the total value for each pixel the difference value from its neighbor is stored reducing the image storage requirements considerably. The absolute value for the pixel is kept at each line of the matrix.

The image matrix depth can be reduced (8 bits) if the pixel density is represented not by a total density value but by a comparative figure obtained by reference to its neighbor. Small relative numbers can then be used to form an image. Following an image profile line by line the next pixel need only be incremented or decremented when comparing it to its neighbor. An example is shown in Fig.12.15 and the list of stored difference values is given in Tab.12.7 showing the significant decrease in stored number values. For this profile a 5-bit (32 decimal) matrix would be needed to store the original signal values whereas, as Tab.12.7 shows, only 3-bit storage is needed for the difference values, representing a 40% space saving or 20% if a sign bit is kept. This method of encoding retains all the original image information.

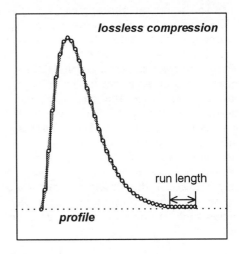

Figure 12.15 Image compression using a difference value technique on a single line of image data.

Pixels in image areas which contain little detail have neighboring pixels with the same value. These can be compressed by storing these values along with the number of pixel locations having this value as a **run length**. Storage areas can be significantly diminished since radiographs contain a significant proportion of black or white pixel values.

Table 12.7   Difference value compression

Image value	Stored difference value
	-
2.7	
8.7	6
14.9	6
20.1	6
23.6	3.5
25.6	2.0
26.2	0.6
25.7	–0.5
24.4	–1.3

Pixel averaging   Images can also be compressed by replacing small pixel regions with single pixels which are the average of all values in the region. Storage can be reduced by 75% using a 2:1 pixel averaging method or 88% using a 3:1 method. There is a slight loss of image detail which may be unacceptable.

Digital subtraction angiography (DSA) only concerns vessel architecture so a computer algorithm can trace the vascular tree and generate a map of data which only belong to the vascular components. **Data mapping** requires only a fraction of the original storage.

There are two major techniques for compressing and decompressing images: they either retain all the original image data or drop some of this information that is deemed diagnostically uncritical (lossy decompression).

No data loss   These algorithms include **run-length encoding**, which is based on the observation that image areas which contain little detail have neighboring pixels with the same value so these locations can be stored as a pixel value and pixel range (a 'run-length'). Storage requirements can be considerably reduced since large areas of radiographs consist of black background. The radiograph can be further cropped by using electronic shutters so only areas of diagnostic importance are saved.

Lossy compression   Pixel averaging techniques selectively reduce image information by replacing numbers of pixels with single pixels which are the average of all values in the region. Storage requirements can be significantly reduced by using 2:1 or 3:1 pixel averaging however image quality is degraded (information loss) which may result in loss of diagnostic information. Other lossy methods can be employed to retain only those features of importance in an image. For instance cardiac or DSA images where vessel detail is only required can retain image information about the vascular tree, rejecting background detail which may be of no diagnostic importance. This vessel map requires only a fraction of storage space. **Fractal compression** (see Chapter 1) offers the greatest efficiency for image storage however the time taken for compressing each image imposes a serious limitation.

12.5.3   Image transmission

A high resolution image typically contains in excess of 1 million bytes (Table 12.6). These require immediate storage for display and diagnosis (processor semiconductor memory) and then intermediate (magnetic disk) and permanent storage (optical disc).

The practical transmission (downloading) of this data from intermediate or permanent storage to other localities (clinics or hospitals) depends on the speed of data transmission; two or three seconds may be tolerable for each image. More than 10 seconds would not acceptable, unless it was accomplished prior to requirements (downloading during lunchbreaks or outside work time) anticipating reporting requirements.

High speed data transmission is achieved by using high grade co-axial or (better) fiber optic cable for networking the image communication system. Such a network would give transmission rates of 10M-bits to over 100M-bits per second. These speeds would transmit a $1024 \times 1024 \times 10$bit image (10M-bit) in 1s or 10ms respectively.

Box 12.2

Image transmission times

Using a 9600 baud telephone line
Transmitting a CT image of 512×512×12 bits.
Image size $2.09×10^6$ bits.
Transmission time:
$$2.09×10^6/9600 = 3.6 \text{ minutes.}$$

Using a co-axial or wireless link giving
10M-bit s^{-1}
Transmission time:
$$2.09×10^6/10×10^6 = 0.3 \text{ seconds}$$
Transmitting a 2048×2048×12 bit chest radiograph.
Transmission time:
$$5.0×10^7/10×10^6 = 5.0 \text{ seconds}$$

Using a fiber optic cable giving 1G-bit s^{-1}
Transmission time:
$$5.0×10^7/10×10^9 = 0.05 \text{ seconds}$$

12.5.4 Display stations

In order to display the images on a PAC system a large fast access display memory is necessary. This feature allows quick access to the image bank. For maximum resolution of multiple images the video display should be 2000 to 3000 lines non-interlaced. A limited amount of image processing such as smoothing, edge enhancement, pixel shifting and image subtraction should also be available.

Radiology information systems (RIS) should use the PAC system so that patient data along with the relevant images can be displayed. Each radiology image would then carry related clinical information including:

- patient name
- sex, age
- reason for examination
- date of examination, exam time
- total dose received by the patient
- formatted text regarding examination
- free text for clinical comments

A RIS and PACS facility is networked so information can be appended to the images during patient investigations.

12.5.5 Teleradiology

The transmission of images over a WAN involves telephone or radio communication links between hospitals or clinics; the term teleradiology describes this branch of a PACS design.

Conventional voice telephone links are unsuitable for long distance image transmission due to data speed limitations so dedicated digital links have been developed; dedicated microwave frequencies have also been allocated.

A teleradiology system consists of two or more sites connected as a wide area network (WAN). Video teleconferencing facilities may also be incorporated into such a system using a small CCD camera situated on the display station so that face-to-face contact can be established for security purposes. The essential points to be considered with a teleradiology system are:

- image transmission speed
- individual workstation display quality
- communication links
- number of patient studies to be transmitted
- security

12.5.6   PACS Implementation

Picture archiving and communication systems attempt to overcome the limitations of film based systems: storage retrieval and cost. PACS technology has been limited by capital costs, display resolution and accessibility. Many points of a PACS image storage depend on a single laser recording device (optical discs). If this laser should fail then an entire radiology department could be seriously compromised. Clearly a backup contingency plan is essential involving system redundancy which increases system costs. Figure 12.16 contains the basic components for a PACS design that connects radiology and hospital information systems (RIS and HIS).

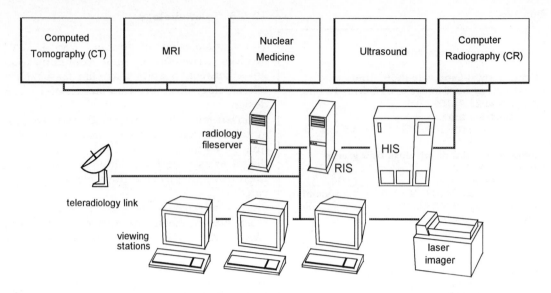

Figure 12.16   An outline design for a basic PACS for radiology. Gateways connect the PACS fileserver to the radiology (RIS) and hospital (HIS) information system. A teleradiology microwave link is also indicated. Telephone modem links are also common between other systems.

The input to a system must obviously be in digital format: computed radiography (image phosphor or selenium plate), MRI, CT, ultrasonography, fluoroscopy and nuclear medicine. Analog film/screen images can be digitized. A good film scanner must be able to avoid geometric distortion. A number of film scanners cannot achieve the level of resolution necessary for mammography which would require a pixel size of between 20 and 40μm. CCD camera digitizers at the moment are inferior to flat-bed scanning devices.

While ACR/NEMA have produced a DICOM standard for radiology image communications several problems still exist. PACS must be justified largely on the basis of cost saving. Displays of digital images on a high resolution video monitor are still technically inferior to back-lighted film. Video displays are also less portable than a film envelope and since the introduction of dry laser (non-photographic) imagers the film image itself is more reliable for archiving and may last longer than optical disks. The film image is also immune to changes in recording and replay electronic standards that may occur over quite short time intervals (remember 78, 45 and 33$\frac{1}{3}$ rpm vinyl audio records!). Many manufacturers have introduced mini-PACS subsystems where CT, MRI, ultrasound and nuclear medicine images are incorporated into a PACS network and use teleradiology features.

Computed radiography is acquiring importance as a general recording medium even though its resolution (2000×2000 pixels) is inferior to film. This is being developed as a PAC subsystem having archive and image database facilities.

The capacity of a PACS is measured by the number of images that may be accessed. An optical disk holding 2.6G-bytes (10^9) can hold 1650 images in 1024^2 12 bit format (1.5M-bytes) or 9,900 512^2 8 bit format. Data compression, as discussed above, can increase this storage capacity and PACS facilities commonly incorporate data compression. Box 12.2 gives examples of the time taken to transmit a 512×512 and a 2048×2048 image over telephone, coaxial cable and fiber optic cable lines. The problems associated with PACS can be demonstrated by taking a example which devotes itself to digitizing a mammogram and investigates transmission, storage and retrieval. Box 12.3 calculates storage requirements for two image examples.

Comparison of image storage systems No single storage medium possesses the requirements of a large storage capacity and high image transfer rate combined with short access times. As a result of this most digital imaging systems comprise a combination of different storage devices. They contain a fast semiconductor memory capable of storing digitized images in real time. However because of the relatively high cost per bit of semiconductor memory this type of storage is limited. The semiconductor memory is used again for the next exposure so if the data already stored is to be retained it must be transferred to the auxiliary memory: magnetic disk. The magnetic disk serves as intermediate storage and will retain its data if the power is lost. However older studies can be erased after a period of time or when the disk runs out of memory space.

If the images are to be archived then the optical disk is the most suitable medium. The optical disk has the lowest specific storage costs but does not enjoy very fast data transfer times. If a number of archived studies were requested by the Radiologist then this data stored on optical disk would first be transferred to magnetic disk. From the disk it would be placed in solid state semiconductor memory for viewing purposes. During a viewing or reporting session the data stored in the semiconductor memory would constantly be updated and replaced as a new patient study is requested from the digital magnetic memory.

As mentioned in chapter 11 analog magnetic tape (video tape) can be used as a storage medium for diagnostic images. The information to be stored would be acquired prior to digitization and stored in real-time. Video tapes have a very large capacity (about 500,000 images) and low specific storage costs. However video recorders suffer from lengthy access times, poor signal-to-noise ratios and limited bandwidth, particularly when attempting to record high-resolution images (1024×1024). Limited bandwidth effectively means a lack of spatial resolution.

Box 12.3

Image storage

Chest
Required resolution (L) is 2Lp mm^{-1} on a 430×430mm field of view ($14''\times14''$). $430\times2\times L = 1720\times1720$ matrix
A standard matrix of 2048×2048 would be used having a 10-bit pixel depth.
The size of this matrix is: $2048\times2048\times1.25/1048 = 5$M-byte
A low density CD of 2G-bytes would store 400 of these matrices. A department producing 50,000 chest radiograph a year would require 125 CD's.

Mammography

A digital mammogram having a 10Lp mm^{-1} resolution on a 200×200mm field size would require: $200\times2\times10 = 4000\times4000$ matrix
A standard matrix of $4096\times4096\times10$bits would need 20M-bytes of storage.
A 4-view breast screening program dealing with 10,000 women a year would require 800G-byte storage facility for uncompressed storage.

Further reading

The Image Processing Handbook
John C. Russ (CRC 1992)

Explorations in Signal Processing
(Mathsoft CD-ROM)

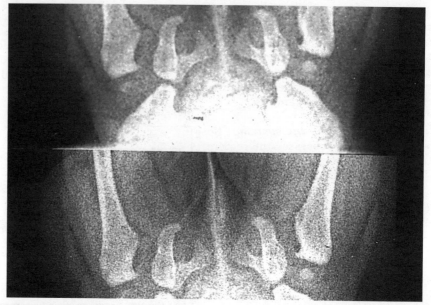

Figure 12.17(a)(b) noisy and smoothed images.

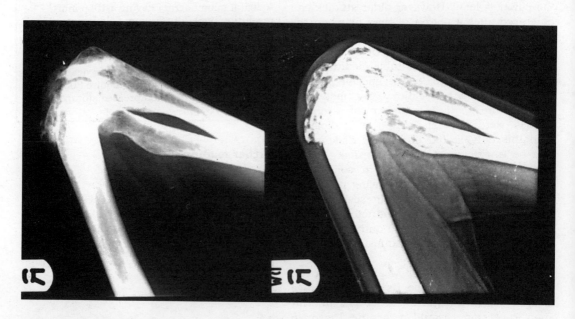

Figure 12.18(a)(b) smoothed and edge enhanced images.

KEYWORDS

ACR-NEMA: American College of Radiology/National Electrical Manufacturer's Association. A standard which specifies communication and image format between computer systems.

bandwidth: measures the capacity of the network expressed in bits per second.

bridge: a connection between two similar networks.

contention: when two or more computers try to use a network simultaneously.

DICOM: Digital Imaging and Communications in Medicine. Specify the items necessary to interface medical equipment to networks.

Ethernet: A network where every message is broadcast to all systems but only the destination node actions it. Messages sent simultaneously causes collision and then requires re-transmission.

FDDI: Fiber Distributed Data Interface. A fiber optic based ring network with faster performance than Ethernet or token ring networks.

fileserver: A centralized large disk store on a network holding database or program material. A fast and reliable computer controls access.

gateway: A connection between two dissimilar computers.

HIS: Hospital Information System

ISDN: Integrated Services Digital Network refers to any network that meets an industry standard.

LAN: Local Area Network

Multiplexer (MUX): A device that enables multiple signal transmission.

Node: A device attached to a network; either a computer or peripheral.

PACS: Picture Archiving and Communication Systems. An attempt to provide practical storage and rapid retrieval of images at multiple sites

Repeater: Receives data on one network link and retransmitts them onto another network link so extending transmission distance.

RIS: Radiology Information System

Router: A complex hardware device connecting dissimilar networks: LANs WANs that have different protocols.

TCP/IP: Transmission Control Protocol/Internet Protocol. The most common network protocol making networking between machines possible.

Teleradiology: Long distance transmission of radiographs between computer stations.

Token: A special bit pattern used on a network. The node must seize the token before it can be activated.

Token ring: A bit string "token" is transmitted from one node to anther activating a system on the ring network.

Topology, Bus: Extension of computer bus for limited networking.

Topology, Ring: Closed loop network using token transmission principle.

Topology, Star: All nodes connected to central exchange.

WAN: Wide area network cable or wireless.

Wireless-LAN: Digital microwave connection using 2.5 to 3.0GHz radio band.

13

Digital Fluorography (DF) and Digital Subtraction Angiography (DSA)

13.1 Basic components
13.2 Digital fluorography
13.3 Digital subtraction angiography

13.4 Digital subtraction programs
13.5 Machine performance

13.1 BASIC COMPONENTS

Initial attempts used for storing fluorographic images used video techniques. The video image from the camera tube was captured on a video disk which was then displayed without further irradiation of the patient. This gave great benefits regarding reduction of patient dose but had limitations regarding image quality, speed of display and image storage. The development of digital fluorography allowed much faster image acquisition and storage and more importantly digital image manipulation. The patient dose reduction was significant. The machines used for digital fluorography commonly use C-arm geometry although under and over-table designs now use digital acquisition. A digital imaging system offers the following advantages:

- Dose reduction
- Wide dynamic range
- Image storage
- Instant imaging (filmless)
- Dynamic imaging (up to 30fps)
- Image copying without loss of quality
- Image data transfer (PACS)

13.1.1 Imaging chain

The imaging chain of a modern DF system is shown in Fig.13.1. The important component parts are:

- The image intensifier
- Input phosphor
- Photo-cathode
- Output phosphor
- Coupling optics
- The video camera: Plumbicon, CCD
- The amplifier
- The analog to digital converter
- The signal conversion circuit and look-up-table

Image intensifier These have previously been described in Chapter 10. A large field of view (40cm) image intensifier is commonly used for DSA so that both legs can be imaged during 'bolus-chasing' or serial studies. Specifications for a typical image intensifier suitable for digital fluorography are given in Table 13.1.

Video camera The video camera quantum efficiency is 0.05 for a vidicon or 0.3 for a plumbicon. A semiconductor charge-coupled device (CCD) used for a video camera offers several advantages: it has a very high signal to noise ratio and absence of persistence (lag). The disadvantage of a 1024×1024 matrix is its restricted resolution when compared to plumbicons which can give a high resolution line standard of 2498 lines/100Hz for 50 cycle supplies and 2046 lines/120Hz for 60 cycles, displaying higher resolution matrices.

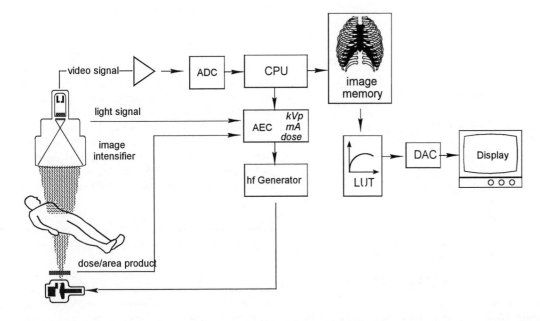

Figure 13.1 Basic components for a DF imaging system. The image intensifier output influences exposure settings maintaining a fixed exposure rate at the image intensifier face. Image data are digitized and stored in memory. LUT's are used for controlling automatic control and display settings.

Table 13.1 Standard specifications for a 40cm image intensifier used for DSA studies.

FOV	40cm 16"	28cm 11"	20cm 8"	14cm 5½"
Resolution (Lp mm^{-1})	3.6	4.0	4.6	6.0
Intensification factor	20k	10k	5k	2.5k

Conversion factor :	23cd m^2 µGy^{-1} s (200cd m^2 mR^{-1} s)
LFD	9%
Contrast ratio	20:1

Noise The limiting factor for the detection of small contrast differences is the measurement of the transmitted x-ray intensity. Low contrast visibility improves with increasing x-ray fluence but this itself is limited by patient dose restrictions. An expression for the noise variance δ^2 in a logarithmically amplified video image, including contributions from both x-ray quantum noise and the image intensifier signal to noise ratio is given by the formula:

$$\delta^2 = \frac{e^{+\mu x}}{N_o} + \frac{e^{+2\mu x}}{(SNR)^2} \qquad (13.1)$$

The first half of this expression describes the noise from x-ray photon statistics. N_o in the first half of the equation is the detected photon fluence whilst the second half is given by the imaging chain, principally the image intensifier signal to noise ratio (SNR). The exponent in each contains the standard thickness x and attenuation coefficient μ. Both noise sources increase with absorber (patient) thickness but the video noise increases at a faster rate so this is the greater limiting factor to dynamic range. Figure 13.2 shows the improvement in dynamic range as the image intensifier SNR increases. An SNR figure of 1:1000 is a minimum expected value exceeded by most DF systems.

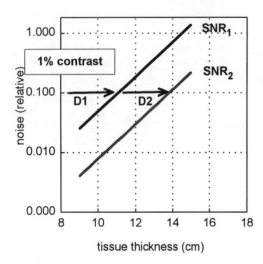

Figure 13.2 The improvement in dynamic range (D1 to D2) with increasing image intensifier signal to noise ratio from SNR_1 to SNR_2. A threshold low contrast level of 1% can be visualized over a wider tissue thickness using SNR_2.

From Fig.13.2 it is clear that image quality degrades with patient thickness principally due to video noise. Improvement in the video SNR therefore extends the dynamic range of the subtraction process.

Iris control This is a light aperture positioned between the image intensifier and video camera. Its action is similar to those found in ordinary 35mm cameras. A small aperture decreases the efficiency of light capture by the video camera so a greater x-radiation density is required at the image intensifier face. This will:

- Increase photon density
- Decrease quantum noise so improving SNR but
- Increase patient dose

Increasing the iris aperture would have the converse effect.

13.1.2   Video scanning modes

In the description of the video system in Chapter 7 the conventional TV raster scanning mode was presented. It is well known that the eye will perceive as a continuous event an optical stimulus with a repetition rate over 50 flashes per second. Therefore the frame repetition rate in a video system should not lie below 50 frames per second for flicker-free reproduction but fast frame rates above 50Hz increases the bandwidth and cost. High resolution displays use 100-120Hz scan frequencies.

Interlaced scanning This was introduced to give the impression of a frame repetition rate of 50 frames per second in domestic television. The two video fields which comprise the video frame are repeated at a rate of 50 per second. This gives an effective frame repetition rate of 25 per second, i.e. each frame lasts 40 ms. Although each individual pixel does not light up 50 times per second, pixels on two neighboring lines are scanned alternately. The eye merges the two adja-cent pixels together and gets the impression of 50 frames per second.

Progressive scanning This method of video scanning was introduced to cope with fluoroscopic imaging systems using pulsed operation. Conventional interlaced scanning, using pulsed systems, gives a flickering image display. This occurs because charge is applied only once to the target of the TV camera. When the charge on the target is read using interlaced scanning it results in the amplitudes of the two fields having different levels. This occurs because some charge from the neighboring line will be read out as part of the first field. This produces the flicker as there will be much less than about half the original amount of charge left on the target for the second field.

Camera targets have a certain amount of lag so it takes several 20ms video fields (Fig.13.3(a) field 1 and 2) before the output video signal is stable (fields 3, 4, 5 and 6). This wastes x-ray exposure so increasing patient dose unnecessarily. However using progressive or non-interlaced scanning the whole image is read line by line in 40 ms. A direct read-out would also produce flicker as a repetition rate of 50 frames per second is required for flicker-free display. The problem is solved by using a digital memory device as a standard converter. The sequence of pixels read in differs from the read out sequence. Data from the video camera is written into memory line by line in 40 milliseconds. The data in memory is read from memory using the interlaced procedure at 20 milliseconds per field. Therefore the image observed on the monitor appears continuous although the data is read from the camera at half the required rate. This allows efficient use of the x-ray beam which is applied in pulses (Figure 13.3(b)).

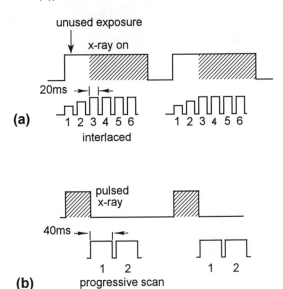

(a)

(b)

Figure 13.3 **(a)** An interlaced scan mode showing the first frames are not used so wasting x-ray exposure. **(b)** a progressive scan mode combines two 20ms fields and stores these as 40ms which are then displayed.

Slow progressive scanning If a large radiation dose is used to produce the image then the SNR will be high. It is appropriate in these situations to attempt to increase the electronic SNR. The electronic noise increases as the bandwidth increases therefore an improvement in the signal to noise ratio is obtained when the bandwidth is limited. In Chapter 10 it was shown the bandwidth was directly responsible for the horizontal resolution and indirectly for the vertical resolution due to the choice of lines per frame. In order to reduce the bandwidth but yet preserve the spatial resolution the horizontal and vertical deflection frequency must be reduced. The frame repetition rate is reduced by a factor of two to five so this technique can only be successfully used with static imaging or when using a low framing rate. Flicker-free images are displayed on the monitor as the memory is again read using interlaced scanning. The system SNR can be increased to 6000:1 using slow scanning.

Look up tables (LUTs) These play an important role in DSA during acquisition, exposure control and display. An LUT can be stored in ROM or RAM depending on whether the signal is to follow a fixed or variable program.

The **transmission** characteristics of the video imaging chain can be altered from its linear response to a non-linear one (e.g. logarithmic). The **automatic exposure** control determines the optimum exposure required for the chosen acquisition protocol (frame rate and dose etc.). LUT's then set generator voltage, current and timing (pulse width). The iris diaphragm on the video tube input is also adjusted for optimum display brightness. The video **display** itself is also controlled by an LUT. The table is operator selected to give linear or a variety of non-linear scales. This is used in conjunction with the windowing facility.

13.2 DIGITAL FLUOROGRAPHY

Small mobile C-arm system These are the simplest DF units and are used for:

- Orthopedic intervention
- Foreign body localization
- Cholangiography, cystography, pyelography
- Cardiac pacemaker implantation

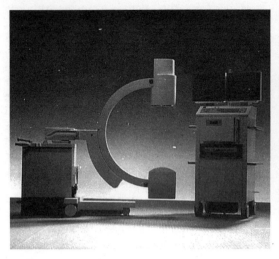 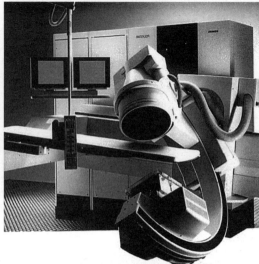

Figure 13.4   **(a)** A small mobile C-arm used for small field of view interventional work. (Courtesy Siemens) **(b)** a large 40cm image intensifier on a cantilevered C-arm which replaces under/over table fluoroscopy units. (Courtesy Siemens)

A general design is shown in Fig.13.4(a). The image intensifier is typically 17cm with a 10cm zoom setting (7″ and 4″) and the x-ray tube uses a stationary anode having a 0.5mm focal spot since only small currents are required during the investigation. A high frequency generator gives 40-106kV at 8mA and digital image storage can hold 2 to 20 1024^2 images.

Large field C-arm   High output fixed units use cantilevered C-arms holding a large image intensifier and x-ray tube, suitable for vascular intervention studies with or without DSA facilities.   Figure 13.4(b) shows a common design. A typical large C-arm DSA machine specification would have an image intensifier giving field sizes of 14, 20, 28, 40cm, a heavy duty x-ray tube (metal/ceramic) capable of over 2kW in continuous operation and having a heat capacity of up to 3 to 5MHU with dual focal spot of 0.6 and 1.0mm. The generator would be 80kW high frequency. This would give a system performance allowing an acquisition of up to 8 fps for a 1024×1024×10 matrix.

Table 13.2 Specifications for DF

Feature	
Image	
CCD or plumbicon	$1024^2 \times 10$, $512^2 \times 10$
Frame rate	7.5 - 30fps
Image storage	
Image memory	64-320Mb
Magnetic disk	1024^2 (100 frames)
Image processing	spatial filtering
Clinical analysis	vessel diameter

The image storage of the system decides its extended capabilities and a full specification for a DSA system using a large diameter image intensifier cantilevered C-arm system is listed in Tab.13.2   In most digital fluorography systems it is common practice to sum more than one image in order to improve the image SNR (recursive filtering). This averaging is accomplished by a data loop where the incoming image is added to the previously stored image. This requires at least 14 to 16 bits per pixel and many image processors have up to 3 image memories in order to speed this averaging process. Where a sequence of images is acquired they are stored in the main memory which can be 64Mb or larger. After image subtraction however the images are stored on disk which should be at least 1-2G-bytes.

13.2.1 Image storage

Image data transfer Transfer rates and storage times are listed in Tab.13.3 for these two matrix sizes. The large storage requirements should be accommodated by fast cache-memory and then transferred to disk for post acquisition processing. Memory size is therefore critical in DF systems.

No single storage medium possesses the requirements of a large storage capacity and high image transfer rate combined with short access times. As a result of this most digital imaging systems comprise a combination of different storage devices. They contain a fast semiconductor memory capable of storing digitized images in real time. However because of the relatively high cost per bit of semiconductor memory this type of storage is limited. The semiconductor memory is used again for the next exposure so if the data already stored is to be retained it must be transferred to the auxiliary memory which is a magnetic disk. The magnetic disk serves as intermediate storage and will retain its data if the power is lost. However older studies can be erased after a period of time or when the disk runs out of memory space.

If the images are to be archived then the optical disk is the most suitable medium. The optical disk has the lowest specific storage costs but does not enjoy very fast data transfer times. If a number of archived studies were requested by the radiologist then this data stored on optical disk would first be transferred to magnetic disk. From the disk it would be placed in solid state semiconductor memory for viewing purposes. During a viewing or reporting session the data stored

in the semiconductor memory would constantly be updated and replaced as a new patient study is requested from the digital magnetic memory.

Table 13.3 Image data transfer M-bytes s^{-1} and storage (M-byte).

	512×512×10	1024×1024×10
Transfer time		
7.5 fps	2.4	9.4
30fps	9.6	37.5
60fps	19.2	
Storage (5s duration)		
7.5fps	12	47
30fps	48	187
60fps	96	

Analog magnetic tape (video tape) can be used as a storage medium for diagnostic images. The information stored would be acquired prior to digitization and stored in real-time. Video tapes have a very large capacity, about half a million images and low specific storage costs. However video recorders suffer from lengthy access times, poor SNR and limited bandwidth, particularly when attempting to record high-resolution images (1024×1024) since limited bandwidth effectively means a lack of spatial resolution; as a consequence tape is not now used as a storage medium.

13.2.2   Image resolution

The theoretical attainable resolution given by an image intensifier has been listed in Tab.13.1 this is usually not a limiting factor since digitization can cause a major resolution loss. Table 13.4 shows how resolution can be improved by increasing the contrast ratio of an image intensifier.

Table 13.4 The improved resolution given by an image intensifier with increased contrast ratio.

Contrast ratio			
20:1			
Diameter (cm)	21	17	13
Resolution Lp mm^{-1}	5.2	5.8	6.2
30:1			
Diameter (cm)	30	23	15	11
Resolution Lp mm^{-1}	5.0	5.6	6.8	7.5

Image matrix size   A general formula relating matrix size M and image intensifier field size D with resolution R in Lp mm^{-1} is:

$$R = \frac{M \cdot m}{20D} \tag{13.2}$$

Where m is the image magnification, usually taken as 1.25 due to patient offset from the image intensifier face. This is plotted in Fig.13.5 for three matrix sizes 512^2, 1024^2 and 2048^2 showing the combined effect of image intensifier size and expected resolution given by these three matrix sizes.

Cardiac investigations require the greatest resolution and a rough indication of a system's ability to resolve small vessels r is given by the formula:

$$r = \frac{2D}{M} \tag{13.3}$$

For a 512^2 matrix which may represent an image intensifier field size of 200mm, it will resolve 0.78mm or 1.25Lp mm^{-1}. A 1024^2 matrix using the same intensifier will resolve 0.4mm or 2.5Lp mm^{-1} but for the same noise content the higher resolution 1024^2 matrix will require ×4 the dose of a 512^2 matrix.

The spatial resolution of a digital fluorography system depends on the setting of the image intensifier decreasing from 0.27, 0.19 and 0.14mm for field sizes 33, 23 and 17cm respectively representing matrix resolutions from 1.8, 2.6 and 3.5 Lp mm^{-1} respectively. For comparison a film screen resolution is approximately 5Lp mm^{-1} at 200 speed.

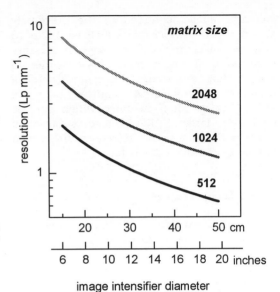

Figure 13.5   Combine plot of the image resolution given for image intensifier sizes and three matrix sizes.

Focal spot and image resolution   The digital image matrix rather than the image intensifier limits the spatial resolution, although the limitations are reasonably well matched. At higher magnifications geometrical unsharpness becomes a problem which can be reduced by utilizing smaller focal spot sizes (switching from 1mm to 0.6mm). The dependence of image resolution R on the x-ray tube focal spot is described by:

$$R = \frac{m}{F(m-1)} \tag{13.4}$$

Where F is the x-ray tube focal spot size and m the image magnification (typically 1.25 as before).

13.2.3 Image data processing

After the initial processing of the acquired image data (amplification and log transformation) and before producing the clinical image the image data is subjected to a series of post-processing measures which are used to improve image quality. These are:

- windowing
- spatial filtering
- temporal or recursive filtering

Windowing The digitized image is held in a matrix of 512^2, 1024^2 or 2048^2 pixels each pixel represented by 10 or 12 bits. Theoretically this can give 2048 or 4096 gray levels but since the eye can only appreciate about 35 gray levels only a fraction of the stored information can be displayed at any one time. This post processing procedure is called windowing and allows small contrast changes to be amplified. Chapter 12 describes how stored values from 0 to 4096 can be displayed as a 256 level gray scale (window width) and placed, by operator control, at different levels of the stored range.

Spatial filtering This is a post processing procedure where raw data images obtained from the image intensifier contain noise due to quantum effects and electronic noise. The effect of this noise can be reduced by subjecting the data to **low pass filtering** or **smoothing**. This has already been demonstrated in Chapter 12. **High pass filtering** is used for emphasizing edge detail in the picture; this is important for enhancing small vessel detail in contrast angiography: this is commonly called **edge enhancement**.

Temporal (recursive) filtering Image noise reduction using spatial filtering techniques is limited to individual images. Reduction of noise is particularly important in digital fluorography owing to low dose imaging which has a low signal to noise ratio.

A very effective method for removing noise is to average several image frames, where stored image D_{old} is incorporated into the acquired image producing a matrix of average values D_{new}; the schematic in Fig.13.6 shows the data flow. This is a pre-processing procedure when several images are summed (typically four). The useful signal strength increases linearly whereas the noise component, because of its random nature, does not show any

correlation between images and its presence is reduced. This is best seen by studying the standard deviation of the image noise. Comparing the individual image noise value σ with the average noise σ_n obtained by summing n images:

$$\sigma_n = \frac{\sigma}{\sqrt{n}} \qquad (13.5)$$

There is an improvement in noise by a factor $\sqrt{n}$, so averaging over 4 images halves the noise content. A continuous process for temporal smoothing uses a moving weighted average where noise reduction is calculated, not from a fixed number of images but from all the part images. An example of moving weighted averaging is given in Box 13.1.

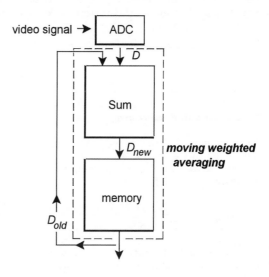

Fig.13.6 Moving weighted averaging which is incorporated into a DSA system.

Temporal filtering exaggerates image lag since it combines video camera lag over the image number summed. For this reason the number of images being summed at any one time is small. **Motion correction** can be used if the difference signal between images is used as a motion detector and the contrast of a moving object is emphasized above the noise component.

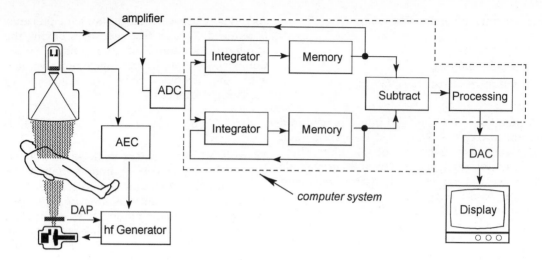

Figure 13.7 A basic DSA system design showing the log amplification of the video signal and the temporal smoothing feedback in dual memory circuits before subtraction and display. A post-processing module allows the operator to choose image manipulation routines.

Box 13.1

Moving weighted averaging

The averaging technique used in Fig.13.6 is applied to five samples: 8, 12, 8, 10, 8, 12 collected at set time intervals and temporally smoothed using the formula:

$$D_{new} = \frac{D_{old}}{K} + \frac{D}{K}$$

When a smoothing factor K of 1 is used then the values do not change. If K = 1.5 then at the start:

(a) $D_{new} = 0 - \dfrac{0}{1.5} + \dfrac{8}{1.5} = 5.3$

(b) $D_{new} = 5.3 - \dfrac{5.3}{1.5} + \dfrac{12}{1.5} = 9.76$

The temporally smoothed values then become:

5.3, 9.76, 8.58, 9.52, 8.5, 10.8

The contribution from each sample, from 8 through to 12 in this example, decreases proportionally with time giving the running or moving weighted averaging.

13.3 DIGITAL SUBTRACTION ANGIOGRAPHY

The is a technique for producing images of the blood vessels isolated from overlying structures. To achieve this, two images of the same region, separated in time, are acquired.

- The first image, called the **mask**, is taken prior to the injection of a contrast agent.
- The second image, called the **contrast** image, is the mask but now containing the contrast agent.

An image frame of vessels just containing iodine-contrast is obtained when the mask image is subtracted from the contrast image. The subtracted image contains any differences which exist between the two images, i.e. the addition of the contrast media and any movement artifact.

13.3.1 The DSA system
The component parts of a DSA system are outlined in Fig.13.7. The starting point in any DSA system is the video signal from the image intensifier.

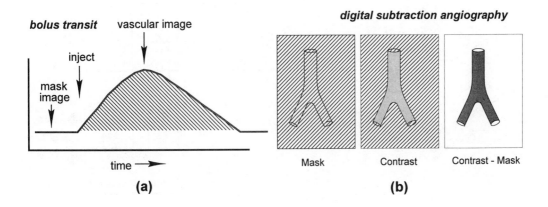

Figure 13.8 **(a)** The arterial and venous phases of a DSA study **(b)** Basic DSA technique: a mask image is first stored then the relevant vessels are injected with contrast medium and a second image stored. Subtracting these images yields the difference image free of surrounding anatomy.

The video signal, after amplification, is converted into digital format using the ADC. Two memories are used for the subtraction process; one holds the mask image and the other the contrast image. The memory contents are subtracted in a separate arithmetic unit and then undergo windowing before being converted back into a video analog voltage using a digital to analog converter (DAC). They are then displayed on a high resolution monitor. Multiple images of the investigation are stored on a magnetic disk. A very large computer memory (RAM) is essential for image manipulation; its size can vary between 30 and 300M-bytes. A fast CPU controls data acquisition and processing.

Digital subtraction presents images of vessels in isolation from their background (soft tissue and bone). Two images are acquired from exactly the same anatomical region before and after injection of a contrast medium. The contrast density/time curve of Fig.13.8(a) shows the timing which coincides with the peak arrival of the iodine-contrast bolus.

Figure 13.8(b) illustrates the subtraction process. The first pre-contrast image is called the mask M containing background anatomy. The post-contrast image contains the vessels together with the background C. After some data processing (smoothing, edge enhancement etc.), the mask is subtracted from the contrast image to reveal the vessels in the difference image D:

$$C - M = D \qquad (13.6)$$

The improved SNR that this imaging process yields over plain film contrast imaging and the benefits of image storage and transmission has made DSA the technique of choice for contrast angiography.

The noise component of each image (M and C), being random, does not subtract but adds so the noise component increases in the subtracted frame D. This is not serious in the high photon flux images of DSA but can become a problem in low photon/low dose techniques.

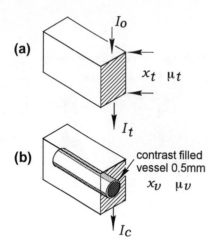

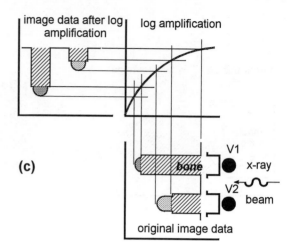

Figure 13.9 (a) the parameters used in the calculation in Box 13.2. (b) Log subtraction graphically demonstrated showing that after log amplification the contrast filled vessels V1 and V2 lying behind bony tissue (shown as steps) are represented without distortion in the log amplified data. The graphed log values are stored as a look-up-table.

13.3.2 Logarithmic subtraction

An essential requirement for DSA is that the contrast signal obtained by subtraction corresponds linearly with the concentration of the contrast medium. Direct subtraction of the two sets of images will not produce an image that is independent of the overlying structures, e.g. the contrast signal would be reduced in regions overlying a bone compared with soft tissue regions.

Logarithmic subtraction is used to insure that an artery of uniform diameter that traverses regions of varying thickness appears in the subtracted image with uniform contrast. The logarithm of the video signals is obtained prior to subtraction. The reason that log amplification is used prior to subtraction can be explained using the simple Beer-Lambert formula for the transmission of monochromatic radiation through matter. Figure 13.9(a) identifies the various parameters used in the calculation:

- I_o is the incident radiation fluence
- I_t the transmitted intensity before contrast

- I_c the transmitted intensity after iodine contrast.
- x_t and μ_t are the tissue thickness and attenuation coefficient respectively
- x_v and μ_v are the vessel thickness and iodine attenuation.

For the **mask image**, if the intensity of radiation incident on a tissue thickness x_t is I_o then the transmitted intensity is I_t

$$I_t = I_o \cdot e^{-\mu_t x_t} \qquad (13.7)$$

If contrast media, e.g. iodine, is added to a vessel overlying the tissue then the equation for the transmission after iodine contrast I_c is modified to include the extra vessel thickness x_v of iodine which has an attenuation coefficient μ_v:

$$I_c = I_o \cdot e^{-(\mu_t x_t + \mu_v x_v)} \qquad (13.8)$$

The subtraction image is obtained by subtracting the mask image from the contrast image. Direct subtraction of the transmitted intensities I_s produces a complex expression which is not independent of the overlying structures and which is directly related to the input intensity I_0 :

$$I_s = I_c - I_t$$
$$= I_0 \cdot e^{-(\mu_t x_t + \mu_v x_v)} - e^{-\mu_t x_t} \qquad (13.9)$$

However subtracting the logs of the transmission:

$$I_s = \log(I_c) - \log(I_t)$$
$$= -(\mu_t x_t + \mu_v x_v) - (-\mu_t x_t)$$

$$I_s = -\mu_t x_t \qquad (13.10)$$

In comparison to linear subtraction the logarithmic method does not retain stationary anatomical structure which may obscure small signal levels from the opacified vessel. In this way the resulting signal forming the DSA display is not influenced by patient size and produces an output pattern of intensities which depend only on the product of the thickness and attenuation coefficient of the injected contrast medium. Box 13.2 compares the linear and logarithmic methods.

The logarithmic transformation can be implemented either in an analog fashion using logarithmic amplifiers prior to analog to digital conversion, or using a 'look-up table' (LUT), after digitization. The latter is the preferred approach as log amplifiers can present stability problems and add noise to the signals. The digital arrangement can be fine-tuned to the dynamic range of the input data, however quantization errors can still occur.

In spite of logarithmic amplification tissue variation still gives irregular attenuation of vessels in the image field of view. Some form of extra compensation is necessary in the form of either tissue equivalent material or some form of shaped filtration. DSA wedge filters have been developed which can be adjusted to compensate for object thickness differences and, under operator control, these significantly reduce non-uniformities in the image.

13.3.3 Misregistration (movement artifact)

This is a major limiting factor in DF. Small movements in bone-tissue interfaces can give edges that far exceed that given by the vessels themselves. This is demonstrated in Fig.13.10 where a profile across a soft-tissue/bone interface is shown with the same profile a short time later plus the vessel contrast signal. The boundary between soft-tissue and bone has changed however.

The magnitude of this misregistration artifact C is given by:

$$C = \frac{\Delta b}{n\,\tau} \cdot \Delta t \qquad (13.11)$$

Where Δb is the brightness change at the bone/tissue boundary, t is the image pixel interval (sampling period in the ADC) and n is the number of pixels in the boundary region. The difference Δt is the magnitude of the misregistration.

Several methods have been devised for dealing with misregistration. Re-masking by retrospective selection of an alternate mask (time-interval difference) often reduces misregistration artifacts and in practice misregistration in temporal subtraction studies can be either improved or salvaged by re-masking.

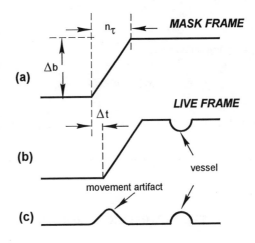

Figure 13.10 Misregistration across a bone/soft-tissue interface during subtraction angiography. The parameters are identified in the text.

308 *Physics of Diagnostic Imaging*

Pixel shift   If movement artifacts cannot be corrected by alternative mask selection then the image pixels *in-toto* can be shifted vertically or horizontally. This provides better alignment of the two images so improving subtraction.

Box.13.2

Comparing linear and logarithmic subtraction.

Using parameters identified in Fig.13.9(a) and derivations in eqns.13.7 to 13.10

Tissue thickness x_t of 5cm μ_t is 0.018 cm^{-1}
Vessel diameter x_v of 0.5cm μ_v is 0.03cm^{-1}
The incident photon density I_o is 1.0

The Mask Signal I_t is $I_o \cdot e^{-(\mu_t \cdot x_t)}$
The Contrast Signal I_c is $I_o \cdot e^{-(\mu_t \cdot x_t - \mu_v \cdot x_v)}$

Using Linear Subtraction:
DSA Image $= I_{lin} = I_c - I_t$

$= (-\mu_v \cdot x_v) \cdot I_o \cdot e^{-(\mu_t \cdot x_t)}$

$= -0.015 \times e^{-0.09}$

$= 0.0137$

For increased tissue thickness (say 8cm) similarly:

$I_{lin} = -0.015 \times e^{-0.144}$

$= 0.0129$

Using log subtraction:
DSA Image $= I_{log} = \ln(I_t) - \ln(I_c)$

$= -(\mu_t \cdot x_t) - (\mu_t \cdot x_t - \mu_v \cdot x_v)$

$= \mu_v \cdot x_v$

which is 0.015 regardless of tissue component $\mu_t \cdot x_t$

13.4 DIGITAL SUBTRACTION PROGRAMS

The exact procedures used for producing the highest quality subtracted image vary from manufacturer to manufacturer but they all contain the same basic principles described here. The signal to noise ratio of the subtracted image decreases since during the subtraction process although the unwanted image data is removed the noise content of each image is summed. Owing to its random nature noise cannot be reduced by image subtraction.

The signal to noise ratio of the final DSA image *SNR* depends also on the concentration of contrast medium *C* (iodine or barium) and the radiation dose *D* (photon density) so that:

$$SNR = C \times \sqrt{D} \qquad (13.12)$$

Increasing the concentration of contrast material is therefore a more effective improvement than increasing patient dose.

An effective way to improve image SNR is to integrate (add) image frames. Noise reduction depends on the number of similar frames added. If *N* frames are integrated, each having a noise value of σ, then the noise in the summed image is:

$$\frac{\sigma}{\sqrt{N}} \qquad (13.13)$$

Image integration reduces both quantum and electronic noise sources whereas increasing dose only affects quantum noise.

13.4.1 Snap-shot imaging

This uses digitally enhanced single images utilizing one mask and one contrast image, it is the basic DSA technique and is also called digital spot imaging previously illustrated in Fig.13.8(a).

Remasking   If a series of contrast images are taken and a single mask used for constructing the subtracted image then patient movement (voluntary or involuntary) will lead to misregistration errors. These errors can be reduced by selecting images from the acquisition series that can be used for suitable updated masks.

Extending the snap-shot example shown in Fig.13.8, a series of contrast images taken during bolus transit $C_1, C_2, C_3 ..C_n$ would provide the subtracted images:

$$C_1 - M = D_1, \quad C_2 - M = D_2 \dots C_n - M = D_n$$

If during this series there is patient movement during (say) contrast image C_8, which contains peak contrast together with some misregistration errors yielding a suboptimum subtraction image D_8, then a new mask can be obtained from C_{10} (a frame which matched the shifted anatomy). The desired image would be equivalent to $C_8 - C_6$. If D_8 and D_{10} are subtracted the result would be equivalent to:

$$D_8 - D_6 = (C_8 - M) - (C_6 - M) = C_8 - C_6 \quad (13.14)$$

So although the difference images D_6 and D_8 are the stored images an updated remasked difference image can be derived from them since the original mask image M cancels out in the equation yielding the required image which is $C_8 - C_6$.

subtraction facility which provides a continuous orientation aid for selective catheterisation procedures and is illustrated in Fig.13.11. Using this facility the operator can observe the position of the catheter in relation to the path of the vessel. The technique involves:

- Injecting a small quantity of the contrast medium into the area of interest.
- An image of the filled vessel is then stored in memory as the mask for the rest of the procedure.
- During catheter movement the mask is continuously subtracted from the fluoroscopic image.
- The resulting subtraction image contains both the vessels and the advancing catheter superimposed on the subtraction image.

road mapping

(a)   **(b)**   **(c)**

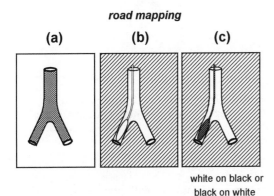

white on black or
black on white

Figure 13.11   Roadmapping   used   for presenting a real-time image of the catheter position **(a)** A vessel contrast image is taken which is then continuously subtracted **(b)** after catheter insertion to give the real-time image **(c)**

13.4.2 Road-mapping

Road-mapping involves super-imposing real time images onto a previously acquired mask so that intra-luminal manipulation of the catheter can be followed. This is a digital

13.4.3 Dual energy and hybrid subtraction subtraction

Using two x-ray energies for acquiring image data is a technique that can be used to eliminate either bone or soft tissue detail. The technique depends on the energy dependence of x-ray attenuation through matter. In Chapter 5 it was shown that in the diagnostic range as the energy of the incident radiation increases the linear attenuation coefficient μ decreases. The decrease in μ is much greater for bone than the decrease for soft tissue. To obtain soft tissue cancellation which will produce a bone enhanced image two radiographs, one with a low kVp and one with a high kVp, are acquired of the same anatomical region. When the low energy image is subtracted from the high energy image the soft tissue detail cancels leaving mainly bony detail. Bone cancellation is obtained by subtracting this bony image from the original low energy image. Table 13.5 identifies the high and low energy masks and contrast image series.

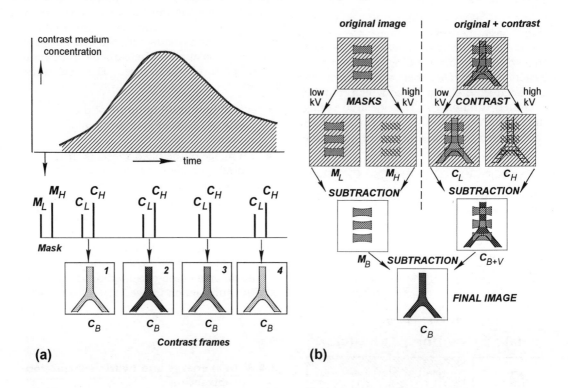

Figure 13.12 **(a)** The hybrid subtraction sequence representing passage of contrast medium through the vessel and the series of temporal frames C_L C_H taken at low and high kilovoltage. **(b)** The image series formed during a dual energy subtraction series ending with the final image which contains only the vessel detail free from bone interference.

Table 13.5 Dual energy subtraction image series

	Bone	Soft-tissue	Iodine
Mask			
M_L low kV mask	high	medium	NA
M_H high kV mask	medium	medium	NA
Contrast			
C_L low kV image	high	medium	high
C_H high kV image	medium	medium	high

Patient motion is the main limitation to vascular imaging using temporal subtraction methods. Artifacts caused by involuntary motion, usually of soft tissue, e.g. due to bowel gas, peristaltic or cardiac movement, are very difficult to suppress. Dual energy sub-traction is relatively insensitive to this motion as attenuation coefficients of either gas or soft tissue change little between the two energies.

Thus subtraction of the dual energy images removes effects due to involuntary motion due to bowel gas. However, only one material can be eliminated using dual energy subtraction. If a iodine contrast is introduced between the low and high energy images, while motion artifacts will be alleviated the image obtained by subtraction will now contain the vessels containing iodine contrast but also any overlying bone.

The image acquisition sequence during bolus transit for dual energy subtraction is detailed in Fig.13.12(a). A pictorial sequence in Fig.13.12(b) shows a pair of images is acquired at both low and high x-ray energies prior to the arrival of the contrast agent into the region of interest. Using energy subtraction these two images are combined to eliminate soft tissue and leave only bone structures as a pre-contrast mask:

$$M_L - M_H \rightarrow \text{bone image } M_B$$

A series of low and high energy image pairs is then acquired as the contrast bolus flows through the region of interest. Each of these pairs is processed to suppress soft tissue components and to yield a post-contrast image of iodinated vessels plus bone residuals:

$$C_L - C_H \rightarrow \text{bone + iodine } C_{(B+V)}$$

Finally a temporal subtraction of the dual-energy mask and post-contrast images removes the bone structures and successfully isolates the iodine-filled vasculature:

$$C_{(B+V)} - M_B \rightarrow \text{iodine image } C_V$$

Hybrid subtraction combines dual energy techniques and temporal subtraction and successfully cures both overlying bone obscuring vessel detail and movement misregistration problems. The advantage of hybrid subtraction in comparison to temporal subtraction is that it eliminates artifacts caused by soft tissue motion and its ability to eliminate both soft tissues and bone. However because of the extra subtraction involved in the hybrid method there is increased noise in the final subtracted image. Hybrid subtraction also involves increased radiation exposure for the patient. However elimination of motion artifacts may lead to a lower over all dose caused by repeat examinations.

13.5 MACHINE PERFORMANCE

13.5.1 Equipment specification

Hybrid subtraction requires two essential components. The first is that of timing since the interval between x-ray exposures must be minimized and the pulse widths are short in order to minimize residual motion artifacts. The second requirement is an energy constraint that requires separation of the two x-ray energies (typically 60 and 110kVp) in order to minimize noise in subtracted hybrid image. The short exposure times and relatively high exposure rates require tube currents of 1000mA so the x-ray tube must be able to tolerate this high loading.

A suitable x-ray tube would be grid controlled and have a heat storage capacity approaching 2MJ and a long term anode loadability figure of 3kW depending on focal spot size.

13.5.2 Cardiac DSA

Storage Digital cardiac angiography can capture non-subtracted images in 512×512×8 format at 50fps. Digital cardiac imaging produces considerable image storage problems as shown in Tab.13.6 and image frame rates can be reduced to alleviate this problem. The major advantage with digital cardiac imaging is that the images can be retrieved immediately after acquisition (unlike cine-angiography).

Table 13.6 System specification for digital cardiology.

Feature	Cardiac DF
Video	$1024^2 \times 10$, $512^2 \times 10$
CCD or plumbicon	
Frame rate	30 - 60fps
Image storage	
Image memory	320M-byte
Magnetic disk	1 - 2G-byte
Image processing	cardiac subtraction
Clinical analysis	cardiac ejection fraction

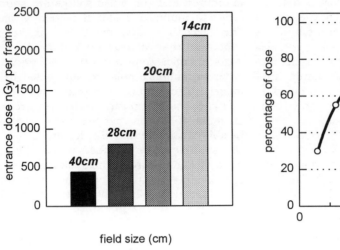
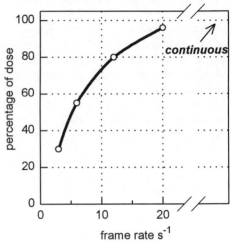

Figure 13.13 (a) Entrance dose varying with field size (b) Radiation dose increases with frame rate.

Image analysis Edge enhancement, windowing and magnification are a few of the image post-processing features that can improve the diagnostic quality of the images. Quantitative analysis programs are also available in the form of ejection fraction calculation and wall motion measurements.

Pulsed beam   A standard feature found in cardio-angiography is a pulsed x-ray delivery which provides short repetitive pulses which serve to decrease motion unsharpness.

The x-ray beam is pulsed by using a grid controlled x-ray tube. This cuts out inductive/capacitive delays introduced by the high voltage cable as would be given by electronically switching the high frequency generator so providing very sharp cut-off pulses.

13.4.5 Patient dose

Most digital fluorography units employ extra beam filtering. Copper filtration is commonly employed (0.1-0.2mm) which hardens the x-ray beam both reducing patient dose and improving image quality.

A typical intensifier entrance dose of $0.9\mu Gy$ s^{-1} is required using the full image intensifier size in general angiography. DSA requires a higher dose technique in order to reduce image noise at a set concentration of contrast material; this is typically between 1.8 to $4.4\mu Gy$ s^{-1}. Peripheral angiography using snap-shot DSA, where a complete run of contrast is followed along extremities (legs), has reduced dose requirements to approximately $0.4\mu Gys^{-1}$ for a 40cm image intensifier. This dose requirement increases as the field size decreases as indicated by Fig.13.13(a).

Since the digital imaging system is a more sensitive detection method than cine-film a significant reduction in patient dose rates is possible. Frame rate selection is typically available between 5 and 30 fps, depending on application; significant dose reductions are achieved at the slower frame rates as shown in Fig.13.13(a). Fast frame rates matching cine-camera runs are not yet possible however in digital systems so cineangiography is still the choice for pediatric investigations.

Further reading

Medical X-ray imaging. B.H. Hasegawa
Medical Physics Publishing (2nd Edition)

KEYWORDS

bi-planar a system using two C-arm fluoroscopy units which have independent positioning. Commonly used in cardiac studies.

C-arm a fluoroscopy design found both in small mobile and large fixed units. The image intensifier is fixed in-line with the x-ray tube on a C structure which is sometimes cantilevered giving oblique views.

dual energy subtraction a method for removing hard and soft tissue contributing to a subtracted image. X-ray energies of 60 and 110kVp are commonly employed.

filtering (spatial) simple filters are smoothing or edge enhancement.

filtering (temporal) frame averaging or recursive filtering takes the average value from a small series (typically four) which reduces image noise.

hybrid subtraction this combines the advantages of both dual energy subtraction and temporal filtering to remove interfering tissue (bone) and vessel movement.

look-up-table a series of stored values in memory which is used for mathematical transformations (log or non-linear image processing).

mask an early image containing tissue detail which is subtracted from later images.

progressive scanning a non-interlaced video display giving higher definition and less flicker.

road mapping subtraction of a contrast filled reference image continuously from the display to reveal catheter placement.

windowing displaying only part (usually 256 levels) of the complete pixel depth (usually 4096 levels).

14

Linear and Computed Tomography

14.1 Introduction
14.2 Linear tomography
14.3 Computed Axial Tomography (CAT or CT
14.4 CT image signals and data handling

14.5 CT image reconstruction
14.6 CT equipment and Image quality
14.7 CT image artifacts
14.8 Radiation exposure

14.1 INTRODUCTION

One of the major disadvantages associated with conventional planar radiography is its inability to produce sectional information. The image produced on film represents the total attenuation of the x-ray beam as it passes through the patient. It is impossible to distinguish any depth information on the film image.

Tomographic techniques have been developed which will separate these superimposed anatomical details and produce slice images which convey depth information.

There are two general classes of tomography in radiographic imaging:

- **Linear** or conventional tomography producing longitudinal sections and
- **Computed axial tomography** (CAT or CT scan) producing sectional or axial slices.

Linear tomography gives longitudinal sectional information by moving the x-ray tube and film in synchrony about a fulcrum or axis. This fulcrum defines the sectional plane of the patient. The images produced are degraded to some extent by blurring caused by interfering absorption on either side of the plane of interest.

Computed tomography is a digital imaging process which produces separate axial sectional images (transverse slices) having no intersection interference.

14.2 LINEAR TOMOGRAPHY

Linear tomographs are produced by making an x-ray exposure during tube and film movement. Figure 14.1 shows a basic system. Both x-ray source and film cassette are connected and move about a fulcrum or axis of rotation *O*. The location of this axis determines the position of the tomographic plane.

The tube and the film cassette carrier are linked so during exposure the tube and cassette moves a distance *S* from *X* to *Y* at an angle θ. The distance from the tube to the cassette (FFD) can be altered. The tomographic plane is at a point *O* and the width of the slice is *T*. Slice depth *a* can be altered by moving the fulcrum point. The parameters shown in Fig.14.1 are used for the demonstration calculation in Box.14.1. using the formulas for cut thickness as:

$$T = \frac{2B \times a^2}{FFD \times S} \text{ or } \frac{2B \times a}{FFD \times \tan\theta} \qquad (14.1)$$

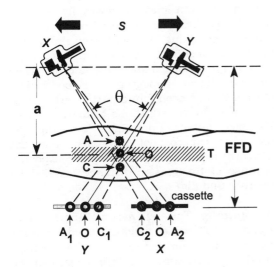

Figure 14.1 Basic linear tomography system showing the x-ray tube connected to the film cassette and swinging through an angle θ.

Where *B* is the acceptable blurring for the overlying sections *A* and *C* in the diagram. Any image point in the **tomographic plane** *O* is projected onto the film and moves exactly as *O* marked on the cassette in the diagram remaining fairly sharply defined.

Image points not in the tomographic plane (A and C) change their position on the film (A_1, A_2 and C_1, C_2) and are therefore misregistered as the cassette moves so producing a streaked or blurred image along the direction of the tube film movement. The blurring increases the further the image point is from the tomographic plane. The thickness or width of the tomographic plane *T* decreases with increasing rotation angle θ.

After several traverses only shadows from *O* and other objects on the tomographic plane remain sharp since their positions on the film do not move. *A* and *C* positions are moving and will be smeared over the film in the direction of the tube-film movement. In practice there is a region on either side of the fulcrum plane where blurring is minimal. Visually this region or thickness seems in focus and is known as the 'in focus layer'; *T* in the diagram. The width of this layer:

- Decreases as the angle of swing of the tube-film combination increases.
- Decreases if the tube to fulcrum distance is decreased or the fulcrum to film distance increases.

There is a minimum practical thickness for this layer of about 1 to 2mm since the subject contrast depends on the difference in x-ray transmission for any two areas in the focus layer, either due to thickness differences or relative attenuation rates μ per unit thickness (bone and soft tissue). A very thin layer will exhibit small differences in x-ray transmission. Increasing the angle of swing (thinner section) will also increase the radiation dose to organs outside the plane of interest, e.g. breast exposure during a kidney examination. The effect of tube swing distance and angle is demonstrated in Box.14.1.

Box.14.1

Slice thickness and depth

The influence of varying tube to film distance, slice depth and swing angle. From Figure 14.1:

FFD	x-ray tube to film distance
S	tube movement
a	tube to arm pivot distance (slice depth)
θ	swing angle
B	acceptable blurring value for overlaying sections (0.7mm).

The formulas in eqn. 14.1 are used

Example: (A)
For a FFD of 90cm and a tube movement *S* of 66cm what will the slice thickness be?
For *S* of 109cm what is the slice thickness?

$$T = \frac{(2 \times 0.7) \times 75^2}{90 \times 66} = 6.6\text{cm}$$

For a tube movement of 109cm the slice thickness would be 4mm

Example (B):
For the above 6.6mm and 4mm slices what will the swing angles θ be? Rearranging the formula

$$\tan \theta = \frac{(2 \times 0.7) \times 75}{90 \times 0.66} = 60°$$

for a 4mm slice the angle would be 70°

14.2.2 Tomography configurations

The tube movement for linear tomography can have various shapes and those that are available in commercial tomographic machines (Fig. 14.2)

Linear   The simplest and cheapest movement but having serious limitations:

- When the angle of swing is increased inverse square law problems are introduced as the tube and film are further away from the fulcrum at the extremities of swing than at the central portion
- Overlying structures which are parallel to the plane of swing are not sufficiently blurred in the final image. Blurring is directional.

Plan view of movement

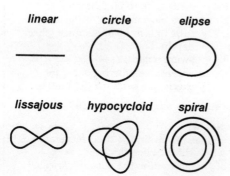

Figure 14.2 Tomographic patterns available from commercial machines.

Non-linear movement   These limitations can be overcome to some extent by employing non-linear movements of tube and film such as circular, elliptical, Lissajous, hypocycloidal and spiral. Non-linear tomography ensures that image blurring is not directional and removes streaking artifacts seen in simple linear movements. Tube and film movements are still synchronized about the fulcrum plane as with linear tomography. Hypocycloidal movement has been found particularly useful for fine detail investigations of the inner ear. The disadvantage of non-linear tomography is the increased cost of equipment and the increase in the time taken for the exposure because of the greater distance traveled by the tube and film.

Zonography   This is narrow angle tomography (<10° swing) which is used for thick section high contrast tomographic images. Overlying structures i.e. rib cage can be removed from the image to reveal soft tissue lung detail.

Linear tomography is rapidly being replaced by computed tomography as its only advantage now seems to be cheapness. Linear tomography is retained as a clinical tool by those who have functioning equipment. It will rapidly lose favor however to more modern approaches (both CT and MRI) with their multi-planar reconstruction giving axial, coronal, sagittal and oblique sections.

Summary

- Linear tomography depends on linked x-ray tube and film cassette system.
- Slice thickness depends on tube movement S or angle of movement θ
- Thicker slices (in focus layer) with smaller θ or S and vice-versa.
- FFD increase will decrease slice thickness
- Slice thickness increases if the blurring value increases.
- Complex scanning motions maintain image sharpness in x and y planes of the slice.
- There are both linear and non-linear movements.

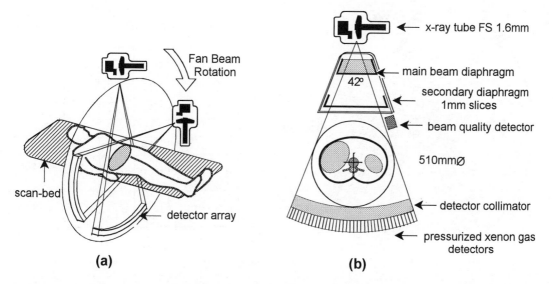

Figure 14.3 **(a)** Basic CT design showing an x-ray source collimated to a fan beam rotating around a patient and **(b)** the fan beam assembly showing collimator and detector geometry. The x-ray tube and detectors are fixed together as a single rotating unit.

14.3 COMPUTED AXIAL TOMOGRAPHY (CAT or CT)

Computed axial tomography is entirely different from longitudinal tomography and produces radiological images as transaxial sections of the body without any intersectional interference or blurring. The method was first developed in a commercial x-ray machine by Godfrey Hounsfield (UK) in 1973. It was immediately successful as a diagnostic imaging technique since much smaller contrast differences are evident in the CT image revealing subtle differences between normal and abnormal soft tissue. For example visible contrast is about 2% on a good radiograph but this is extended to 0.1-0.3% for a typical CT image.

14.3.1 The fan beam geometry

The basic design for a modern transaxial tomographic machine is illustrated in Fig. 14.3(a). A rotating x-ray source collimated as

a fan beam is subtended by a group of up to 800 detectors. The fan arrangement is rotated in a series of **projections** or angles covering the full 360° round the patient. At each projection (up to 1000 is typical for recent machines) measurements are made of the beam attenuation. A typical fan beam geometry, with tube collimators and detectors, is shown in Fig.14.3(b). The primary and secondary beam diaphragms (collimators) control the slice thickness. The beam monitor detector measures the beam quality at each projection.

Machine design Early CT systems used a mixed rotation and rectilinear scan movement (translation) for their data acquisition, which was very slow; these were the first and second generation machines. **Third generation** machines use fan beam **rotate only** designs and have very fast data acquisition times; approximately 1-2 seconds per slice is common. Image data is obtained by rotating the fan beam around the patient in a series of projections completing a 360° sweep (360 projection

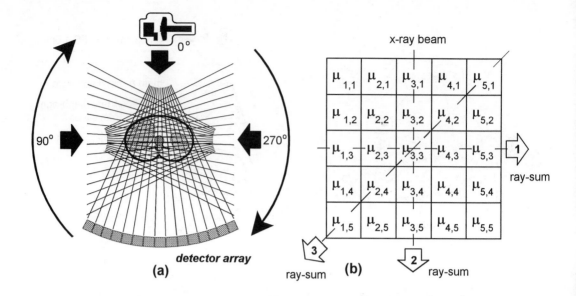

Fig. 14.4   **(a)** Image matrix projections for a fan-beam showing construction of matrix cells during fan-beam rotation. **(b)** a small section of the final matrix showing individual attenuation values combined as a ray-sum.

≡1° per projection; 720 projections≡0.5° etc.). Figure 14.4(a) shows how the rotating fan-beam spatially constructs a matrix of data cells over the patient slice during its 360° rotation; these are stored in computer memory as a data matrix or attenuation values. Machine precision in this movement influences the finest resolution of the matrix. The entire fan-beam mechanism (x-ray tube, detectors and electronics) weighs about 500kg and must move with a precision better than 0.01mm.

A small matrix of 5×5 elements in Fig. 14.4(b) represents a central area of this data set which contains the individual attenuation coefficients μ. The sum of these is available during data collection as the **ray-sum**. The transaxial image is formed by calculating individual μ values within the matrix using image reconstruction techniques. The final result is a complete digital matrix whose elements represent the individual linear attenuation coefficients for the section or slice in the plane of the x-ray beam. The fundamental mathematics involved was first presented by J. Radon in 1913.

An alternative CT design was available that used a fixed 360° detector ring and is shown in Fig.14.5. This is the so called **fourth generation** design but the development was somewhat premature showing serious disadvantages since the x-ray tube assembly moved inside this detector circle.   Very fast scan times were possible but the design suffered from the limited packing density of its detectors and geometrical misalignment problems between the detector ring radius and the x-ray beam origin.

This geometrical misalignment restricted detector size and depth which was not the case in third generation designs using fan beam geometry. For both 3rd and 4th generation designs the x-ray tube must return to its starting (home) position after each rotation; high voltage cable and signal leads connected to the rotating mechanism make this essential. Spiral/ helical scan machines address this problem.

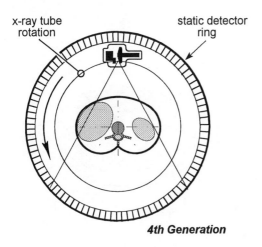

4th Generation

Figure 14.5 Fourth generation design showing geometrical misalignment between x-ray source and center of detector gantry. Shallow solid detectors are necessary.

Sampling frequency During each projection the detector signals give information about the total tissue attenuation between the source and detector. High resolution CT requires high density samples. If an insufficient number of projections are taken then streaking is seen. A total of 500 projections are sufficient for a 256×256 matrix with 1mm resolution whereas 1000 projections require a 512×512 matrix to see 0.5mm. Detector density and the speed of image reconstruction time is listed in Table 14.1.

Table 14.1 Machine configuration: number of detectors, detectors per degree and image reconstruction time (seconds)

Machine	Detector No.	Detec. per °	Reconstr. time (s).
Stepped fan beam			
Low Spec.	384	8.3	9
Medium Spec.	704	18	real time
4th Generation	2304	6.4	24
Continuous rotation	768 (×2)	18.3	4

14.3.2 Slice thickness

The spatial resolution of a CT system must consider both the resolution in the slice plane together with that perpendicular to it, which is determined by the slice thickness. A high resolution in the slice plane can only be achieved if it is matched by a thin slice, so resolution should be balanced between the slice plane and slice thickness.

The slice thickness is determined by the collimation shown in Fig.14.6(a) and (b) applied to both the emerging x-ray beam and the entrance to the detectors (see also Fig. 14.3(b)). The slice thickness is measured from its profile as the full width at half maximum (FWHM); this is demonstrated in the profiles in the figure.

Sensitivity profile The sensitivity profile is an important factor of a CT machine since it determines the image quality. The steeper the profile slope the less interference from adjacent slices which would cause partial volume effects (Fig.14.6). The perfect sensitivity profile would be rectangular and for a point source of x-rays this could be achieved by simple colli-mation; however for a practical system where the focal spot has a finite size geometrical unsharpness causes penumbra effects and tight collimation at the detector entrance is necessary as shown in Fig.14.7(a).

sensitivity slice profiles

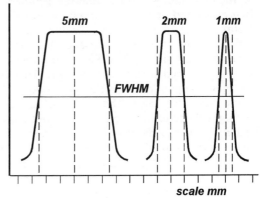

Figure 14.6 Sensitivity profiles for 5, 2 and 1mm slice thicknesses. The dose profiles for these slices thicknesses are slightly larger.

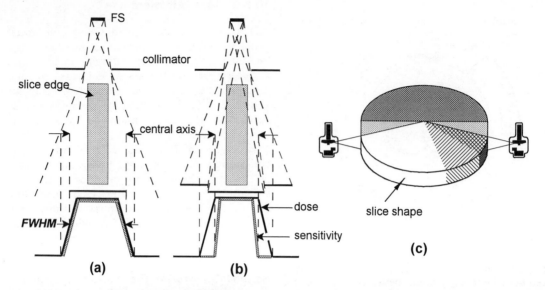

Figure 14.7 **(a)** The comparison of sensitivity and dose profiles. The slice is viewed edge on and with this simple collimation the dose and sensitivity profiles coincide. **(b)** In order to obtain a sharp sensitivity profile some detector collimation is necessary; the dose and sensitivity profiles are then different. **(c)** The diverging shape of the x-ray beam causes the center of the slice to be thicker than the periphery. This is more pronounced in thin section slices.

Dose profile Since there are two sets of collimators shaping the beam, one at the exit of the x-ray tube and the other at the entrance to the detectors, the object or patient plane (axis in diagram) experiences the radiation burden from the penumbra even though this is blocked by the detector collimation. Consequently the sensitivity profile and the dose profile have a different geometry when measured at the axis, as shown in Fig. 14.6(a). The larger dose profile in (b) contributes to increased surface dose if a series of image slices are taken, compared to the dose received from a single slice. This is due to overlapping dose profiles and causes a pile-up factor. Owing to the design of certain xenon gas detectors, which offer in built collimation, extra detector collimation is unnecessary and there is good agreement between sensitivity and dose profiles giving very little pile up factor; a typical set of profiles from 5mm to 1mm is shown in Fig.14.6.

The dose pile up factor is only part of the overall picture of patient dose in computed tomography. A more comprehensive dose measure is given by the CT dose index calculation (CTDI) described later.

When opposing beam shapes are super-imposed as would be seen in a full 360° data collection series the two diverging beams give a slice section which departs from a true rectangle. The middle of the slice is thicker than the periphery. This is particularly noticeable for thin slices. The general bi-conical shape of a CT slice is indicated in Fig.14.7(b).

14.3.3 Fan beam x-ray production

X-ray tube CT x-ray tubes have a very high standard of performance since they must deliver a stable, intense pulse of x-ray photons for each projection. The x-ray beam is highly filtered by both aluminum and copper to produce a high effective photon energy. X-ray tube specifications are listed in Tab.14.2 for two x-ray tubes, one suitable for a low to medium use machine and the other a high throughput or rapid scan machine.

Table 14.2   CT x-ray tube specifications

Design feature	Low-medium	High
Focal spot	1.6mm	0.8 - 1.2mm
Anode loading	1MJ (1.35MHU)	2.7MJ (3.5MHU)
Thermal diss.	350kHU	730kHU
Max. power	30kW	40kW

The x-ray intensity or output must not vary over the image acquisition cycle as any variation would be treated as absorption differences in the image; generator stability is typically better than 1%. The linear attenuation coefficient μ is kV dependent so variations in the effective kV energy of the beam will produce variations in the image. In addition it is necessary to maintain the x-ray spectrum to within very narrow limits so that μ does not alter. For large object thicknesses a slice energy of about 30kWs and a pulse power of 40kW is necessary in order to generate the necessary minimum number of x-ray photons. The heat capacity of the anode (in excess of 5MHU) allows a large volume scan consisting of up to 20 to 30 slices.

The **focal spot size** of the x-ray tube determines the minimum point size in the center of the scanned field which is projected onto the detector array. This determines the amount of information distributed over the detector array. As the focal spot increases the point information is spread over a larger number of detectors; this limits resolution. Typical focal spot sizes are between 0.6 and 1.6 mm.

The **anode angles** in CT x-ray tubes are smaller than normal and a common design feature is a completely flat anode surface with an angled cathode/filament assembly. The flat anode ensures more uniform heat transfer and dissipation. The **heel effect** is minimized by setting the cathode-anode axis perpendicular to the detector axis.

Modern machines using a continuously ro-

tating fan beam design can also switch the position of the focal spot (Fig.14.8(a)). This has the effect of doubling the number of projections during a scan. The direction of the electron beam in the x-ray tube is magnetically shifted so altering the position of the focal spot on the anode. This small movement effectively halves the detector width for a given number of fan beam projections and doubles the number of ray projections for each sectional image.

High frequency power supplies are used exclusively in CT machines; these provide extremely stable tube current and voltages controlled by a dedicated microprocessor. The x-ray tubes are operated in a fast pulse mode by switching the grids of the x-ray tube. Pulse duration of between 2-4ms and a pulse power of over 40kW is necessary to give optimum speed of data acquisition and the x-ray tube currents can be up to 800mA. The small generator size can be judged from the photograph in Fig.14.8(b).

14.3.4 Beam attenuation

Computed tomography operates at about 125kVp, a little higher in some machines. This is at least 50% higher than conventional radiography and extra beam filtration (2.5mm aluminum with 0.4mm copper) ensures that the effective energy is also high (70-80keV). This reduces the effect of beam hardening by the tissues.

Subject contrast of soft tissue detail from this high effective energy does not depend on photoelectric absorption (in common with most conventional radiography) but the dominant interaction is due to inelastic or Compton scattering which removes x-ray photons from the main beam. Since the fan-beam system has a narrow, highly collimated x-ray source and the detector array is also carefully collimated, the amount of scattered radiation that reaches the detectors is minimized so the image information is carried by the emerging unscattered x-ray beam.

Photoelectric absorption is dependent on atomic number Z and density but Compton

x-ray tube anode

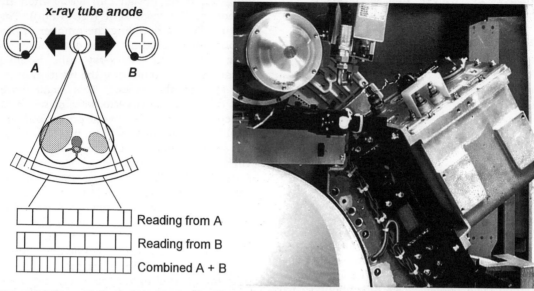

Figure 14.8 **(a)** X-ray beam switching from one focal spot to another which effectively doubles the resolving power of the detector array. **(b)** The small high frequency generator attached to the x-ray tube and fan-beam assembly (courtesy GE Medical Inc.)

scattering depends on tissue electron density (see Chapter 5). Although the electron density per gram of soft tissue is very consistent over a fixed volume of tissue the electrons per unit volume (electrons cm^{-3}) does vary. This gives the tissue differentiation in CT images.

Beam hardening As the incident beam passes through the patient lower energy photons are preferentially removed; the effective energy of the x-ray spectrum increases and thus the values of the linear attenuation coefficients decrease. The increase in effective energy causes beam hardening which is influenced by the patient thickness and tissue material; it is worse for bone.

Absorption of a monochromatic x-ray beam with increasing depth of water will give a straight line for I_{in} divided by I_{out} as shown in Fig.14.9(a). However a typical polychromatic x-ray beam will give a curved response as the lower energies are filtered by the thicker absorption pathway. This non-linear response is predictable and provides corrections for

beam hardening in CT images. The computation of CT numbers is given in section 14.4.1 and the effect of beam hardening on these is demonstrated in Box.14.2.

The **cupping effect** caused by uncorrected beam hardening is seen in profile across a uniform absorber in Fig.14.9(b). Both tube filtration and correction algorithms reduce beam hardening artifacts in the final CT image. The corrections work well for soft tissue (water equivalent) but problems can occur in images containing a large amount of bone (head sections). In order to minimize beam hardening it is heavily filtered, using 0.25mm to 0.4mm copper foil; this reduces spectrum width and also x-ray photon intensity. The tube current must be large to compensate for this photon reduction, consequently the heat rating of modern CT tubes must be high as the anode cooling rate limits the number and duration of CT scans. High power output requires oil cooled tubes which often have heat capacities up to 5 MHU.

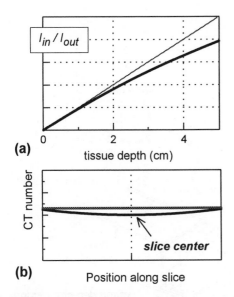

(a)

(b)

Position along slice

Figure 14.9 (a) the loss of photon intensity from a polychromatic beam with tissue depth leading to (b) The cupping profile (reduction of CT number value) across the field of view compared to the corrected level profile.

14.3.5 X-ray detection

Three types of detector systems are suitable for CT machines:

- Multiple scintillation detectors with photo multipliers
- Multiple scintillation detectors with photo diodes
- A single multi-chamber inert gas (xenon) detector.

Current designs favor gas detectors in spite of their lower quantum efficiency.

Scintillation Detectors Early CT machines used scintillation crystals (thallium doped NaI) and photo-multiplier tubes as x-ray detectors. The photo-multiplier tubes could not provide the packing density that was necessary with fan beam designs so photo-diode detectors were substituted. Cesium iodide superseded sodium iodide as a detector since it gives light photons in the visible range (sodium iodide gives ultra-violet) which can

be detected by a simple photo-diode which packs into a very small volume array (example sketched in Fig.14.10(a)). A complete photo-detector array is shown in Fig.14.10(b). Major problems with scintillation detectors are:

- Relatively long after-glow following the detection of an x-ray photon.
- Stable output signals depend on a very stable high-voltage supply.
- Multi-detector uniformity of response is difficult to maintain.

In spite of their high quantum efficiency solid state devices have been replaced by gas detectors which have several advantages.

Gas proportional detectors The common detector uses xenon-gas filled chambers which are less dependent on stable high voltage supplies, are inherently uniform and provide in-built collimation as an added bonus. Fig.14.10(c) gives a design for an integral 768 detector array using pressurized xenon. The xenon gas used to fill the chambers has a high atomic number which increases photo-electric absorption in the detector. Absorption is further increased by keeping the gas under high pressure (up to 20 atmospheres or 20×10^5Pa) and increasing the length of the chambers. Under these circumstances the sensitivity can be about 50% of the scintill-ation detector. The complete detector array (Fig.14.10(d)) is subdivided, using electrode plates, into a large number of chambers (up to 1000). Each one shares the same gas volume minimizing variation in sensitivity between the chambers. The signal strength is not influenced by small supply voltage vari-ations, unlike the crystal/photo-multiplier or crystal/photo-diode systems. The electrode plates forming the chambers also act as collimators so added collimation is minimal between patient and detector. Each detector anode feeds a dedicated amplifier which is switched to a common A/D converter. The detector electrodes are aligned with the focal spot of the x-ray tube. This is the acceptance angle of the detector decided by the detector collimation and detector aperture size.

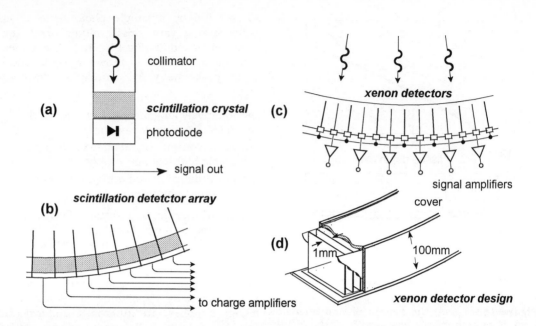

Figure 14.10 **(a)** Separate solid state (scintillation) detectors combined with their photo-diodes require separate collimation **(b)** to form a detector array. **(c)** xenon gas detectors have deep chambers, have a common compressed xenon gas fill and because of their depth provide their own collimation. **(d)** The complete detector array consists of over 700 separate 1mm detector elements

Typical detector aperture sizes are between 1 and 2mm for a detector depth of 100mm. The fixed detector design of the fourth generation machine has two geometrical centers, that of the gantry-patient and that of the x-ray focal spot. This geometric misalignment between x-ray beam and the center of the detector array gives misaligned beam angles at the detector surface so only shallow depth detectors (photo-diodes) can be used to accommodate this differing geometry and the packing density of the detectors (influencing resolution) is restricted. For this reason the fixed detector design has become unpopular in spite of its fast scan times.

Detector signals These are analog voltage pulses which vary in height according to the level of absorption. They are digitized for processing by a fast analog to digital converter (ADC) which is switched to serve the complete detector array. The requirements for an ideal detection system are:

- High efficiency for recording radiation
- Fast response time recording all the detected radiation.
- Linear and stable
- Large dynamic range of the detector which is dependent on the accuracy and precision of the ADC.

In practice the detector system is a compromise between quantum efficiency which influences patient dose, packing density which influences resolution and response which influences image contrast.

14.3.6 Spiral / Helical CT

There are certain limitations to collecting data as contiguous axial slices particularly when small lesions are being imaged since these can be missed if they happen to be located between adjacent slices. The contiguous slice protocol, although giving complete disk-like sections as shown in Fig.14.11(a) and (b),

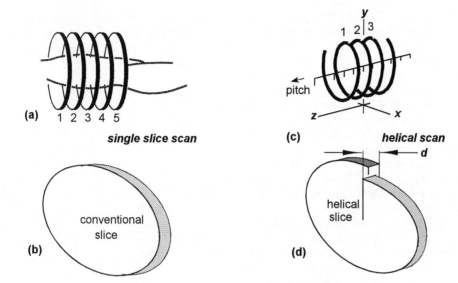

(a) 1 2 3 4 5

single slice scan

(c) *helical scan*

Figure 14.11 **(a)** Contiguous separate slice acquisition which is not continuous showing **(b)** the complete slice periphery. **(c)** spiral acquisition where the table moves during continuous acquisition at different pitch settings giving a continuous helical acquisition but the slice periphery **(d)** is incomplete.

includes delays between slices since the process consists of:

- Fan beam assembly accelerated to scan speed
- X-ray tube pulsed and data collected
- Fan beam assembly halts and returns to its home position
- Table indexed to next longitudinal position while x-ray tube cools.

This series of events constitutes the inter-scan delay time (ISD) and adds a significant time to the clinical study causing problems if the patient must hold their breath or patient movement is present. The missing data between slices also give inconsistencies (jagged edges) to 3D reconstruction images. Following an iodine contrast bolus through a section of anatomy also produces an incomplete data set due to ISD.

For these reasons spiral or helical scanning was introduced in 1989 for continuous CT data collection while at the same time moving the patient through the gantry as shown in

Fig.14.11(c). Helical scanning imposes certain limitations on the CT machine:

- a cable-free method for connecting x-ray tube and detectors must be installed
- x-ray tube power must be substantially increased
- image reconstruction algorithms must consider the spiral shape of the resulting section shown in Fig.14.11(d)

The problems associated with this latter point is further illustrated in Fig.14.12 where two pitch settings are shown (a) and (b).

Since the patient is moved at a constant rate through the gantry during data acquisition the slice shape will not be a simple disk shape as shown in Fig.14.11(b) but will resemble that sketched in (d) which will cause overlap between slices in any 360° section of scan sequence. The degree of overlap depends on the scan pitch d shown in Fig.14.12, which is controlled by the table feed-rate in the z-axis relative to the rotational speed. This is the difference between pitch ×1 where table feed is the same as the slice thickness compared to pitch ×1.5 or ×2 where the movement is greater than the slice width. The larger pitch settings increase the slice distortion however the effective slice width increases and a faster tissue volume is covered with a consequent smaller radiation dose to the patient. In order to overcome this distortion a form of data interpolation is required. Initially this was a 360° **linear interpolation** (LI). This procedure is indicated in Fig. 14.12(a) and (b) interpolation being made between movement z and $z+d$ so correcting for the data offset imposed by the table movement.

The full 360° LI has now been replaced by a 180° LI where interpolation from opposing 180° points reduces the spiral range used for re-construction the offset now being $d/2$. This procedure decreases slice width broadening; even scanning at pitch 1.5 does not increase slice width adversely.

Slip-ring technology The first requirement for spiral acquisition for a third generation machine is a continuously rotating fan beam assembly or a fourth generation machine the x-ray tube must rotate continuously. Some form of brush and slip-ring mechanism must be present operating either at low voltages (200-300 volts), when the generator and x-ray tube must rotate together, or high voltages (up to 140kV) supplying just the x-ray tube alone. Both low and high voltage techniques have their advantages and disadvantages.Low voltage slip rings have the x-ray high voltage generator as part of the tube assembly. The tank unit containing the high frequency transformers and control electronics is associated with the x- ray tube as shown in Fig.14.8(b).

Slip-ring designs can give very fast section times without the need for relocating the fan-beam assembly after each section. Spiral or helical CT acquisition utilizes this continuous rotation by incrementing the patient couch for each rotation which then gives a spiral scan motion producing a rapid acquisition of axial slices (Fig. 14.11(c)). In the case of the third generation machine a method must be devised for collecting the detector signals; this is usually achieved photo-electrically by using infra-red laser diodes on the edge of the fan beam assembly which align with detectors on the fixed gantry.

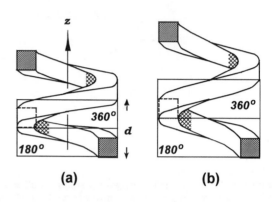

Figure 14.12 Helical scan showing movement of fan-beam assembly over object from a top-view for two pitch settings **(a)** and **(b)** by altering distance z. Reconstruction using 360° and 180° LI demonstrate reduction in d

X-ray generator A major limitation to early spiral systems was the thermal loadability of the x-ray tube which restricted acquisition times allowing only a small area to be covered by the spiral sequence. Increased x-ray tube power from 3.5 to 5.0MHU has now removed this restriction allowing multiple spiral acquisitions without lengthy tube cooling delays. The generator and x-ray tube must be capable of providing high photon flux and fast cycle times. Typical minimum power ratings would be 125kW at 120 or 140kVp.

Since x-ray output has been increased to accommodate larger scanned volumes and reduce image noise the dose rate has increased particularly for studies using a table pitch of one. Patient dose is improved when a higher pitch value is selected but for a reduced image quality if thin slices are required for multi-planar reconstruction (3-D).

The geometry of the fan beam itself can contribute significantly to increased patient dose. Figure 14.13 shows two fan beams one from a small CT gantry (a) which has the x-ray tube close to the object (patient) axis in order to achieve a small gantry size. The other belongs to a 'regular' sized CT gantry (b) where the x-ray tube is at a greater distance. The exposure factor difference between the two designs is obtained from the ratio of the squares of the focus to gantry center distance. For the example shown the increase in exposure is the ratio between 50^2 and 70^2 which is approximately ×2.

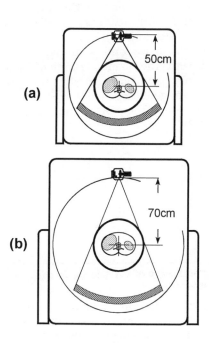

Figure 14.13 Geometry and dose due to varying source to detector distances from a small and a large gantry calculated in text.

Data storage Multiple spiral acquisitions together with 3D reconstruction has meant the need for very large memory sizes, in many cases exceeding 32M-bytes. A thirty second spiral acquisition sequence capturing data as a 512×512×12 matrix would use approximately 20M-bytes of memory.

14.4 CT IMAGE SIGNALS AND DATA HANDLING

The CT machine must be capable of acquiring a large number of data samples from its detector array over a very short time to give fast scan times and reduce motion artifacts. Signals from each detector are digitized and transferred to the array processor. The stepped fan beam has a limited travel where ribbon cables carry the detector signals (just over 360°). Detector signals from machines having continuously rotating detectors are picked up from optical sensors placed at locations around the gantry. Data transmission rates of 200M-bytes s^{-1} are common.

For each scan projection a number of mathematical operations is performed on the raw data from the detectors. Separate very fast circuits perform one operation on the signal data and then pass it on to the next circuit using a **pipe-line** process. Image reconstruction is an example of pipe-line processing.

While filtering is being performed on one profile, say *P*, back projection is occurring with the last profile *P*+1 and log amplification is occurring with the next profile *P*−1 etc. The fact that many different processes are occurring simultaneously increases the speed of image reconstruction and presentation.

14.4.1 CT numbers

The absorption coefficient μ depends on the kV. However if the tissue absorption coefficient is related to that of water at the same kV a reference number insensitive to kV change can be obtained. A CT number or **Hounsfield Unit** can now be used which is:

$$1000 \times \frac{\mu_{tissue} - \mu_{water}}{\mu_{water}} \quad (14.2)$$

Box 14.2 shows calculations for three different kV values; the CT value remains constant since the water reference also matches the kV value.

Box 14.2

CT number calculation
(Using eqn. 14.2 for the data)

	80kV	*100kV*	*150kV*
μmuscle	0.1892	0.1760	0.1550
μwater	0.1835	0.1707	0.1504

At 80keV: $1000 \times \dfrac{0.1892 - 0.1835}{0.1835} = 31$

At 100keV: $1000 \times \dfrac{0.1760 - 0.1707}{0.1707} = 31$

At 150keV: $1000 \times \dfrac{0.1550 - 0.1504}{0.1504} = 31$

Beam hardening At 100kV the reference for water is 0.1707 but if the beam effective energy changes to 105kV in the center of the profile, the μ for tissue changes to 0.1750 then:

$$\text{New CT value} = \frac{0.1750 - 0.1707}{0.1707} = 25$$

and not 31 which it should be. This gives the cupping effect seen in Fig.14.9(b).

In practice a range of CT values are produced from −1000 for air, 0 for water and between 2000 to 3000 for bone, some machines producing an even wider range. Figure 14.14 shows values for common tissues. These values are approximately the same between different machines since they are always referenced to water.

The Dynamic Range The ADC must be capable of responding to a wide variation of attenuation in the patient. This is usually mare than 1,000,000 to 1. The dynamic range reflects the ratio of the largest signal (no attenuation) to the smallest signal (maximum attenuation) that can be detected. This allows obese and slim patients to be imaged with the same definition including dense bone and low density soft- tissue. Dynamic range is dependent on the accuracy and precision of the ADC of the voltage signal (Box 14.3).

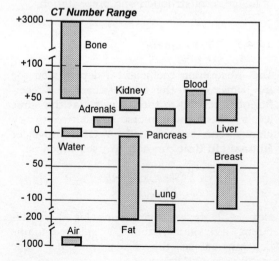

Figure 14.14 A bar plot of common CT value ranges for tissues and reference materials.

Box 14.3

Dynamic Range of an Analog to Digital Converter (ADC)

Analog voltage level for 20 bit binary number as 2^{20} gives a range of 1:1,000,000. Uncertainty in voltage measurement is therefore $\sqrt{10^6}$ or 1000 which represents 0.1%. At 150keV μ value for muscle is 0.155 (0.1% of this value is therefore 0.000155) A positive or negative 0.1% variation in μ gives:

$$\frac{0.155155 - 0.1504}{0.1504} \times 1000 = 32$$

$$\frac{0.154845 - 0.1504}{0.1504} \times 1000 = 30$$

Conclusion: A greater than a 0.1% variation in voltage measurement will influence CT number calculation

---

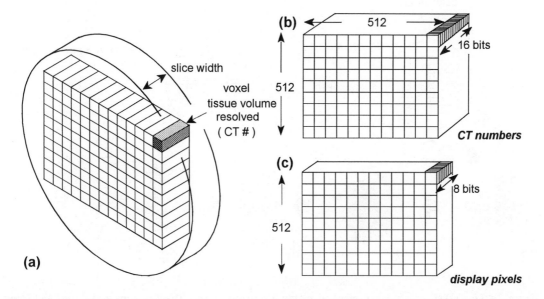

Figure 14.15 **(a)** The body slice represented as a digital matrix stored as CT numbers. Each small tissue volume resolved by the matrix is a 'voxel' or volume element **(b)** The voxel information is stored in memory by typically a 512×512 matrix each voxel occupying a 12 to 16 bit word **(c)** The windowed display pixel is stored as a 512×512 matrix which can be 4 to 8 bits deep.

14.4.2 Data matrices

These CT numbers are stored in computer memory and represent a volume slice element or **voxel**. The matrix store must be able to hold a range of voxel values of over 4000. A single voxel is represented in Fig.14.15(a) situated in a CT slice. The primary storage matrix for the computed CT numbers must be able to handle values from 0 to 3000, (both positive and negative figures). This requires a memory location of at least 12 bits which is 2^{12} or 4096, plus a 'sign' bit positive or negative. Figure 14.15(b) represents part of a 512×512 voxel memory 16 bits deep. This represents a total storage of 500k-bytes.

The entire CT information in a data matrix (as CT numbers) cannot be displayed, since video monitors have limited dynamic range and are usually driven by 8-bit DAC's giving 256 gray levels; the entire contents of a raw data matrix, representing CT numbers from +3000 for bone to –1000 for lungs would require 4000 gray levels which is not practical

for electronic display devices. The display matrix represented in Fig.14.8(c) is therefore restricted to only 8 bits deep and a sampling method called windowing has been devised for representing the full 12 bit data on the 8 bit display (described in Chapter 12 and later in this chapter).

14.5 CT IMAGE RECONSTRUCTION

Absorption signals that have been collected as single-dimensional values must now be displayed as a two dimensional image. The matrix of absorption coefficients is obtained from the scanning pattern of the fan beam previously shown in Fig.14.4 and is commonly represented in a 512×512 format. A small portion of such a matrix is shown in Fig.14.4(b) where the line source of x-rays (1,2,3 etc.) has undergone absorption and the attenuated beam is measured using a detector array opposite the x-ray beam. Only the

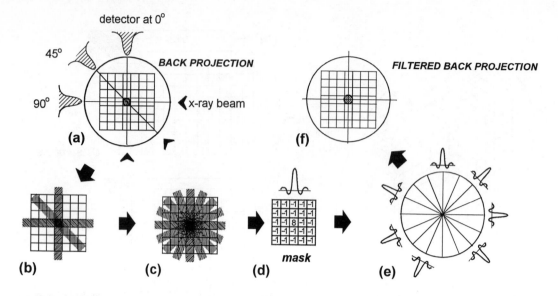

Figure 14.16 (a) Simple back projection yields a blurred image. The ray sum signals are collected and the totals back-projected onto a matrix shown in (b). After all the projections have been collected and stored the star-burst pattern in (c) is then filtered (d) and (e) to reveal the true signal displayed in (f)

total absorption figure is known: this is the ray sum. The separate matrix values shown in the diagram: $\mu_{(1-1)}$, $\mu_{(1-2)}$ ········ $\mu_{(5-5)}$ are found by mathematical reconstruction. The individual values in the matrix can be calculated by using either:

- an **iterative technique** or
- **back-projection** (or its derivatives).

The calculations are performed in a dedicated array processor in order to provide almost instantaneous image display.

14.5.1 Reconstruction algorithms

Iterative technique   This uses an exact mathematical solution for reconstructing the image slice from the attenuation data. This was the original method for image recon-struction used by Godfrey Hounsfield in the first CT machine. Its disadvantages are that

it takes a considerable amount of computer time and is slow. It also suffers from round-ing errors (0.95=1.0, etc.) which give imprecise CT values and all the data must be collected before reconstruction can begin.

Back projection   The principle is shown in Fig.14.16. A tightly collimated x-ray beam is used and provides the total absorption signal. The total ray sum value is inserted along the matching matrix row, which is the computer or array processor image memory. This is shown in the diagram (a) for 0°, 45° and 90° scan positions (b). If other projections are added (c) the total image is obtained (c). The central high uptake, from the original, is now distinguishable but it has a star-burst inter-ference pattern.   Early attempts at this form of reconstruction used photographic methods and the final images contained star artifacts (there is only one star-artifact shown here matching the single high data point in the original image). The artifacts can be removed by just accepting the high values. This is not a satisfactory solution however.

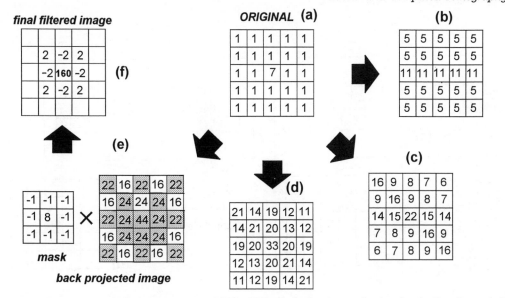

Figure 14.17 A numerical example of filtered back-projection using a simple 9 point matrix. The process starts from the matrix in **(a)** following a simple back-projected process to **(e)** until a filter, mask or kernel is applied to retrieve the true point source data in **(f)**.

Filtered back projection Figure 14.16(d), (e) and (f) continues the process to show how this interference may be removed. A mask signal (d) with negative going edges (e) acts as high pass filter and removing the low frequency interference pattern (f).

A numerical example for filtered back projection is also shown in Fig.14.17 which resembles the previous pictorial example in Fig.14.16 having a high central value (7) surrounded by lower values (1) in Fig. 14.17(a). Horizontal back-projection in (b) stores the total ray-sum in each row of (a). The right diagonal ray sums (c) are then added followed by the vertical (d) and left diagonal ray sums, giving the final image in Fig.14.17(e). The star interference pattern is emphasized by the shaded area in this final back-projected matrix.

Convolution The back projected matrix is subjected to a small 3×3 filter mask, or convolution kernel whose contents are multiplied with the back projected image. The filter mask con-sists of a small sym-

metrical matrix containing a set of numbers. These can have positive or negative values. The filter mask shown in Fig.14.17(e) is shifted over the back projected matrix a row at a time multiplying the image pixel by the corresponding filter value e.g. 22 × –1, 16 × –1 .... etc. until all 9 values under the filter have been multiplied giving the filtered back projection image in (f) with the central value 160 exaggerated by the edge enhancement filter, surrounded by cells of very small numbers (2 and –2). Figure 14.18 shows the filter mask in action for a selected corner of this matrix, 24 being the central value. All the values are summed and the result placed in the central pixel of the image array. The filter mask is then shifted one column and the complete process repeated. The central region of the back-projected matrix (Fig.14.18(b)) is similarly treated giving an enhanced value of 160.

In practice the signal data from the CT detector array are first logarithmically amplified to correct for transmission absorption, then beam hardening corrections are made.

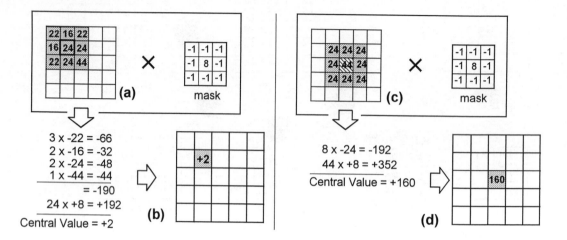

Figure 14.18   Filtering selected regions of the image shown in Fig.14.17. The edge of the matrix is shown filtered in (**a**) yielding a central value of +2 in (**b**) and the central region filtered in (**c**) to give the high positive value in (**d**). This action removes the shadowing artifact associated with back-projection.

Each projection then undergoes the convolution process <u>before</u> back projection (unlike this simple numerical example). The type of convolution filter can be chosen by the user, either smoothing or edge enhancement.

14.5.2   Pre- and post-processing

The raw signal data undergoes processing before taking part in image reconstruction and then the reconstructed image itself can be processed to enhance features or remove artifacts.

Signal data processing   A balancing procedure corrects slight sensitivity differences between individual detector channels so that overlying ring artifacts are not seen. This is a common feature of scintillation detector machines. Extended balancing can help to remove streaking caused by sudden density changes (bone to soft tissue). Beam hardening corrections are also applied at this stage. A sampling error is seen in all reconstructive techniques, where the diagonal x-ray beams do not sample complete volume elements (Fig.14.19(a)). This is corrected by applying chosen weighting factors to each matrix element; the missing sections have a constant area for a fixed beam width and known angle.

Image processing   Secondary or retrospective reconstruction is performed on an image to enlarge or zoom a smaller portion of the scan view. This causes a real improvement in image resolution, up to the machine's maximum dictated by the physical characteristics of the detectors and collimators. A zoom factor of 1 (real size) may give an image resolution of 1mm, increasing the zoom to 10 can increase the image resolution to 0.1mm. Simple magnification of the image does not however involve reconstruction; it merely enlarges the area of interest to fill the display screen.

Multi-planar reconstruction is also a post-processing technique for combining contiguous axial slices into a three dimensional view. This 3-D data set can then be displayed either as a complete image or as a series of sagittal, coronal and oblique cuts.

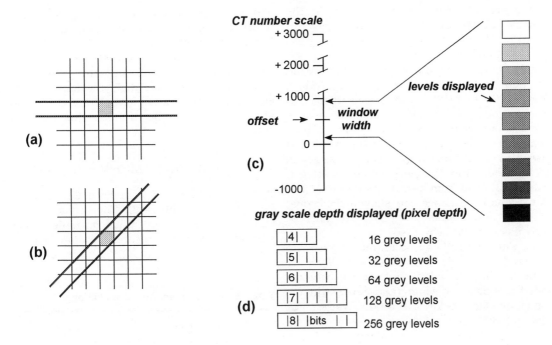

Figure 14.19 **(a)** Diagonal sampling cuts off the corners of the matrix cells causing ray-sum errors. A weighting factor is applied during calculation which corrects for this. **(b)** The entire data set stored as CT numbers from +3000 to −1000 occupying 12bits can only be displayed as separate 4 to 8bit 'windows' (window width). The window can be moved throughout the data (offset) to display different tissue types.

Planar projection view (topogram or scout-view) These are the names given by different manufacturers to 2-D planar projection views. The scanning system remains in a fixed position with the x-ray tube either above and the detectors underneath the patient or occupying a lateral or posterior aspect. The patient is then moved through the gantry. The line profiles are then combined to give a longitudinal radiograph These images are used for determining slice plane position. Slice position is decided and the computer immediately positions the body in the gantry at the chosen point by moving the scan bed. The radiation dose required for these longitudinal views is very low, unlike the CT slice dose itself.

Fast Fourier Transforms this is the preferred method for the reconstruction algorithm for filtered back projection. The data in each profile are treated as a mixed frequency and the entire image reconstruction then takes place as a series of amplitudes in the frequency domain. (Fourier Analysis is explained in Chapter 1.). After filtering each modified projection is added to the sum of the previous filtered back projections.

14.5.3 Windowing and image display

Under ideal conditions the eye can distinguish between 50 to 80 gray levels on a good quality computer monitor. Routinely this range is reduced to nearer 35 to 40. Since the full CT data-set of 4000 levels cannot be displayed at one time the user must select, or **window**, a range of CT values for display; this was discussed in Chapter 12.

The range of displayed CT values is the **window width** and Fig.14.19(b) shows different window widths (4-8 bits) that are used for sampling the available range of CT numbers. The position of the window within the data is the **offset**. If a broad window, from −1000 to +1000 is displayed using 256 gray levels, a CT number difference of 8 is represented by one gray level, giving a poor contrast image. Such an image would be useful as an overview only. Small changes in CT number, and therefore greater contrast, can be obtained from narrower windows. If it is too small the image can show a great deal of noise and details in bony structures or fatty tissue could be missed.

The window itself can be moved or offset up or down the scale to include soft tissue or bone detail. CT values outside the window will be shown as white (above the window value) or black (below the window value). For the differentiation of bony or soft tissues certain window offsets are recommended. For most soft tissue images a window offset of between 35 to 40 and a window width of 200 to 450 covers most detail. For thorax-lung the offset should be −700 and for the inner ear +200.

Double windowing is available on some machines where two different density ranges can be displayed together i.e. negative lung tissue alongside positive detail of the mediastinum. An entire gray scale is available for each of the window widths and, for clarity, a bright contour separates them.

Look-up tables (LUT) The CT numbers can be displayed on a linear or non-linear scale. Each CT number is referenced to a scale held in the computer display memory as a table of values: this scale is the **look-up table**. It normally contains a linear set of gray scale values, so the CT numbers are represented by a linear density scale. However it can be tailored as a non-uniform table where tissues of very similar density can be distinguished by allocating steeply changing non-linear display values. For example a logarithmic scale is often used.

Image filtering The convolution kernel or filter influences the appearance of the image

depending on whether a smoothing (low-pass filter) or edge enhancement (high-pass filter), has been chosen. In most CT machines a variety of convolution kernels are available giving standard, light smoothing, extreme smoothing or special high resolution (edge enhancement). Special kernels are also available for reducing beam hardening in head scans.

14.6 CT EQUIPMENT AND IMAGE QUALITY

The specifications of a modern CT machine are given in Tab.14.3. The choice of a machine depends very much on patient type (neurology, cardiac etc.) and the work-load.

Table 14.3 CT machine specifications

Parameter	Value
Fan beam assembly	
Detectors	512 to 768 Xenon
Detectors/Degree	15 to 18
Fan beam projections	1242 (0.3° per step)
Flying spot acquisition rate	768×2×1242 $=1907712$ s^{-1}
Scan Time	0.7, 1, 2, 4, 8 s
Scan Field	50 - 500mm
Slice Width	1, 2, 5, 10mm
Gantry Aperture	700mm
X-ray tube	
High voltage	137kV
Tube current	70 - 320 mA
Maximum exposure	1250 mAs
Thermal rating	3 - 5MHU
Cooling rate.	200-700 kHU min^{-1}
Filtration	0.2 to 0.4mm Cu
Continuous rotation	60rpm
Image quality	
Reconstruction Matrix	512 × 512
Display Matrix	1024 × 1024
Resolution	14 Lp cm^{-1} (0.35mm)
Contrast	2.5mm at 0.3%
Uniformity	± 2 CT numbers
Reconstruction time	< 3 s
Pixel size	0.032 to 0.52 mm
CT scale	−1024 to +3071

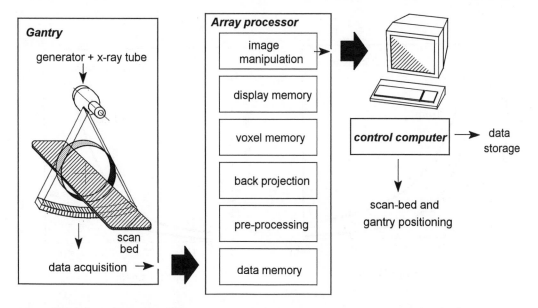

Figure 14.20 CT system data collection and control showing pipe-line processing in the array processor to give fast image display.

For a busy or specialist department a machine capable of a high quality imaging (thin sections, fast scan time etc.) should be considered. Fast scan times (<1 second) will reduce motion artifact (useful in pediatrics). A busy general department would specify a machine with a high power generator and high heat rating x-ray tube giving a large number of sections per unit time. Three dimensional reconstruction or vascular imaging (bolus transit) may require a spiral acquisition mode.

A smaller department would not require a high rated machine, and costs can be significantly reduced by choosing a low or medium rated design. Reconstruction matrices should be 512×512 interpolated to 1024× 1024 for best display; reconstruction times should be less than 5 seconds. Magnification views enlarge image detail but do not improve the overall image resolution. However, image resolution can be improved by zooming a section of the matrix and reconstructing this data. This improves image resolution up to the machine's minimum. Spatial resolution in zoom mode should be less than 0.5mm.

14.6.1 Computed tomography system

A block diagram of a typical CT machine installation is shown in Fig.14.20. The main components are the gantry with its x-ray tube and detector array connected to a computer, image array processor and control console with display. These are linked by a common data bus which transfers information and control signals between the central processor, which holds the acquisition and display programs and the peripheral systems which collect and process the detector signal data. The array processor reconstructs the section images and displays the final results at the console. Patient positioning is also under computer control, and the overall data flow allows a fully automatic patient handling program to be set-up for a particular imaging sequence i.e. zoomed image sequence of the spine between chosen lumbar vertebrae or a complete set of sectional images following a contrast bolus injection.

Calibration An uncalibrated system will have significant influence on overall image

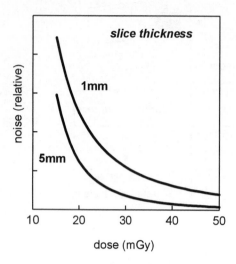 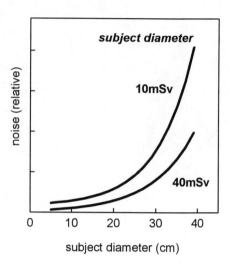

Figure 14.21 **(a)** The relative measure of noise versus dose for 1mm and 5mm slices; the latter give a better contrast **(b)** Noise increases quite rapidly with increasing subject diameter (head versus abdomen for instance).

quality (resolution, contrast and noise) so calibration of the system components (x-ray tube, detectors and electronics) must be carried out prior to imaging. The calibration is usually carried out by performing a single scan of a water phantom and inspecting it for inhomogeneity.

14.6.2 Noise

Noise, in a CT image, is defined as the standard deviation of CT numbers in a uniform image (usually water bath). For a given CT system noise is inversely proportional to resolution. Generally image noise is proportional to $1/\sqrt{mAs}$ when mAs is doubled the noise decreases by $1/\sqrt{2}$ (×0.707). Dose versus noise is plotted in Fig.14.21(a) for two slice thicknesses. Factors affecting noise and low contrast detectability depends on:

- Photon flux reaching the detector: influenced by kVp, filtration, mAs and patient size. This latter point is demonstrated in Fig.14.21(b) showing increasing noise with subject size.

- System noise: mechanical or electrical noise within the CT system
- Detector efficiency
- Reconstruction algorithm.
- X-ray tube age

Slice thickness Thin slices are noisier but this is not important for bone detail reconstruction where greater image contrast already exists. Soft tissue contrast is lost however if the sections are too thin. Structures which are at an angle to the slice plane suffer volume artifact which degrades spatial resolution. Visibility of these structures can be improved by using thin slices which separates overlying detail.

14.6.3 Resolution

This is characterized by the ability to distinguish high contrast small objects (high CT number: bony detail) as well as to differentiate close objects (small vessels). Factors influencing resolution are:

- Display matrix and pixel size

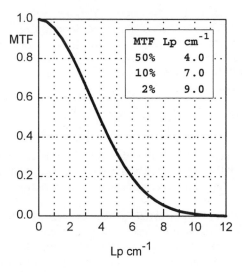

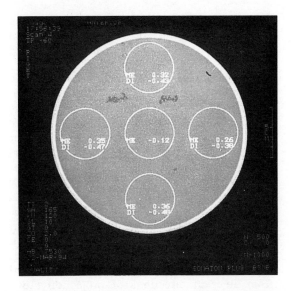

Figure 14.22 (a) An MTF measurement using a point spread function given by a thin wire. (b) A uniformity check giving mean and standard deviation figures for selected areas of a water bath across the field of view

- Field of view (FOV) which can be chosen by zooming.

The size of the display pixel can limit image resolution if it is larger than the intrinsic resolution (measured by the MTF). This is true for whole sections where each matrix pixel represents quite coarse resolution. Interpolation from 512×512 to 1024×1024 is purely a cosmetic exercise and does not affect true resolution. Reconstructed pixel size can be derived from:

$$\frac{Reconstructed\ Field\ of\ View}{Matrix\ Size} \quad (14.3)$$

Typical values of displayed pixel size are ~0.15mm for a 512×512 matrix representing a restricted FOV of 7.5cm. (head scan), and 0.3mm for a 512×512 representing a 15cm FOV (body scan). Spatial resolution is significantly influenced by the kernel used for reconstruction but data reconstruction beyond a certain zoom factor cannot improve on intrinsic resolution.

Figure 14.22(b) is an MTF example obtained by imaging a 10μm wire and using standard reconstruction protocols. This together with the uniformity check would be part of a routine quality control program. The values given by this curve can be translated into appropriate resolution figures. The 2% value of 9Lp cm^{-1} represents high resolution contrast, a single line or point being the reciprocal of this value: 0.6mm. Similarly the 50% low contrast resolution value of 4Lp cm^{-1} translates as 1.3mm. The 512×512 matrix is therefore sufficient for displaying this detail.

Aliasing This has already been discussed in Chapter 7 under Image Quality. If the discrete sampling frequency of the CT system is too low for the frequency of the object then the high frequencies will be distorted. The sampling frequency must be at least twice that of the object frequencies to prevent aliasing. This is particularly important in the petrous bone area.

The x-ray beam width and detector dimensions limit the sampling frequency but this is overcome by introducing a ¼ detector shift where the detector array is shifted with respect to the center of the fan beam. This will achieve beam interlacing on opposing projections (0° and 180°, 90° and 270° etc.) and so double the frequency sampling rate.

Uniformity An important characteristic for assessing image quality is the homogeneity or uniformity over the entire cross section of a homogeneous phantom. Figure 14.22(a) shows measurements on a water phantom. The degree of homogeneity determines the accuracy of CT number measurement for the same tissue (e.g. liver) at various points across the field of view. Owing to beam hardening artifacts due to different attenuation through the object the reconstruction algorithm contains correction factors (as a look-up-table) which adjust for these variations. This is important since data measured from different directions of projection (180° opposed ray-sums) would not match. Since beam filtration is already severe in current makes of CT scanner (between 0.25 and 0.4mm copper) the hardening effect is not pronounced so computer correction can be carried out for a wide range of object diameters.

14.6.4 Contrast

Low contrast detectability is defined as the smallest object size visible at a given percentage contrast level. Image contrast is measured as differences between the object density (in CT numbers) and its background.

$$\Delta CT\% = \left(\frac{CT_2 - CT_1}{1000} \right) \times 100 \qquad (14.4)$$

Low contrast detectability involves both image noise and spatial information. Image reconstruction kernels influence low contrast detectability and resolution. A standard kernel with some smoothing would give a resolution of just under 1mm detecting a 5mm object having a ΔCT of 0.3% an example is shown in Fig.14.26(a). Reconstruction for edge detection such as bony detail relinquishes contrast information in favor of higher resolution

as shown in the petrous bone region of Fig.14.26(b). Object contrast depends on the attenuation property of the tissues and is measured as the difference in attenuation between adjacent structures compared to water:

$$1000 \times \frac{\mu_1 - \mu_2}{\mu_{H_2O}} = 1000 \times \frac{\Delta\mu}{\mu_{H_2O}} \qquad (14.5)$$

If this attenuation difference in the body is fixed then the contrast in the image ΔCT is only dependent on the size of the structures

The contrast detail diagram (CDD) The plot enables both resolution and contrast to be represented on a single graph Fig14.23(a) and is a convenient method for specifying low contrast detectability. The curve plots detectable diameter as a function of measured contrast. The closer the curve is to the vertical line the better the resolution for low contrast objects. The top of the curve represents high contrast detail (i.e. bone). The CT difference ΔCT is a measure of the contrast. The ΔCT range 1 - 100 also represents a contrast difference of 1 - 100%. The region of the curve above the 10% object contrast line, indicates the resolution for contrast capability of the system. A difference below 1% describes the noise limits of the system. The 1 to 10% region is the **transition zone** and detect-ability depends strongly on radiation dose.

A family of curves can be derived for various Dose/mAs rates (Fig.14.28(a)) or slice thicknesses (b). and projections number when the intrinsic resolution can be improved (c). Field of view diameters or reconstruction algorithms can also be compared using CDD curves.

14.7 CT IMAGE ARTIFACTS

14.7.1 Sampling accuracy

Mechanical accuracy to high tolerances are essential to prevent loss of resolution. Misalignment by one-tenth of a detector area can give aliasing. The number of pixels in the image may be set prior to image acquisition.

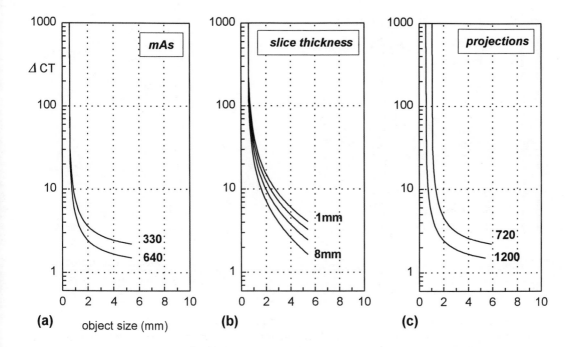

Fig. 14.23 Contrast detail diagrams **(a)** the basic CCD identifying the resolution limit as the vertical line from 1mm. **(b)** improvement in low contrast detail with thicker slice sections and **(c)** improved overall resolution (curve moves to the left) with increased number of projections.

Usually the choice is between a matrix size of 256 or 512. The latter may provide higher spatial resolution but with a cost of increased radiation dose if image quality is to be preserved. The larger matrix images contain more pixels and therefore will take longer to store and retrieve and any image manipulation will also require more time.

14.7.2 Partial volume

High attenuating objects projecting partly into a slice will cause a mixed attenuation value. It is assumed that tissue within the voxel is uniform. However if the slice thickness is large then it might contain a second material, e.g. bone and soft tissue. Therefore the attenuation coefficient that will be calculated for that voxel will be a weighted average of that for soft tissue and bone based on the relative volumes occupied by both in the voxel.. Thinner slice thicknesses reduce this artifact as demonstrated in Fig.14.24(a) and (b).

14.7.3 Beam hardening

Filtration of the beam by tissue (bone) removes the lower energy x-ray component. Attenuation then decreases as the effective x-ray energy increases so distorting the CT number values. This has been demonstrated in Fig.14.9.

14.7.4 Detector non-uniformity

A non-uniform response by the array of detectors leads to the production of 'ring' artifacts or a type of halo effect about objects in

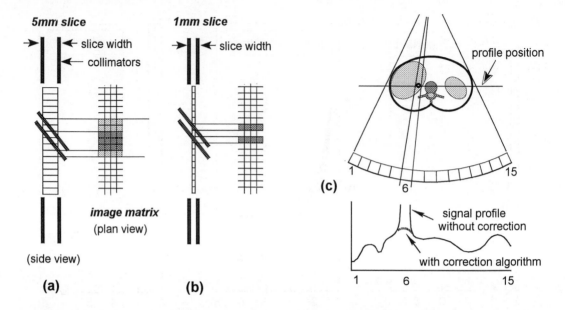

Figure 14.24 (a) Partial volume and slice thickness. The 5mm slice cannot separate fine bone detail as the voxels include both soft tissue and bone anatomy. The image matrix shows this as a single unsharp object **(b)** The thinner slice of 1mm can separate the closely spaced bone; the image matrix now shows the twin bone detail. **(c)** Metal artifact reduction by interpolation before and after spike profile due to abnormal high CT values for metal.

the image. This usually isn't a problem with modern gas detector based equipment. However when first switching on the equipment in the morning sufficient time must be allocated for the system to reach its operating temperature and for the amounts of gas in each detector to equilibrate.

14.7.5 Metal artifact interference
This causes star-burst radiating lines from the metal object in the field of view.
Corrections to these abnormally high absorption values can be made during reconstruction by placing a threshold on the peak values.(Fig.14.25(c))

14.8 RADIATION EXPOSURE

Patient dose   Patient radiation dose is related to the x-ray energy absorbed by the patient. It is usually specified by patient surface dose or as the central dose for a series of scans. Decreasing radiation dose can increase the level of image noise unless this is achieved with increase in detector sensitivity. In a series of contiguous slices the peak dose delivered to the patient is greater than the peak dose for a single slice; this is due to overlap of the radiation profiles. Fig.14.25(a).

CTDI   A better measure of patient dose is the CT Dose Index CTDI. This is more representative than just the skin dose and allows for the profile overlap mentioned above. Since patient examinations generally consist of more than one slice the CTDI is a more representative patient dose figure and is expressed as the total dose for 14 slices multiplied by the slice thickness T. The formula devised by the US Food and Drug

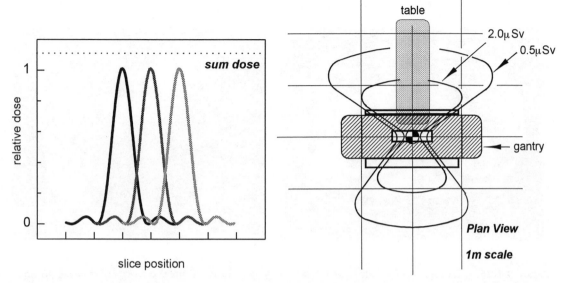

Figure 14.25 **(a)** Dose profiles from contiguous slices sum to give a higher sum dose than the individual dose profiles due to slice overlap **(b)** typical dose contours surrounding a CT machine shown on a meter square scale.

Administration (FDA) is :

$$CTDI = \frac{1}{T} \int_{-7T}^{+7T} D_z dz \qquad (14.6)$$

Where D_z is the measured dose for location z. Typical values for the central dose of a water phantom would be 12mGy 100mAs^{-1} for a 8mm slice on a 16cm water phantom and 10mGy 100mAs^{-1} for a 1mm slice. This compares with 8mGy and 7.5mGy for the surface dose respectively. These values would be correspondingly less for a 32cm diameter phantom. Typical routine scanning protocols use ~400mAs which would give a central dose of 48mGy (4.8rad) and 32mGy (3.2rad) surface dose

Staff dose The scatter radiation from a modern CT Machine is extremely restricted owing to the tight collimation of the x-ray beam. A typical dose contour pattern is shown in Fig.14.25(b). Staff exposure is estimated from the machine use; this is expressed in μGy 1000mAs^{-1}. A typical worked example is given in Box 14.4.

Box 14.4

CT Dose contours

What is the expected exposure/week at the 10μSv/1000mAs contour in Fig.14.26(b)

A typical exposure per slice for 70mA at 3 s. would be 210mAs.

Average slices per patient = 20
Total mAs per patient 4200mAs
5 patients per day (25 per week) = 105,000mAs
The total exposure per week at the 10μSv contour would be ~1mSv

---

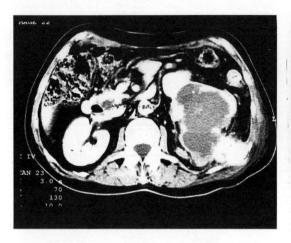 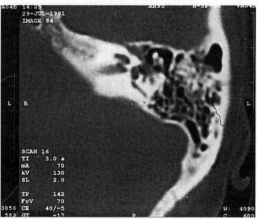

Figure 14.26   Examples of CT images for **(a)** soft tissue taken from the liver region and **(b)** bone detail from the petrous bones of the skull emphasized by choosing an edge enhancement algorithm.

Further reading

Computed Tomography. Physical Principles and clinical applications. E. Seeram (W.B. Saunders Co. 1994)

GLOSSARY

back projection   A method for reconstructing a sectional display from a series of radial projections.

CT number (see Hounsfield Unit)

effective focal spot   This decides the size of a point at iso-center as projected onto the detector

fan beam   The geometry of a 3rd generation machine describing the fixed assembly between x-ray tube and detector array which rotates together.

helical scan   Continuous rotation of a fan beam assembly while the scan bed moves incrementally.

Housfield Unit (HU)   The CT value or number relating $\mu_{unknown}$ to μ_{water}

iso-center   Center of gantry

kernel   A discrete filter for image reconstruction

look-up table (LUT)   Controls displayed gray scale. Either linear or non-linear.

magnification   Image enlargement re-displaying to full display dimensions. No improvement in resolution

pixel   Picture element matrix holding a narrow range of CT numbers. Can be 4 to 8 bits deep

topogram ⎫
scoutview ⎬ Longitudinal scan with the fan beam assembly fixed in AP, PA or lateral position.

system magnification   Focal spot to detector distance divided by focal spot to iso-center distance

voxel Volume element matrix holding the complete range of CT values from −1000 to +3000.

windowing Displaying a selected range of CT numbers stored in a voxel array.

zonography Narrow angle linear tomography.

zooming Image enlargement with reconstruction giving improved resolution

Nuclear medicine: Basic principles

15.1 Nuclear parameters
15.2 Decay schemes
15.3 Specific activity
15.4 Radionuclide production

15.5 Laboratory instrumentation
15.6 The gamma camera
15.7 Camera performance
15.8 Collimator properties

15.1 NUCLEAR PARAMETERS

15.1.1 Nuclear Structure

The nucleus of any atom consists of a mixture of protons and neutrons (see Chapter 2). A simple nuclear model therefore consists of Z protons and N neutrons, making a total of A **nucleons**. Each element 'X' can therefore be defined uniquely in terms of these 3 components:

$$_Z^A X_N$$

Where Z is the atomic number (proton number), N the neutron number and A the mass number $(Z + N)$. Some common elements, iodine, potassium, carbon are described using this coding:

131		40		14	
Iodine		Potassium		Carbon	
19	21	53	78	6	8

In practice a nucleus can be identified by reducing these parameters to only Z and A. The atomic number Z is redundant, since the element name defines the value of Z; change the number of protons and the element changes.

Therefore the mass number A is commonly used as a single identifier:

$$^{131}\text{Iodine} \quad ^{40}\text{Potassium} \quad ^{14}\text{Carbon}$$

This is sufficient to identify a nuclear species or **nuclide** exactly. This model of the nucleus, using only neutrons and protons, fits all practical requirements in nuclear medicine. In the early days of chemistry most naturally occurring elements i.e. iron, were found to have atomic mass values that were not whole numbers. This problem was solved when it was found that most chemical elements consist of a mixture of two or more species having different neutron numbers; iron has four stable species making up the common metal.

$^{54}_{26}\text{Fe}_{28}$	$^{56}_{26}\text{Fe}_{30}$	$^{57}_{26}\text{Fe}_{31}$	$^{58}_{26}\text{Fe}_{32}$	$^{59}_{26}\text{Fe}_{33}$
(5.84%)	(91.7%)	(2.17%)	(0.31%)	(45d)

Since the Z value remains constant the chemical element itself did not change. The increasing number of neutrons, having no electrical charge, just adds mass without changing the element.

The percentages shown in this series are the relative abundance of each species in the natural element mixture but ^{59}Fe is unstable with a half-life (T½) of 45 days. Figure 15.1 shows a section of the nuclide chart from the more familiar Periodic Table. This particular section identifies 3 stable isotopes of iron showing their percentage abundance and the unstable isotope ^{59}Fe. Stable and unstable isotopes of cobalt and nickel are also shown.

Nuclides with a constant Z (proton number) but varying N (neutron number) are called **isotopes**. The iron series shown above are isotopes. Nuclides with a constant N but varying Z are called **isotones**. The diagonal arrow in Fig.15.1 indicates the series:

$^{57}_{26}Fe_{31}$ $^{58}_{27}Co_{31}$ $^{59}_{28}Ni_{31}$

Nuclides having a constant mass but varying Z and N values are called **isobars** or isobaric nuclides identified by the vertical arrow:

$^{59}_{26}Fe_{33}$ $^{59}_{27}Co_{32}$ $^{59}_{28}Ni_{31}$

Three of the stable iron isotopes are shown in Fig. 15.1 but the other iron isotope ^{59}Fe is unstable having a stated T½ of only 45 days. Similarly other unstable isotopes or **radio-nuclides**, indicated by their decay rate as half-lives T½, in brackets, are:

^{60}Co ^{58}Co ^{57}Co ^{59}Ni

$^{59}Nickel$ has a very long T½ of 80,000 years.

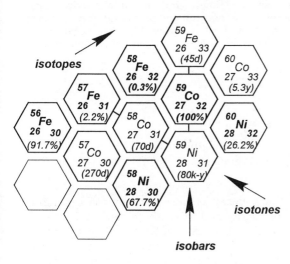

Figure 15.1   Examples of isotope, isotone and isobar series, identified by arrows, for cobalt, iron and nickel

15.1.2 Nuclear decay rate

The decay, or transformation, of an unstable nuclide is a statistical process which is expressed in mathematical form as the rate of transformation of N nuclei changing per unit time (dN/dt) and is proportional to the number of nuclei N present at that moment:

$dN/dt = \lambda N$ where λ is the decay constant. The rate or activity A at which the nucleus decays is measured in disintegrations per second (dps). This is the **becquerel** (Bq), which is a measure of activity: $A = dN/dt$. It is named after Henri Bequerel (1852-1908, French physicist) who, in 1895, discovered radioactivity. Prior to the adoption of the becquerel as the System Internationale (S.I.) unit of activity, the common measurement was the **curie** (Ci). This is 3.7×10^{10} dps and was related to the activity of 1mg of pure $^{226}Radium$, named after Marie Curie (1867-1934, Polish-born French chemist), the discoverer of radium. Since the adoption of the SI Units this measure has been superseded by the becquerel. The becquerel, since it is a small unit, carries the common prefixes of: giga- G, mega- M and kilo- k. The relationship between the curie and becquerel is:

1 curie (Ci)	37×10^9 dps	37GBq
1 millicurie (mCi)	37×10^6 dps	37MBq
1 microcurie (μCi)	37×10^3 dps	37kBq
1 nanocurie (nCi)	37 dps	37Bq

The half-life   Since unstable nuclides decay exponentially their total life-span cannot be measured. The rate of decay is therefore measured as a half-life.   Half lives of radionuclides are determined by measuring the amount of activity in a sample over a period of time; since radionuclides emit ionizing radiation, the intensity of this can be measured by a radiation detector. The semi-log plot in Fig.15.2(a) shows the decay with time for $^{131}Iodine$ over a 30 day period. The slope shows that the intensity decreases as an exponential and since it is an asymptote the total life-span of a radionuclide cannot be given exactly (see Chapter 1). The stability is thus expressed as a **half-life** 'the time taken for a given activity to reach half its initial value'. Examples of half-lives for various isotopes used in nuclear medicine are given in Tab. 15.1.

Biological and Effective Half Life   The time taken for a substance (chemical, drug, radiopharmaceutical, isotope etc.) to undergo biological excretion often follows an exponential pattern,   so the biological retention of an

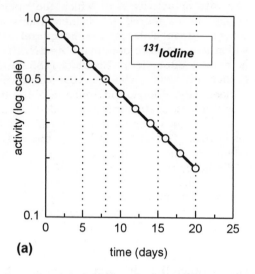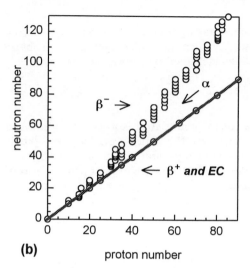

Figure 15.2 **(a)** Decay graph plotted on semi-log scale for ^{131}Iodine. Half the initial activity remains at about 8 days. **(b)** Some of the nuclides plotted according to neutron and proton number. The stable nuclides have excess neutron numbers and break away from the 1:1 relationship. Beta negative decay gains proton number, beta plus loses protons. Alpha decay loses equal numbers of protons and neutrons.

isotope or labeled compound is also expressed in terms of its half life. The overall or **effective half-life** of a substance in a patient's body depends on both its **physical half-life** and its **biological half-life**. The effective rate constant is the sum of rate constants for physical and biological disapearance so that:

effective half life =
physical half life + biological half life

The biological half-life of a substance is difficult to measure; it is commonly derived from the measured effective half-life (excretion rate) and the known physical half-life of the nuclide.

15.1.3 Energy of emissions

There are three basic modes of decay associated with unstable nuclei, these decay processes are:

- Alpha (α),
- Beta (β^- and β^+)
- Gamma (γ)

Each decay process involves the expenditure of energy and in all three cases this is measured in **electron volts** (eV) (see Chapter 2). Since the energy emitted from radioactive materials usually involves energies of thousands or millions of eV the common prefixes are kilo-electron volts (keV) or mega-electron volts (MeV). Alpha emissions are always given in MeV. This is mostly true for β^- and β^+ radiation also, except for very low energies e.g.

Tritium (^{3}H)	18.6 keV β^-
^{14}Carbon	156.0 keV β^-

Gamma radiation, from radionuclides, used in nuclear medicine, mostly has energies measured in keV.

Table 15.1 Physical half-lives of common clinical nuclides

Isotope	T½	Clinical use
^{191m} Iridium	5s	vascular imaging
^{81m}Krypton	13s	lung ventilation
^{82} Rubidium	1.3min	cardiac imaging
^{99m} Technetium	6h	universal imaging
^{111} Indium	2.8d	imaging sepsis
^{125} Iodine	60d	in vitro analysis
^{241} Americium	500y	marker source

15.2 DECAY SCHEMES

Figure 15.2(b) plots a succession of nuclides according to their **neutron : proton ratio**. The straight line indicates equal numbers of neutrons and protons but since the stable nuclei have more neutrons than protons these form a distribution curve above this line. Alpha decay results in a loss of an equal number of neutrons and protons; the nuclear mass therefore decreases down the nuclide curve. Beta negative decay occurs only in 'neutron excess' isotopes so a neutron is lost and the decayed nucleus will take up a position to the right of the line. Beta positive decay and electron capture position the nucleus to the left of the line.

15.2.1 Alpha decay

This mode of decay involves an alpha particle or helium nucleus and causes the greatest loss of energy from an unstable nucleus since it loses 4 nucleons in the form of 2 neutrons and 2 protons. All naturally occurring helium is formed from alpha particle decay; the alpha particle eventually captures an electron to form an atom of helium gas. The formula for alpha decay is:

$$ {}^{A}_{Z}X \rightarrow {}^{A-4}_{Z-2}Y + {}^{4}_{2}\alpha \qquad (15.1) $$

where X and Y represent the parent and daughter elements respectively. Since the proton number changes so does the element. A particular alpha decay may involve the si-

multaneous emission of gamma radiation. Common examples of alpha decay are shown by sections of the natural ^{238}Uranium decay series. This is a very complex decay chain involving many different elements. Radium decaying to radon gives a short half-life gas (T½ 3.8d) that is a natural radioactive contaminant of buildings:

$$ {}^{226}_{88}Ra \rightarrow {}^{222}_{86}Rn + \alpha \ (4.78 \ MeV) + \gamma\text{'s} $$

In this equation the alpha particle energy is shown in brackets, 4.78MeV. The ^{222}Rn decays further in the lung tissue to ^{218}Polonium and ^{214}Lead each giving an alpha emission:

$$ {}^{222}_{86}Rn \rightarrow {}^{218}_{84}Po + \alpha \ (5.49 \ MeV) $$

$$ \rightarrow {}^{214}_{82}Pb + \alpha \ (6.0 \ MeV) $$

This decay scheme is part of the ^{238}Uranium decay series, a section of which is shown in Fig.15.3 starting from ^{226}Radium. Following accepted convention α–particle emission is illustrated in decay schemes by showing arrows sloping to the left. Beta decay from ^{214}Pb is represented by right sloping arrows. Many alpha emitters decay in chains shown in Fig.15.3: these are called **collateral series**. Table 15.2 shows some natural α–emitters; their α–energy decreases as T½ increases.

$$ {}^{226}_{88}Ra \quad 1600 \ y \quad (\alpha \ 4.78 \ MeV) $$
$$ {}^{222}_{86}Rn \quad 3.8 \ d \quad (\alpha \ 5.49 \ MeV) $$
$$ {}^{218}_{84}Po \quad 1600 \ y \quad (\alpha \ 6.0 \ MeV) $$
$$ {}^{214}_{82}Pb \quad 26 \ min \quad (\beta \ 0.67, \ 0.73 \ MeV) $$
$$ {}^{214}_{83}Bi \quad 20.0 \ min \quad (\text{etc. etc.}) $$

Figure 15.3 Alpha and beta decay from radium which is part of the natural ^{238}U decay series.

Clinical value of alpha decay   Alpha emitters are rarely met in clinical work. They sometimes form useful therapy sources; ^{211}Astatine with a half-life of 7 hours and an α–energy of 5.8MeV has been used for labeling monoclonal antibodies for tumor therapy. The common anatomical marker source for gamma cameras is ^{241}Americium, an α–emitter which also has a useful 60keV gamma ray emission.

15.2.2 Beta decay

The unstable nucleus can lose energy by neutron decay, proton decay or electron capture. A beta particle, or high-energy electron, is ejected. The beta particle can carry either a negative or a positive charge.

- $n \rightarrow p + e^-$ (β$^-$ decay)
- $p \rightarrow n + e^+$ (β$^+$, positron decay)
- $p + e^- \rightarrow n$ (electron capture, EC)

These nuclear transformations are accompanied by an electrically uncharged neutrino or antineutrino. This particle was initially postulated to explain the continuous beta spectrum; it plays no part in nuclear medicine imaging or dosimetry.

Negative beta particle emission (β$^-$)   For those unstable nuclei with excess neutrons a negative β–particle is produced by neutron decay forming a proton; the nucleon number (atomic mass) does not change:

$$_0^1 n_1 \rightarrow {}_1^1 P_0 + e^- \qquad (15.2)$$

The equation for β$^-$ decay is:

$$_Z^A X \rightarrow {}_{Z+1}^A Y + \beta^- (\gamma\text{'s}) \qquad (15.3)$$

Since the mass number A does not change the parent and daughter nuclei are **isobars**. The proton number Z increases so the element changes from X to Y. Gamma emission (γ's) commonly accompany β$^-$ decay although pure β$^-$ emitters do occur. The decay scheme of a negatron emitter is depicted by an arrow drawn sloping to the right.   Figure 15.4 shows two important pure beta emitters commonly employed in nuclear medicine as therapy agents.

During beta decay a further small energy loss is observed in the form of an anti-neutrino (a neutral and massless emission similar to a photon). The random nature of neutrino ejection (angle of emission) gives a variable small energy loss for each beta decay so β$^-$ particles from the same decay process have a range of energies and are therefore seen as a continuous spectrum. The curve plotted in Fig.15.4(c) shows the beta spectrum for ^{32}P which has a maximum β$^-$ particle energy of 1.7MeV. The continuous energy distribution of β$^-$ emissions is of importance when calculating the radiation dose delivered to the patient from a β$^-$ emitter.

Table 15.2   Alpha nuclides from natural decay chain of uranium.

Nuclide	Energy (MeV)	Half life	Remarks
^{222}Rn	5.4	3.8 d	Radon gas from ^{232}Th
^{240}Pu	5.1	6537 y	Nuclear fall-out
^{239}Pu	4.9	2.4×10^4 y	Nuclear material
^{226}Ra	4.8	1600 y	Natural radium
^{235}U	4.6	7×10^6 y	1% natural uranium
^{238}U	4.2	4.5×10^9 y	99% natural uranium
^{232}Th	4.0	14×10^9 y	natural thorium

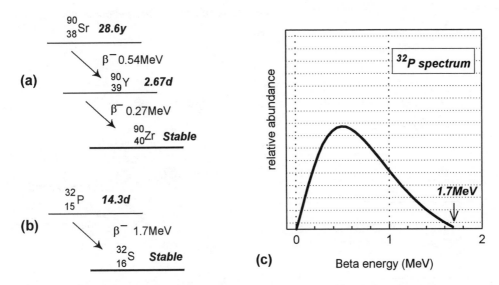

Figure 15.4 **(a) (b)** Radionuclides of strontium and phosphorus showing pure β⁻ decay to a stable isotope. **(c)** Plot of the ^{32}P β⁻ spectrum showing a spread of energies rather like an x-ray spectrum with a peak or maximum energy point.

Clinical value of* β⁻ *decay Very few β⁻ emitters are used for imaging since the β⁻ particle contributes a high patient radiation dose. Pure β⁻ emitters ^{90}Y and ^{32}P are commonly used for therapy. Thyroid investigations sometimes use ^{131}Iodine for imaging as well as therapy since its β⁻ decay is accompanied by a gamma emission (364keV). It has also been used for labeling antibodies since iodine chemistry is mild and does not disrupt complex molecules. Lung ventilation is commonly performed using ^{133}Xe which is a gamma emitter; the β⁻ decay similarly increases the patient radiation dose. In spite of their increased patient radiation burden these two isotopes continue to be used since they are cheap and readily available.

Positive beta particle (positron* β⁺) A positive beta particle is produced by proton decay in the nucleus:

$$_1^1 P_0 + e^- \rightarrow {}_0^1 n_1 + e+ \qquad (15.4)$$

$$_Z^A X + e^- \rightarrow {}_{Z-1}^A X + \beta^+ \qquad (15.5)$$

As with negatron (β⁻) decay in eqn.15.3 the total number of nucleons remains constant, parent and daughter are **isobars**. The proton Z has decreased by one, so the element changes and again a continuous β⁺ energy spectrum is seen since simultaneous neutrino emissions are also involved. The positron (a member of the antimatter world) can exist only as long as it has kinetic energy. At rest it undergoes mutual annihilation with any nearby electron. This electron reacts with the β⁺ forming a positron/negatron pair; the two masses each having an equivalent rest mass of 0.511Mev disappear releasing two gamma photons of this energy. The two γ–photons are ejected from the center of the reaction at 180°

$$\beta^+ + \beta^- \rightarrow 2\,\gamma\text{'s } (0.511\text{MeV each}) \quad (15.6)$$

This reaction has important applications in **positron emission tomography** (PET), described in Chapter 16.

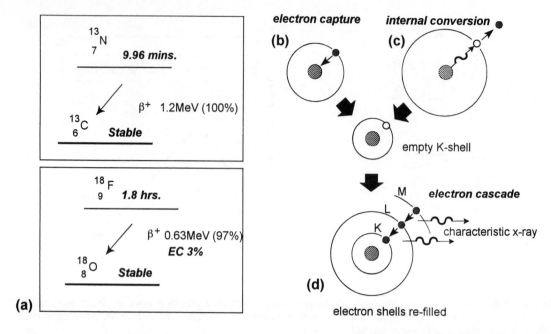

Figure 15.5 **(a)** The decay schemes for two nuclides produced by an on-site clinical cyclotron: ^{13}Nitrogen and ^{18}Fluorine **(b)** Orbital electron involvement with nuclear decay. The nucleus can either capture a K-shell electron or **(c)** K- and L-shell electrons absorb energy during internal conversion. Both interactions result in electron loss and subsequent filling of electron shells **(d)** producing characteristic x-radiation.

Positron decay for ^{13}N and ^{18}F, used in PET studies, is shown in Fig.15.5(a); β^+ decay adopts a left pointing arrow similar to $\alpha-$ decay schemes. Positron annihilation is a practical demonstration of Einstein's equation relating energy and mass: **$E = mc^2$** (see Box 15.1).

Clinical value of β^+ decay Positron emission tomographic imaging relies on β^+ decay which produces opposed 0.511MeV gamma radiation. The physiologically important elements have isotopes that are pure β^+ emitters. The two isotopes ^{13}N and ^{18}F shown in Fig.15.5(a) must be produced by an on-site cyclotron because of their short half-lives. The other two nuclides used in PET are:

^{11}C $\rightarrow$ T½ 20 minutes β^+ 1.97 MeV
^{15}O $\rightarrow$ T½ 2 minutes β^+ 1.74 MeV

Box 15.1

Positron annihilation

Creation of gamma radiation energy from matter (electron and positron). Basic formula: $E = mc^2$ where m is the sum of the rest mass of electron and the rest mass of positron:

$$= 9.1 \times 10^{-31} + 9.1 \times 10^{-31}$$
$$= 1.82 \times 10^{-30} \text{ kg}$$

c is speed of light = 3×10^8 m s^{-1}
$$c^2 = 9 \times 10^{16} \text{ m s}^{-1}$$
therefore $mc^2 = (1.82 \times 10^{-30}) \times (9 \times 10^{16})$ J
$$= 1.638 \times 10^{-13}$$
since 1 J = 6.24×10^{12} MeV then:

E = $1.638 \times 10^{-13} \times 6.24 \times 10^{12}$ MeV
    = 1.022MeV

This energy appears as two opposed gamma rays each of **0.511MeV**

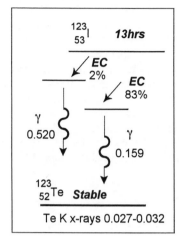 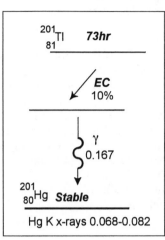 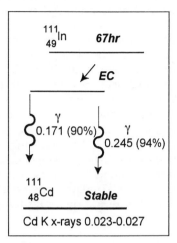

Figure 15.6   Electron capture **(a)** ^{123}Iodine showing a useful gamma photon and **(b)** ^{201}Thallium which has a small (11%) abundance 167keV gamma, not used for imaging; but the 93% abundant Hg K x-rays are useful. Electron capture in ^{111}Indium **(c)** yields two useful gamma energies.

15.2.3 Electron capture

In the neutron poor region, below the line of stability seen in Fig.15.2(b) nuclear instability can be satisfied by the capture of an orbital electron. This can be seen as the equivalent of positron emission since it achieves the same end result as a decaying proton seen in eqn.15.4:

$$_1^1 \mathrm{P_0} + e^- \;\rightarrow\; {_0^1}\mathrm{n}_1 \qquad (15.7)$$

Figure 15.5(b), (c) illustrates the two important interactions that involve the nucleus and closely bound electrons. Interactions with both K and L shell electrons are possible. Figure 15.5(b) shows the nucleus absorbing a K-electron in **electron capture**. An alternative reaction is (c) where the K-shell electron absorbs all the energy during gamma emission resulting in a photon loss due to **internal conversion**. Both electron capture and internal conversion result in electron loss from a K or L-shell. The resulting vacancy in the K shell is quickly filled by an outer shell elec-tron L; this vacancy in turn is filled by an electron from the M shell and so on until all the electron vacancies are filled causing an **electron cascade** and the emission of characteristic x-radiation; they are characteristic of the daughter element (d).

Clinical nuclides that undergo electron capture are ^{201}Thallium which produces x-rays characteristic of mercury and ^{125}Iodine giving tellurium x-rays. The overall equation for electron capture is similar to eqn.15.5 for β^+ decay:

$$_Z^A \mathrm{X} + e^- \rightarrow {_{Z-1}^A}\mathrm{Y} + \mathrm{Y}\ \textit{characteristic x-rays} \qquad (15.8)$$

Electron capture by the nucleus produces a form of **bremsstrahlung** radiation owing to the electron orbital disturbance. The resulting x-ray photons are termed **internal bremsstrahlung** to distinguish them from similar x-ray tube radiation which is **external bremsstrahlung**; these join the characteristic x-rays to produce a burst of x-ray photons.

352 *Physics of Diagnostic Imaging*

Clinical importance of electron capture
Common nuclear medicine isotopes that are not generator produced (see later), decay by EC. This mode of decay produces low patient radiation dose. Examples are ^{123}I ^{201}Tl ^{111}In and ^{67}Ga. The decay schemes for the first three are shown in Fig.15.6. Nuclides undergoing electron capture are represented by a left sloping arrow similar to α–decay. ^{123}Iodine and ^{111}Indium have useful γ–photons at energies suitable for imaging. The 520keV of ^{123}I however only contributes to image noise. The nuclide ^{67}Gallium has three useful gamma energies at 93, 185 and 300keV. ^{201}Thallium has poor gamma abundance but useful Hg x-rays for imaging.

15.2.4 Gamma radiation.

Radionuclides emitting gamma radiation during their decay are potential imaging agents for nuclear medicine providing their gamma energies are between 80 and 200keV. This is the ideal energy range for gamma cameras since lower energies undergo tissue absorption and higher energies are not absorbed by the thin NaI(Tl) detector used in gamma camera construction. Certain high energy gamma radio-nuclides (^{131}Iodine; γ–energy 364keV) are useful for non-imaging tracer studies where their activity levels are measured with thicker single crystal scintillation detectors (probes).

Isomeric transition In the decay processes previously described for α and β–emitting nuclides, any gamma radiation that was emitted came from an excited nuclear state. These excited states usually last for extremely short times (pico-seconds) but others can last for

relatively long periods (many seconds or even hours) and are called **metastable states** these can be considered as transition processes. The transition from a metastable state involves the emission of a gamma photon and since no other decay process (i.e. β⁻) is involved, they impart a low radiation dose to the patient. Consequently these nuclides have become most popular for imaging in nuclear medicine. Three examples of metastable states are listed in Tab.15.3, the most widely used being ^{99}Mo/^{99m}Tc ; its decay scheme is fully explored in Fig.15.7 and discussed later.

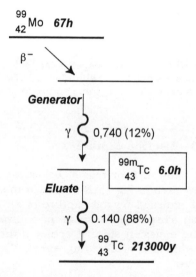

Figure 15.7 Isomeric transition of molybdenum where ^{99}Mo decays to a metastable state. This then decays to give a pure gamma photon uncontaminated by beta decay.

Table 15.3   Isomeric Transition giving metastable states.

^{99}Mo	(β⁻ 67 h)	→	**^{99m}Tc**	(140keV, T½ 6h)	→ ^{99}Tc
^{81}Rb	(EC 4.5h)	→	**^{81m}Kr**	(190keV, T½ 13s)	→ ^{81}Kr
^{195}Hg	(EC 42hr)	→	**^{195m}Au**	(262keV, T½ 30s)	→^{195}Au

Isometric transition can be represented by:

$$_Z^A X^* \rightarrow \,_Z^A X + \gamma \qquad (15.9)$$

where X^* denotes an excited state. There is no change in proton or neutron number so X^* and X are identical elements or **isomers**.

Internal conversion A nucleus in an excited state may also interact with K or L shell electrons and transfer excess energy to these electrons. This is the process of internal conversion mentioned together with electron capture and illustrated in Fig. 15.5(c) where the converted electron is ejected from the atom with an energy minus its binding energy. This is a competing process with gamma ray emission and an **internal conversion coefficient** is used for describing the proportion of internal conversion events in a gamma decay process which blocks gamma emission and is measured as:

$$\frac{Internal\ Conversion\ Process}{Gamma\ Emission} \qquad (15.10)$$

This ratio can range from zero (all transitions result in gamma emission) to infinity (all transitions are internally converted: no gamma emission). The process of internal conversion makes the decay scheme for ^{99m}Tc more complex. It has been measured that 10.4% of all ^{99m}Tc nuclear transformations involve internal conversions by the K, L and, to a lesser extent, M shell electrons. Gamma emissions therefore occur in 89.6% of nuclear transformations and not 100% that would seem likely from the ^{99m}Tc decay scheme. Similarly 40% of transformations involve internal conversion in the decay of ^{81m}Kr.

Clinical value of gamma decay: Gamma radiation within the energies 90 to 200 keV are optimal for gamma camera imaging. Those isotopes that decay by isomeric transition provide a source of activity that is short lived yielding a pure gamma emitter; both of these factors which lead to low patient radiation dose. A summary of α and β–radiation properties is given in Tab.15.4, listing their range

Table 15.4 Summary of α, β and γ–radiation properties

Property	Alpha	Beta	Gamma
Type	$[He^4]^{++}$	High speed electrons	Electromagnetic
Specific Ionization	4×10^7 for 5MeV	6×10^4 for 1MeV	
Range in Air, cm			
0.5MeV	0.3	140	infinite
2.0MeV	1	840	infinite
4.0MeV	2.5	1600	infinite
Range in Tissue, cm			
1.0MeV	0.0006	0.42	infinite
5.0MeV	0.0037	2.2	infinite
Range in Al, mgcm^{-2}			
0.5MeV	0.5	111	infinite
2.0MeV	1.6	926	infinite
H V L in Tissue, cm			
1.0MeV	-	0.04	10
5.0MeV	-	0.4	24

in various materials. In the case of β and γ–radiation a half-value layer is given for tissue; α–radiation is stopped completely.

Auger electrons Since electron capture and internal conversion create electron vacancies in the inner orbits, an electron cascade starting from the outer electron orbits commences to fill the vacancies (Fig.15.5(d)) causing characteristic radiation to be emitted. An alternative process instead of this energy being released as characteristic x-rays it can be transferred to another orbital electron ejecting it from the atom. These ejected electrons are Auger electrons and are important in patient dosimetry since they impart damage to surrounding tissue.

Table 15.5 Specific activity and impurity levels for some important clinical nuclides.

Nuclide	Specific activity	Impurity levels
^{67}Ga	370MBq μg^{-1}	^{65}Zn <0.1%
^{111}In	1.8GBq μg^{-1}	^{114m}In <0.1%
^{123}I	74MBq mg^{-1}	^{125}I <0.01% ^{124}I none
^{131}I	185kBq mg^{-1}	none
^{201}Tl	3.7GBq μg^{-1}	^{202}Tl 2% ^{200}Tl 1.0% ^{203}Pb 0.25%

15.3 SPECIFIC ACTIVITY

Activity concentration can be used to describe several different terms in nuclear medicine but it commonly refers to the concentration of the nuclide, expressed as either activity by volume or activity by weight. This form of specific activity is measured in:

- becquerels per milliliter
- becquerels per mole
- becquerels per milligram

Since the becquerel is a small unit practical activities are expressed in mega- or giga- becquerels; the non-SI units are curies and milli-curies as mCi mg^{-1}. Table 15.5 shows the specific activity of some important nuclear medicine isotopes in Bq mg^{-1} and their impurities. In practice specific activity is commonly used for describing:

- weight of a given activity
- impurity concentration
- residual activity

Descriptions of these and the formulas involved are given by the worked examples in Boxes 15.2 to 15.5.

15.3.1 Activity and concentration of a substance

It is sometimes necessary to calculate the activity of a known weight of radionuclide for contamination reasons. This is most often used for compounds containing long lived radionuclides (i.e. ^{238}U) but is sometimes required for clinical purposes. The weight of a known activity can also be calculated for toxicity reasons. If the weight W of a given activity A is required then the decay constant λ is $0.693/T\frac{1}{2}$ and if N is the number of radioactive atoms per gram of material then $A = \lambda N$ and $N = A/\lambda$. The **weight of a given activity** is then:

$$W = \frac{M \times N}{k} \qquad (15.11)$$

where M is the atomic mass and k is Avogadro's number: 6.0×10^{23}. Box 15.2 uses this formula in an example calculation.

Activity per unit weight Equation 15.11 can be rearranged to give:

$$A = \frac{k \times W \times \lambda}{M} \qquad (15.12)$$

This formula is useful when considering contamination levels, an example is given in Box 15.3.

15.3.2 Residual activity after decay.

Specific activity per unit volume This is given by the basic formula:

$$A_t = A_o \times e^{\frac{-0.693\,T}{T\frac{1}{2}}} \qquad (15.13)$$

Box 15.2

Weight of a given activity and toxicity

A patient professes to be iodine sensitive. What is the weight W of iodine in 550MBq of ^{131}Iodine used as a therapy dose? Using eqn. 15.11 and converting all parameters to seconds:
T½ (8.04 days) = 6.94×10^5 s $\lambda = 9.985 \times 10^{-7}$
The number of atoms in 550MBq is:

$$\frac{550 \times 10^6}{9.985 \times 10^{-7}} = 5.5 \times 10^{14} \text{ atoms}$$

$$W = \frac{131 \times (5.5 \times 10^{14})}{k} = 1.2 \times 10^{-7} \text{g}$$

or approximately 120ngm which is far below any toxicity level. Since daily iodine intake is 150µg, chemical toxicity and iodine sensitivity are not a problem. Similarly 70MBq of ^{201}Tl is equivalent to 9ng; also way below toxicity level.

Box 15.3

Activity per unit weight : contamination

Equation 15.13 can calculate the activity from certain naturally occurring nuclides i.e. ^{40}K in sea water where T½ = 1.25×10^9 years or 3.942×10^{16}s so $\lambda = 1.758 \times 10^{-17}$
Calculating the activity of 1g ^{40}K:

$$A = \frac{(6 \times 10^{23}) \times (1.758 \times 10^{-17})}{40} = 2.34 \times 10^5 \text{Bq}$$

Abundance of ^{40}K is 0.012% of total natural potassium. Concentration of potassium in seawater is 380mgm L^{-1} of which 0.0456mg is ^{40}K which has an activity:

$$(2.34 \times 10^5) \times (4.56 \times 10^{-5}) = 12 \text{Bq}$$

The same calculation can be used to estimate the natural activity due to ^{40}K in the human body and the amount of activity introduced by spreading artificial potash fertilizer on agricultural land.

---

where A_t is the activity after time T and A_o is the original activity. An example of its use is given in Box.15.4. Certain radiopharmaceuticals are sensitive to aluminum whose concentration reduces labeling effectiveness or when acidity (low pH) will be a biological hazard (i.e. white cell labeling). In both instances

high specific activities are essential so that contaminants are present in small concentrations. An example is given in the second half of Box.15.4.

Box 15.4

Specific activity per unit volume

A solution of ^{131}I solution on day 1 is 4.22GBq (100mCi) per 10 ml. On day 13 a 600MBq aliquot is required (13.5mCi). T½ is 8.05 days. From eqn.15.13: $A_t/A_o = e^{-\lambda T} = 0.356$. So **35.6 %** of the original activity remains in 10ml (150MBq ml^{-1}) Required activity is 600MBq contained in 4ml.

Concentration levels There is 185MBq ml^{-1} (5mCi) of ^{111}Indium chloride on day 1. T½ = 2.8 days, 20MBq is used for labeling in 0.1ml. (0.9ml remaining), what volume will 20MBq occupy on day 4 ? $e^{-\lambda T}$ is 37% so on day 4 there is 61MBq in 0.9ml. The volume required for 20MBq would be 0.3ml

NB This larger volume may require extra buffering when labeling white cells, etc.

Equation 15.11 is useful for calculating decayed levels of activity prior to disposal as low-activity waste; an example is given in Box. 15.5.

Box 15.5

Residual Activity for Waste Disposal

The permitted activity of ^{125}Iodine for waste discharge is 4.5×10^4Bq (45kBq). A sealed bag of contaminated waste measures 185×10^6Bq (185MBq). How long must it be stored before safe discharge? (T½= 60days, λ = 0.0115) Rearranging the basic formula in eqn.15.13:

$$\ln \frac{A_t}{A_o} = -\lambda T$$

Inserting the above values:

$$\ln \frac{4.5 \times 10^4}{185 \times 10^6} = -0.01155 \times T$$

$$T = \frac{8.3214}{0.01155}$$

Which is 720 days or approximately 2 years

15.4 RADIONUCLIDE PRODUCTION

Three methods are available for producing nuclear medicine radionuclides :

1. Bombardment of stable elements with charged beams.
2. Irradiation of stable elements with neutrons in a nuclear reactor.
3. Generator production.

The first method uses a considerable amount of electrical power so these isotopes are costly. The nuclear reactor since it is continuously working is the cheapest method for nuclide production. Both charged beams and nuclear reactors can provide parent
isotopes that decay to give short half-life daughters which may be removed or **eluted** from time to time; this forms the basis of the isotope generator. These three methods produce quite different products.

15.4.1 Production rate

The first two procedures mentioned above obey the same basic equation for the rate of isotope production:

$$A = C(1 - e^{-\lambda t}) \qquad (15.14)$$

Where A is the amount of activity and C is a **saturation constant**, since it is the maximum amount of activity that can be produced for the given conditions; t is the irradiation time and λ the decay coefficient for the nuclide. At a certain time, during irradiation, a production limit is reached: the number of atoms being produced are balanced by those decaying. This point is the **saturation limit**. For short half-life isotopes the saturation limit is reached quickly (ideal for expensive cyclotron operation), or can take minutes, hours or days for high activity long T½ nuclides so production is only practical by using high current cyclotron or reactor production methods.

15.4.2 Cyclotron production

Charged particles, (i.e. protons or ions) can be accelerated to sufficiently high energies so when they collide with target materials nuclear reactions are induced. This is an important method for the commercial production of radionuclides for nuclear medicine. Since charged particles are used in these reactions the nuclides tend to be relatively **neutron deficient** and in order to gain a stable neutron : proton ratio they decay by creating a neutron from a proton by one of two reactions:

- **Positron emission** (β+) by proton decay:
  p → n + e+ + *neutrino*
- **Orbital electron capture** by a nuclear proton: p + e− → n + *anti-neutrino*

An electron gun acts as an ion source, similar in design to an x-ray or cathode ray tube. The ions produced are accelerated towards the target by a high voltage. The acceleration of the charged particles takes place in an evacuated chamber by an applied electric field; the design of the field depends on the choice of accelerator. Particle beams are commonly derived from a light gas; hydrogen, deuterium or helium which produce respectively **protons**, **deuterons** and α–**particles**. The primary gases are ionized by either an electron beam or a radio-frequency field. Several forms of linear accelerator were developed for the early investigation of nuclear reactions but they required a great deal of space and still remain essentially research tools. Accelerators having circular orbits are more popular: these are called **cyclotrons**. A practical cyclotron was developed at the University of California at Berkley by Ernest Lawrence and M Stanley Livingston in 1931.

Cyclotron design   The cyclotron design restricts a beam of accelerated charged particles within a circular orbit contained in a strong magnetic field. Figure 15.8(a) shows the basic cyclotron design and a plan view of the spiral beam path. The charged particles are generated from an ion source located in the center of the machine. From here they are accelerated in a circular path by a high frequency field applied across two hollow metal D-plate electrodes placed in a strong perpendicular magnetic field. On each orbit the charged particles receive increments of energy which increase their orbit-diameters until they reach

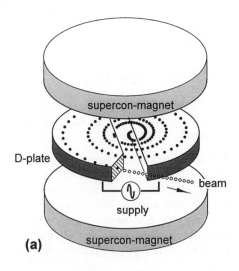

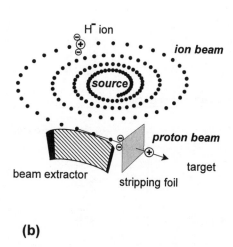

Figure 15.8 **(a)** Basic design of a clinical cyclotron showing superconducting magnets, D-plate electrodes in a vacuum housing and the alternating power supply for accelerating the charged particle beam. **(b)** The spiral path of the negative ions (H^{-1}) are deflected then stripped of their electrons to give a proton beam which bombards the target.

the periphery of the D-plates. Here they are deflected from their spiral path by either a change in magnetic field or a momentary charge on a **beam deflector**. They are then steered through a thin metal **stripping-foil** which removes electrons from the ions leaving a **proton beam** which bombards the target as shown in Fig. 15.8(b).

Small cyclotrons are now available for a hospital environment that can produce quantities of useful isotopes (positron emitters and electron capture isotopes i.e. ^{18}F and ^{123}I). They commonly use negative ion acceleration (H^{-1}) which is eventually stripped of electrons by a stripping-foil to provide a proton (H^{+1}) beam. **Neutrons** can be generated by using a beryllium or lithium target.

Cyclotron performance A compact hospital cyclotron can accelerate protons to 16MeV and deuterons to 8MeV energy. The extracted beam currents are between 50 to 100μA.

Typical specifications for a small superconducting cyclotron (Oxford Instruments) are shown in Table 15.6.

Table 15.6 Specifications of a small cyclotron

Proton energy	12MeV
External beam current	100μA
Ion source	H^{-1}
Magnet field strength	2.35 Tesla
Beam radius	220mm
Radio frequency	108MHz
Concrete shielding	1 m thick

Clinical radionuclides that are manufactured by cyclotrons are listed in Tab. 15.6. Short-lived positron emitting isotopes can be produced using a small low current cyclotron on a hospital site.

Table 15.7 Cyclotron nuclide production

Small current (p,n) reactions

Product	Target	Abundance	Yield GBq (mCi)
^{15}O	^{15}N	0.36%	90 (2500)
^{11}C	^{14}N	99%	10 (270)
^{13}N	^{13}C	1.1%	18 (500)
^{18}F	^{18}O	0.2%	3 (66)

Large current reactions

Product	$T\frac{1}{2}$	Target	Reaction
^{201}Tl	73h	^{203}Tl	$(p,3n)$
^{67}Ga	78h	^{68}Zn	$(p,2n)$
^{111}In	67h	^{110}Cd	(p,γ)
^{123}I	13h	^{127}I	$*(p,5n)$
^{81}Rb	4.5h	^{82}Kr	$(d,3n)$

*see text

The early production of ^{123}I relied on the reaction: $^{122}Te\ (d,n)^{123}I$ but this was contaminated with long lived ^{124}I giving radiation dosimetry problems. This reaction has now been superseded in the US by:

$$^{124}Xe\ (p,pn)\ ^{123}Xe\ -(T\frac{1}{2}\ 2h) \rightarrow\ ^{123}I$$

and in Europe the ^{123}Xe is obtained from:

$$^{127}I\ (p,5n)\ ^{123}Xe$$

Both reactions yield uncontaminated ^{123}I. Typical production rates for radionuclides at 12MeV using a low beam current of 50μA are given in the table. The natural abundance of the stable target material and the half-life of the daughter nuclide are given. A dual particle feature (protons and deuterons) is advantageous since inexpensive target gases can be used. Radionuclides produced by large commercial cyclotrons with larger beam currents use more efficient higher energy reactions; a list is shown in the second part of Tab.15.7. These are the commercially available nuclides with longer half-lives. Since parent (carrier element) and daughter are mostly different elements the daughter product can be separated chemically to give a **carrier free state**.

Radiation shielding If acceleration potentials are kept to within 10-12MeV in a small hospital cyclotron then the cyclotron shielding can be easily manufactured to restrict surface dose rates to 25μSv h⁻¹ (2.5mR h⁻¹) which simplifies safety requirements.

15.4.3 Reactor production

Neutron bombardment of stable elements in a nuclear reactor produces radionuclides by two different reactions:

- **Neutron capture** where the nucleus accepts an additional neutron. The nucleus then has an excess of neutrons and decays as eqn.15.2.
- **Fission** where a large nucleus accepts an additional neutron, becomes unstable and splits into two smaller nuclei.

Reactor design The basic design for a nuclear reactor is given in Fig.15.9. This type of reactor is specifically designed for the production of medical radioisotopes and is smaller than the reactors used for power generation. The neutron field of a typical reactor would be 10^{14} neutrons s⁻¹. Nuclear reactions take place according to neutron energy. The energy bands are:

- Thermal neutrons with energies up to 0.025eV
- Medium energy neutrons of up to 10keV
- Fast neutrons up to 100MeV

The moderator material is usually graphite; which slows the neutrons so that neutron capture reactions can take place.

Neutron capture reactions: These involve a neutron/gamma (n,γ) reaction. The neutron is the bombarding particle and the γ-ray is emitted as a consequence. The gamma radiation from this event is called a **prompt gamma**.

Since the products of irradiation have excess neutrons these nuclides usually undergo β⁻ negative decay, converting a neutron into a proton (eqn.15.2) n → p + e⁻. Since parent and daughter elements are the same chemically, separation is not possible and reactor products contain small amounts of their stable parent (carrier) elements as impurities so they are not entirely carrier free. Nuclear medicine isotopes produced by neutron capture (n,γ) reaction are listed in Table 15.8.

Fission produced radionuclides are carrier free but small amounts of other radioactive contaminants are sometimes present. The fission reaction for ^{235}U is outlined in Fig.15.10 and shows some of the products that are formed. Table 15.9 lists important medical nuclides manufactured by the fission process.

$$^{99}_{43}Mo \rightarrow\ ^{99m}_{42}Tc$$

$$\nearrow$$

$$^{235}_{92}U +\ ^{1}_{0}n \rightarrow\ ^{236}_{92}U + 4\ ^{1}_{0}n$$

$$\searrow$$

$$^{133}_{50}Sn \cdots \rightarrow\ ^{133}_{53}I \rightarrow\ ^{133}_{54}Xe$$

Figure 15.10 The production of ^{99}Mo from fission products. The individual elements are separated chemically.

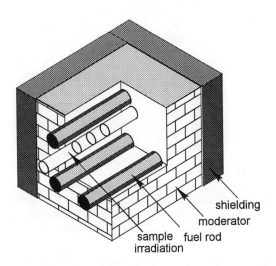

shielding
moderator
sample fuel rod
irradiation

Figure 15.9 Simplified reactor design for the production of radio-nuclides. In this design the enriched fuel $^{238/235}$U is held in graphite blocks which acts as the moderator. Cadmium control rods regulate the reaction (not shown) and the whole assembly is shielded with thick ferroconcrete. A sample tube holds the material for irradiation.

Table 15.8 Products from (n,γ) reactions.

Target	Product	Comments
^{31}P	^{32}P ⎤	therapy isotope
^{32}S	^{32}P ⎦	
^{124}Xe	^{125}Xe	decays to ^{125}I
^{74}Se	^{75}Se	imaging
^{59}Co	^{60}Co	external therapy
^{112}Sn	^{113}Sn	parent for ^{113m}In generator

Fission reactions Fast neutron absorption can induce fission in such nuclides as ^{235}U which leads to a mixture of nuclides that can be chemically separated and then purified.

Table 15.9 Nuclides from fission reactions.

Isotope	γ– (keV)	Half-life	Fission yield (%)
^{90}Sr	pure β^-	28.6 y	6.0%
^{99}Mo	740	66 h	6.0%
^{131}I	364	8.0 d	3.0%
^{133}Xe	81	5.3 d	6.5%
^{137}Cs	662	30 y	6.0%

Originally ^{131}Iodine production was produced by a neutron capture reaction:

$$^{130}Te\ (n,\gamma)\ ^{131}Te \rightarrow\ ^{131}I$$

but a fission process is now used:

$$^{235}U\ (n,f)\ ^{131}Te \rightarrow\ ^{131}I$$

The ^{131}Tellurium quickly decays to ^{131}Iodine which now has a much higher purity and specific activity.

The early ^{98}Mo (n,γ) ^{99}Mo reaction, which yielded ^{99m}Tc-generator grade molybdenum, has also been superseded by the fission reaction:

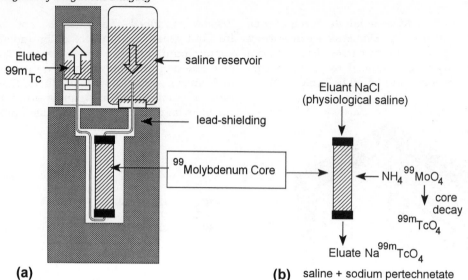

Figure 15.11   **(a)** The basic components of a ^{99m}Tc generator showing the alumina core on which the ^{99}molybdate anion is absorbed. An evacuated vial sucks saline through the system so eluting the soluble ^{99m}pertechnetate. **(b)** Ammonium ^{99}molybdate adsorbed onto the alumina core decays to ^{99m}pertechnetate which undergoes ion-exchange with Cl$^-$ to form sodium ^{99m}pertechnetate.

$$^{235}U\,(n,f)\,^{99}Mo$$

The fission sequence shown in the upper half of Fig. 15.10 yields ^{99}Mo. The ^{99}Mo is 6% of the fission product and after separation, is much cleaner than the (n,γ) reaction, which was previously used. It has a much higher specific activity; the (n,γ) production gives 400GBq g^{-1} (10Ci g^{-1}) whereas the fission product, after separation, gives 370TBq g^{-1} (10^4Ci g^{-1}). The radioactive gas ^{133}Xe is produced eventually from the second fission path in this reaction which is a clinical radionuclide used for lung ventilation studies.

15.4.4 Generator production.

It has already been seen (Fig.15.7) that radioactive decay can lead to the formation of intermediate or **metastable states**, which decay by **isomeric transition**. The metastable state can exist for periods of time covering seconds (^{81m}Kr and ^{185m}Au) to hours (^{99m}Tc and ^{113m}In). Metastable products form useful imaging nuclides if their gamma energies are in the range of 100-200keV and the parent isotope has a sufficiently long half-life to allow for generator construction and shipment. The

production of metastable isotopes by generator systems has been central to the growth of nuclear medicine. New generator systems are constantly under development and will form important future advances in nuclear medicine.

Generator design   The basic design involves a long lived parent which is adsorbed onto a column of alumina, silica or ion-exchange resin. As the parent decays the activity of the daughter rises. The carrier free daughter is then eluted from the generator by passing a solvent over the column; this is often saline (^{81m}Kr uses air). The basic construction of a typical generator system is shown in Fig.15.11 which represents a ^{99}Mo/^{99m}Tc generator and is essentially a heavily shielded core holding the parent isotope ^{99}Mo with a system for eluting the daughter product ^{99m}Tc with saline.

Bateman equation   The isomeric **parent: metastable-daughter** transition is exploited to produce a radionuclide generator for clinical use. The parent has a longer half-life than the daughter in a clinically useful generator.

The basic equation describing the ratio of parent: daughter activity in a generator is given by the Bateman equation, a simplified version of which is:

$$A_d = \frac{\lambda_d}{\lambda_d - \lambda_p} \times A_p \times (e^{-\lambda_p t} - e^{-\lambda_d t}) \quad (15.15)$$

where A_d is the daughter activity at time t and λ_d is the decay constant for the daughter, A_p is the initial activity of the parent and λ_p is the decay constant of the parent. This equation can be applied to any parent:metatstable-daughter system. Figure 15.12 gives two practical examples ^{99m}Tc and ^{81m}Kr. The decay constants for these are given in Tab. 15.10.

Table 15.10 Decay constants (λ) for equation

Generator	$T\frac{1}{2}$	$\lambda = \frac{0.693}{T_{0.5}}$
Technetium		
Parent ^{99}Mo	67.2h	0.0103
Daughter ^{99m}Tc	6.0h	0.1155
Krypton		
Parent ^{81}Rb	16488s	0.000042
Daughter ^{81m}Kr	13s	0.0533

Transient equilibrium When the parent has a longer half-life than the daughter and $\lambda_d > \lambda_p$ then the generator has a transient equilibrium. In the example plotted in Fig. 15.12(a) the ^{99m}Tc content grows to about half the ^{99}Mo content after 6 hours (T½ ^{99m}Tc). As time progresses the ^{99m}Tc activity is a function of the ^{99}Mo half-life only and at about 23 hours in an uneluted generator there is actually more ^{99m}Tc activity than ^{99}Mo. This is shown as a crossover in Fig. 15.12(a).

Secular equilibrium The second case demonstrates the condition where the half-life of the parent is much longer than that of the daughter ($\lambda_d \gg \lambda_p$); ultimately the activities of the parent and daughter are equal. This de-

scribes a generator having secular equilibrium. The example in Fig. 15.12(b) is a ^{91}Rb-^{91m}Kr generator; the ^{91m}Kr, being a gas, is used for lung ventilation studies.

Impurity levels A certain concentration of chemical impurities is present in generator eluant. The list given in Tab. 15.11 is for the common ^{99m}Tc generator where a list of impurities and their acceptable levels is given. Significant quantities of aluminum can seriously influence the effectiveness of labeling chemistry so in order to reduce aluminum concentration fresh, high specific activity eluate should be used.

^{99}Molybdenum 'breakthrough' from the core material into the elute also occurs and is calculated in Box 15.6. This should not be greater than 0.1% of the total eluate activity which is equivalent to 1µCi/mCi or 1kBq/MBq. Recent limits put this figure at 0.015%.

Molybdenum breakthrough is measured by comparing eluate activity levels with and without 6mm Pb shielding (shielded vial container).

Table 15.11 Impurity limits for ^{99}Mo/^{99m}Tc

Impurity	Typical level	Limit
pH	5.5	4 to 8
Aluminum	<1µg ml^{-1}	10µg ml^{-1}
^{131}Iodine	0.0002nCi	50nCi
^{103}Ru	0.0001nCi	50nCi
*^{99}Mo	3.0nCi	1µCi/mCi ^{99m}Tc (see Box 15.6)
^{99}Tc	0.3×10^{-5} µCi	
H$_2$O$_2$	As radiolysis product	

*<900Bq ^{99}Mo per 37MBq ^{99}Tc ≦ 25nCi per mCi

Only about one millionth of the 140keV gamma activity penetrates 6mm of lead (HVL 140keV is 0.25mm Pb) so this can be ignored whereas 54% of the 740keV gamma photon of ^{99}Mo can be counted (HVL 740keV ~8mm). Box 15.6 gives an example.

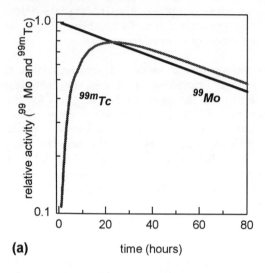

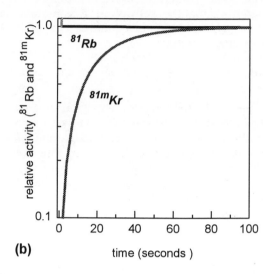

Figure 15.12 **(a)** Transient equilibrium shown by ^{99m}Tc where the daughter activity depends on the parent activity decay and **(b)** secular equilibrium demonstrated by the growth and decay of ^{81m}Kr and 81Rb. The daughter activity reaches a maximum a very short time after elution and is virtually constant.

Box 15.6

Molybdenum breakthrough

Two readings are taken with and without heavy lead shielding around the vial.
(i) Shielded S = 0.28MBq and background B is 0.02MBq
(ii) the unshielded U activity reading is 10GBq

^{99}Mo activity is $k(S-B)$ where k is a constant specific to the generator (3.5 in this case). The percent ^{99}Mo breakthrough is:

$$\frac{k(S-B)}{U} = \frac{0.91 \times 10^6}{10 \times 10^9} = \textbf{0.01\%}$$

Recognized limits vary between 1 and 0.15μCi ^{99}Mo per mCi ^{99m}Tc, equivalent to 0.1 and 0.015%

Nuclear medicine generators Several potential generator combinations are listed in Table 15.13 where the parent T½ (*pt T½*) is long enough for shipment and the daughter T½ (*dt T½*) is short enough for low radiation dose imaging. Current commercially produced generators are marked. The gamma energies

(except for ^{113m}In) are ideal for imaging. The β+ generators would be useful for PET imaging.

15.4.5 Ideal clinical properties

Tab.15.12(a) lists the properties of an ideal isotope for nuclear medicine imaging.

Table 15.12(a) The ideal medical nuclide

Requirement	Comment
Reasonable cost	reactor made
Pure gamma	generator or E .C.
Decays to stable state	stable or long lived.
Single gamma energy	energy 120 to 200keV
Good shelf life	T½ 2 days (or generator)
Short half life	generator produced
High specific activity	generator produced
Easy chemistry	no damage to substrate
Robust labeling	stable in-vivo
Single target organ	free isotope trapped
Rapid excretion	low biological T½

The most common isotope used in nuclear medicine ^{99m}Tc satisfies most of the requirements but has a major drawback with its complex chemistry, which can damage sensitive substrates (hippuran, proteins etc.). The nuclide ^{123}Iodine has a simpler labeling chemistry but has serious practical drawbacks of cost, transport and shelf-life.

Some commonly used clinical radionuclides are listed in Tab.15.12(b). Most of them have suitable γ or x-photon energies for imaging various organs. The non-imaging nuclides are ^{51}Cr, which is a red blood cell label for in-vitro cell mass measurements, ^{125}I is a radio-immunoassay label, and ^{131}I for therapy. ^{18}F produces 0.511MeV gamma photons used for positron tomography.

Table 15.12(b) Clinical radionuclides

Isotope	$T\frac{1}{2}$	Useful photons (γ)
^{18}F	1.83 h	511keV (β^+)
^{51}Cr	27.7 d	320keV
^{67}Ga	78.2 h	93 185 300keV
^{81m}Kr	13 s	159keV
^{90}Mo	66h	740keV
^{99m}Tc	6.0 h	140keV
^{111}In	2.8d	171, 245keV
^{123}I	13.2 h	159keV
^{125}I	59.6 d	27-32keV (x-rays)
^{131}I	8.0 d	364keV
^{133}Xe	5.2 d	81keV
^{201}Tl	73 h	68-82keV (x-rays)

Summary Isotope production techniques

Charged particles	Neutral particles
protons p deuterons d tritons t alpha particle α	neutrons
Production: • using a charged particle accelerator: cyclotron	***Production:*** • nuclear reactor having a very high neutron flux, fast or thermal neutrons • cyclotron giving low/medium thermal neutron flux.
Produces: • proton excess nucleus • daughter product decays by electron capture or positron emission.	***Produces:*** • neutron excess nucleus • daughter product decays by beta emission or by fission.
Nuclide: • mostly carrier free • expensive nuclides • expensive target material for small cyclotrons • short shelf life	***Nuclide:*** • not carrier free • some require chemical separation • cheap nuclides • long shelf life

Reaction choice depends on: nearest stable isotope, highest specific activity, contaminants, cost.

Table 15.13 Clinically useful generators showing parent *pt* and daughter *dt* properties

$pt \rightarrow dt$	Production	pt-$T\frac{1}{2}$	dt-$T\frac{1}{2}$	γ–energy
*^{81}Rb $\rightarrow$ ^{81m}Kr	Cyclotron	4.6 h	13 s	190 keV
*^{99}Mo $\rightarrow$ ^{99m}Tc	Reactor	66 h	6.0 h	140keV
*^{113}Sn $\rightarrow$ ^{113m}In	Reactor	115 d	99 m	390keV
^{62}Zn $\rightarrow$ ^{62}Cu	Cyclotron	9.3 h	9.7 m	511 keV (β^+)
^{68}Ge $\rightarrow$ ^{68}Ga	Cyclotron	270 d	68 m	511 keV (β^+)
^{72}Se $\rightarrow$ ^{72}As	Cyclotron	8.4 d	26 h	511 keV (β^+)
*^{82}Sr $\rightarrow$ ^{82}Rb	Cyclotron	25 d	1.3 m	511 keV (β^+)
^{178}W $\rightarrow$ ^{178}Ta	Cyclotron	21 d	9.3 m	93keV
*^{191}Os $\rightarrow$ ^{191m}Ir	Reactor	15 d	5 s	130 keV
*^{195m}Hg $\rightarrow$ ^{195m}Au	Cyclotron	41 h	30 s	190 keV

* *Commercially available*

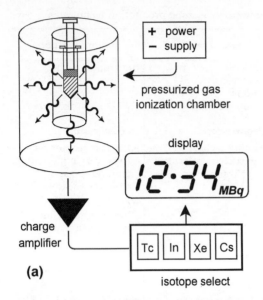

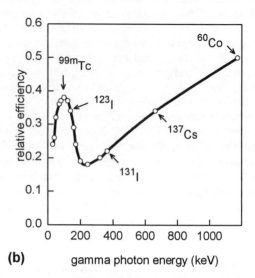

Figure 15.13 **(a)** A basic dose calibrator design showing free standing ionization chamber connected to a high impedance charge amplifier or electrometer which leads to a digital display. Switched amplification levels give choice of radionuclide (gamma energy). **(b)** Dose calibrator sensitivity show that photoelectric events predominate below 200keV. Sensitivity increases due to Compton interactions. This non-linear response is corrected by adjusting charge amplifier gain.

Generator radionuclides

- pure gamma emitters
- low patient radiation dose
- high specific activity
- comparatively long shelf life
- cheap
- difficult chemistry

15.5 LABORATORY INSTRUMENTATION

The emission of radiation from a radioactive source is **isotropic** so a planar (flat) detector surface can only capture a small proportion of the total activity (see Chapter 2). The geometrical efficiency can be represented as:

$$\frac{Detector\ Area}{Area\ of\ Sphere} = \frac{\pi r^2}{4\pi R^2} \qquad (15.16)$$

Where r is the detector radius and R the distance from the source. As the detector gets closer to the source the spherical area decreases, so more radiation is captured. Two types of counting geometry can be identified:

- 2π: a flat detector surface,
- 4π: the detector surface surrounds the entire source.

Inverse square law (see Chapter 2) This describes the change in radiation intensity as a square of the distance D. As the detector moves away from the source the counts I decrease as:

$$I = \frac{1}{D^2} \qquad (15.17)$$

but this only applies to a point source of activity   If the distance is reduced to zero the count rate will not be infinite. A better law for flat detectors is the **Cosine Law** where the geometrical efficiency is represented as:

$$\frac{1}{2}(1 - \cos \theta) \qquad (15.18)$$

Where θ is half the angle subtended by the detector surface. At zero distance θ becomes 90° and as cosine 90° = 0   the efficiency becomes 50%; a 2π detector will capture 50% of the activity placed on its surface.

15.5.1   Dose calibrator

The ionization chamber is a gas filled detector and was described in Chapter 6. An important application is the isotope dose calibrator as used for measuring isotope activities. The dose calibrator drawn in Fig.15.13(a) shows the sealed plastic cylinder forming the first electrode and filled with an inert gas, either argon or xenon pressurized to about 10 atmospheres. The high density gas improves radiation absorption efficiency. In the middle of the chamber there is a smaller cylindrical sample holder which forms the other electrode. The plastic material used in its construction is coated with a conductive surface.

The radioactive sample is placed in this central hollow electrode and the emitted radiation (beta, gamma or x-ray) interacts with the gas atoms causing ionization. Both photoelectric and Compton interactions play a part, producing free ions and electrons. For beta radiation and low energy photons (<200keV) the photoelectric effect in the gas predominates. Above this energy the Compton process plays a more important role and the scattered electrons have sufficient energy for further secondary ionizations.

A voltage applied between the two electrodes (usually about 300 volts) attracts the ions formed by the radiation event, the positive ions to the central negative electrode (cathode) and the free electrons to the positive outer electrode (anode). The current generated by the ionizing events within the chamber is proportional to the activity of the source. The current is very small; 40MBq of ^{99m}Tc produces 1×10^{-10} amps (0.1 nano-amps) so is measured by a very high input impedance electrometer or charge amplifier. The time taken for the dose calibrator to reach 95% of its reading is typically 2 to 3 seconds and the detector achieves very nearly 4π counting geometry.

The dose calibrator, being an ionization chamber, has a very slow response. It cannot separate individual events and distinguish different gamma energies so it can only be used for measuring single isotope activities.

The dose calibrator can measure activities from 4kBq to 40GBq (0.1 millicuries to 10 curies); the lower limit depends on the level of low-background activity, so the dose calibrator should be adequately shielded. The chamber sensitivity for different photon energies is plotted in Fig.15.13(b); low energies are efficiently absorbed by the photo-electric effect. The efficiency then decreases until the energies are sufficient to cause multiplication of electrons by the Compton process when the sensitivity is seen to increase. In order to adjust for this changing energy sensitivity the amplifier gain is varied in step with the photon energy; these settings are the calibration values for the detector; the values are pre-set for the most common isotopes. The dose calibrator is ideal for measuring ^{99}Mo breakthrough from the generator column.

15.5.2.   The well counter

This is essentially a scintillation crystal with a hole or 'well' drilled to accept a sample tube. Figure15.14(a) shows the basic design of a laboratory well counter commonly used for counting radioactive tracer samples having very low activity. Positioning the sample within the crystal achieves a high counting efficiency and 95% of photons emitted by a small (1cm^3) sample can be captured achieving nearly 4π geometry.

Good counting geometry and high sensitivity of NaI(Tl) allows activities of a few hundred becquerels (nano-curies) to be measured, depending on background activity. Unlike the dose calibrator mixtures of nuclides can be separately analyzed since each nuclide energy in the mixture can be identified using the pulse height analyzer. There are count rate limitations since the NaI(Tl) detector **saturates** at high count rates owing to its finite decay time of 240ns; pulses overlap from high activities causing pulse-pileup. The typical upper counting limit is 5000 counts per second; above this there is count loss and poor accuracy. The lower limit of this counter is decided by the interfering background activity.

Background activity can be reduced by ensuring the counter is placed away from other active sources (other samples and patients) and surrounded by a lead-brick castle (5cm thick) built up so the castle rim is about 1-2cm above the well counter itself. The lead should be from an old stock since naturally occurring ^{210}Pb (T½ 22y) occurs in recently mined metal contributing to gamma background activity. For this reason lead based paint should not be used in very low background environments.

Effect of sample volume Counting geometry alters significantly with changing sample volumes for both dose calibrator and well counter. The escape angle becomes broader with larger volumes, and therefore the counter is less efficient. Identical small volumes should consequently always be used.

Theoretically any mixture of nuclides can be counted using a well counter but in practice this is restricted to 4 since good separation is required between gamma energies to minimize cross-talk between photo-peaks and scatter.

Calibration of the well counter and other laboratory instruments is essential if accurate measurements are to be taken. A series of various gamma emitting calibrated sources are available for this purpose; a list is given in Tab.15.14.

Table 15.14 Calibration isotopes for laboratory counters.

Isotope	T½ (years)	Principal γ energies (MeV)
^{129}Iodine	1.57×10^7	0.03
^{241}Americium	500	0.060
^{57}Cobalt	271 days	0.122
^{133}Barium	11	0.356, 0.276, 0.081
^{137}Cesium	30	0.662
^{60}Cobalt	5.3	1.173, 1.332

15.5.3 Organ uptake probes

Single large scintillation detectors, from 5 to 8cm diameter (3″ to 5″), are commonly used for measuring organ uptakes of various radionuclides. The most common detector probe is the thyroid uptake probe, used for measuring the concentration of radio-iodine (either ^{131}I or ^{125}I) in the thyroid gland. The basic design is shown in Fig.15.14(b). It carries a specially shaped collimator which covers the area of the thyroid excluding other activities. It also serves as a sensitive personnel contamination monitor for measuring accidental iodine ingestion in laboratory workers.

Detector efficiency The overall efficiency for the NaI(Tl) detector depends on the crystal thickness. Table 15.15 lists efficiencies of 5×5 and 8×8cm NaI(Tl) crystal detectors for a selection of gamma energies.

Table 15.15 Crystal efficiencies (%) for two sizes.

Nuclide	Photon energy(s) (keV)	5×5cm	8×8cm
^{125}I	28	72	72
^{57}Co	122	86	88
^{99m}Tc	140	85	87
^{111}In	175, 243	70	78
^{51}Cr	320	36	64
^{131}I	364	28	55
^{60}Co	1175, 1333	5.2	17

The low energy photon from ^{125}I is absorbed almost entirely but so also is the relatively weak light emission which also reduces detector efficiency. Several large probe assemblies can be used for low activity whole body counting when placed in a specially shielded low background environment. Very small tracer activities of ^{40}K, ^{59}Fe, ^{57}Co etc. can be measured with this **whole body counter**.

15.5.4 Specific gamma ray constant

The specific gamma ray constant Γ for a point source gives the dose rate in mSv h^{-1} at 1 meter from a point emission.

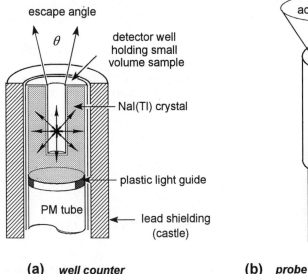

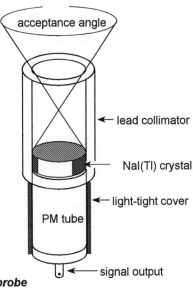

(a) *well counter*   **(b)** *probe*

Figure 15.14 **(a)** The well counter used for counting small samples. It is heavily shielded from background radiation with a lead castle. **(b)** A basic scintillation probe for organ uptake investigations. The crystal is typically 5 to 8 cm thick. The collimator is specifically designed to cover the appropriate organ area.

The calculation in Box 15.7 would be used for calibrating a gamma radiation monitor in terms of dose rate from a particular nuclide commonly used in the laboratory or clinic. Equation 15.19 adjusts the reading for different source distances.

Box 15.7

> ***Specific gamma ray constant* Γ**
>
> From Tab.15.16 the Γ for ^{99m}Tc is 17μSv h^{-1} GBq^{-1} at 1m ($d = 100$cm). What is the dose D for an activity A of 500MBq at a new distance d_n of 30cm ?
>
> $$D = \frac{G \times A \times d^2}{d_n^2} \qquad (15.19)$$
>
> $$= 94\mu\text{Sv h}^{-1} \text{ at 30cm}$$

Table 15.16 Specific gamma ray constants (mSv h^{-1} GBq^{-1} at 1 m)

Nuclide	Gamma energy (keV)	Dose rate
^{241}Am	60	0.004
^{201}Tl	68-82 (x-ray)	0.012
^{57}Co	122	0.016
^{99m}Tc	140	0.017
^{99}Mo	740	0.041
^{131}I	364	0.057
^{111}In	171, 245	0.084
^{137}Cs	662	0.087
^{60}Co	1.173, 1.333	0.360

Contamination monitoring Portable contamination monitors are an important accessory in the nuclear medicine department for detecting and localizing radio-active spills and contaminated areas. The sensitivity of three typical contamination monitors is given in Tab.15.17. It can be seen that a large area scintillation detector has the greatest sensitivity.

Table 15.17 Specification and sensitivity of large area contamination monitors

Detector	^{90}Sr	^{35}Cl	^{14}C	^{125}I	$^{57}Co/$ ^{99m}Tc
100cm^3 argon Al window (3mg cm^{-2})	15	13	5.0	1.0	3.0
100cm^3 xenon Ti window (5mg cm^{-2})	25	20	5.4	3.5	5.4
100cm^{3}NaI(Tl) Al window (0.9mg cm^{-2})	33	25	7.6	50	16

In summary monitoring equipment is used for measuring **absolute activities** of radio-isotopes (in GBq, MBq, kBq or curies, millicuries and microcuries) prior to radiopharmaceutical preparation or patient injection (a 4π **dose calibrator**). The slow response of the counter integrates the ionization events, giving an ion current measured by an electrometer. It cannot distinguish separate gamma energies so only single isotope activities can be measured.

Small activity samples use a well counter in the form of a small volume 4π scintillation detector. The fast response of the counter allows individual gamma events to be recorded; pulse height discrimination can be used to isolate multi-isotope samples.

Either a Geiger counter or scintillation detector or large field gas proportional counter can be used for identifying **contaminated areas** depending on isotope type and concentration. Alpha beta and gamma radiation can be monitored depending on design.

Organ uptake requires a suitably collimated scintillation detector. Examples are thyroid and kidney probes. Multiple large sized de-

tectors, in a properly shielded environment, can measure whole body uptakes of tracer isotopes.

For all these detectors shape, volume and position of samples are critical parameters when comparing activities between different sources of radioactivity; this also applies to imaging systems as well as laboratory counting instrumentation.

15.6 THE GAMMA CAMERA

The basic design of a modern gamma camera shown in Fig.15.15 identifies the major components and shows the detector crystal backed by an array of photomultiplier tubes which feed separate charge amplifiers. A collimator is fixed to the front of this assembly. The basic gamma camera was first constructed by H.O. Anger (US physicist/ engineer) in 1956.

15.6.1 The crystal detector

A large NaI(Tl) scintillation crystal 300 to 500mm (12-20 inches) in diameter either 6 or 10 mm ($^1/_4''$ or $^3/_8''$) thick forms the gamma camera detector. Radiation absorption for various energies (detector efficiency) versus crystal detector thickness is shown in Tab. 15.18. Thinner crystals give better spatial resolution at the cost of reduced absorption efficiency.

As the scintillator crystal is hygroscopic it is hermetically sealed using thin aluminum at the front and sides and glass or transparent plastic at the rear; this transparent window acts as a light guide. Gamma radiation, absorbed by the sodium iodide scintillator, is converted to ultraviolet light events (see Chapter 5) the photons of which are then detected by a set of closely matched photomultiplier tubes (PM-tubes) attached to the light guide.

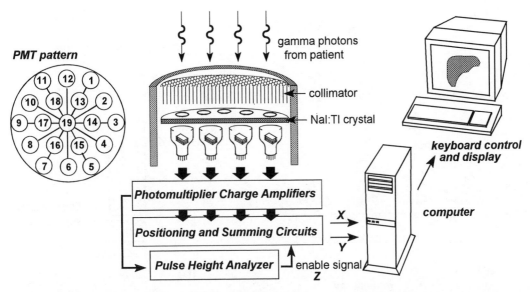

Figure 15.15 Basic gamma camera design. The collimator accepts orthogonal radiation from the patient which is detected by the positional sensitive detector. X and Y spatial information is computed by the positional and summing circuits. If the detected event is within the photo-peak window a Z pulse enables the positional information which is then stored in an image matrix by the computer/array processor. The array pattern of the PM-tubes on the surface of the crystal is shown top-left.

Table 15.18 Percent absorption for various gamma energies (keV)

Depth	80	140	200	350	500keV
1/4″	97	75	45	16	8
3/8″	98	84	58	23	12
1/2″	99	90	70	32	18

15.6.2 Camera electronics

The PM tubes are arranged in 37, 61, 75 or 91 hexagonal arrays depending on the gamma camera model. A simple hexagonal PMT pattern is shown in Fig.15.15 for a circular detector. Rectangular detectors typically have 55 or 59 detectors.

Positional or summation circuitry This receives the signals from all the PM tubes and is usually situated with the amplifiers in the camera head itself. Each photo-multiplier signal contributes to the computation of the positional signal. The summation circuitry accepts signals from the PM amplifiers and computes the spatial coordinates (x and y) of the gamma event in the scintillator. The positional x, y signals can be further processed to correct for imperfections in both the crystal and photo-multiplier interface and also the summing network itself.

Spatial information The light emitted by the gamma event in the detector crystal is dispersed throughout the large scintillator and is seen by all the photo-multipliers. The diagram in Fig.15.16(a) shows a simplified one dimensional example where five PM-tubes detect the light event with varying degrees of intensity. These signals undergo logarithmic amplification illustrated in Fig.15.16(b) so that:

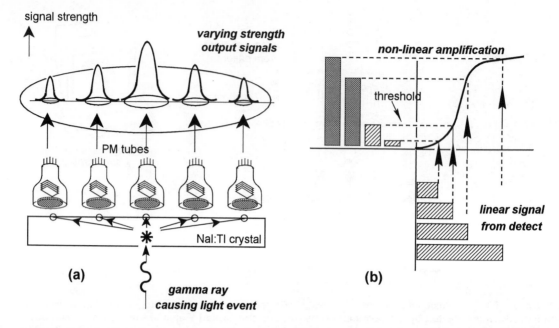

Figure 15.16   (a) A group of 5 PM-tubes responding to a single light event. Their signal amplitudes and those of their surrounding neighbors determine the event position on the crystal surface. (b) non-linear amplification of these signals removes low amplitude signals that do not exceed a certain threshold. These do not carry important spatial information.

- Smaller photo-multiplier signals, which carry very little positional information, are eliminated.
- Large signals are reduced so that the position of the light event on the photo-multiplier face itself has only a small effect on PM signal amplitude.

The logarithmic response can be achieved using either analog or digital circuitry; the latter is now favored since digital processing can be specifically tailored to suit the camera.

Pulse height analysis (energy discrimination)   (see Chapter 6) This circuit accepts signals from all the PM tubes and measures the maximum signal height seen. If this is within the photo-peak energy window, then a Z or energy signal is generated that enables (opens) the x, y signals and gates them to the image display computer shown in Fig 15.15.

All the photo-multipliers take part in the energy analysis. Efficient energy discrimination is essential for removing scatter events and maintaining optimum image quality.

Display   The final x and y signals, generated by the positional circuitry, are accepted by either an analog film formatter or digitized (analog to digital converter) to take part in a computer display system.

The analog film formatter, since it is a simple x, y recorder, uses a cathode ray tube that has an extremely fine dot dimension. The light from this dot is recorded on the film directly to produce an image. On inspection the fine dots can be distinguished, each one represents a single gamma photon within the chosen energy window. A good quality image requires at least 1 million of these dots, equivalent to 1 million accepted gamma events.

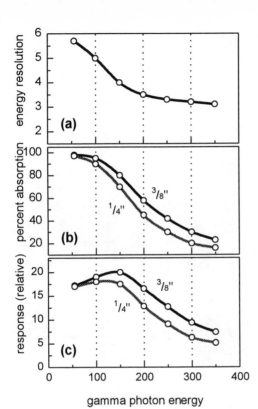

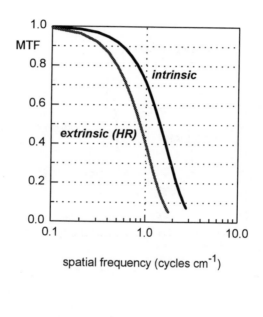

Figure 15.17 Three graphs showing gamma camera performance versus photon energy for **(a)** camera resolution (FWHM), **(b)** photon absorption for two crystal thicknesses ($^3/_8''$ or 1cm and $^1/_4''$ or 0.6cm). **(c)** Graph combines the data revealing optimum efficiency for resolution and absorption in the energy range 100 to 200keV **(d)** The MTF for both intrinsic and extrinsic resolution taken with a high resolution collimator.

Summary The gamma camera is an imaging device for nuclear medicine it consists of:

- A collimator accepting orthogonal gamma events from the patient . A large NaI(Tl) crystal is the scintillation detector usually $^1/_4''$ or $^3/_8''$ thick.
- Photo-multiplier tubes form an hexagonal (circular detector) or rectangular array on its surface.
- The signals from these go to charge amplifiers.
- The signals are logarithmically amplified and accepted by the positional circuitry which computes x and y axes of the gamma event.
- The pulse height analyzer enables this signal if the x, y signal is a photo-peak event.
- The x, y signal forms the display

15.7 CAMERA PERFORMANCE

The three graphs in Fig.15.17(a),(b),(c) compare camera spatial resolution and absorption efficiency for 6 and 10mm ($^1/_4''$ $^3/_8''$) crystals with gamma photon energy. Combining (a) and (b) yields an overall performance curve (c) which peaks between 140-200keV, confirming this as the optimum energy for gamma cameras.

15.7.1 Intrinsic resolution

The resolving power of the gamma camera system without any collimation is obtained by exposing the uncovered crystal to a point or line source of activity. In practice the crystal is covered by a lead-sheet in which fine points or a thin single line has been cut.

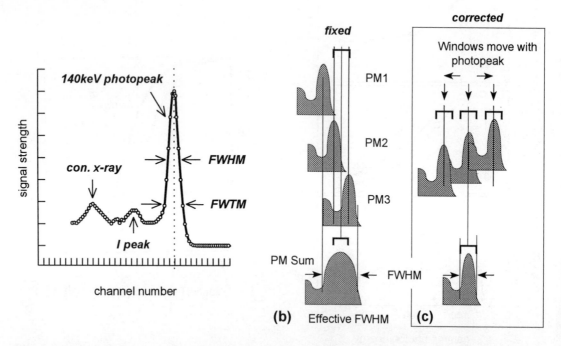

Figure 15.18   **(a)** The spectrum for ^{99m}Tc collected over 100 channels. The 140keV photopeak is centered over channel 70 and the FWHM is 9 channels wide. The smaller peaks represent the conversion x-ray at 18keV caused by the characteristic x-rays of Tc due to internal conversion process. The iodine escape peak at 110keV marks the escape of the K fluorescent x-ray of iodine (NaI detector) . **(b)** Correction for energy window drift. A fixed window leads to loss of energy resolution. **(c)** A moving window follows the energy peak drift and overcomes this problem.

A specially engineered source is then placed on these and a profile obtained. A modulation transfer function (MTF) is then obtained from the point spread or line spread function which gives the camera **intrinsic resolution**. An example is shown in Fig.15.17(d) where the 10% MTF value is approximately 2.5Lp cm^{-1} representing a FWHM value of 4mm. The extrinsic MTF represents the system resolution which includes a high resolution collimator (HR).

The computer display also introduces distortions due to digitization errors placing random events into a fixed image matrix. Since nuclear medicine images are low resolution, when compared to other radiographic images, this is not a serious problem and fairly coarse

matrices are acceptable i.e. 64×64, 128×128 or 256×256, depending on detail required; larger matrices are not necessary except perhaps for large area whole body imaging.

15.7.2 Energy resolution

This is measured as the full-width of the photopeak at half-maximum height (FWHM) and is about 10% for most current cameras (140keV gamma). This setting directly affects spatial resolution of the camera since the accuracy of positional computation improves with decreasing photopeak width. In order to cover the majority area of the photopeak the energy window setting is typically 15%.

Energy resolution is perhaps the most valuable fundamental measure of overall gamma camera performance.

Figure 15.18(a) represents a gamma camera photopeak displayed using the multi-channel analyzer. From the channel measurements made from this spectrum the energy resolution can be calculated as:

$$\frac{FWHM\ channel\ width}{keV\ per\ channel \times 140} \qquad (15.20)$$

The calculation requires a calibration 'keV per channel' which is derived from the number of analyzer channels representing 140keV, which is 70 in this example giving 0.5 channels per keV. The photopeak half-height width is 9 channels so the energy resolution (FWHM) is 12.8%. Since this percentage figure decreases as the photopeak energy increases both percentage and energy values should be stated when quoting FWHM. The full-width-at-tenth-maximum (FWTM) is also shown on the energy spectrum. This is a measure of scatter acceptance, commonly caused by collimator septa penetration, and becomes very broad if higher gamma energies are experienced.

Uniformity correction Variations in sensitivity across the crystal face are mainly caused by the variation in the energy window placed over each PMT photo-peak. This is due to small variations in photo-multiplier gain together with drift. Variations in optical collection efficiency over the camera face can also contribute. If these variations are not corrected then:

- The energy resolution of the camera system will be the sum of the misaligned energy windows of all the PM tubes represented in Fig.15.18(b) and will be subjected to continuous drift.
- Camera sensitivity will consequently vary over the camera face due to the energy window shifting from the photo-peaks.
- Contrast and resolution performance will likewise vary.

Correction procedures have been introduced into recent camera designs (Siemens ZLC and GE Autotune); a simplified correction process is shown in Fig.15.18(c). Since the photopeak variations are quite slow the camera computer system can continuously alter individual PM performance during data collection. The varying position of the photo-peak window is corrected by either moving the window or adjusting the PM supply voltage to shift the peak to the optimum position. This energy correction procedure can be used for a wide range of gamma energies. The correction process for detector/PM optical imperfections usually takes the form of a 64×64 matrix of correction values representing crystal areas seen by each PM tube.

15.7.3 Dead time

Owing to detection dead time (see Chapter 6) the measured count rates from a gamma camera fall short of expected count rate. Gamma camera count rate is therefore expressed as a figure representing a 10%, 20% or 30% count loss. The common value is taken at 20%. The count rate capability is limited by the decay time of the scintillator, about 240nS for NaI(Tl), its charge amplifier and associated converter electronics. Figure.15.19 shows a typical gamma camera response to increasing count rate. The shape of the curve depends on the width of the energy spectrum and the scatter present; both of these factors should be minimized. If N_i is the incident number of gamma photons and N_a is the photon counts recorded then the dead time τ is given as:

$$\tau = \frac{ln\frac{N_i}{N_a}}{N_a} \qquad (15.21)$$

The dead time calculated from eqn. 15.21 for a 20% loss at 200,000 cps in Fig. 15.19 gives a value of just over 1μs. There are two types of detector dead time **paralysable**, where further photon events serve to increase the total dead time and **non-paralysable** where further events are ignored, the detector operating again after a set time. Most gamma cameras behave as paralysable detectors over the clinical count range.

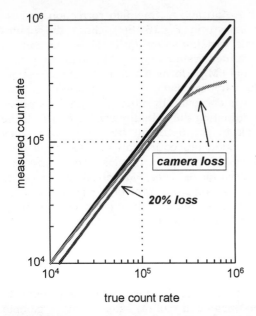

Figure 15.19   System count losses plotting incident versus recorded count rate. The drop in recorded count rate is commonly measured at the 20% line. This camera has a maximum count rate of 200,000 for a 20% loss.

Fast count modes

Fast count modes   High activities of short lived isotopes and high bolus-activity heart studies require high count rate capabilities. Each gamma ray interaction with the scintillator requires about 1mS for complete light collection. Since non-useful scattered radiation is similarly analyzed along with the photo-peak events the total dead time for the camera is longer. Faster count rates can be handled if the positional computation uses only the first part of the light signal, but accepting only a fraction of the light output; the drawback is a small loss in resolution. So pulse shortening can increase count rate capability but with a corresponding reduction in intrinsic resolution.

15.7.4 Field of view

The **useful field of view** (UFOV) is defined as the practical or collimated area available for imaging. The uniformity and general response of a gamma camera deteriorates toward the edge of the crystal however and this can be seen as a bright periphery in Fig.15.20. The **central field of view** (CFOV) represents the central 75% of the camera field of view which commonly holds image clinical detail. Figures for resolution and uniformity are commonly quoted for both these areas; Table 15.19 lists typical values for two camera types along with spatial and energy resolution.

Table 15.19 Intrinsic camera specifications

Parameter	CFOV (0.75×UFOV)	UFOV
Spatial resolution		
FWHM	3.9mm	4.1mm
FWTM	7.6mm	7.8mm
Energy resolution		10.6%
Field Uniformity		
Integral	±2.5%	±4.5%
Differential	±2.0%	±3.0%

15.7.5 Field uniformity

The uniformity of camera sensitivity for both UFOV and CFOV is measured by placing a point source of activity at a distance at least ×5 the crystal diameter (2m).This provides a photon flux with <1% variation. Any irregularities in the image obtained are caused mainly by variations in spatial linearity and energy response. The flood image should contain 10 million counts for planar work and 30 million for tomography. A uniformity image is shown in Fig.15.20 together with a spatial linearity multiple line source. Camera non uniformity of response for both UFOV and CFOV can be described as either **integral** or **differential**.

Integral non-uniformity   This can be measured as the percentage difference between the maximum and minimum pixel counts in a sampling area (UFOV or CFOV):

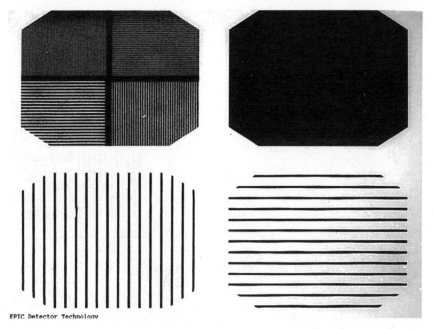

EPIC Detector Technology

Figure 15.20 A rectangular field of view camera showing a flood field uniformity picture and a multiple line source showing position linearity in both x and y directions.

$$U_i(+) = \frac{(C_{max} - C_x)}{C_x} \times 100\%$$

$$(15.22)$$

$$U_i(-) = \frac{(C_{min} - C_x)}{C_x} \times 100\%$$

Where $U_i(+)$ and $U_i(-)$ are the measured extreme values for non-uniformity. C_{max} and C_{min} are the maximum and minimum pixel counts and C_x is the mean pixel count within the sampled area of an image matrix. The NEMA (1980) definition for integral non-uniformity is simply:

$$\frac{C_{max} - C_{min}}{C_{max} + C_{min}}$$

$$(15.23)$$

Both eqn.15.22 and 15.23 give the same result.

Differential non-uniformity The percentage maximum difference between two adjacent pixels in an image matrix is the differential non-uniformity and is defined by NEMA as:

$$\frac{high - low \ pixel}{high + low \ pixel}$$

$$(15.24)$$

The high and low values are obtained from image matrix pixel values measured over a range of five pixels in all rows and columns.

15.7.6 Spatial resolution

The intrinsic resolution described earlier is the best resolution that the camera is capable of giving without considering the degradation offered by collimation (extrinsic or system resolution). The total amount of light emitted by the crystal is proportional to the energy of the gamma ray and this influences the intrinsic resolution figure which increases with gamma energy. However, since absorption decreases (Figure 15.17) an optimum energy for gamma cameras is reached which is seen to be between 100 and 150keV. For high count rate acceptance **pulse shortening** or reduction in pulse density would reduce intrinsic resolution.

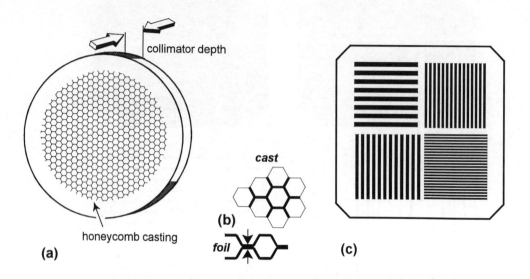

Figure 15.21   **(a)** A typical cast collimator design for a gamma camera showing honeycomb pattern for the holes.   **(b)** A thumb-nail sketch shows the difference between cast and foil designs, the latter has non-uniform septa thicknesses (arrows).   **(c)** Bar-phantom used for estimating the resolution of a camera /collimator system. Bar dimensions are typically 0.25, 0.19, 0.13 and 0.08 inches.

In summary the two resolution measurements describing gamma camera performance: **energy resolution** and **spatial resolution** should not be confused. Energy resolution measures the ability of the detector system (crystal plus PM tube electronics) to resolve the small variation in photon signal events (pulse height discrimination) and is measured as the width of the photopeak spectrum at half its height (FWHM): this is a **percentage** figure. Spatial resolution describes the 2D positional accuracy of the camera detector which is measured with a point of line source of activity placed directly on the crystal surface (intrinsic resolution) or collimator face (extrinsic resolution). The point spread or line spread function also yields a FWHM measurement but this time it represents **distance** in millimeters.

Spatial distortion This is due to mis-registration of an image event on the display so that its true position on the crystal is distorted. This is commonly due to un-matched PM tubes or variation over the face of the PM tube itself.

The overall effect produces positional deviations at regular positions on the crystal face. The visibility of the PM tube locations on a flood field picture is partly caused by this. A measure of spatial linearity as a deviation from a line source is typically 0.35mm CFOV and 0.7mm UFOV.

Typical performance specifications for current gamma cameras are :

Detector size	60×45cm
UFOV	53×38cm
PM tubes	59 3″ diameter
Count rate	200 000 at 20% loss

Intrinsic resolution:

75 000cps	5mm
150 000cps	5.7mm

Performance factors A number of factors have improved overall system performance:

- Increased number of photo-multipliers (from 19, 37, 75, 91)
- Thinner crystals ($^3/_8$" or $^1/_4$")
- Uniformity correction by continuous energy window adjustment .
- Large field of view (from 10" to 30")

15.8 COLLIMATOR PROPERTIES

The collimator is a lead honeycomb plate containing a large number of holes (Fig.15.21(a)). The plate can be constructed from either solid lead cast in a honeycomb pattern or made from lead-sheet bent to form a honeycomb or cell-like system, illustrated in (b). The important directional properties of the collimator are responsible for rejecting oblique radiation and only accepting radiation orthogonal to the detector face. Without a collimator the camera would not be able to register spatial information since oblique radiation would saturate the detector. The collimator serves the same basic purpose as antiscatter grid described in Chapter 8 although the radionuclide source is isotropic and not uni-directional like an x-ray source.

Common collimator designs use parallel hole patterns but degrees of image magnification or minification can be obtained from non-orthogonal collimators with angles holes. The hole dimensions and lead content decide the efficiency and resolving power of the collimator. With a collimator in place only a small photon fraction reaches the detector face (1 in 10,000 gamma events from the source). Collimator sensitivity varies inversely with resolution so collimator design is always a compromise between these two factors.

15.8.1 Extrinsic resolution

This is a measure of the camera system resolution with the collimator in place, frequently referred to as the system resolution. Again a subjective measurement can be made

with a bar phantom (an Anger or pie phantom used with the collimator would create moiré or interference patterns with the collimator holes). Figure15.21(c) shows a typical bar phantom with bar dimensions.

Resolution can be more precisely measured with a line source placed on the collimator face and a modulation transfer function derived (see Fig.15.17(d)). The bar phantom or line source can be placed either on the collimator surface or at a distance with scattering medium (water or plastic) interposed to gain information about resolution with depth. From the original work by Anger an index of collimator resolution is given by:

$$R = \frac{a + b + c}{a} \times d \qquad (15.25)$$

Where a is the collimator length or thickness, b is the distance from source to collimator, c is the distance from the collimator to the interaction within the crystal and d is the hole diameter. For the same camera and parallel LE collimator design both c and d can be ignored and the formula simplified to:

$$R = (a+b)/a$$

Some useful practical information can now be derived.

Resolution change with collimator length
If the distance from the collimator to the source (b) is constant then for collimator length a = 2, 4 and 6cm the resolution improves as 1.5, 1.25 and 1.16. Notice that the change from 2 to 4cm improves the resolution by 16% but from 4 to 6cm only a 7% improvement is obtained for the same hole density.

Resolution change with depth of organ
For a 2cm collimator length (high sensitivity design) with the source 8cm from the collimator face (b) then R = 5. If the source is now 12cm from the face then R = 7; a 40% decrease in resolution. For a 6cm collimator length (high resolution design) the resolution decrease is smaller, 28%. The camera should always be positioned as close to the patient as possible and a high resolution collimator used for imaging deep organs. Collimator properties are

further demonstrated by the graphs in Fig.15.22 showing that resolution is significantly affected by length of collimator or distance of source from the collimator face.

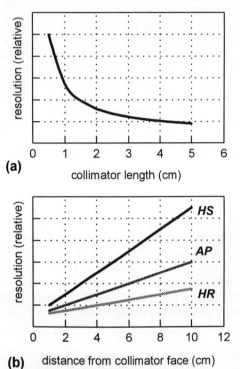

(a)

(b)

Figure 15.22 The effect on system resolution by altering collimator depth *a* for the same value *b* (top graph) and using high sensitivity, an all purpose and a high resolution collimator to visualize an organ at various depths (varying *b*).

Overall resolution An expression for system total resolution r_t combines intrinsic r_i and collimator r_c resolution so that:

$$r_t = \sqrt{r_i^2 + r_c^2}$$ (15.26)

Crystal thickness alters r_i to some extent but these changes to intrinsic resolution have less effect than changes in extrinsic resolution due to collimator design and position relative to the source. For instance an intrinsic resolution change from 4 to 5mm will only have a small effect on the image resolution with a collimator resolution of 8mm (r_t in eqn.15.26

increases from 8.9mm compared to 9.4mm). If a scattering medium (the patient) is placed between the source and the collimator face the effect of small changes to intrinsic resolution would not be visible. When scatter is considered a third factor representing scatter resolution r_s should be added to eqn.15.26.

15.8.2 Collimator types

Collimator design optimizes sensitivity and resolution which are inversely related. **High sensitivity** collimators are used for high count rate studies when organ resolution is not important or unobtainable due to involuntary movement for instance kidney or heart dynamic studies or lung ventilation perfusion. **High resolution** collimators are used when definition is important i.e. bone and brain studies but patient movement must be controlled for best performance. Low energy all purpose or general purpose collimators (LEAP or LEGP collimators) try to combine the attributes of resolution and sensitivity for routine use.

Some common collimators are illustrated in Fig.15.23(a),(b). A complete gamma camera installation should include high sensitivity and high resolution parallel hole collimators; and a low energy all purpose (LEAP) collimator for general static imaging (soft tissue pathology) and improved resolution dynamic studies.

Parallel This is the most common design for collimators in nuclear medicine since it does not distort the source shape with depth having a 1:1 magnification. Designs for high sensitivity (Fig.15.23(a)) and high resolution (b) cover all clinical applications.

Converging (Figure 15.23(c)) When a large field of view camera is the only one available in a nuclear medicine department a converging collimator is essential for providing practical sized images of small organs including the brain, single kidney or thyroid otherwise electronic zooming is the other option which will not improve image resolution which the converging collimator does.

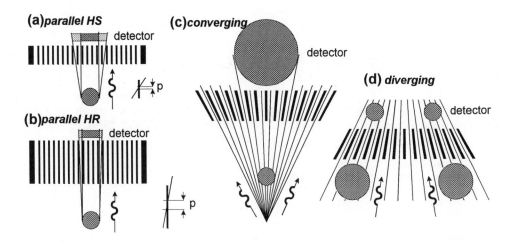

Figure 15.23 Two parallel hole collimators. **(a)** The high sensitivity (HS) gives a large penumbra (unsharpness). **(b)** The high resolution collimator has a greater depth and smaller penumbra. **(c)** A converging collimator magnifies the image in the focal plane. Since it is focused there is distortion with depth **(d)** the diverging collimator minifies the image. Septa penetration by the gamma photon. The angular thickness p increases with hole length.

It will give magnification of about 3:1 but unfortunately since it has a focal point it will give distortion with depth. The extreme version of the converging collimator is the pinhole collimator but this gives considerable distortion with depth and is difficult to align with the source and should be treated with the utmost caution.

Diverging This collimator design is the converse of the previous collimator: it minifies the image, as shown in Fig.15.23(d). This is useful if a small field of view camera is required to image both lungs or kidneys. It also gives distortion with depth which causes problems with large areas of anatomy.

15.8.3 Collimator efficiency

System sensitivity This is a measure of the ratio of count rate within the photopeak to the known activity of a source placed on the collimator and is commonly expressed as either counts per minute per μCi or counts per second per MBq. The conversion is cpm $\mu Ci^{-1} \times 0.45 = cps\ MBq^{-1}$. System sensitivity is influenced by collimator design and gamma spectrum. There is also a trade off between collimator sensitivity and resolution; they are inversely proportional to each other. Table 15.20 lists the properties of some modern commercial collimators using an hexagonal design. In general LEAP collimators have sensitivity figures from 86 to 180cps MBq^{-1}, LEHS from 180 to 290, LEHR from 51 to 145 and 'super' LEHR <60.

Collimator septa penetration Collimators for low energy radiation (^{201}Tl, ^{99m}Tc) are made of very thin lead. Septa penetration is not a problem and high resolutions can either be obtained by keeping the hole pattern the same and increasing the collimator depth (hole length) or maintaining a constant hole length but increasing the hole number (see second half of Tab.15.19). Increasing the collimator depth also increases the oblique angle p in Fig.15.23(a), (b) so high resolution collimators can have thinner septa with corresponding improvements in sensitivity for resolution.

Table 15.19 Collimator specifications for ^{99m}Tc, the source at three depths.

Type	FWHM at 5	10	20cm	cps/MBq	Septa pen. %
LEAP	6	9	15	148	0.8
LEHS	7	11	18	225	1.7
LEHR	5.5	8	13	103	0.4
LEHR(S)	5	6.6	10	63	0.2

Type	Hole #	Hole length mm	Septa thickness mm
LEHS	28	24	0.36
LEHR	148	24	0.16

Collimators for medium/ high energy radiation (^{111}In,^{131}I) suffer from septa penetration. The hole pattern is coarse and they give poor resolution. The thickness of lead separating the holes in a collimator depends on the energy of the gamma radiation being imaged. The septa thickness required to minimize penetration changes significantly over the energy ranges seen in nuclear medicine. Septa penetration makes the design of a high energy radiation collimators difficult since the hole pattern and septa thickness could have a worse impact on image quality than the septa penetration that is being minimized. Septa penetration can be generally expressed as the penetration fraction f_p

$$f_p = \frac{Photons\ penetrating\ septa}{Photons\ passing\ through\ holes} \quad (15.27)$$

As the absorption of radiation is exponential a certain amount of radiation always penetrates the septa. Table 15.19 shows that high resolution collimators (LEHR and LEHR(S))

have much lower septa penetration figures since the oblique photon has a longer pathway p than the LEHS. However because of their tighter scatter rejection the sensitivity (cps MBq^{-1}) decreases.

Further reading

National Electrical Manufacturers' Association 1986 Performance measurements of scintillation cameras NEMA NUI-1986 (NEMA Washington)

KEYWORDS

alpha-decay: nucleus loses 2 neutrons and 2 protons in the form of a helium nucleus

Bateman equation: describes parent:daughter decay in a radionuclide generator

beta-decay: the unstable nucleus loses a positive or negative beta particle.

collimator: a device which fits onto a probe or gamma camera accepting only gamma photons from a particular direction. Parallel hole gamma camera collimators only accept radiation perpendicular to the detector surface.

cyclotron: a charged particle accelerator where the beam travels in a circular path. Used for manufacturing short-lived positron emitters.

dead-time: the point at which measured count rates fall short of incident count rates for a detector.

electron cascade: the successive filling of empty orbit locations after electron loss leading to characteristic x-ray photons.

generator: a device for generating clinically useful daughter products from a long lived parent. i.e. ^{99}Mo/^{99m}Tc and ^{81}Rb/^{81m}Kr.

half-life (biological): the time taken for half the activity of a substance to be excreted.

half-life (effective): the sum of the biological and physical half-lives.

half-life (physical): the time taken for a given activity of a radionuclide to reach half its initial value. This is abbreviated to T½.

internal conversion: excess nuclear energy is transferred to a K or L shell electron. This is a competing process with gamma emission and reduces the incidence of gamma photon emission.

isobar: nuclides having a constant mass A (a constant) but varying proton Z and neutron N values. i.e. ^{201}Hg, ^{201}Tl, ^{201}Pb

isomeric transition: the decay of a metastable state yielding a single gamma photon only (pure gamma emitter). Isomers would be ^{99m}Tc and ^{99}Tc

isotone: nuclides with a constant neutron number N (a constant) but varying proton number. The stable isotones with N = 1 are ^2H and ^3H.

isotope: nuclides with the same proton number (Z constant) but different neutron numbers. The three stable isotopes of oxygen are ^{16}O, ^{17}O, ^{18}O. Radioactive isotopes would be ^{14}O (T½ 1.2m), ^{15}O (T½ 2m).

metastable state: a excited nuclear state existing after α or β decay lasting for seconds, minutes, hours or days. Sometimes called isomeric state. Indicated as $^{99}Tc^m$ or ^{99m}Tc.

moderator: a material used in nuclear reactors to slow down neutron velocities. Typical moderators are graphite or heavy water (D_2O).

neutron capture: slow and thermal neutron reaction of the form (n,γ) indicating gamma photon emission. A common method for preparing clinical nuclides i.e. ^{60}Co, ^{125}I

Non-uniformity (differential): percentage maximum difference between two adjacent pixels. Typical value ≤ ±1.5%

Non-uniformity (integral): the percentage difference between maximum and minimum pixel counts in a sampling area. Typical value ≤ ±2.0%.

nuclide: a specific nuclear species identified by the form $^A_ZX_N$ where A is the atomic mass, Z the proton number and N the neutron number. Consist of stable and unstable nuclides.

photopeak: the peak in an energy spectrum (e.g. scintillation detector) corresponding to complete photoelectric absorption.

positron: β+ the antiparticle to β⁻ or negatron (electron). The two mutually annihilate producing 180° opposed 0.511MeV gamma photons.

pulse height analyzer: an electronic circuit that can threshold the lower and upper limits of the photopeak energy and accept signals just within these limits.

radionuclide: an unstable nuclide

reactor: a critical assembly of fissile material (^{235}U, ^{239}Pu) capable of a sustained chain reaction.

resolution (energy): the FWHM dimension of a photopeak, the energy spread at this level expressed as a percentage of the peak energy. Typical value for a single NaI(Tl) detector would be 8%. A gamma camera value would be 11%

resolution (extrinsic): the spatial resolution of a gamma camera with the collimator in place. Measured in mm. Typical high resolution collimator gives 5mm FWHM.

resolution (intrinsic): the spatial resolution of a gamma camera with the collimator removed and using a line source. Typical value would be 3mm FWHM.

resolution (spatial): see extrinsic and intrinsic resolution.

secular equilibrium: a parent:daughter decay series where $\lambda_d \ggg \lambda_p$

transient equilibrium: a parent:daughter decay series where $\lambda_d > \lambda_p$.

16

Nuclear Medicine: Radiopharmaceuticals and Imaging equipment

16.1 Radiopharmaceuticals

16.2 Dosimetry

16.3 Planar imaging

16.4 Tomography: single photon emission (SPECT)

16.5 Tomography: positron emission (PET)

16.6 Comparison of other tomographic techniques

16.1 RADIOPHARMACEUTICALS

The parallel development of instrumentation and the chemistry of clinically useful isotopes has maintained nuclear medicine as a premier diagnostic imaging service. The distribution of labeled radiopharmaceuticals in the body allows imaging of organ function since these chemical substances are actively accumulated (i.e. MDP bone agents, liver colloid) or excreted (i.e. DTPA, EHIDA) by the target organ.

Although several radionuclides are available for nuclear medicine the predominant one is ^{99m}Technetium; it complies with most of the requirements for an ideal clinical isotope. It is generator produced which can be kept in the nuclear medicine radiopharmacy and renewed at weekly intervals. It is immediately available allowing a nuclear medicine clinic to offer a continuous service.

16.1.1 ^{99m}Tc Generator Specifications

Chapter 15 gave basic information on generator construction. The Technetium genertor used for routine nuclear medicine purposes is commonly eluted each morning; Fig.16.1 shows the decreasing activity of available ^{99m}Tc A in equilibrium with ^{99}Mo and eluted

^{99m}Tc over a 3 day period (curves B and C).

Partial elution of the generator gives high activity in a small volume which is useful for efficient labeling of small samples (white cells and complex molecules). Specific concentration for small volumes is plotted in Fig.16.2.

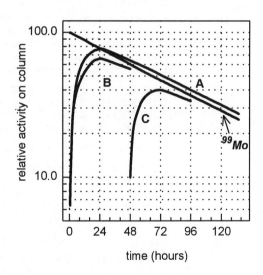

Figure 16.1   The straight line represents the ^{99}Mo decay (T½ 67h). Curve A is the ^{99m}Tc activity if the column is left undisturbed in equilibrium. ^{99m}Tc activity-time curves B and C reach a peak at about 23 hours after each elution.

Choice of the correct generator size is critical to the efficiency of a nuclear medicine department; if it is too small then not enough activity is available on a day-to-day basis, too large and it is unnecessarily expensive. Box 16.1 calculates a specific generator size using the decay constants for ^{99}Mo and ^{99m}Tc in Table 16.1, which gives both ^{99}Mo and ^{99m}Tc decay factors (bold integers). ^{99}Molybdenum decay factors (left most column) in days and ^{99m}Tc decay factors in hours with fractions of 15, 30 and 45 minutes. The calculation requires a knowledge of :

- Patient numbers over the working week
- The type of investigations to be performed and their scheduling.

The particular activities required in Box 16.1

require a standard generator of 3.7GBq (100mCi). Generators are sized according to their activity on a reference or calibration day; this is always quoted with their specification. Typical commercially available generator sizes for most nuclear medicine department patient requirements are:

2	3.7	7.4	11	15	18	**GBq**
50	100	200	300	400	500	**mCi**

Table 16.1 ^{99}Mo and ^{99m}Tc Decay Factors

Box. 16.1

Calculating suitable generator size

Choose the minimum size ^{99m}Tc generator that will fulfill the following requirements using ^{99}Mo and ^{99m}Tc decay factors in Table 16.1

1. Generator for use on Monday Morning
2. Generator referenced for 09:00 on following Thursday
3. Eluted once a day at 09:00.
4. On the Wednesday before reference day there should be activity for an 8 patient clinic requiring the following activities:

2 × 550MBq @ 09:30.	(Total 1166MBq eluted at 09:00)
2 × 550MBq @ 10:30	(Total 1309MBq eluted at 09:00)
2 × 75MBq @ 10:00	(Total 168MBq eluted at 09:00)
2 × 500MBq @ 14:00	(Total 1780MBq eluted at 09:00)

So total activity **4423MBq** required 09:00 on Wednesday

Size of generator: (see Tab. 16.1 ^{99}Mo Decay)
Reference Activity for Thursday at 09:00
$$4423 \times 0.78 \text{ (24h decay)} = 3449\text{MBq}$$
The minimum size of the Generator that will supply the Wednesday activities.

Using ^{99m}Tc decay factors (Table 16.1)

Available activities through the week are then:

Monday (R−3)	(3449 × 2.12)	= 7311MBq
Tuesday	(3449 × 1.66)	= 5725MBq
Wednesday	(3449 × 1.28)	= 4414MBq
Thursday	(Reference Day)	= 3449MBq
Friday (R+1)	(3449 × 0.78)	= 2690MBq

^{99}Mo	Period	^{99m}Tc	15 min.	30 min.	45 min.
Days		**Hours**			
3.45	-5	1.78	1.83	1.89	1.94
2.70	-4	1.59	1.63	1.68	1.73
2.12	-3	1.41	1.46	1.50	1.54
1.66	-2	1.26	1.30	1.33	1.37
1.28	-1	1.12	1.16	1.19	1.22
1.00	0	1.00	1.03	1.06	1.09
1.00	0	1.00	0.97	0.94	0.92
0.78	1	0.89	0.87	0.84	0.82
0.61	2	0.79	0.77	0.75	0.73
0.47	3	0.71	0.69	0.67	0.65
0.37	4	0.63	0.61	0.59	0.58
0.29	5	0.56	0.54	0.53	0.51

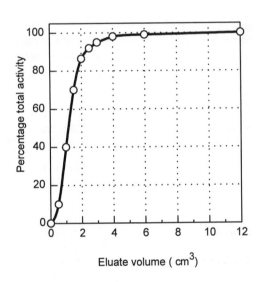

Figure 16.2 Activity in a small volume elution (partial elution) gives a high specific activity: $5cm^3$ contains approximately 90% of the available activity.

16.1.2 Oxidation states and labeling ^{99m}Tc

The chemistry of technetium involves seven oxidation or valency states. These are listed in Table 16.2 and play major roles in the labeling of radiopharmaceuticals.

The eluted technetium has an oxidation state of [VII] and must interact with a reducing agent (Sn^{++} stannous ion) in order to produce an oxidation state of [IV] which is necessary for radiopharmaceutical kit labeling. Other oxidation states are listed; some are important but others play a minor role in kit labeling. It is important to note that the reduced state of Tc[IV] is easily oxidized by atmospheric oxygen back to Tc[VII]; the labeled compound (DTPA, MAA, MDP etc.) becomes detached leaving free ^{99m}Tc which will concentrate in extraneous target organs (thyroid, stomach etc.).

Table 16.2 Technetium oxidation states

TECHNETIUM [I]
Exists in certain Organic Complexes :
$^{99m}Tc[I]$-(t-Butyl-isonitrile) $^{99m}Tc[I]$-MIBI
Good in-vivo stability

TECHNETIUM [II]   Not important

TECHNETIUM [III]
Compounds labeled with this undergo in-vivo reduction:
Tc[III] → Tc[II]   giving liver activity
Tc[III] may be the active form of ^{99m}Tc-HIDA

TECHNETIUM [IV]
This is the most stable state used for Kit preparation
Tc[VII] + 3 E++ → $^{99m}Tc[IV]$-KIT + 3 E+++
'E' is commonly Stannous ion (Sn++)
It oxidizes to: Tc[IV] + Oxygen → Tc[VII]
(see Tc[VII] below)

TECHNETIUM [V]
Modified reduction reaction increasing the pH produces this oxidation state. Mostly seen as $^{99m}Tc[V]$-DMSA for tumor targeting

TECHNETIUM [VI]   Not important

TECHNETIUM [VII]
This is the most stable oxidation state represented by the eluted technetium.
Labeled kits degrade to Tc[VII] with atmospheric or blood borne O_2 and disassociate producing free Tc[VII] with the pharmaceutical.

16.1.3   Radiopharmaceuticals

The properties of an ideal isotope for nuclear medicine imaging have already been described in Chapter 15. If ^{99m}Tc is accepted as a practical example of an ideal isotope (with some limitations) then the properties of an ideal radiopharmaceutical are listed in Tab. 16.3. Most of these points are satisfied by commercially available compounds and radiopharmaceuticals except the requirement for positive uptake in pathology (both liver colloid and lung MAA show pathology as a 'negative' uptake). Certain radiopharmaceuticals still need heating for optimum labeling (MAG3). All radiopharmaceuticals are non-toxic in the very low concentrations used although pediatric applications may need careful scrutiny.

Some radiopharmaceuticals used in routine applications and their typical activities for each adult study are listed in Table 16.4

Table 16.3   The ideal radiopharmaceutical

1. Easy labeling: single procedure
2. Short reaction time
3. Single target organ
4. Room temperature reconstitution: (no boiling water bath)
5. Useful reconstituted life.
6. Multiple patients per vial
7. Non toxic or allergic response
8. Good shelf life (unreconstituted)
9. Stable in-vivo (minimum free isotope)
10. Pathology seen as increased activity

Table 16.4   Radiopharmaceuticals in routine applications

Organ	Agent	Application	Activity (MBq)
Bone	MDP	Metastases	500-700
	HMDP	Fractures	
Brain	DTPA	Tumor	500-700
	HMPAO*	Perfusion	400-600
Cardiac	MIBI**	Myocardium	400 -600
	Pyrophosphate.	Infarct	400
Kidney	DTPA	GFR	75 - 100
	MAG3***	Function	120
	DMSA	Function	80 - 200
Lung	MAA	Perfusion	80 - 100
	Aerosols	Ventilation	40 - 60
Liver/Spleen	Colloid	Function	80 - 100
	EHIDA	Biliary	70 - 150
Bone marrow	Nano-Colloid ****	Metastases	200
Lymph	Nano-Colloid	Function	200-400
Whole body	HMPAO white cells	Infection	400-600
Whole body	Tc[V]-DMSA	Tumor sites	80 - 100

* Commercially available as Ceretec® (Amersham)
** Commercially available as Cardiolite® (DuPont)
***Commercially available as MAG3® (Mallinckrodt)
**** Commercially available as NanoColloid® (Solco)

16.1.4 Quality control

Tests for the in-vitro stability of labeled compounds should be carried out on a regular basis. Figure 16.3 shows a measuring cylinder fitted with a plastic sealing lid which is suitable for radiopharmaceutical quality control using chromatographic techniques.

A drop of the labeled radiopharmaceutical is placed onto a strip of absorbent gel (thin layer chromatography strips: Gelman Instrument Co.) approximately 0.5cm from the bottom. The gel-paper is carefully dried and placed upright in the solvent. For most ^{99m}Tc agents acetone is a suitable solvent. The cap is replaced to keep a saturated atmosphere in the container.

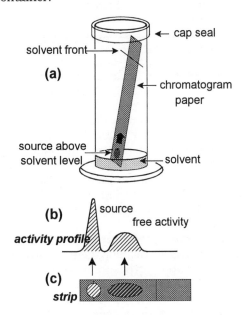

Figure 16.3 (a) Radiopharmaceutical quality control equipment consisting of a glass measuring cylinder holding a small volume of solvent. Detail of the activity profile (b) and the position of fractions on the thin-layer strip is shown (c).

The solvent front advances up the paper quite slowly and when it reaches almost to the top it is removed, dried, and placed on a gamma camera with a high resolution collimator (protecting this with a polythene sheet). A direct image is then obtained and activity profiles taken through the active areas on the strip. Alternatively the paper can be divided and each half counted using a well-scintillation counter. The quality control result gives a measure of:

- Bound ^{99m}Tc
- Free ^{99m}Tc (TcO$_4$)
- Hydrolyzed ^{99m}Tc (TcO$_2$)

Other radionuclides Radionuclides other than ^{99m}Tc have less than ideal properties but they have either specific targeting (^{67}Ga, ^{201}Tl), easier chemistry (^{123}I) or longer half lives for observing longer physiological phenomena (^{111}In). These are listed in Table 16.5.

16.2 DOSIMETRY

Radiation exposure to nuclear medicine staff and patients is generally much lower than investigations using conventional x-rays. Most radiation exposure to staff occurs in the radiopharmacy and with close handling of patients injected with high activities (i.e. bone and cardiac investigations). In most nuclear medicine studies patient exposure is highest for non-^{99m}Tc isotopes so these activity levels are carefully controlled as would be with, for example ^{201}Thallium and ^{131}Iodine.

16.2.1 External exposure

The limit for surface exposure levels in a controlled area from sealed sources is 7.5µSv h^{-1}. Exposure levels from giga-becquerel activities of common isotopes as specific gamma ray constants have already been introduced in Chapter 15.

External dose levels Shielding and storage of radioactive substances must conform to international regulations (ICRP, NRPB) and feature in the hospital local rules for radiation safety. Some suggested limits for surface doses and dose rates 5cm from the surface are:

Table 16.5   Other radionuclides and their applications

Nuclide	Half-life	γ–Energy(s) keV	Compound	Target tissue or application
^{67}Gallium	3.2 d	93, 185, 300	Citrate	Inflammatory lesions and tumor location
^{111}Indium	2.8 d	171, 245	Chloride DTPA	Biological labeling Cisternography
^{75}Selenium	120 d	136, 265, 280	nor-Cholesterol Methionine	Adrenal cortex Pancreas
^{201}Thallium	3.0 d	*68 - 82	Chloride	Myocardium
^{133}Xenon	5.3 d	81	Gas	Lung ventilation
^{127}Xenon	36 d	172, 203, 375	Gas	Lung ventilation
^{81m}Krypton	13 s	190	Gas	Lung ventilation
^{123}Iodine	13 h	159	Hippurate or MIBG	Kidney function Adrenal medulla

*x-rays

Surface activity	7.5µSv h^{-1}
5cm distance (long term storage)	0.2mSv h^{-1}
5cm distance (short-term storage)	2.0mSv h^{-1}

These levels are constantly revised; the most recent limits should be observed. In the USA the areas containing radiation-producing sources must be labeled according to their exposure levels. A **radiation area** is defined as an area accessible to staff where radiation levels could approach 50µSv h^{-1} at 30cm, either from the source itself or any surface that the radiation penetrates. A **high radiation area** is an area where radiation levels to staff could approach 1mSv h^{-1} at 30cm.

Generator shielding   Radiation levels from a medium size technetium generator would be:

- Unshielded core of 18.5GBq (500mCi) generator 6mSv h^{-1} at 0.5m
- For 7.5µSv h^{-1} this would require **6.8cm** Pb
  (HVL for ^{99}Mo 740keV γ 7mm Pb)
- A typical shielded core with 5.0cm Pb additional lead shielding 4.5cm Pb total lead shielding : 9.5cm Pb

The total shielding supplied by the manufacturer typically exceeds the minimum levels.

Syringe shielding   Lead or tungsten syringe shields of about 3mm thickness reduce finger and body doses by about ×200 from syringe activities. The dose rate from an unshielded vial containing 4GBq (100mCi) ^{99m}Tc would be 800µSv h^{-1} at 30cm; the suggested shielding is based on an HVL of 0.25mm Pb (140keV γ). To maintain a surface dose level of 7.5µSv h^{-1} it would require 1.67mm Pb. A typical vial lead-pot supplies 3mm to 10mm

Radiation dose from patients   Close proximity to nuclear medicine patients contributes to staff radiation exposure and reasonable distances should be kept (Table 16.6). As a consequence waiting rooms for patients who have received a radionuclide injection should be separate areas in the department.

Table 16.6 Staff exposure from patients

Nuclide	T½	Activity (MBq)	Exposure (µSv h^{-1} @ 1m)
^{67}Ga	78h	150	1.6
^{111}In	2.8d	80	2.4
^{99m}Tc	6.0h	800	6.0
^{131}I	8.0d	40	0.9
^{201}Tl	73h	80	0.3

The reduction of staff exposure from nuclear medicine patients can be significantly reduced by taking sensible precautions. Table 16.7 lists the reduction possible if certain safety measures are maintained.

Table 16.7 Radiation reduction from ^{99m}Tc study

Conditions	Exposure
Patient activity (^{99m}Tc)	800MBq (20mCi)
Exposure to staff at 30cm	160µSv h^{-1}
Exposure to staff at 1m	6µSv h^{-1}
Complete 15min study at 30cm	20µSv total
Complete 15min study at 60cm	5µSv total
Wearing 0.25mm Pb Apron	80µSv h^{-1} at 30cm
Natural radiation 2-5mSv y^{-1}	8 - 20µSv d^{-1}

Guidelines of activity limits for patients leaving hospital   Nuclear medicine offers a very useful out-patient service as the patient can normally be discharged. Certain precautions however should be observed depending on isotope and activity. Table 16.8 identifies **restricted** contact where the patient is likely to mix with children, so the activity levels are kept low. **No-restriction** applies where children are unlikely to be involved so the patient activity levels can be higher.

Patients should be given an instruction leaflet detailing contact with other people and appropriate action if clothing becomes contaminated.

Table 16.8 Patient activity levels.

Radionuclide	Restricted	No restriction
^{131}Iodine	30MBq	150MBq
^{99m}Tc	80MBq	400MBq

16.2.2   Internal dosimetry

In order to maintain the patient radiation dose within acceptable limits various procedures have been developed for estimating dose to the patient from internally administered isotopes and radiopharmaceuticals.

Marinelli formula   This was an early attempt at calculating internal dosimetry estimating organ and whole body radiation dose from beta, non-penetrating radiation D_β and gamma D_γ penetrating radiation. It uses a rough geometric factor g allowing for simple variations in organ shape (liver, lungs, kidney etc.).

$$D_\beta = 21 \times C \times E_\beta \times T_e \qquad \text{mSv} \qquad (16.1)$$
$$D_\gamma = 0.3225 \times C \times \Gamma \times g \times T_e \quad \text{mSv} \qquad (16.2)$$

Where T_e is the effective T½ in days, Γ in mSv GBq^{-1} h^{-1} at 1m (the gamma ray constant) and C is the percentage of activity retained by the target organ. E_β is the mean beta energy and the constants 21 and 0.3225 express D_β and D_γ as mSv. Box 16.2 calculates the radiation dose from a ^{99m}Tc-Liver colloid study using eqns. 16.1 and 16.2.

The limitations of the Marinelli method are:

- The geometry factor g only covers simple spheroids which do not relate to real organ shapes.
- No allowance is given for radiation exposure to adjacent organs from the target organ (liver or bladder to uterus, etc.)
- Unequal distribution of the tracer within the target organ cannot be included or distribution times within the organ.

MIRD formula   A more accurate approach to internal dosimetry was proposed by the Medical Internal Radiation Dose (MIRD) Committee in the USA. The MIRD technique:

- Groups both penetrating and non-penetrating radiations together.
- Considers biological and physical data regarding distribution and resident time

Box 16.2

Marinelli example

A liver investigation uses 74MBq (2mCi) ^{99m}Tc-Colloid. 85% is trapped and its weight is 1.8 kg.

$$C = \frac{total\ activity \times fraction\ absorbed}{weight\ of\ organ}$$

The radiation dose to the liver from Auger electrons and gamma photons (eqns.16.1 and 16.2) where T_e is 6h and Γ is 0.017:

$$D_\beta = 21 \times \frac{74 \times 0.85}{1.8} \times 0.016 \times 0.25$$

$$= 2.9mSv$$

$$D_\gamma = 0.3225 \times \frac{74 \times 0.85}{1.8} \times 0.017 \times 50 \times 0.25$$

$$= 2.39mSv$$

The total dose to the Liver is **5.29mSv**

Box 16.3

MIRD example

The same details as given in Box 16.2 but using eqn.16.3

$$\bar{D}\ Liver = A_o \tau\ S$$

Where:
The activity (A_o) is still 74MBq
Calculated resident time $\tau = 0.85/\lambda = 7.4$ h.

Non-SI example:
The S value in rad mCi^{-1}h^{-1} = 4.6 ×10^{-5}
$$\bar{D}\ Liver = 2000 \times 7.4 \times 4.6 \times 10^{-5}$$
$$= 0.68\ rad$$

SI example:
The S value in Gy MBq^{-1} s^{-1} = 1.2 ×10^{-5}
$$\bar{D}\ Liver = 74 \times (1.2 \times 10^{-5}) \times 7.4$$
$$\mathbf{= 6.57mGy}$$

NB
This is a higher value than the Marinelli result in Box 16.2

- The irradiation of adjacent organs by the target organ.

Dose calculations can be solved for:

- Radio-tracers that accumulate mostly in one organ (liver colloid, lung perfusion)
- Tracers that are distributed in a number of organs (vascular, hepatobiliary system)
- Time varying distribution (bolus studies)
- Dose variations to selected organs (the bladder depending on voiding frequency)

The parameters used in the MIRD formula (eqn.16.3) are listed in Table 16.9. Absorbed dose per unit of administered activity is therefore:

$$\bar{D} = A_o \tau\ S \qquad (16.3)$$

Where

$$\tau = \frac{fraction\ retained\ by\ organ}{\lambda} \qquad (\lambda = \frac{0.693}{6.02})$$

A simple example is used in Box 16.3 to recalculate the liver investigation of Box 16.2

Contribution to other organs and irradiation of other organs would complete the dose calculation i.e.:

- Contribution from the spleen to the total liver dose: Spleen → D_∞ Liver
- Contribution from the skeleton to the total liver dose: Bone → D_∞ Liver
- Dose to specific organs from the liver: Liver → D_∞ Uterus

Since organ to organ radiation exposure values can be incorporated into the formula the MIRD dose rate is higher than the Marinelli formula. Other organs such as the spleen and bone marrow can also be included into the overall dose to the patient, a factor which is missing in other calculations.

Limitations Although the MIRD calculations have solved a number of problems, there can be large uncertainty in some of the calculated parameters e.g. absorbed fraction.

The coefficient of variation (a measure of uncertainty for the radiation dose) can be as much as 20-50% in some cases. Other weaknesses are:

- Models for certain organs, such as the kidney do not allow for cortex and medulla
- Bone marrow is not well represented.
- The MIRD formula assumes a uniform distribution of activity within any organ, which is not always the case (i.e. transit of DTPA in the kidney, gas clearance in the lung).

Patient dose reduction   When deciding radionuclide activities used for clinical studies the following points should be considered:

- Good counting statistics in laboratory tests (GFR etc.)
- A diagnostic image in a reasonable time.
- Acceptable radiation dose to the patient from the target organ and excretion pathway.
- Cost of expensive isotopes (^{123}Iodine, ^{111}Indium)

The common activity levels used for various studies are listed in Table 16.20 at the back of this chapter. The activities listed in MBq give optimal results (best counting statistics or image quality) the ranges of whole body dose (H_E) given by ^{99m}Tc-DTPA, MDP, EDTA etc. are due to variations in bladder retention/voiding times. World Health Organization (WHO) category groups approximate low, medium and high radiation dose rates. As a

comparison with conventional x-ray investigations a urogram using iodine contrast materials will give:

Ovarian dose	30mSv
Bladder wall dose	43mSv
Whole-body dose (typical)	30mSv

The patient radiation dose from nuclear medicine studies are therefore much lower than the equivalent functional radiology investigation and incidentally far less invasive.

16.2.3 Pediatric exposure

The injected activity level for determining adult radiation dose usually depends on the weight and age of the patient. Guidelines are given on the radiopharmaceutical package insert for a standard man. There are several different multiplication factors used for obtaining children's doses from the adult dose including:

1. Body surface area (BSA) $\div 1.73$
2. Child's age + 1 divided by age + 7 years
3. Child's weight divided by 70kg
4. Child's height divided by 174cm

For static studies multiplication factors based on 1, 2 and 3 are used. For dynamic studies where imaging time and image quality is of primary importance factor 4 is recommended.

Table 16.9 MIRD symbol definition.

Parameter	Symbol	Non-SI	SI
Activity	A_o	$1mCi = 3.7 \times 10^4 Bq$	$1MBq = 27.03mCi$
Absorbed dose	D	$1rad = 10mGy$	$1Gy = 100rad$
Mean dose	$\overline{D}$	same	same
Mean dose per unit of cumulated activity	S	$\dfrac{rad}{\mu Ci.h}$	$\dfrac{Gy}{MBq.s}$
Residence time	τ	hour	

Box 16.4 gives an example of each for the same child size. Doses should be increased for 'large-for-age' children.

Box 16.4

Children's injected activity

An example for a 6 year, 20kg, 110cm child using an agent having a 200MBq adult activity. Using the multiplication factors given in the text the injected activity for this child would be:

Factor 1.   BSA* = 0.77/1.73   89MBq
Factor 2.   (7/13) will give   107MBq.
Factor 3.   (20/70) will give   57MBq
Factor 4.   (110/174) will give   126MBq

* Body Surface Area formula where Weight (kg) Height (cm) is $W^{0.425} \times H^{0.725} \times 0.0072$ m^2

$$= 0.77 \text{ m}^2 \text{ for this child.}$$

Most radio nuclides used for nuclear medicine investigations are concentrated in breast milk (^{131}Iodine and ^{99m}Tc particularly). A neonate thyroid gland can receive a high radiation dose from these nuclides in the mother's milk therefore either nuclear medicine investigations should be avoided or the mother instructed to bottle feed after the investigation for a suitable period. Over 90% of the ^{99m}Tc activity appears in the breast milk over 24 hours and breast feeding can continue after this term. The trauma imposed on the child and mother by restricting contact should be seriously weighed against the radiation risk.

16.2.4   Radiopharmacy

The management of radioactive materials is governed by local, national and international regulations. The following recommendations are based on ICRP and IAEA reports detailed at the end of this chapter.

The classification of a laboratory space for a radiopharmacy depends on the expected workload and the isotopes used (Group type). Table 16.10 lists the maximum activity levels that each radiopharmacy class should carry at any one time. Most radiopharmacies would be classified as medium, where the majority of work uses ^{99m}Tc for imaging (as the Group 4 isotope), with small quantities of Group 2 and 3 isotopes.

High levels of ^{99}Mo (Group 2) contained in the ^{99m}Tc generator would require a separate location classified as a high radiation or controlled area. Suggested requirements would be:

- Isolated from radiopharmacy
- Dispensing bench shielded with 3cm lead bricks
- Barrier essential (door)
- 10m^2 minimum area
- Hand monitoring (large area counter)
- Room monitoring (wall mounted TLD's)

A fume hood and extractor fan would not be essential since this radionuclide is not volatile. Disposable rubber-gloves should always be used for preventing hand contamination. The radiopharmacy would also be treated as a **controlled area** and available access restricted to designated staff only.

Disposal of radioactive waste   Radioactive waste may be identified as:

- Decayed sealed sources
- Spent Radio-nuclide generators (^{99m}Tc, ^{81m}Kr, ^{185m}Au etc.)
- Laboratory solutions of low activity
- Low activity liquid washings from vials
- Liquid scintillants immiscible with water
- Biologically contaminated solid waste i.e. syringes, vials.
- Radioactive gases.

Table 16.10 Classification of nuclear medicine laboratories in terms of activity areas (ICRP 25)

Classification	Low	Medium	High
Group 2 nuclides ^{125} and ^{131}Iodine	<500kBq	500k-500MBq	500MBq-5GBq
Group 3 nuclides ^{51}Cr,^{32}P,^{99}Mo,^{201}Tl	<5MBq	5M-5GBq	**5GBq-500GBq
Group 4 nuclides ^{99m}Tc,^{133}Xe	<500MBq	*500MBq-500GBq	500GBq-50TBq

* Supervised Areas
** Generator Room

Table 16.11 Discharged activity limits Bq (µCi)

Classification	No control	Controlled
GROUP 1	Not used	Not used
GROUP 2		
^{125}I, ^{131}I	5×10^4 Bq (1.4µCi) (USA 1.0µCi)	1×10^7 Bq (270µCi) (USA10.0µCi)
GROUP 3		
^{201}Tl, ^{32}P, ^{67}Ga, ^{51}Cr, ^{111}In, ^{57}Co, ^{58}Co, ^{99}Mo, ^{90}Y	5×10^5 Bq (14µCi) (USA10.0µCi)	5×10^6 Bq (140µCi) (USA 100µCi)
GROUP 4		
^{99m}Tc, ^{133}Xe	5×10^6 Bq (140µCi) (USA 100µCi)	5×10^7 Bq (1.4mCi) (USA 1mCi)

Each of these requires special consideration since biological contamination (e.g. blood) may be a more serious hazard. Accepted levels for disposal of radioactive waste under controlled and non-controlled conditions are given in Table 16.11; activities are given in becquerels (µCi in brackets).

Controlled disposal is defined as disposal with permission from the regulatory authority (government or state body). Records should be kept listing initial activities and recommended disposal dates for medium and long half-life nuclides. ^{99m}Tc waste should be kept for an appropriate decay period before disposal (24 hours); no records are normally required for decayed ^{99m}Tc contaminated items.

Exhausted ^{99m}Tc generators A 12.5GBq (345mCi) ^{99}Mo generator core decays to 5×10^6Bq after 31 days so could undergo disposal under controlled conditions with proper authorization. Spent generators awaiting disposal should be removed to a separate storeroom or bunker for the requisite decay period. Shielding should be provided so that exposure does not exceed 7.5µSv h^{-1}.

Patient waste Special toilets should be available to nuclear medicine patients. The toilet should have direct access to the sewage system and should not run under the nuclear medicine department since high activities will affect the performance of counters and imaging devices by increasing background activity levels. Patient excreta are exempt from disposal restrictions. Urine and feces should be discharged using a toilet connected directly to a main sewer. Legislation exists which governs the handling, use, storage, administration, disposal and transportation of isotopes and labeled radiopharmaceuticals. Local regulations and codes of practice should be consulted.

Transport of radioactive material Certain conditions have been defined by the International Atomic Energy Authority (IAEA) for the packaging and transport of radioactive material. They include a transport index which is the maximum dose rate at a distance of 1m from the package surface in µSv divided by 10. These Transport indices are indicated on the three types of package label given in Table 16.12. The package category depends on both the transport index and the surface radiation level. An example label is shown in Fig.16.4.

Table 16.12 Package category

Category label	Surface dose $\mu Sv\ h^{-1}$	Transport index
I White Low level	5	0
II Yellow Moderate level	5-500	$\leqslant 1$
III Yellow High level	500-2000	1-10

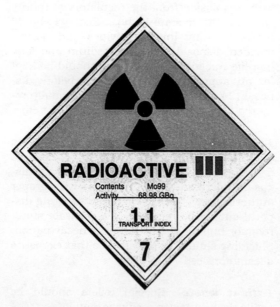

Figure 16.4 An identifying label used on the transportation packaging of radioactive materials. The three types of labels are listed in Tab.16.12

16.3   PLANAR IMAGING

Nuclear medicine planar images represent a volume activity so the activity from overlying tissue degrades image contrast from pathology within the organ volume. Circulating activity (blood) also adds background noise and also obscure pathology. Planar examples routinely collected in nuclear medicine are liver images (oncology), lung images (pulmonary embolism), DMSA (kidney function) and myocardial activity (^{201}Thallium).

16.3.1   Static planar

This is the conventional procedure for following radiopharmaceutical distribution. Image acquisition normally provides anterior, posterior and several lateral views with oblique views.

Table 16.13 lists common collimator types and their application for planar clinical studies. High sensitivity collimators are used where count rate is more important than resolution (moving organs i.e. lungs, or dynamic studies). High resolution gives best detail (bone). Converging gives magnified, detailed images but gives depth distortion.

Table 16.13 Collimator selection

Collimator	Application
Low Energy (^{99m}Tc ^{201}Tl ^{123}I) High sensitivity,	Planar lungs, planar myocardium, dynamic renography, MIBG adrenals.
All purpose (LEAP)	Planar liver pediatric ^{81m}Kr lungs.
High Resolution	SPECT brain, SPECT heart, planar DMSA kidney.
Converging (magnification)	Planar brain, planar thyroid
Medium Energy (^{111}In, ^{67}Ga) All purpose	labeled white cells, tumor marking
High energy (^{131}I and positron emitters) All purpose	thyroid metastases, PET (non-coincidence)

matrices, assuming a required visible contrast difference 1.5 times the background activity. In order to maintain the noise equivalent of 6% seen in 64×64 matrix (1), the total counts collected must increase for the 3 matrix sizes in (2) and (3); note the increased time necessary for a 256×256 matrix. **Time equivalent noise** is the increased time that must be spent to achieve the same noise content of the reference matrix (64×64 pixels) for a fixed value of radioactivity given; for 256×256 this is ×16.

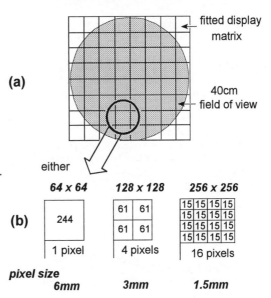

Figure 16.5 Three sizes of matrix 64×64, 128×128 and 256×256, each holding a total of 1 million counts. The individual pixel count is given for the 3 matrix sizes along with the pixel size.

Matrix size The gamma camera image is commonly represented as a matrix; common matrix sizes are 64×64, 128×128 and 256×256. It is recommended, for visual acuity, that the displayed pixel size should be smaller than the data pixel size and 256×256 would be used for displaying static images from present day gamma cameras; 64 gray levels seems optimum. Figure 16.5 illustrates three examples used in Box 16.5 where a circular field-of-view, holding a uniform 10^6 counts, is digitized to 64×64, 128×128 and 256×256 matrices. There is a drop in individual pixel counts for the same total count. Pixel depth would be 8-bits (256 decimal) although for clinical studies with high count rates 16-bits would prevent data overflow in a 64×64 matrix.

Noisy images will result if the pixel count density is not sufficient as Box 16.5 demonstrates, for 64×64, 128×128, and 256×256

The time taken to acquire a reasonably diagnostic image is a critical factor in a busy nuclear medicine department with a large patient load. A suggested maximum patient load for a single gamma camera facility taking static images would be about six to eight patients per day depending on study type. Beyond this a second camera should be considered or a multi-head camera installed. Speeding up image acquisition by increasing injected activity is usually not acceptable due to patient radiation dose restrictions.

Box 16.5

Matrix size and noise

Conditions:

Matrix size M and count density N from Fig.16.5. FOV 38cm, pixel size $380/M$

Pixel noise = $\sqrt{N}$

Visible Contrast Difference = $1.5 \times \sqrt{N}$

1) 64 × 64 matrix

(This is the **equivalent noise** reference)

Pixel Size	= 6mm
Events per pixel	= 244
Noise	= $\sqrt{244}$ = 6%
ΔContrast limit	= $1.5 \times \sqrt{244}$ = 10%
Total counts	= **1 million**

Collimator Used : High Sensitivity

Suggested Applications:

Renography, lung, cardiac (^{201}Tl). SPECT. MUGA, ^{111}In white cell, ^{67}Ga tumor/infection study

2) 128×128 matrix

Pixel Size	= 3mm
Events per pixel	= 61 Noise = 12.5%
ΔContrast limit	= 20% difference
Total counts (Equivalent Noise)	= **4 million**

Collimator Used : High Sensitivity LEAP

Suggested Application:

Liver, cardiac (^{99m}Tc Agent). MUGA, white cell (^{99m}Tc label)

3) 256×256 matrix

Pixel Size	= 1.5mm
Events per pixel	= 15 Noise = 25%
ΔContrast limit	= 40% difference
Total counts (Equivalent Noise)	= **16 million**

Collimator Used High Resolution LEHR

Suggested Application:

Bone detail, vascular blood pool, ^{99m}Tc-RBC intestinal blood loss, kidney DMSA

Contrast and resolution Both contrast and resolution in a nuclear medicine image depends on whether the lesion shows as a negative or positive uptake, e.g. pulmonary

emboli and liver metastases are identified as negative uptakes, a bony metastasis as a positive uptake. Figure 16.6 demonstrates that a 'cold' or negative lesion has a limited range whereas a positive uptake has no theoretical limit. As a consequence only large sized negative lesions are visible whereas very 'hot' lesions can be quite small.

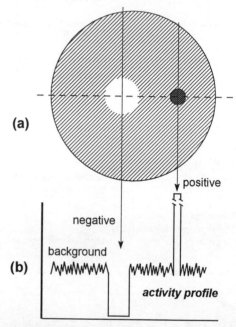

Figure 16.6 The detectability of a negative uptake or 'hole' compared to a positive uptake or 'hot-spot'. The contrast difference is limited for negative uptakes and sensitivity for hole detection is dependent on image background noise (high count density required) and size of lesion.

The imaging chain Figure16.7 shows a gradual degradation of contrast as the data passes through the imaging sequence. A general equation describing the low count difference detectability ΔC for a known signal S and background activity B uses the signal to noise ratio S/B :

$$\Delta C = \gamma \log \left(1 + \frac{S}{B}\right) \qquad (16.4)$$

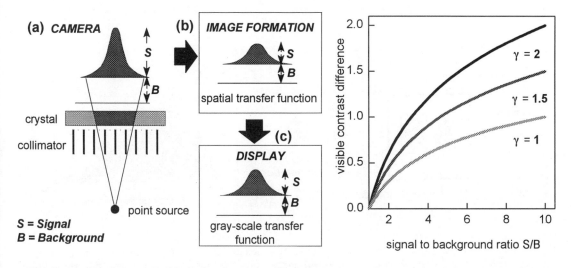

Figure 16.7 Loss of visible contrast through the imaging chain from (**a**) the gamma camera detector through to (**b**) image formation and then (**c**) the display system. The general eqn.16.4 describes low contrast detectability and the plot of contrast differences in (**d**) uses different γ values. Gamma is a measure of response to count density change; a color display would have a high gamma value.

For the imaging chain in Fig.16.7 the signal is high at the detector (a) but digitization (b) reduces *S:B* which can be improved slightly by using emphasis in the display (c) such as a color scale.

The display contrast is demonstrated in Fig. 16.7(d) where increased display contrast shows that small count differences (*y*-axis) are more easily seen with a high signal to background ratio and high contrast (γ values). A color display gives a higher contrast than a gray-scale and film contrast will also play a significant role.

16.3.2 Dynamic planar

Dynamic studies almost always use high activities of 99mTc labeled agents. Rapidly changing distributions of this radionuclide (kidney studies) or moving organs (heart) can be captured as a sequence of image frames (frame mode).

The kidney renogram, as an example, usually is a series of at least 60 image frames (byte mode 64×64), each frame taking between 10 and 20 seconds. Multiphase studies are possible where the fast vascular phase of the bolus through the kidney is captured at 0.5 or 1.0s intervals for say 30 frames then the clearance phase is captured at a slower 10s frame rate, ending with the excretion phase of 60 frames at 20 seconds per frame.

Very rapid sequences can be captured in list mode where the individual counts (coded for positional information) are stored directly in memory or disk and are reconstructed into matrices after the study. Matrix timing (0.5s 5.0s 30s etc.) can be chosen after the study, unlike frame collection. Table 16.14 lists common protocols for frame mode dynamic studies.

Regions of Interest (ROIs) Regions of Interest are used for identifying whole organs (kidneys) or specific regions (lung transit studies). Having selected a single or series of

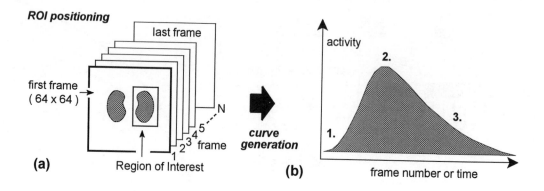

Figure 16.8   **(a)** A dynamic study showing several frames and a single ROI placed over the organ (kidney) which gives a time/activity curve in **(b)**. Point 1. on the curve marks the injection time. Point 2. shows peak activity and 3. indicates wash-out.

ROIs the computer program then sums all the counts over these regions for all the frames collected in the study (see Fig.16.8(a)) The results are then presented as a time/activity curve which is the renogram shown in (b).

Table 16.14   Dynamic protocols

Study	Frame Rate	Activity
Fast		
Lung Transit (vascular)	100 at 0.5s	800MBq
Kidney Transit (vascular)		
Medium		
Renography (vascular)	30 at 5s	100MBq
Renography (excretion)	60 at 20s	
Slow		
Gastric Emptying	60 at 60s	40MBq

ROIs can cause major problems since the organ itself represents a 3-dimensional volume source over which the 2-dimensional ROI area is placed for quantification. This is not serious in the case of homogeneous organs (liver, lung) but can cause errors in non-uniform distributions (heart, brain).

16.3.3 First pass and gated acquisition cardiac studies

The problem of capturing the motion of the moving heart and measuring wall motion and ejection fraction can be solved by either:

- A first pass bolus study
- Gating the cardiac cycle

First pass bolus study   This involves collecting fast dynamic frames while a bolus is in transit through the major heart chambers. Figure 16.9(a) represents a time activity curve for a 'first-pass-study', showing the swings between end diastole and end systole. The LV mean point is used to calculate Left Ventricular Fraction (LVEF). A normal value would be 30 to 50%

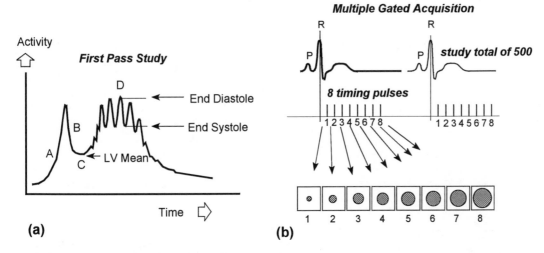

(a)

(b)

Figure 16.9 **(a)** A representation of a first pass bolus study showing (A) bolus entry into the right ventricle (B) wash-out from right ventricle (C) pulmonary activity (D) left ventricular peak activity with end-systole and end-diastole. **(b)** The timing sequence for a multi-gated acquisition (MUGA) study. In this example eight cardiac images are stored in computer memory representing a phase of the cardiac cycle. About 500 QRS events are required for a complete study.

Cardiac gating The data acquisition is gated with the ECG (EKG) giving a multiple gated acquisition (MUGA). Figure 16.9(b) shows how the image count data from the gamma camera is steered by the timing pulses (1 to 8 for simplicity) from the ECG, into the 8 image matrices (64×64) initiated by each QRS complex. About 500-600 QRS events are necessary to give a good series of diagnostic quality images.

In practice between 14 and 32 frames are collected. Irregular timing due to ectopic heart beats leads to data steering problems in MUGA programs but a certain amount of ectopic rejection tolerance is built into the program and gated list-mode acquisition can overcome errors associated with ectopic beats by rejecting these count data when reformatting.

The first pass dynamic acquisition gives information on both left and right heart ejection fractions which is not usually available in gated studies.

16.4 TOMOGRAPHY: SINGLE PHOTON EMISSION (SPECT)

The first Single Photon Emission Computed Tomography (SPECT) images were obtained in the early 1960's using separate scanning detectors (David Kuhl USA); this was before the development of x-ray computed tomography. In the 1980's improvements to gamma camera design (field uniformity) confirmed these as the tomographic machines of choice, since they gave multiple slices in multiple orientations (axial, saggital, coronal and oblique sectional views).

SPECT has many advantages, perhaps the main one being the separation of overlapping interference that is the problem on planar views. By removing overlying background activity image contrast can be significantly improved. Figure 16.10 illustrates how contrast can be improved by viewing separate slices rather than a volume source given by the planar image.

In this example the differences between planar image counts of 420, 450 and 400 would only just be visible (1.5×√400 = 30) but pixel differences in the separate slices would be easily visible (1.5×√100 = 15).

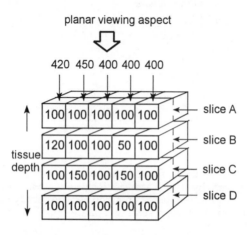

planar viewing aspect

420 450 400 400 400

| | | | | | |
|100|100|100|100|100| ← slice A |

tissue depth

120	100	100	50	100	← slice B
100	150	100	150	100	← slice C
100	100	100	100	100	← slice D

Figure 16.10   The improvement in image contrast possible with tomographic sectioning. A planar view of this volume distribution of activity (420, 450, 400, 400, 400 in arrow direction), however separate slices will indicate the obscured contrast differences.

16.4.1   Principles of operation

Single head rotating gamma camera tomographic systems are mounted on special gantries that allow the detector head to rotate 360° around the patient (Fig.16.11(a)). The camera takes a series of images at equal angular spacing called projections during its rotational movement. The detector usually stops at each projection during data collection using a step-and-shoot mode. Either a complete 360° or partial 180° rotation can be chosen. Image quality is improved by reducing the camera/patient distance so elliptical or non-circular orbits which follow patient contours improve image quality. Improvement in sensitivity can be significantly increased by using a 2 or 3 head camera (Fig.16.11(b)).

Dedicated systems   These use multiple fixed-detectors and have been exclusively developed for head scanning, giving single or multi-slice axial images. They have superior resolution to the rotating gamma camera but are restricted to axial tomographic planes. Some designs have 4 banks each of 16 NaI(Tl) detectors. The entire array rotates giving 40 projections in 180° rotation; this takes about 5 seconds and 3 slices are usually obtained simultaneously.

16.4.2   Machine requirements

Machine performance is critical for acceptable SPECT images. Careful choice of acquisition programs for each organ study is necessary before embarking on a clinical study.

Step-and-Shoot   versus   Continuous Data Collection   There are two methods for collecting data from a rotating gamma camera

- **Step and shoot**   The camera steps around the patient, (stops to collect counts over a fixed time), then moves to the next projection and collects count data. It progresses around the patient until a full 360° (or 180°) data set has been collected. The data consists of 64 or 128 separate image matrices (size 64×64 or 128×128) which represent each projection.

- **Continuous rotation**   The camera moves continuously collecting count data as it rotates for a complete 360°.

Angular sampling   This is determined by the resolution of the camera system. For gamma cameras with resolutions of 5-10mm equivalent to a spatial frequency of $1cm^{-1}$ then the sampling frequency should be at least 2 cm^{-1}. An angular sampling interval of 3° should be maintained (120 projections). When a full 360° coverage has been made using an inadequate number of views the data distortion shows as image streaking due to aliasing problems. A sampling interval greater than 5° gives aliasing artifacts due to insufficient sampling points.

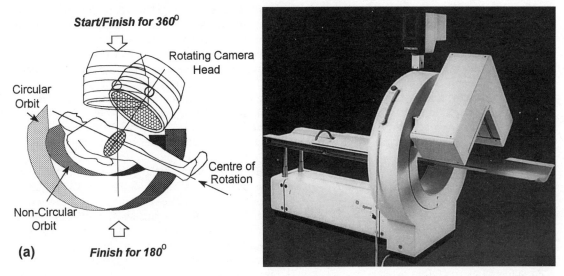

Figure 16.11 **(a)** A single head rotating camera SPECT system using either a complete 360° or 180° collection. Circular and non-circular rotation is represented and the center of rotation. **(b)** commercially available dual head SPECT system showing V opposed detectors for cardiac studies (courtesy GE Medical Inc.).

Step-and-shoot uses a considerable proportion of the scan time moving the camera between data acquisition points and waiting for the head to come to rest before collecting count data. Continuous rotation causes image blurring but as SPECT resolution is 10-15mm (at best), the blurring on a 64 projection 360° study is not significant. The speed of acquisition is much improved.

Center of rotation (COR) If a parallel hole collimator is positioned around an object first at 0° then at 90° and again at 180° then 270° the collimator at 0° should exactly align with the 180° position and again at 90° and 270°. The cells of the reconstructed matrix will then exactly coincide and a point source at the center of camera rotation will be situated exactly at the matrix center. In practice there is always a slight misalignment due to mechanical errors and corrections must be made for this off-set error. Camera SPECT phantoms are available that allow COR to be identified before data collection.

Non circular orbits The patient in cross section is essentially ellipsoid so that the distance between the camera face and the patient will vary drastically with a circular camera orbit. Resolution deteriorates with distance, so the resulting tomographic image will show unsharpness. Non-circular orbits, illustrated in Fig.16.11(a) and Fig.16.12(a), can be achieved by either moving the detector in an elliptical path or by moving the table towards and away from the camera face while the camera itself traces a circular orbit. With the moving table technique image reconstruction is simpler than with elliptical orbiting of the camera head.

360° or 180° acquisition Most SPECT imaging procedures collect data from a full 360° orbit. Cardiac studies however lend themselves to 180° data collection since the heart is partially shielded by the liver on the right side; this organ contributes a high activity particularly with ^{99m}Tc heart agents. Collecting data over 180° can save substantial time and improve image contrast; the camera can also be kept closer to the heart. Incomplete sampling can introduce artifacts and in the case of cardiac studies reduce information from the posterior wall of the ventricle.

Uniformity This is most important in
SPECT imaging since a central non-
uniformity of 3% can generate SPECT errors
of 30%. Accurate non-uniformity correction
must be applied before data collection, and
measured for each collimator used. The reason for high count densities in the uniformity
measurement is explained in Box.16.6 and in
order to achieve the necessary accuracy when
using a 64×64 matrix a total of 30 million
counts must be collected.

Box 16.6

SPECT field uniformity QC

Matrix count density and noise.

For a 64×64 matrix (4096 pixels)

   5 million total counts gives 1220/pixel
   $\sqrt{pixel} = 35$ 3% variation

   10 million total counts gives 2441/pixel
   $\sqrt{pixel} = 49$ 2% variation

   30 million total counts gives 7324/pixel
   $\sqrt{pixel} = 85$ 1% variation

NB A 30 million count density image matrix
gives a noise figure suitable for SPECT calibration.

16.4.3 Machine performance and image quality

The resolution given by SPECT images is
worse than planar, due to count limitation,
however contrast levels are much improved.

Resolution This is simply measured by using a thin line source parallel to the image
plane and measuring the Full Width at Half
Maximum (FWHM) from this or the MTF (see
Chapter 8). Resolution measurements should
be taken at different distances from the detector face(s).

Variable spatial resolution SPECT gives
non-uniformity of resolution with depth; this

is illustrated in Fig.16.12(b). Positron emission tomography has a uniform resolution
across the detector field of view (c).

The loss of SPECT resolution with depth
using two collimator types (general purpose
and high resolution) is plotted in Fig.16.13(a)
and emphasizes the value of the high resolution collimator if resolution is to be maintained. A double headed SPECT system reduces this resolution loss still further.

SPECT contrast Using an asymmetric window over the photo-peak set at 135-160keV
improves the image contrast by between 5
and 20% by decreasing scatter events. There
are problems however with computing the
attenuation correction for asymmetric windows which leads to additional image non-
uniformity.

Different composite phantoms can be used for
pictorial displays of both resolution and contrast performance. A typical QC phantom,
drawn in Fig.16.13(b), has a series of hollow
and solid rods of various diameters placed
within a cylindrical plastic container filled
with about 400MBq ^{99m}Tc. The hollow rods
can be filled with varying activities of ^{99m}Tc
and give low contrast information.

Slice thickness This can be measured by
using a known dimension grid source. The
minimum slice thickness will be determined
by the camera resolution. Thin slices will
have maximum noise so image quality can be
improved by choosing an optimum slice
thickness before reconstruction or summing
slices together after reconstruction.

Choosing a large slice thickness will reduce
image contrast and increase partial volume
effects (see Chapter 14). Since the resolution
of a parallel hole collimator decreases with
distance the reconstructed slice thickness increases toward the center of rotation; multi-
head camera SPECT designs reduce this effect.

SPECT sensitivity This is defined as
counts per second per MBq and is measured
by imaging a 20cm diameter cylindrical water
phantom containing about 400MBq ^{99m}Tc. It

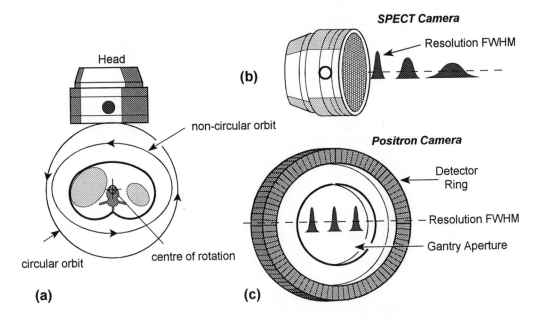

Figure 16.12   (**a**) Circular and non-circular orbit showing how the non-circular data acquisition closely follows body contours. (**b**)   Comparison between SPECT and (**c**) PET for resolution with depth. A PET scanner maintains uniform resolution with depth.

is important to quote the total number of axial slices being collected. Step-and-shoot systems show the poorest sensitivity, since they are not collecting count data between projections. Long scan times using step and shoot improve sensitivity since more time is spent acquiring data than moving to the next projection.

16.4.4 Attenuation correction

Since the gamma camera collects data in a 2 dimensional form calculation of a 3 dimensional distribution from this data poses problems. A single slice through a volume source will present data as a single row of pixels across the camera face (ray-sum). Tissue activity near the surface contribute stronger signals than tissue of equal activity at the center of this row due to tissue attenuation. This leads to a cupping or depression of central values (similar to beam hardening in computed tomography).

If a uniform flood source is imaged without attenuation correction then this would show cupped images and profiles.   In practice attenuation leads to both spatial distortion in the final reconstruction and significant errors in quantitative accuracy. Correction is difficult and is commonly applied by assuming uniform distribution and knowing the dimensions of the object being imaged. Count data from opposing projections are averaged and to this modified projection a hyperbolic function is commonly added in order to boost the central regions of the projection.

Attenuation distortion influences the image in the following ways:

- Surface detail emphasized while deeper detail in the center of the image is lost
- Pixel count density depends on position within the section preventing quantification of uptake

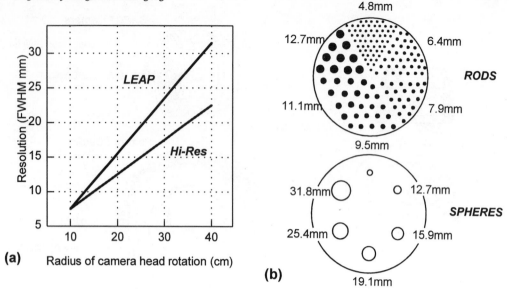

Figure 16.13 **(a)** The loss of resolution from the face of the collimator in a SPECT study. A high resolution collimator maintains resolution but the study time is extended due to low sensitivity. **(b)** The test objects in a commercially available SPECT phantom. The rods are solid plastic which give negative 'holes' in an active background. The spheres are filled with different activities for high and low contrast levels.

- Photon scattering from attenuation events destroys positional information
- Absolute uptake values cannot be obtained from a specific region of interest.

Attenuation varies according to gamma energy, Fig.16.14(a) compares 140keV gamma photons (SPECT) with 511keV (used in PET). Tissue attenuation is much less with the higher energy. Methods commonly applied for **attenuation correction** are:

Geometric mean where opposing ray sums are multiplied together and the square root taken.

Iterative (Chang) method where the image is reconstructed without correction then each pixel is corrected for attenuation according to its position within the matrix. Attenuation correction is usually standardized at 0.12 cm^{-1} from the accepted value of 0.15cm^{-1} for 140keV γ–radiation so that over-correction is prevented. The projection values, before reconstruction, are modified by a special filter whose shape compensates for attenuation. This is a very rapid correction process.

Transmission scans (uniform activity on one side of the subject creating a shadow image on the camera) are useful for assessing true attenuation. Hardware and software are available for transmission correction and a commercial design is shown in Fig.16.14(b) using a long lived nuclide (^{153}Gd; 97 and 103keV; T½ 242d)

SPECT scatter problems Scattered photons can contribute to a significant number of events (up to 50%) and lesions which are seen as decreased areas of uptake (myocardial perfusion defects) suffer loss of contrast in the central regions of the image. Unless scattered correction is applied before attenuation correction an amplification of background noise will occur.

If scatter is assumed to be uniform then a background subtraction can be made before reconstruction. With a standard 20% photo peak window for ^{99m}Tc about 30% of the photons forming the image come from scattered events.

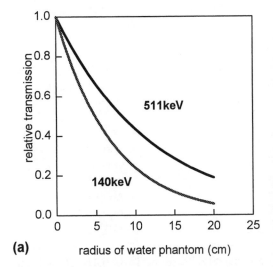
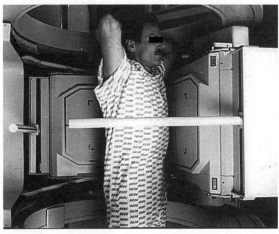

(a)   radius of water phantom (cm)

Figure 16.14 **(a)** Photon absorption with depth in water for SPECT and PET imaging. Attenuation is less with 511keV photons and correction is simpler since two photons are emitted. **(b)** Attenuation correction obtained by reference to a radionuclide source contained in the white rod which is scanned across the field of view (courtesy ADAC Inc.)

Some compensation can be obtained by selecting an energy window that overshoots the photo peak by about 5%. (asymmetric windowing)

16.4.5 Pre- and post-reconstruction filters

Pre-image filtration reduces noise content of the data set so preventing artifacts from appearing in the reconstructed tomographic images. High frequency noise in the projection image degrades the reconstructed image. Post-image filtration can be applied that will smooth or edge enhance images.

Ramp filter This would produce a mathematically exact solution to the reconstruction problem but the data would need to be collected over an infinite number of angles with infinitely small pixels and maximum counts. It retains the highest spatial frequencies but,

of course, would amplify any noise. Although this filter has very limited practical application it is basic to all filters used in SPECT. The following filters use a ramp for the lower frequency spectrum in the image and then modify or roll-off at the higher frequency component by combining a second filter; this is called filter windowing. The window can be set to 'cut-off' at a certain frequency so tailoring the filter to specific conditions.

Figure 16.15 demonstrates how windowed filters differ from the basic ramp. The common window functions that can be applied to SPECT data are the ***Butterworth and Hamming*** filters which give varying degrees of smoothing with the Hamming filter giving the greatest. Both the cut off frequency and the slope of the roll off can be varied. The ***Hanning*** filter reduces higher spatial frequencies so fine detail is lost. The filter choice should reflect both the frequency content of the noise and the diagnostic frequency content of the organ.

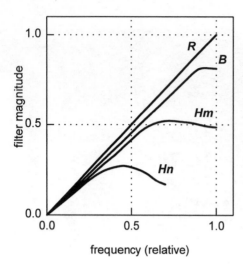

Figure 16.15   Some SPECT filter responses, Butterworth *B*, Hamming *Hm* and Hanning *Hn*, compared to a simple ramp filter *R*. (Courtesy ADAC Inc)

16.4.6   Practical aspects

Several important parameters must be considered before acquiring a SPECT study. A trial acquisition should be taken using a phantom holding about 200MBq ^{99m}Tc. This can either be a commercially available phantom (seen in Fig.16.13(b)) or a simple drum of uniform activity.

Summary

Advantage	Disadvantage
• Improved contrast	• Non-uniform sensitivity
• Multiplanar reconstruction matching CT and MRI	• Slow so fast dynamic events cannot be followed
	• Low photon density
	• Poorer resolution
	• variable resolution with depth
	• Accurate attenuation correction essential

Recommended protocols   Common SPECT protocols are listed in Tab.16.15. Before setting up a SPECT protocol the following choices should be made:

- Quality control
- Uniformity reference
- Center of rotation reference
- Size of image matrix
- Collimator choice
- Number of projections or angular increments
- 360° or 180° orbit
- Time per projection
- Total counts collected

Table 16.15 SPECT protocols

Study	^{99m}Tc-Agent	Collimator	Projections	Counts per projection	Time projection (seconds)
Cerebral	HMPAO (700MBq)	High Resolution	64- 128 over 360°	50k	20-10
Cardiac	MIBI (500MBq)	High Resolution	64- 128 over 180°	30k	40-20
Lumbar Spine	MDP	High Resolution	64 - 128 over 360°	50k	40-20
Liver	Colloid	LEAP	64- 128 over 180°	50k	40-20
Lungs	MAA Aerosol	High Sensitivity	64 over 360°	20k	20

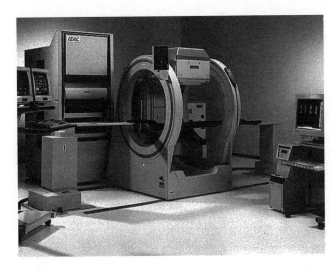
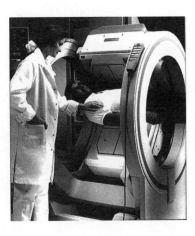

Figure 16.16 Two rectangular field of view gamma cameras showing **(a)** ring gantry with a single head and **(b)** close up of the same design showing a double head design (courtesy ADAC Inc.)

During reconstruction the filter type should be selected and attenuation correction applied. Commercially available camera designs for SPECT are shown in Fig.16.16

16.5 TOMOGRAPHY: POSITRON EMISSION (PET)

Cyclotron production of positron emitting isotopes has been described in Chapter 15. Recent cyclotron models using super conducting magnets have dramatically reduced cyclotron size so that small, department based positron imaging systems are now commercially available with their own integral shielding.

Positron Emission Tomography PET uses cyclotron produced β^+ isotopes to provide an imaging procedure that takes advantage of the unique coincident gamma radiation. This provides 'self-collimation' which significantly improves detection sensitivity. Attenuation correction is simplified owing to the paired gamma events, and resolution loss with depth is much reduced.

PET offers the greatest sensitivity of all diagnostic imaging techniques. Table 16.16 indicates the tissue concentration of labeled compounds necessary for imaging; they range through milli-, micro- and nano-gram amounts.

Table 16.16 Applications and concentrations

Pharmaceutical	Specific activity MBq/mole	Tissue conc. g/g tissue
Metabolites (glucose etc.)	2.5×10^{-3} to 2.5×10^{-2}	0.2 to 1.0×10^{-3}
Neurotransmitters (adrenaline etc.)	2.5 to 25	0.2 to 2.0×10^{-6}
Receptor sites (morphine, DOPA etc.)	2.5×10^{3} to 2.5×10^{5}	0.04 to 4.0×10^{-9}

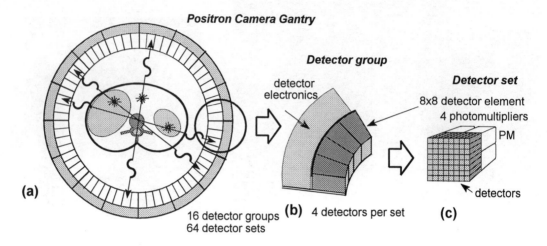

Figure 16.17   **(a)** A basic positron section scanner with circular detector array of 16 sets of 4 detectors made from (typically) Na(Tl) or bismuth germanate. **(b)** Each group of four is made up from 8×8 separate detectors © which give 8 slices simultaneously.

16.5.1 Cyclotron specifications

Most hospital cyclotrons accelerate negative hydrogen ions (H⁻) which are stripped to protons by a carbon stripper foil prior to bombarding the target.

$$H^- \rightarrow p + e^- \qquad (16.5)$$

Chapter 15 gives the general design. There are no neutrons produced that would require heavy shielding and beam currents are intentionally restricted to 100μA. Practical currents are usually 50μA which limits the surface dose on the cyclotron surface to 25μSv h⁻¹; this simplifies protective shielding requirements.   The target area itself is surrounded by 90cm of boronated polyethylene which effectively stops scattered neutrons formed during the reactions.

A typical small cyclotron would have a 12MeV proton beam designed to produce ^{11}C, ^{13}N, ^{15}O and ^{18}F. Higher beam energies require larger shielding thicknesses.   Different positron isotopes can be chosen by selecting a particular target on a remote changer. In some instances less abundant (and so more expensive) stable isotopes are used as target material for (p, n) reactions.

Modern small cyclotrons use super conducting magnets to give high intensity magnetic fields. This further reduces the size and weight of the installation and consumes less power. The whole cyclotron sits inside its own integral shielding forming a complete unit.

16.5.2   Imaging equipment

There are three major requirements for positron imaging:

1. Distinguishing the opposed 180° γ–radiation from background non-positron gamma photons.
2. Identifying the angle of travel
3. Reconstruction of the activity distribution

The positron imaging device   A basic design in Figure 16.17 contains 64 NaI(Tl) detectors in a polygon array giving a single transaxial plane. Each detector can operate in coincidence with a number of detectors that oppose it on the array. Spatial resolution is independent of depth within the section provided the coincidence detectors are sufficiently far apart and occupy about 60% of the detector diameter. Restricting the detection solid angle reduces the probability of two uncorrelated events occurring in opposing detectors within the coincidence resolving time (usually 12 nanoseconds) and adding to image noise. Heavy detector shielding limits the axial field of view to approximately the coincidence field of view.

Time of flight (TOF) estimation Incorporating the time of flight into image reconstruction can significantly improve resolution. If the coincident radiation originates from the center of the source (patient's head) then the 2 gammas will reach the opposing detectors at the same time. However if the positron anihilation is at the surface of the source then the coincident gammas will arrive at different times. Since they are traveling at the speed of light very fast timing circuits are needed. Commercial systems are capable of resolving events less than 200picoseconds apart (200×10^{-12} s). Several detector materials are used for PET scanners:

- Sodium Iodide   NaI(Tl)
- Bismuth germanate   BGO
- Barium Fluoride BaF_2
- Gadolinium orthosilicate   GSO

Detector material should have a high absorption coefficient for 511keV gammas and BGO has ×2.4 greater efficiency than NaI(Tl). The block detector design shown in Fig. 16.17(b) uses an encoding system with 4 photo multipliers viewing 64 BGO scintillation detectors arranged in an 8×8 matrix, (Fig. 16.17(c)). This gives effectively 8 rings to the detector so multiple sections can be taken without moving the patient. Maximum data acquisition is typically 1 million events per second.

Image processing typically takes less than 10 seconds. The signals are decoded for position, time and energy of the detected event.

The time encoder defines the time of the 511 keV event to within 2 nanoseconds of its appearance. The events recorded by the coincident detectors are used in a similar manner to computer tomography for reconstructing an axial slice of activity. The accuracy of reconstruction depends on the number of detectors in the detector ring; a typical PET system can contain 300 detectors.

The detectors translate stepwise by a total of one inter detector distance along the side of the polygon. The polygon arrays also rotate in steps through 60° (hexagon) or 45° (octagon) for each rotational step (5°) a complete inter-crystal translation scan is performed. This translation/rotation scanning provides the necessary angular sampling. Unlike SPECT absolute corrections for the effects of tissue attenuation can be made. Thus PET can be calibrated to give absolute levels of radioactive tracer concentration in tissue. It is possible to solve equations that define the isotope's fate and derive absolute values for tissue function, blood flow in ml. blood tissue cm^{-3} min^{-1} or mg metabolic substrate consumed tissue cm^{-3} min^{-1}.

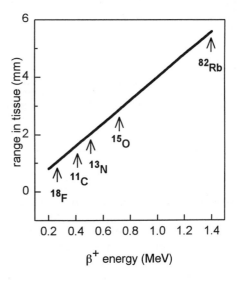

Figure 16.18 The distance traveled by positron particles in tissue. This will degrade image resolution since positron origin and eventual annihilation radiation will not coincide.

16.5.3   Positron nuclides

Figure 16.18 plots the β^+ energy and the mean distance traveled before an annihilation event. The emitted positron loses most of its energy after traveling a few millimeters in tissue before undergoing annihilation with a free electron and emitting the characteristic radiation.   This positron movement from its source of formation is a limiting factor for image resolution and as the energy of the positron increases (comparing ^{18}F and ^{82}Rb) the distance between origin and eventual annihilation can be considerable. Table 16.17 lists useful cyclotron and generator derived positron emitters. Each one has a good yield but their half-lives differ considerably.

Table 16.17   Cyclotron and generators

Nuclide	$T\frac{1}{2}$ (min.)	β^+ yield (%)	β^+ energy (MeV)
Cyclotron			
^{15}O	2.04	99.9	0.735
^{13}N	9.96	99.8	0.491
^{11}C	20.4	99.8	0.385
^{18}F	109.80	96.9	0.242
Generator			
^{68}Ga	68.1	89	0.740
^{82}Rb	76.4	95	1.409
^{62}Cu	9.74	97	1.280
^{52m}Mn	21.1	97	1.130
^{122}I	3.62	77	1.087

Automated chemistry modules These are provided by most small cyclotron manufacturers in order to simplify production of labeled compounds. Some common compounds that can be rapidly manufactured 'on-line' are listed in Table 16.18. Some of them are precursors for other more complex compounds while compounds such as carbon monoxide, carbon dioxide and water are used directly for regional blood flow measurement.

Table 16.18   Positron compounds

Positron emitter	Labeled compounds	Dose (H_F) mSv / 40MBq
^{11}Carbon	^{11}CO $^{11}CO_2$ $^{11}CN-$ $^{11}CH_3I$ $H^{11}CHO$	0.05 - 0.2
^{13}Nitrogen	$^{13}N-N_2$ $^{13}NH_3$	0.002 - 0.05
^{15}Oxygen	$^{15}O-O_2$ $H_2^{15}O$ $C^{15}O$ $^{15}O-CO_2$	0.02 - 0.2
^{18}Fluorine	$^{18}F-F_2$ $H^{18}F$ $^{18}F-$ $^{18}F-$ FDG	0.5

Image quality   Resolution and contrast are superior to SPECT images and recent software developments have enabled both coronal and sagittal sections to accompany the familiar high quality axial images. Figure 16.19 shows examples. Advantages over conventional nuclear medicine imaging:

- A selection of biologically important isotopes: Carbon, Nitrogen, Oxygen
- Isotopes can be incorporated into complex biological molecules without distorting them: Glucose, DOPA, alkaloids etc.
- Extreme sensitivity (approximately ×1000 that of SPECT) means that dangerous, addictive or toxic materials can be labeled and target organs and receptor sites identified with picogram (10^{-12}g) quantities of agent.
- Very short half lives give very small patient dose however a cyclotron must be on-site for continuous delivery.
- More precise localization of event gives superior resolution (theoretically 3mm). In practice about 5mm; far superior to SPECT images.
- Accurate attenuation correction can be applied to the data so that quantification of activity can be made.

16.6 COMPARISON OF OTHER TOMOGRAPHIC TECHNIQUES

Positron Emission Tomography (PET), Single Photon Emission Computed Tomography (SPECT) and Nuclear Magnetic Resonance Imaging (MRI) have now reached a degree of maturity where it is possible to assess where, if at all, any overlap occurs in their clinical usefulness. The early expectations that MRI would provide similar information as SPECT or PET in measuring regional metabolic processes has not been realized. The sensitivity of these three imaging processes is given in Table 16.19. The normal composition of living tissues includes, in addition to hydrogen, other elements that can generate NMR signals (see Chapter 19 and 20 on MRI). Unfortunately because of their low concentration in soft tissues and their lower NMR sensitivity (compared to hydrogen) their image gives a very high signal-to-noise ratio. At the present time the MRI image of ^{31}Phosphorus is poorer than conventional nuclear medicine imaging.

The application of tracer techniques in MRI is severely limited by the low signal-to-noise ratio which requires high concentrations of stable NMR isotope to give a good image. This invalidates tracer techniques in MRI for studying metabolic processes: compare the concentrations required for imaging drug receptor sites in PET and the use of sub-toxic levels of ^{201}Thallium for cardiac imaging in nuclear medicine. The present MRI resolution for protons is about 1mm. The best achievable PET resolution is 3mm but with a sensitivity about 10^{12} times greater than MRI. SPECT has a best resolution figure of about 5mm with a similar sensitivity as PET but over a much limited range of useful metabolic tracers. MRI is recognized as a valuable investigation not involving ionizing radiation. It also gives multisection planes, (axial, sagittal, coronal and oblique), although CI, SPECT and PET can also give these. Disadvantages are length of study time limiting good quality studies to the head and extremities at a distance from respiratory movement, cost and lack of sensitivity. The usefulness of PET has become established mostly for investigating physiological processes.

A certain number of clinical investigations have been identified particularly brain receptor sites of psycotropic drugs (morphine, LDOPA) and metabolic agents (glucose) for cardiac function (perfusion, metabolism and blood pool). With a sufficiently large population of patient material the cost per examination decreases to the level of MRI and complex nuclear medicine studies (cardiac and labeled white cell imaging). The usefulness of SPECT is more varied. Its resolution and contrast is lower than PET.

Multiple section acquisition leads to section overlap and interference. The isotopes available are more limited but have become wider since the introduction of ^{99m}Tc labeled brain perfusion (HMPAO) and cardiac (MIBI) agents.

Table 16.19 Comparing CT, MRI, SPECT and PET

System	Specific details
CAT Collimated Source and Detector	Multiple-axes. Fixed source to detector position. No attenuation problems. Good signal strength.
SPECT Collimated Detector Internal source (γ -nuclides) Energy windowed	Multiple-axes. Attenuation problems. Good signal strength.
PET Coincident Detectors Internal Source (β^+ Nuclides) Fixed Energy (511keV)	Multiple-axes. No attenuation problems. Good signal strength. At Least ×2 sensitivity of SPECT.
MRI General/Local Coils Magnetic Field ^{1}H,^{31}P,^{23}Na Images	Radio Signals. Multiple Axes. Attenuation. Poor signal strength.

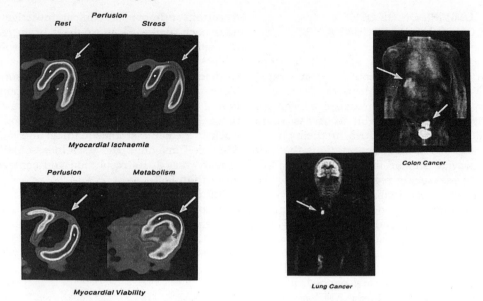

Figure 16.19   Axial sections of the brain and heart using positron emission tomography. (Courtesy Guy's and St Thomas's PET Centre)

Other radio pharmaceuticals specifically developed for SPECT imaging would increase the usefulness and more routine application of SPECT. The complementary nature of MRI, PET and SPECT seems to reduce competition among the three imaging methods. MRI gives superb morphological information which allows integration with the functional images of PET and SPECT.

CT images are purely anatomical in character with no physiological information but, because they provide valuable ana-tomical information, the combination of CT and PET or SPECT becomes a potentially powerful imaging set.

Further reading

International Commission on Radiological Protection 1977: The Handling Storage, Use and Disposal of Unsealed Radionuclides in Hospitals and Medical Research Establishments. Publication 25 (Pergamon Press, Oxford UK)

Management of Radioactive Wastes produced by users of radioactive materials IAEA Safety Series (IAEA Vienna)

Radiation Protection in Nuclear Medicine and Pathology. Report No. 63. The Institute of Physical Sciences in Medicine, UK.

Sources and Magnitude of Occupational and Public Exposures from Nuclear Medicine. NCRP Report 124. Bethesda 1996

Clinical Nuclear Medicine. Maisey, Britton and Gilday. Chapman and Hall 1991

The MIRD Primer. Loevinger et al. Society of Nuclear Medicine 1988.

KEYWORDS

angular sampling   The sampling interval for SPECT imaging.

body surface area   This is computed for dose or GFR calculations. Combines individual's weight and height as:

$$W^{0.425} \times H^{0.725} \times 0.0072 \text{m}^2$$

center of rotation Adjusted so that 0° and 90° and 180° and 360° positions align before SPECT data acquisition

collimator The device in front of the camera crystal that accepts gamma photons only from a particular angle. Common collimators have a parallel hole design that only accepts gamma photons perpendicular to the crystal face.

controlled area A room or location where maximum exposure level is 7.5µSv h^{-1}

dynamic study A study where a certain number of timed frames are collected (see renogram).

field uniformity Acceptable planar imaging non-uniformity in the central field of view is about 3% but SPECT requires uniformity <1%.

filters Image data is filtered pre and post-reconstruction to reduce noise. There are also smoothing and edge enhancement filters.

first pass A fast dynamic study which follows transit of a bolus of activity (i.e. heart/lungs).

gated acquisition Image data acquisition under the control of a gating signal either ECG or respiration.

group classification A radionuclide toxicity classification ranging from Group 1. (most toxic) to Group 4. (least toxic). Group classification determines limits for safe disposal.

Marinelli formula An early method for calculating internal dose rates using a simple organ geometry estimation but with no organ to organ contribution.

MIRD formula An improved internal dose estimation with better organ geometry factor and the addition of contributing organ activity.

MUGA Multi-gated-acquisition using the ECG for gating heart images according to their position in the cardiac cycle.

multiphase study A dynamic study using a mixture of frame timings.

oxidation state This is related to the valency state of an ion which influences chemical combination. Iron has two oxidation states: ferrous Fe[II] and ferric Fe[III] whereas technetium has seven.

PET Positron emission tomography using the 180° opposed 511keV gamma photons from positron annihilation.

planar imaging Acquiring the volume activity image of an organ either as a static or dynamic sequence.

radiation area (USA) a staff area where radiation levels approach 50µSv h^{-1} at 30cm from the source.

radiation area (high) (USA) an area where levels approach 1mSv h^{-1} at 30cm from the source.

renogram An example of a dynamic study using multi-phase acquisition where (for instance) the vascular phase is collected as 30 frames at 0.5s, GFR phase as 30 at 1s and excretion phase as 30 at 20s.

shelf-life A measure of radionuclide storage, related to half-life. ^{123}I has a poor shelf life (T½ 13h) whereas ^{201}Tl has a good shelf life (T½ 3.0d).

SPECT Single-photon-emission-computed-tomography. Axial tomographic images acquired by rotating a gamma camera 180° or 360° around the patient and reconstructing. multiple slices according to the camera field of view. Coronal and sagittal slices can be obtained from the axial information.

step and shoot as opposed to continuous rotation where the camera stops at each angular projection and acquires data.

target organ the organ receiving most activity (the thyroid is the target organ for iodine radionuclides and ^{99m}Tc)

time of flight improving PET resolution by including time of detection for the coincidence gammas.

WHO category a segregation of labeled radio-pharmaceuticals according to patient dose. There are three groups denoting high, medium and low radiation dose.

Table 16.20 Common investigations, the administered activity and whole body dose.

Investigation	Radiopharmaceutical	MBq	Whole Body Dose H_E (mSv)
WHO CATEGORY I	(< 0.5mSv)		
GFR	^{51}Cr-EDTA	3	0.01- 0.03
Lung Ventilation	^{81m}Kr Gas	37	0.06
ERPF	^{125}I Hippuran	2	0.1- 0.4
Thyroid Uptake	^{123}I Oral	1	0.17
Renography	^{123}I-Hippuran	12	0.2 - 0.4
Gastric Emptying	^{99m}Tc-Colloid Oral	12	0.3
Renography	^{99m}Tc-MAG3	75	0.2 - 0.3
	^{99m}Tc-DTPA	75	0.4 - 0.7
WHO CATEGORY II	(0.5 - 5.0mSv)		
Renography	^{131}I-Hippuran	3	0.5
Thyroid Imaging	^{99m}Tc-Pertechnetate	75	0.8
Lung Perfusion	^{99m}Tc-MAA	75	0.9
Liver Imaging	^{99m}Tc-Colloid	75	1.0
Renal Function	^{99m}Tc-DMSA	70	1.0
Thyroid Imaging	^{123}Iodide	8	1.4
Plasma Volume	^{125}I-albumin	0.2	1.5
Hepatobiliary	^{99m}Tc-EHIDA	100	2
Renal Blood Flow	^{99m}Tc-DTPA	400	2.0-4.0
Meckel's Diverticulum	^{99m}Tc-pertechnetate	200	2.2
Brain perfusion	^{99m}Tc-HMPAO	500	2.5
Myocardial perfusion	^{99m}Tc-MIBI	400	2.7
Thyroid Uptake	^{131}I Oral	0.2	3.2
Cisternography	^{111}In-DTPA	30	3.6
Bone Imaging	^{99m}Tc-MDP	550	3.7-6.0
Bone Marrow	^{99m}Tc-Nanocolloid	300	3.9
WHO CATEGORY III	(5 - 50mSv)		
Abscess	^{111}Indium	30	5.0
Brain	^{99m}Tc-pertechnetate	500	5.5
Gated MUGA	^{99m}Tc-RBC's	800	5.6
Haemodynamics	^{99m}Tc-pertechnetate	600	7.0
Myocardial	^{201}Tl chloride	75	7.0
Abscess Imaging	^{67}Ga citrate	80	9.0

17

Ultrasound principles

17.1 Ultrasound properties
17.2 Interaction of ultrasound
    with matter

17.3 The Ultrasound transducer
17.4 The Ultrasonic field

17.1 ULTRASOUND PROPERTIES

Ultrasound waves have frequencies many times higher than the upper limit for human hearing. A comparative range of common sound frequencies is given in Tab. 17.1 along with the clinical ultrasound range for comparison.

Table 17.1 Common sound frequencies

Audible range	15 to 20,000 Hz
Children's hearing	up to 40,000 Hz
Male speaking voice	100 to 1500 Hz
Female speaking voice	150 to 2500 Hz
Middle C	262 Hz
Concert A	440 Hz
Top C	2093 Hz
Bat sounds	50,000 to 200,000 Hz
Maximum sound frequency	6×10^8 (600MHz)
Medical ultrasound	2.5 to 40 MHz

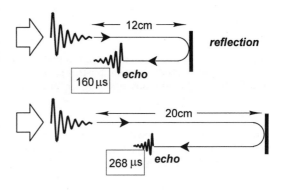

Figure 17.1 Sound waves reflecting from two surfaces at 12 and 20cm depths respectively. Speed of sound is 6.7μs cm^{-1} for soft tissue

High frequency ultrasound can provide information about tissues *in-vivo* by producing a sound image. Rapid image formation can reveal organ movement in real time. Ultrasound differs from most conventional imaging methods in three important ways:

- The ultrasound beam is a non-ionizing longitudinal wave (unlike electromagnetic radiation).
- The signal is recorded in reflection rather than transmission mode (unlike x-ray imaging).

Ultrasound images are constructed by computing the time taken for an ultrasound beam to travel from a transducer, and return from a reflecting surface. Figure 17.1 shows an ultrasound pulse reflected from 2 surfaces at different depths. If the sound velocity in soft tissue is 6.7μs cm^{-1} (1500 m s^{-1}) then from the time of arrival (round-trip) the depth of the reflecting surface can be calculated.

The magnitude of the echo influences (modulates) the brightness of a display and is coded as a gray-scale. An echo image is then built up to give an image of a body slice.

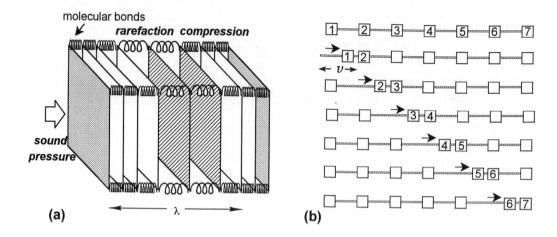

Figure 17.2   **(a)** Three dimensional model of sound pressure being conveyed through a medium consisting of plates (molecules or particles) loosely connected by spring-like bonds. **(b)** Propagation of sound energy as elongation about a center of equilibrium (particle velocity about its center is v)

Clinical ultrasound systems use computer methods for producing images continuously in 'real-time' which has valuable clinical applications.

The ultrasound signal is produced by electrically stimulating a crystalline material to oscillate. Ultrasound waves obey all the conventional laws associated with light waves except they require a medium (gas, solid or liquid) for their transmission, which takes place by a sequence of compressions and rarefactions within the conducting medium (see Chapter 2).

17.1.1   Propagation

Sound waves are **longitudinal waves** and require a medium (gas, liquid, solid) for their transmission. The passage of ultrasound energy through a medium is illustrated in Fig.17.2(a). The material boundaries or molecules are represented as flat plates connected by massless bonds shown as springs. A lon-gitudinal wave transmits its energy through material by causing the molecules in its path to oscillate back and forth parallel to the direction of travel of the wave front; oscillations are shown as compressions traveling along the plates. Sound travel first involves molecular or particle vibration (elongation) at the excitation frequency. Sound particle velocity (elongation velocity v in cm s^{-1}) is the velocity of a particle about its equilibrium position (v in Fig.17.2(b)). The elongation disturbance **propagates** through the medium (tissue) at a specific propagation velocity c in meters s^{-1}, the absolute speed depending on the medium.

A picture of ultrasound transmission is represented in Fig.17.2(b) as a row of connected particles. The sound pressure applies a force from the left hand side to particle '1'. The force exerted on '1' causes it to acquire a velocity and be displaced to the right both stretching and compressing the connecting bonds. Particle '2' now receives the force from '1' and '2' is now displaced.

The force having now been transferred, '1' now returns to its original position. The energy of the sound wave is contained in the compressed bonds or springs.

Ultrasound causes the particles in its path to oscillate back and forth at the particular frequency so mechanical energy is transported across the material. Particle '2' displacement is slightly smaller than '1' due to loss of heat energy within the bond, so the signal energy gradually decays.

   This vibration phenomenon is repeated for the remaining particles, causing the original sound wave to be transported across the particles by compression and rarefaction events, as the particles move to and fro. This can be treated as a sine wave as shown in Fig.17.3(a) which has wavelength λ, frequency f (cycles per second: Hz) and amplitude A depending on the sound pressure characteristics and transmitting medium.

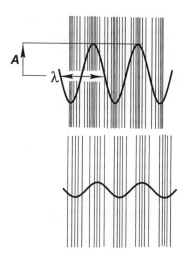

Figure 17.3   Compression and rarefaction in a medium producing a sound wave with wavelength λ and amplitude A emulating a sine-wave. A reduced power level is shown in the lower waveform

17.1.2   Sound characteristics

Sound particle velocity v   is the velocity of the material particles as they oscillate to and fro with the sound pressure. A typical value would be 35mm s^{-1}.

Acoustic pressure p   is caused by the pressure changes induced in the material by the sound energy measured in pascals (Pa). A typical value would be 0.06MPa. Imaging pressures can be ×10 this value and Doppler pressures ×25 which has important safety associations.

Frequency f and wavelength λ   These are identified in Fig.17.3 where compression and rarefaction events in the medium are described as a sine wave having a frequency measured in cycles s^{-1} or Hertz and a wavelength measured in millimeters (mm). Frequency and wavelength are related as $\lambda = c/f$ where c is the speed of sound in the medium (tissue, bone air etc.)

Propagation velocity   This is the speed with which the elongation displacement is transferred across the material and is measured in meters per second (m s^{-1}). The excitation in the medium propagates with a velocity specific to the material. The stiffer the springs in Fig.17.2(a) and the smaller the molecular masses the greater the propagation velocity. The distance between repeated compression states is the wavelength of the propagation event. Propagation velocity, wavelength and frequency (Hz) are related as:

$$wavelength\ (\lambda) = \frac{propagation\ velocity}{frequency} \qquad (17.1)$$

Propagation speeds increase from gases to liquids and are highest in solids. This is not directly related to material density but depends on increasing molecular bond stiffness or 'springiness'. A typical velocity for soft tissue (a mixture of connective tissue and fat) is between 1480 and 1568 m s^{-1}; a rounded value of 1500 m s^{-1} is used in order to simplify calculations. The magnitude of the force produced by each particle shown in Fig. 17.2(b), gradually decreases or **decays** as the wave travels across the medium.

   From eqn.17.1 propagation velocity is related to frequency of oscillation f in cycles s^{-1} (Hz) and its wavelength (λ in meters) as:

$$c = \lambda \cdot f \text{ and } \lambda = \frac{c}{f} \qquad (17.2)$$

If the velocity of the ultrasound wave changes (traveling from one medium to another) then the wavelength and not the frequency changes (see Box 17.1). This is demonstrated in Fig.17.4 for two different materials: soft tissue and bone for a frequency of 2MHz. Change of wavelength is an important consideration for imaging resolution. Examples of frequency and wavelength for ultrasound in soft tissue are given in Tab.17.2. Table 17.3 gives velocity and density for important clinical materials and tissues.

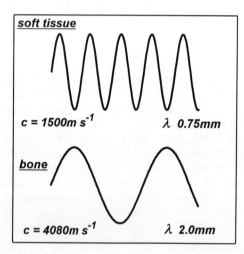

Figure 17.4 Sound waves having the same frequency but different wavelength when traveling in soft tissue and bone

Amplitude   The maximum amplitude coincides with the compression peak. (*A* in Fig.17.3(a)). Reduced power level in Fig.17.3(b) gives a reduced amplitude

Power This is the rate at which work is done or the rate of sound energy transfer. It always contains a time period. Power is measured in watts (W = joules s^{-1}).

Intensity This is a measure of power per unit area and is commonly measured as W cm^{-2}. Comparative power and intensity is measured in decibels.

Box 17.1

Ultrasound wavelength change

From eqn. 17.2
What is the wavelength λ of a 2.0MHz sound wave

- in soft tissue (c = 1500m s^{-1})
- in bone (c = 4080m s^{-1})

Soft tissue: $\dfrac{1500}{2 \times 10^6}$ = 7.5×10^{-4} m or 0.75mm

Bone: $\dfrac{4080}{2 \times 10^6}$ = 2.04×10^{-3} m or 2.04mm

These values are represented by the waveforms in Fig.17.4

Table 17.2 Frequency and wavelength for ultrasound in soft tissue.

frequency (MHz)	wavelength (mm)
2.0	0.74
3.5	0.42
5.0	0.30
7.5	0.20
10.0	0.15

Modulus of Elasticity (E)   The rate of transfer of the molecular displacement (the wave velocity) depends on the molecule's reluctance to motion and the density of the material.   The material elasticity is measured as Young's Modulus (Thomas Young, British physicist/physician 1773-1829), measured as material stress under a given strain: *E* = *stress/strain*.   Stiffer springs (higher modulus) and smaller molecular masses increase the propagation velocity *c* so that:

$$c = \sqrt{\frac{E}{\rho}} \qquad (17.3)$$

where *E* is Young's Modulus and ρ is material density. As *E* increases, signifying stiffer springs, sound propagation velocity also increases.

Modulus of elasticity is inversely proportional to the **deformation** or compressibility $1/E$. The modulus of elasticity is measured in pressure units giga-pascals (GPa). Typical values of E are: fat 2.0GPa, soft tissue 2.2GPa and bone 25GPa. Bone has a larger value of E (less compressibility or deformation) so sound travels faster in bone than in soft tissue.

17.1.3 Acoustic Impedance

When pressure p is applied to a molecule it will move exerting a pressure on an adjacent molecule and so setting up the sequence seen in Fig.17.2(b). Acoustic pressure increases with particle velocity v but it also depends on properties of the medium. The relationship between these parameters is characterized by the **acoustic impedance** Z so that:

$$Z = \frac{p}{v} \qquad (17.4)$$

Acoustic impedance Z, sound pressure p and particle velocity v have certain similarities to electrical units of resistance R, voltage V and current I (see Chapter 2) so the following relationships exist:

$v = p/Z$ (analogous to $I = V/R$)
$p = v \cdot Z$ (analogous to $V = IR$)
$Z = p/v$ (analogous to $R = V/I$)

The acoustic impedance Z, which is measured in kg m^{-2} s^{-1} shortened to **rayl**, is also related to the **modulus of elasticity** E. The stiffer the bonding between molecules (springs) the greater the pressure exerted by a molecule moving at a particular velocity so sound pressure is related as $p = Z \cdot v$, thus acoustic impedance is directly related to sound pressure. A material having a great deal of springiness (low E value) and consequently high molecular motion, will absorb sound energy in the bonds and less will be transferred to the next molecule so impedance Z and modulus of elasticity E are related as :

$$Z = \frac{E}{c} \qquad (17.5)$$

Velocity of sound transfer depends on material elasticity E (modulus of elasticity) and density of the medium ρ shown by eqn.17.3 and combining eqns. 17.3 and 17.5 gives:

$$Z = \rho c = \sqrt{E \times \rho} \qquad (17.6)$$

Z is a material specific constant and is analogous to electrical resistance: as resistance increases it inhibits velocity (current) for a given pressure (voltage). Acoustic impedance is the product of density and propagation velocity: $\rho \cdot c$. Acoustic impedances for various materials are given in Tab.17.3 .

Table 17.3 Velocity, Density and acoustic impedance for clinical materials

Material	Speed of sound c m s^{-1}	Density ρ kg m^{-3}	Acoustic impedance Z kg m^{-2} s^{-1} ($\times 10^{-6}$)
Air	330	1.3	0.00043
Fat	1470	970	1.42
Castor Oil	1500	933	1.40
Water	1492	1000	1.48
Soft tissue	1500	<1000	~1.45
Brain	1530	1020	1.56
Blood	1570	1020	1.60
Kidney	1561	1030	1.61
Liver	1549	1060	1.64
Muscle	1568	1040	1.63
Eye Lens	1620	1130	1.83
Bone	4080	1700	6.12

17.1.4   Power and intensity

Sound energy is measured in joules. Sound power is measured as joules s^{-1} or watts and since it is analogous to the respective electrical unit power can be derived from pressure and particle velocity and is transferred as kinetic energy from one molecule to the next since $P = pv$.

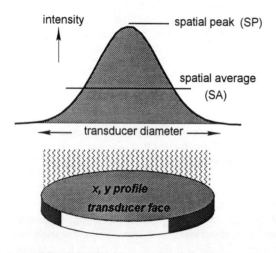

Figure 17.5   Intensity profile across an ultrasound beam.

Increased energy drives the compression bands closer together depositing more energy in the tissue increasing the amplitude of the ultrasound oscillation. During travel through the tissue the oscillations lose energy as heat and the wave amplitude decreases, while frequency and wavelength are unaltered in the same tissue.

Sound or acoustic intensity is measured as watts cm^{-2}. This is the instantaneous power passing through a unit area of material (tissue). A practical measure is mW mm^{-1} and the energy of medical ultrasound is typically between 0.01 and 1mW mm^{-2} for imaging and 0.01 and 0.3mW mm^{-2} for Doppler flow. Acoustic intensity across the ultrasound beam is not uniform but has a **spatial peak intensity** (SP) and **spatial average intensity** (SA) identified in Fig.17.5.

Decibel scale   Comparative sound intensity is measured using the decibel scale (described Chapter 1.). The range of intensity values in clinical ultrasound extends over 100dB. Power or intensity variations (I_1 and I_2) are compared as:

$$dB = 10 \log_{10} \frac{I_2}{I_1} \qquad (17.7)$$

So for an incident power of 1.0 W cm^{-2} and an echo power of 0.1mW cm^{-2} the power loss would be:

$$dB = 10 \log_{10} \frac{0.0001}{1} = 10 \times -4.0$$
$$= -40dB$$

The value minus 40dB is termed '40dB below'.   The **half power distance** (a reduction of 50%) is the distance over which the power is reduced by 3dB, derived from $10 \log_{10} 0.5 = -3.010$.   From the diagram in Fig.17.3 the maximum intensity coincides with maximum pressure in the medium (air). Pressure p and intensity I are related as:

$$I = \frac{p^2}{2\rho c} \qquad (17.8)$$

where ρ is the density of the medium and c the speed of sound in that medium. Substituting eqn.17.8 in eqn.17.7 and canceling the common factor $2\rho c$ gives:

$$10 \log \left[\frac{p_2}{p_1}\right]^2 \quad \text{or} \quad 20 \log \frac{p_1}{p_2} \qquad (17.9)$$

so pressure or amplitude (measured in volts) is described by eqn.17.9 and commonly describes amplification or **amplifier gain**.

The **half amplitude** value (a 50% loss of gain) would be –6dB. Ultrasound **attenuation** is measured per unit length and frequency as dB cm^{-1} MHz^{-1} and will be used later to describe ultrasound absorption. For soft tissue it is approximately 1dB cm^{-1} MHz^{-1}.

7.2 INTERACTION OF ULTRASOUND WITH MATTER

When ultrasound waves interact with matter they exhibit the same phenomena as visible light. They can undergo:

- Reflection (specular and non-specular)
- Refraction
- Diffraction
- Attenuation or absorption.

17.2.1   Reflection

Specular or mirror reflection occurs when the ultrasound beam strikes a smooth boundary between two media having different impedance. Sound reflection is the basis of ultrasound image formation. From Fig.17.6(a) an ultrasound beam incident I_i on a smooth surface (irregularities much smaller than its wavelength) has a proportion of the beam reflected I_r and the remaining transmitted I_t through the surface or interface. The fraction of the transmitted T and reflected R depends on the acoustic impedances of the two media (Z_1 is acoustic impedance of the first tissue and Z_2 the acoustic impedance of the second).

When an ultrasound wave perpendicular to the surface crosses from one medium Z_1 to another Z_2 a change in **velocity** occurs. There is partial reflection of the **incident wave** at the interface between the two materials as shown in Fig.17.6(a). The wavelength of the reflected wave has not changed and remains in phase with the incident wave. The amount of reflection depends on impedance differences Z_1 and Z_2. For a sound wave perpendicular to a smooth surface, the amount of reflection is given by:

$$R = \frac{I_r}{I_i} = \left[\frac{Z_1 - Z_2}{Z_1 + Z_2} \right]^2 \times 100 \qquad (17.10)$$

Where R is the percentage of the beam reflected. This relationship is only valid for incident radiation perpendicular to the surface of the medium. **Reflection** is greatest when the difference in acoustic impedance between materials, Z_1 and Z_2, is large, for example between soft tissue and air, or between bone and soft tissue.   Only small reflections occur between different soft tissues, the echoes from these interfaces have a weak intensity. Box 17.2 gives some worked examples.

Non-specular reflection   If   the   beam strikes a boundary having irregularities or fine structures similar in size to the ultrasound wavelength then non-specular reflection or **scatter** is produced. The same effect occurs when an ultrasound beam passes through a particulate medium e.g. blood corpuscles, which are small compared with the wavelength and have a different impedance from the surroundings. This again gives scatter.

Table 17.4 Common parameters used to describe ultrasound.

Measurement	Symbol	Unit	Clinical range
Velocity	c	m s^{-1}	1480 m s^{-1} (soft tissue)
Wavelength	λ	mm	0.6 to 0.15mm (soft tissue)
Frequency	f	hertz	2.5-10MHz
Elastic Modulus	E	pascal	25GPa (bone)
Acoustic Impedance	Z	kg m^{-2} s^{-1}	1.63×10^6kg m^{-2} s^{-1}
Density	ρ	kg m^{-2}	water = 1000 kg m^{-2}
Power	W	watts cm^{-2}	typically 1 to 10mW cm^{-2}
Elongation	ξ	mm	~2×10^{-6}mm at 3MHz
Pressure	p	pascal or bar	0.6bar or 0.06MPa
Elongation velocity	υ	cm s^{-1}	< 3.5cm s^{-1}

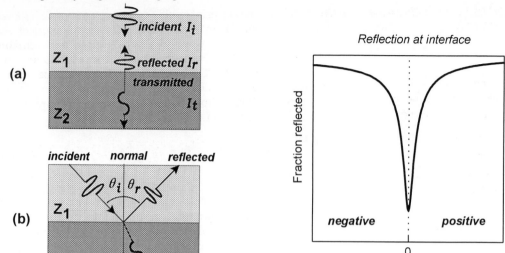

Figure 17.6 (a) A sound wave perpendicular to a reflecting surface showing incident, reflected and transmitted rays and (b) at an angle to a smooth surface θ_i showing angles of reflection θ_r and refraction θ_t. (c) Reflection from interfaces due to mismatch between Z_1 and Z_2 values. The null point (zero reflection) is where $Z_1 = Z_2$; to the left and right of the null point $Z_1 > Z_2$ and $Z_1 < Z_2$ respectively.

Box 17.2

Reflection and transmission

Using the acoustic impedance values from Tab. 17.3 using eqn. 17.10:

$$\text{Reflected} \quad R = \left[\frac{Z_1 - Z_2}{Z_1 + Z_2}\right]^2 \times 100$$

Interface A   *AIR : FAT*

Air Z_1 $= 0.0004 \times 10^6$ Fat $Z_2 = 1.42 \times 10^6$

Reflection = 99.9%

Conclusion: 99.9% of the incident radiation can be reflected from an air/tissue interface.

Interface B   *LIVER: KIDNEY*
Liver Z_1 $= 1.64 \times 10^6$ Kidney $Z_2 = 1.61 \times 10^6$

Reflection = 8.5×10^{-5} = or 0.0085%
(see eqn. 17.11)

$$\text{Transmitted:}\ T = \frac{4 \cdot (Z_1 \times Z_2)}{(Z_1 + Z_2)^2} = 99.9915\%$$

similarly $T = 1 - R$ $= 99.9915\%$

Conclusion Over 99.9% of the incident radiation is transmitted through tissues having similar Z values.

The scattered echoes from the incident beam form a cone about the reflection axis. The spread or the scatter (cone angle) depends on the wavelength of the ultrasound and the magnitude of the roughness. For rough surfaces and small wavelengths (higher frequency) then the scatter angle is wider. Ultrasound scatter assists in the imaging of curved surfaces and of boundaries which are not 90° to the direction of the ultrasound beam. Intensity of scattered ultrasound is related to frequency f decreasing as f^4. The echoes produced by scatter are much smaller than those produced by specular reflection but they can contribute useful information on tissue characteristics inside an organ. Scattering is responsible for a characteristic of diagnostic ultrasound imaging called **speckle** (not to be confused with speculation mirror reflection). Speckle is produced when scattered ultrasound waves from different sites interfere or add together constructively. The pattern produced does not correspond to anatomical detail but disruptions in the pattern may indicate pathology; liver pathology is an example that may be distinguished.

Both specular and non-specular reflection reduce the intensity of ultrasound traveling through different tissue types.

17.2.2 Transmission and refraction

Transmission (T) The unreflected ultrasound passes on as a transmitted beam, and the efficiency of transmission T of an incident sound beam at right angles to a smooth interface (Fig.17.6(a)) is described by the equation:

$$T = \frac{I_t}{I_i} = \frac{4 \cdot (Z_1 \times Z_2)}{(Z_1 + Z_2)^2} \times 100 \qquad (17.11)$$

also $\qquad T = (1 - R)$

The response in Fig.17.6(c) between Z_1 and Z_2 values graphically illustrates the rapid increase in reflection even with small mismatches between Z_1 and Z_2 reaching a null point when $Z_1 = Z_2$.

Refraction When the incident wave strikes a surface at 90° (Fig.17.6(a)) a reflected wave travels back along the incident path. The incident and reflected wave are superimposed additively since they have the same wavelength and phase. An ultrasound wave passing from one medium to another (Z_1 to Z_2) changes its velocity. As the frequency of the beam is not altered the wavelength must change to accommodate the new velocity in the second medium. The transmitted wave therefore has a longer wavelength in the denser medium Z_2.

If the incident beam strikes a smooth boundary at some oblique angle θ, then the reflected beam is projected at the same angle from the surface (Fig.17.6(b)). A boundary is described as smooth if its surface roughness is small compared with the ultrasound wavelength. The non-reflected transmitted wave is now traveling at a new (faster) velocity and so the wavelength increases which changes the direction of the wave front in the second medium causing it to undergo refraction; the main beam deviates from its original pathway. Since the speeds in various soft tissues are very similar refraction only plays a minor role in diagnostic ultrasound imaging but refraction can be used deliberately in a transducer design to construct acoustic lenses which will focus the ultrasound beam.

Snell's Law (W. Snell; Dutch physicist 1591-1626) governs angles of reflection and refraction for ultrasound. If sin θ is the angle the beam makes with the surface and v is the sound velocity then:

$$\frac{sin\ \theta}{v} = constant \qquad (17.12)$$

The **angle of refraction** θ_t in Fig.17.6(b) is described by modifying eqn.17.12 so:

$$\frac{\sin \theta_i}{\sin \theta_t} = \frac{V_i}{V_t} \qquad (17.13)$$

Where θ_1 is the angle of incidence, θ_2 is the angle of refraction, V_i is the wave velocity in the first medium and V_t is the wave velocity in the second medium. The change in direction depends on the change in velocity between the two tissues. When the wave moves from a higher velocity material to another having a lower velocity the angle of refraction is less than the angle of incidence and vice versa. Examples are given in Box 17.3

Diffraction This is the bending of the ultrasound beam into the shadow of a strong absorber. It takes place at the absorber edge and can be seen when a denser material (gall stones, bone, etc.) interrupts the sound beam and a shadow is cast behind the object. Although the ultrasonic intensity in this shadow is less than in the incident field it is not reduced to zero, due to diffraction around the edges of the dense material. This leads to image artifacts.

Box 17.3

Examples of Snell's Law

Referring to the parameters in Fig.17.7(b) and using the sound velocities listed in Tab.17.3. From eqn 17.13 the refracted beam angle θ_t is related as:

$$\sin\theta_t = \frac{\sin\theta_i \times V_t}{V_i}$$

A common incident angle of 20° where $\sin\theta_i$ = 0.3420 is used.

Interface 1.   *WATER: SALINE*
Where: velocity for water is 1492 and for saline is 1540, then θ_i = 20° and θ_t = 20.6°

Conclusion: Small difference between incident and refracted angles with similar tissues

Interface 2.   *LIVER: FAT*
Where: velocity for liver is 1549 for fat is 1470 then θ_i = 20° and θ_t = 18°

Conclusion: The refracted angle is smaller than the incident angle; conversely if the velocity in the second medium is greater then the refraction angle is greater.

17.2.3 Absorption and attenuation

The decrease in the intensity of the ultrasound beam in the direction of propagation is called attenuation. There are two processes which produce attenuation:

- **Absorption** by the tissue. This is the main mechanism for the reduction of beam intensity (accounting for up to 80% of the power loss).
- **Beam divergence** by reflection or scattering.

Absorption Ultrasound absorption is the conversion of ultrasound energy to heat and is produced by the frictional forces which oppose the motion of the particles in the medium. The amount of absorption is determined by the viscosity of the medium, its relaxation time and the frequency of the ultrasound. Increasing the viscosity of a medium decreases the molecular motion and increases the internal friction.

Relaxation frequency The rate of energy loss in a medium depends on the frequency of ultrasound. Ultrasound may be attenuated more strongly in one type of tissue than another if the relaxation frequency of that medium is near the ultrasound frequency. This is illustrated in Fig.17.7(a) where, for a given tissue, maximum absorption occurs at the relaxation frequency ω.

The decrease of the ultrasonic intensity with increasing tissue thickness or path length x can be characterized by an exponential law which has already been used for gamma and x-radiation:

$$\frac{I_x}{I_o} = e^{-\beta x} \tag{17.14}$$

Where I_o is the initial value of ultrasound intensity (at $x=0$) and I_x is the reduced intensity at depth x, and β is an **absorption coefficient** which is not unlike the linear attenuation coefficient in diagnostic radiology. For water the value of β is proportional to frequency as f^2. Instead of the absorption coefficient β a measure of power loss α is often given:

$$\alpha = 10 \log_{10} \frac{I_o}{I_x} \tag{17.15}$$

where α is the attenuation in dB per unit length. Table 17.5 lists the reference absorption values (α dB cm^{-1} for 1MHz) for some common tissues. There is an approximately linear relationship between attenuation α and frequency f as the ratio of α/f is roughly constant for the diagnostic frequency range. In tissue the absorption of ultrasound increases almost linearly with frequency over the range: 0.2 to 100 MHz. Doubling the frequency halves the beam intensity.

Higher frequency ultrasound is attenuated more strongly than lower frequencies. The sharp decline in tissue penetration at frequencies greater than 7.5MHz is shown by the graph in Fig.17.7(b) which shows image depth in millimeters for a 50% attenuation of the signal.

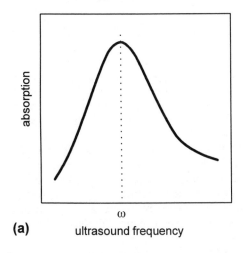

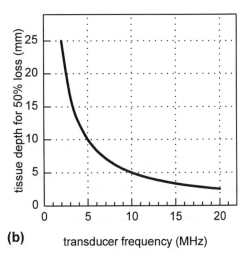

(a) ultrasound frequency

(b) transducer frequency (MHz)

Figure 17.7 (a) Absorption of ultrasound with frequency for a particular tissue showing its relaxation frequency (ω) **(b)** Tissue depth for 50% loss of intensity for a typical frequency range assuming 1dB cm^{-1} MHz^{-1}.

Table 17.5 Sound absorption and acoustic impedance.

Material	α dB cm^{-1} at 1MHz	Z kg m^{-2} s^{-1}
Fat	0.6	1.38
Blood	0.18	1.61
Brain	0.85	1.55
Soft tissue	1.0	1.63
Liver	0.9	1.65
Muscle (along fibers)	1.2	1.65
Muscle (across fibers)	3.3	1.65
Eye lens	2.0	1.85
Bone	20	6.1
Plastic	2.0	3.2

17.3 THE ULTRASOUND TRANSDUCER

Audible sound waves can be produced by hitting a piece of metal and making it ring. The same basic principle is used to produce ultrasound waves but in this case an electric pulse is used as the 'hammer' which causes deformation and vibration of special crystalline material.

A device which converts one form of energy to another is called a **transducer.** Transducers are used in the production and detection of diagnostic ultrasound and convert electrical energy into mechanical energy (producing sound); the returning sound echoes convert their mechanical energy to electrical energy (the signal). This is the **piezoelectric effect** and the materials are piezoelectric crystals. Ultrasound transducers are used in a variety of clinical applications:

- **A-scan.** This displays reflection patterns only as time/depth displays.
- **B-scan.** The transducer is scanned mechanically or electronically. Positional signals give x and y axes for the single slice display.
- **Real time scan.** The beam is swept electronically at fast frame rates. This is the most common form of transducer now available.
- **M-mode.** This transducer records the movement of organ walls particularly cardiac chambers.

17.3.1 Piezoelectricity

Piezoelectric materials experience a change in shape upon the application of an electric field. They have **molecular dipoles** where positive and negative charges are separated. This is represented in the diagram Fig.17.8. When an electrical pulse is applied across the crystal the orientation of these dipoles changes, causing a variation in the thickness of the crystal, **compression** or **expansion.** Conversely, if mechanical force is applied to the crystal the molecular dipoles change their orientation, altering the electric field and producing a small voltage signal. Due to the reciprocal property the same transducer can be used for producing ultrasound pulses (mechanical signal) and detecting the returning sound echoes (electrical signal). Quartz was the first material seen to have piezoelectric properties, but the most commonly used transducer materials in diagnostic ultrasound are synthetic materials e.g. ceramic lead zirconate titanate ($PbZrTiO_4$). These have replaced quartz in transducer manufacture.

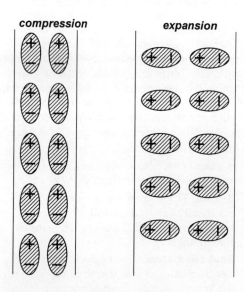

Figure 17.8 Piezoelectric effect showing the electrically charged dipoles positioned during compression and expansion due to either electrical or mechanical effects.

17.3.2 Basic transducer design

Simple, individual transducers are now rarely used in medical ultrasound imaging, but the basic design of a single transducer serves to illustrate the important parts that are common to multiple crystal (multi-element) transducers. The basic design illustrated in Fig.17.9(a) shows a **transducer crystal** with electrical connections to front and back.

Damping material as a **backing block** behind the crystal is composed of a resin/metal powder composite, (Z 3×10^7 kg m^{-2} s^{-1}) damping reverberations in the crystal, absorbing backward radiation and maintaining a forward pulse direction through the tissue (a lower impedance path).

In **transmitting-mode** a high voltage is applied to the transducer. The applied voltage V is related to intensity as:

$$V = \sqrt{intensity} \qquad (17.16)$$

Similarly in **receiving-mode** the crystal experiences changes in pressure from the returning echo signals producing the very small signal voltages.

17.3.3 Wavelength matching

When an ultrasound probe is applied to a patient it is desirable that the majority of sound energy produced in the crystal should penetrate the patient's skin, however there is a very large difference between the acoustic impedance of the transducer crystal and soft tissue. Major mismatch problems are solved by fixing a matching or **transmission layer** on the transducer crystal face. This is a plastic polymer layer which, for optimum transmission, has a thickness equal to a **quarter wavelength** of the sound (¼λ or odd multiples of this value). Its impedance is given by:

$$Z_M = \sqrt{Z_T \times Z_L} \qquad (17.17)$$

where the acoustic impedance: Z_M for the plastic matching layer, Z_T for the crystal and Z_L for the tissue. Figure 17.9(b) identifies the crystal and matching layer thicknesses used

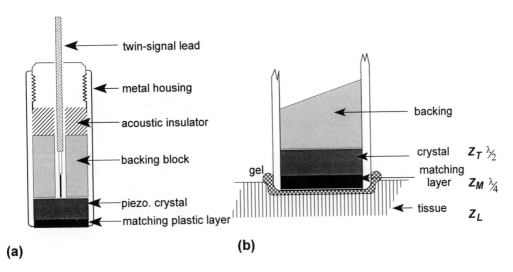

Figure 17.9 **(a)** Basic single transducer design showing the component parts that are also common to transducers having multiple elements (crystals) **(b)** Half and quarter wave matching for the transducer crystal and matching layer

for optimum performance examples and examples are calculated in Box 17.4.

Box 17.4

Matching layer impedance

The basic formula is: $Z_M = \sqrt{Z_T \times Z_L}$

Where: Z_M is the required acoustic impedance for the matching layer.
Z_T transducer acoustic impedance $(30 \times 10^6 \text{ kg m}^{-2} \text{ s}^{-1})$
Z_L the tissue acoustic impedance $(1.5 \times 10^6 \text{ kg m}^{-2} \text{ s}^{-1})$

$$Z_M = \sqrt{(30 \times 1.5)} = 6.7 \times 10^6 \text{ kg m}^{-2}\text{s}^{-1}$$

The matching layer is usually made from plastic material:
Perspex/Plexiglas = $3.2 \times 10^6 \text{ kg m}^{-2} \text{ s}^{-1}$.
This is commonly loaded with aluminum powder to exactly match the calculated Z value.

The primary function of the matching layer is to increase sound transmission into the soft tissues. Applying a layer which has a quarter wavelength thickness or an odd multiple, known as 'quarter-wave matching', provides good transmission through the skin layer. A gel coupling medium between the skin surface and transducer matching layer is used which removes air bubbles which would cause significant signal loss.

Due to a range of frequencies in the ultrasound pulse the matching layer cannot be exactly λ/4 for all wavelengths so matching is less than 100% efficient. Multiple matching layers are sometimes employed to improve efficiency. The frequency of the transmitted ultrasound pulse is determined by the crystal thickness d; the wavelength λ of the ultrasound is equal to twice the thickness of the crystal and from eqn.17.2 as λ = 2d then:

$$f = \frac{c}{2d} \qquad (17.18)$$

where c the velocity of sound in the piezoelectric crystal. If crystal thickness is λ/2 then

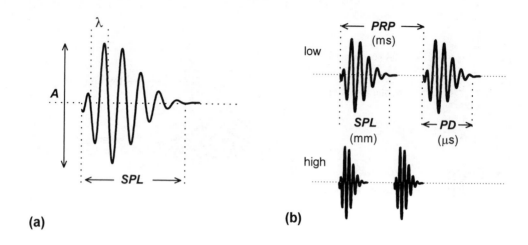

Figure 17.10 **(a)** Ultrasound pulse shape showing 3 cycles having wavelength λ and amplitude *A* and spatial pulse length SPL. **(b)** increasing frequency shortens SPL.

excitation stresses are reinforced and the crystal resonates at that frequency. These formulas are used in the design of ultrasound transducers and worked examples are shown in Box 17.5.

The output from the crystal should fall off quickly once the electrical stimulus is removed. The damping material provides this since the backing block behind the piezoelectric crystal is highly absorbent made of fine tungsten particles suspended in epoxy resin. The tungsten particles act as scattering centers, while the resin absorbs the scattered ultrasound. The backing block should ideally have an acoustic impedance which equals that of the crystal so that no reflection occurs at the crystal/backing block interface.

The transducer and backing block are separated from the casing of the probe by an ultrasonic insulator, e.g. rubberized cork. This minimizes the transmission of the ultrasound energy to the casing vibrations that would be picked up by the transducer in receive mode and registered as image artifacts.

Box 17.5

Transducer design considerations

Transducer Crystal Thickness

Basic formula: $\lambda = \dfrac{c}{f}$

For $PbZrTiO_4$ material $c = 4000$ m s^{-1}
So in order to construct a 1MHz Transducer:

$$\lambda = \frac{4000}{1 \times 10^6} = 4 \times 10^{-3} \text{ m (4mm)}$$

Therefore ½λ = 2mm for a 1MHz transducer
For a 5MHz Transducer this would be :

$$\lambda = 8 \times 10^{-4} \text{ m (0.8mm) } \tfrac{1}{2}\lambda = 0.4\text{mm}$$

Matching Layer thickness
The speed of sound for plastic used for transducer lenses is typically 2680m s^{-1}. The wavelength for a 5MHz transducer would be 0.536mm. A ¼λ matching layer would be 0.134mm or odd multiples of this (i.e. ×3 = 0.402mm)

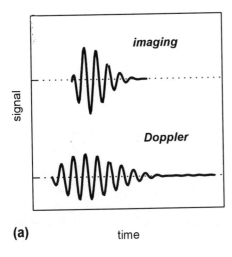 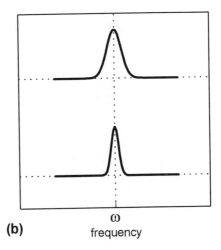

(a)   time   **(b)**   frequency

Figure 17.11 **(a)** Two signals showing the difference between a broad bandwidth short SPL pulse used for imaging and a narrow bandwidth long SPL pulse used for Doppler flow measurements. **(b)** Fourier analysis reveals the frequency component.

17.3.4 Pulse geometry

Once the crystal is pulsed the duration of its output is very short. Ideally the pulse would rise and fall very rapidly and contain only one wavelength, however a pulse usually contains 2 to 3 wavelengths. A typical pulse shape is shown in Fig.17.10(a) identifying wavelength λ, amplitude A and the pulse length.

Spatial pulse length (SPL) This is the length of the pulse in millimeters and is defined as:

$$wavelength \times number\ of\ cycles\ (n)$$

For a 5MHz transducer where λ is 0.3mm the SPL would be 0.9mm for a three cycle pulse ($n=3$). The SPL has a typical range of 0.3 to 1.0mm for diagnostic ultrasound and depends on transducer frequency as shown by the pulses in Fig.17.10(b) for a low and high frequency transducer (e.g. 3.5 and 7.5MHz). The **pulse duration** (PD), measured in µs, is given by n/f and varies typically between 0.4 and 1.5µs. A range of SPL and PD values for a three-cycle pulse is given in Tab. 17.6.

The SPL alters during its transmission through tissue since the process of attenuation resembles a low-frequency (low-pass) filter removing higher frequencies. The higher frequencies of the transmitted pulse are attenuated more strongly during their travel through tissue than the lower frequencies and as a consequence the spatial pulse length increases so degrading image resolution. This filtering of higher frequencies is called **dispersion**. This has a strong influence on **spatial resolution** in the ultrasound image.

Table 17.6 Frequency, SPL and PD for 3λ

Frequency (MHz)	SPL (mm)	PD (µs)
2.5	1.8	1.2
5.0	0.9	0.6
7.5	0.6	0.4
10.0	0.45	0.3

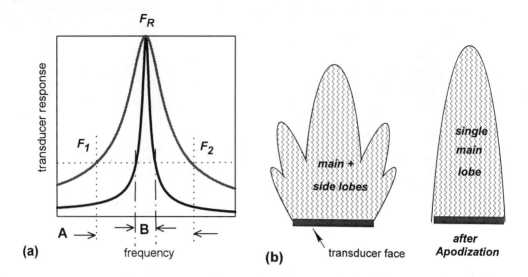

Figure 17.12 **(a)** Two signals having a low(A) and high (B) Q factor. The horizontal line represents a 0.707 reference point (not to scale). **(b)** The ultrasound beam projecting from the transducer face showing side-lobes which can decrease main lobe power unless removed by apodization.

***Pulse repetition frequency* (PRF)** This is the number of pulses per second and set by a master clock in the ultrasound unit. An electrical pulse generator drives the transducer which causes each resonant pulse. For a SPL of about 1μs and a PRF of 1kHz this leaves a period of approximately 999μs between pulses so the transducer is in 'receive-mode' for 99.9% of the time. Increasing the PRF increases the image information rate (echoes received) but shortens receive time so limiting the time for receiving distant echoes in the anatomical region being studied.

Image depth The time between pulses must be greater than the 'return trip' which is equivalent to image depth $D{\times}2$; the maximum PRF is determined by $c/2D$. If a penetration of 150mm is required and c is 1500m s^{-1} then the PRF is about 5kHz. A typical value in practice is 2 to 3kHz

17.3.5 Resonant frequency and Q

The pulse produced by the transducer in Fig.7.11(a) is a mixture of frequencies. The shorter the pulse the greater the frequency mixture and the broader the **bandwidth.** The frequency spectrum of two signals is shown in Fig.17.11(b) for both imaging and Doppler. The Doppler pulse has a greater SPL and gives a tighter frequency spectrum since increasing SPL decreases bandwidth. SPL and bandwidth are related as $1/SPL \propto bandwidth$.

Bandwidth The frequency spectrum shown by curve A in Figure 17.12(a) has a broad bandwidth and curve B a narrow bandwidth. This is measured between F_1 and F_2 in the graph. The frequency cut-off, above and below these limits should be sharp in order to reject noise; this is the case with spectrum B. The efficiency of ultrasound production, its purity of sound (restricted frequency range) and the duration of the pulse are expressed in terms of a Q factor. A high Q transducer produces a pure single frequency with a long duration or ringing time (Doppler waveform in Fig.17.11) A low Q transducer produces a mixed frequency sound pulse of short duration. The two signals B and A shown in Fig.17.12(a) have a high and a low Q factor.

Q is expressed as:

$$Q = \frac{F_R}{F_2 - F_1} \qquad (17.19)$$

where F_R is the resonant or dominant frequency and F_1, F_2 are points below and above the resonance peak where the signal intensity is reduced by $1/\sqrt{2}$ or 0.707; these points are marked as dotted and dashed lines. An increased bandwidth and a decreased spatial pulse length reduces the Q factor. A high Q crystal is used for transmission when a pure ultrasound source is required (e.g. Doppler). A broader Q crystal would be used for imaging where a short SPL gives good image resolution. Transducers for medical imaging have Q factors related to the number of cycles in the pulse typically 2-4.

Side lobes Ideally ultrasound pulse energy appears as a single front traveling in a forward direction from the crystal face however some energy travels off in different directions called grating or side lobes (Fig.17.12(b)). This extraneous energy must be suppressed otherwise the transmitted energy will be dissipated in multiple lobes and degrade image quality (contrast and resolution). **Apodization** means 'removal of the feet' representing removal of subsidiary maximas in the sound pulse. Shaping the acoustic aperture changes the envelope of the transmitted pulse from a square function to a gaussian; this effectively eliminates the side lobes and markedly improves image quality.

17.4   THE ULTRASONIC FIELD

The shape of the ultrasound pulse produced by the transducer crystal determines the resolution of an imaging device. The beam dimensions change as they travel through tissue; this strongly influences image quality with depth.

17.4.1 The beam profile

The ability of the imaging device to distinguish two objects placed very close together in the plane at right angles to the direction of the beam is a measure of its **lateral resolution**. The shape of the ultrasound beam, shown in Fig.17.13(a) is at first narrow and is determined by the size of the transducer and the wavelength of the sound (which depends on the frequency). After a certain distance the beam diverges. The beam shape therefore consists of two distinct regions: the near field or **Fresnel zone** (AJ Fresnel, French phyicist 1788-1827) and the far field or **Fraunhofer zone** (J von Fraunhofer, German physicist 1787-1826). The near field maintains the width of the transducer, the beam then spreads out in the far field or undergoes divergence causing a decrease in lateral resolution and intensity of the beam. The length of the near field Z_f is governed by:

$$Z_f = \frac{\alpha^2}{\lambda} \qquad (17.20)$$

where α is the half width (radius) of the transducer and λ is the wavelength of ultrasound.

As the width of the transducer is increased the length of the Fresnel zone is maintained, (Fig.17.13(b)), so a narrow transducer will provide high resolution over a short distance while a wider probe will maintain lower resolution for greater distances. Equation 17.20 shows that the length of the Fresnel zone is proportional to the square of the transducer radius and inversely proportional to the wavelength. Figure 17.13(c) and (d) demonstrates that length of the near field (and therefore the lateral resolution at depth) is improved as the wavelength is shortened i.e. using a higher ultrasound frequency from 1MHz to 5MHz. But the attenuation of ultrasound increases with frequency, so while the lateral resolution is maintained for greater depths the amplitudes of returning echo signals will be decreased and **image depth** reduced.

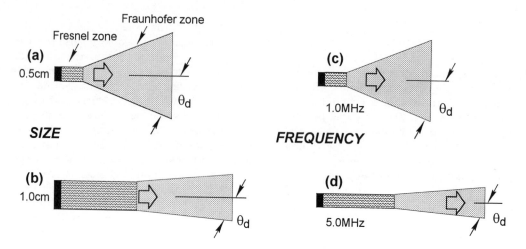

Figure 17.13   The variation of Fresnel and Fraunhofer zones for a single element transducer having sizes **(a)** 0.5 and **(b)** 1.0cm. The beam profile for the 0.5cm transducer is then shown at **(c)** 1MHz and **(d)** 5MHz.

17.4.2 Divergence

At the end of the near field (Fresnel zone) the beam begins to spread out or diverge; this is the far field or Fraunhofer zone. The magnitude of this divergence is given by:

$$\theta = \sin^{-1}(0.61\,\lambda/\alpha) \qquad (17.21)$$

where θ is the **angle of divergence**, λ is the wavelength and α is again the half width of the transducer. Field divergence decreases with increasing transducer width and with decreasing wavelength or increasing frequency; so **resolution at depth** is best with wide transducers and high frequency. Clearly compromises are made to optimize image quality with image depth; this will be a problem as frequencies are increased. Ophthalmology requires high resolution for shallow depths and the frequency of ultrasound is generally higher than for conventional diagnostic imaging.

17.4.3 Resolution

There are two axes of resolution in an ultrasound image: **lateral** resolution which describes resolving power across the beam and **axial** in the path or parallel to the beam. Both the axial and lateral resolution are measures of the system's ability to separate closely placed reflecting surfaces.

Axial resolution   Resolving two closely placed surfaces parallel to the direction of the beam is determined by the spatial pulse length (SPL) so the higher the frequency of the ultrasound the shorter the pulse length (Fig.17.10(b)). Since the high frequency component of the pulse is preferentially absorbed by its passage through tissue (frequency dispersion) the SPL increases and axial resolution becomes degraded. A measure of axial resolution is given by $SPL/2$.

Lateral resolution   The resolution across the beam depends on the focusing ability of the transducer as shown in Fig.17.14. The distance to the focal zone Z_f where the beam starts to diverge is given by eqn. 17.20. The lateral resolution at this point depends on the radius of curvature R determining the focal dimensions. These are usually termed weak focus $Z_f/R < 2$, medium $Z_f/R \simeq 2\text{-}3$ and strong $Z_f/R \approx$3-4. In general ultrasound transducers have better axial than lateral resolution but strongly focused beams can provide symmetrical resolution performance.

Examples of image depth and approximate axial resolution/lateral resolution are listed in Tab. 17.7 for selected frequencies. Examples will be given in the next chapter on ultrasound imaging.

Table 17.7 Transducer resolution

Frequency	Image depth	Axial res.	Lateral res.
2.0	30	0.7	3.0
3.5	17	0.4	1.7
5.0	12	0.3	1.2
7.5	8	0.2	0.8
10.0	6	0.15	0.6

Summary

Where λ is wavelength, c speed of sound in the medium and f the ultrasound frequency and n the number of cycles in the pulse.

- $Intensity = \dfrac{power\ (mW)}{area\ (mm^2)}$

- Wavelength matching:
  Crystal thickness $\lambda/2$ mm
  Matching layer $\lambda/4$ mm

- Matching layer impedance $Z_M = \sqrt{(Z_T \times Z_L)}$
  where Z_T represents the transducer and Z_L the matching layer

- Propagation period = $1/f$ µs
- Pulse wavelength = c/f mm
- Spatial Pulse Length (SPL) = n/λ mm
- Pulse duration (PD) = n/f µs

- Near field length (Fresnel zone) $Z_f = \dfrac{\alpha^2}{\lambda}$

  where α is half width (or radius) of the transducer.

- Diversion angle (Fraunhofer zone)
  $\theta = \sin^{-1}(0.61 \cdot \lambda/\alpha)$

- Axial resolution = SPL/2
- Lateral resolution $R\lambda/\alpha$

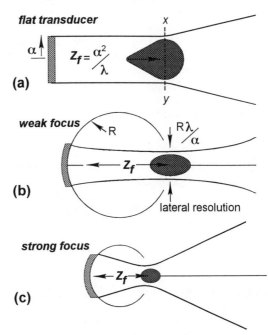

Figure 17.14 The various focal positions for **(a)** flat **(b)** a weakly focused and **(c)** a strongly focused transducer showing the length of the near field (Z_f) and focal zone.

KEYWORDS

acoustic absorption   The loss of sound energy by attenuation and scatter.

acoustic amplitude   This measured from the zero (cross-over) point of the sine-wave to its peak in mV or µV

acoustic frequency f The compression and rarefaction events translated as a sine wave whose frequency range is 2.5 to 15MHz in clinical ultrasound.

acoustic impedance Z is the product of material density and speed of sound.

acoustic intensity   The power per unit area (W cm^{-2})

acoustic parameters   pressure density, temperature, acoustic impedance.

acoustic power   The sound energy per unit time J s^{-1} or watts.

acoustic pressure   The pressure difference from normal pressure induced by sound waves. Units are pascals. $1Pa = 1N\ m^{-2} = 10\mu bar$; a typical range is 0.06 to 1.5MPa

amplitude   wave peak height.

anechoic   echo free

angle of incidence   angle between beam direction and the perpendicular axis

angle of reflection   equals the angle of incidence.

apodization   removal of sound beam side lobes by using gaussian beam profile

continuous wave   indefinite wave not pulsed

coupling gel   soft grease provides continuous interface excluding air.

cycle (Hz)   complete transition of waveform measured from identical points (zero crossing or peaks)

cycles per pulse   typical pulse contains 1 to 3 cycles.

decibel (dB)   the logarithmic comparative measure of power, intensity and amplitude or voltage gain.

diffraction   bending of a beam at the edge of an absorbing surface into the shadow area of the surface.

dispersion   pulse spreads out as it passes through medium. Pulse height decreases as pulse width increases. Depends on the property of the medium.

divergent angle (θ)   the angle describing far field divergence. (see Fraunhofer zone)

duty factor DF :   time fraction that the pulse is on. Typical value 5ms, range 1 to 10ms. $DF = PD/PRP \times 1000$ or $PD \times PRF/1000$ ms.

elongation velocity   velocity of a particle about its equilibrium position. Typical value 35mm s^{-1}

Fraunhofer zone   far field divergence related to wavelength and transducer diameter as $\sin \theta = 0.612 \times \lambda / \alpha$

frequency (Hz)   cycles per second. typical ultrasound values 2 to 10MHz.

Fresnel zone   near zone dependent on transducer diameter d or aperture $d^2/4\lambda$

imaging depth   maximum penetration that will yield image information. Proportional to $75/PRF$

impedance Z   material density × propagation speed. Typical range 1.3×10^6 to 1.7×10^6 rayls

longitudinal wave   compression wave in parallel to wave direction.

modulus of elasticity E   a measurement of material stiffness represented by *stress/strain*. The inverse is compressibility or $1/E$

particle velocity   typically 3.5 cm s^{-1} displacement to and fro from the rest position.

period T   time per cycle. Range 0.1 to 0.5μs. $T = 1/f$

piezoelectric effect   shown by a material whose dimensions change with electric charge. Mechanical deformation produces an electrical charge.

power   work done per unit time J s^{-1}

propagation velocity c   speed of displacement through the medium. Typical value 1500 m s^{-1} for soft tissue.

pulse duration   a typical pulse duration is 0.5 to 3μs. PD = cycles × period or *cycles/f*

pulse repetition frequency PRF   time to repeat ultrasound pulse. Range 2 to 10kHz

pulse repetition period (PRP)   time from one

pulse to the next *PRP* = 1/PRF range 0.1 to 0.5ms.

Rayl a measure of acoustic impedance in kg $m^{-2} s^{-1}$

reflection (specular) reflection of ultrasound from a smooth surface.

reflection (non-specular) reflection of ultrasound from a rough surface.

refraction the bending of the transmitted beam due to change in propagation velocity shown by the change of beam direction when traveling from one medium to another.

relaxation frequencies frequency of maximum absorption in a medium.

resolution (axial) resolving power parallel to the beam travel. Influenced by *SPL*/2

resolution (lateral) resolving power across the beam. Depends on focal dimensions of the beam influenced by aperture size and electronic focusing.

scattering redirection of sound beam in several directions.

side lobes minor sound beams traveling at an angle from the main beam in a single element.

spatial pulse length (SPL) length of a single pulse. Typical values 0.1 to 1.0mm.

specular reflection (mirror reflection) reflection from a large smooth surface.
SPL = cycles × wavelength.

wavelength propagation speed/frequency. Typical ultrasound range 0.1 to 0.5mm depending on medium.

Ultrasound Imaging

18.1 Ultrasound Imaging
18.2 Image Processing
18.3 Transducers

18.4 Image Artifacts
18.5 Blood velocity measurement
18.6 Safety

18.1 ULTRASOUND IMAGING

Since the development of multi-element array technology in the early 1970's mechanical scanning methods have been gradually superseded. Electronically switched transducer arrays are now used exclusively for ultrasound imaging except for annular transducers that still use mechanical methods.

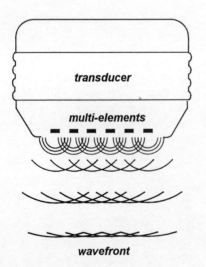

Figure 18.1 Sound wave propagation from multiple transducers forming a wave front according to Huygens principle.

Display modes There are two basic display modes offered by diagnostic ultrasound: brightness modulation or B-mode which gives a gray scale picture and M-mode which instead of a two dimensional spatial image traces out a two dimensional time-versus-movement graphic display, which indicates the motion of cardiac chambers or valves.

The B-mode display gives a brightness scale (gray scale) depending on echo strength. Distinct interfaces between different tissues are seen as white regions. The B-mode picture displays a section through the body anatomy whose image depth depends on transducer parameters (frequency, focusing etc.). The image display, or **frame**, is constructed from **scan lines**, the number depending on the number of individual elements in the transducer. The image is refreshed at regular intervals called the **frame rate**. If the frame rate is fast enough then a 'real-time' display can be observed. Single frames can be held in the computer memory for inspection; this is a 'freeze-frame' display.

Multi-element propagation The array transducer consists of many small elements that combine to give a single ultrasound wave front. Figure 18.1 shows the propagation of a sound front formed in front of a transducer array.

The sound issuing from multiple transducer elements in an array obeys Huygens Principle developed by him to explain the propagation

multi-element transducer

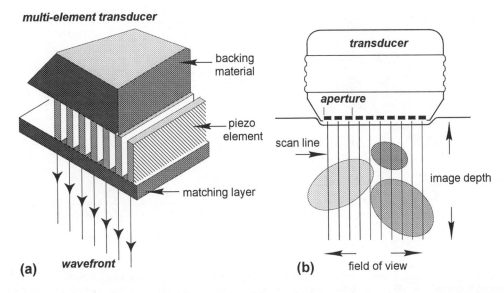

Figure 18.2 **(a)** Three dimensional plan of a multi-element transducer showing individual elements, the common backing material and matching layer. **(b)** Basic multi-element linear transducer showing scan length and field of view and image depth.

of light. (C. Huygens: Dutch physicist 1629-1693). Each transducer element serves as a point sound source radially expanding until they interact with each other and produce a combined **wave front.** The ultrasound from these **real-time** transducers travels as a wave-front through the tissue.

18.1.1 Real time transducer

The ultrasound real-time transducer consists of a series of identical rectangular shaped piezoelectric elements, each element individually pulsed. The general construction is shown in Fig.18.2(a). The width of each element is measured in wavelengths ranging from 1 to 4λ, the absolute dimension decided by transducer frequency (see previous Tab. 17.2).

The wave front issuing from the multi-element transducer has the same dimensions, in the near field (Fresnel zone), as the total transducer surface. The near field converges slightly just before diverging. In the far field elements in an array obey Huygens Principle (Fraunhofer zone described in Chapter 17). The near and far field dimensions are gov-

erned by transducer frequency and array dimensions (**aperture**) and electronic focusing procedures.

Scan lines Figure18.2(b) shows that each element of a linear transducer produces a **scan line** whose length is the **image depth**. Linear arrays produce parallel scan lines while other array designs produce sector shapes. The image depth depends on beam penetration (sound frequency) and pulse timing. The physical size of the array head (area) is its **footprint;** linear arrays have large foot-prints, other array designs have smaller footprints.

Aperture The transducer **aperture** is determined by the group of transducer elements working in unison. Aperture size can vary during data transmission and reception giving the transducer a **dynamic aperture**. A linear transducer produces a 3-dimensional ultrasound beam whose propagation pattern, shown in Fig.18.3(a), gives a rectilinear cover whose area depends on the number of elements in the transducer. The side dimension

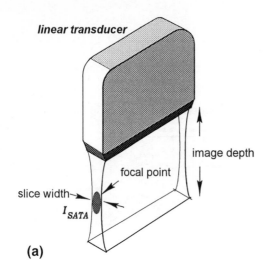

(a)

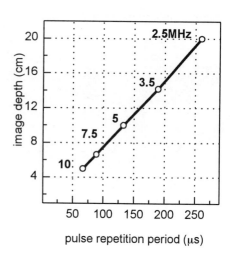

pulse repetition period (μs)

Figure 18.3   **(a)** A linear transducer giving a beam shape which narrows toward the middle.   This is the section thickness. I_{SATA} is a measure of sound intensity referred to in the section on safety. **(b)** The change of image depth with pulse repetition period (PRP). Transducer frequency from 2.5 to 10MHz is also identified on the slope.

of the beam edge is defined by an acoustic lens which determines the **section thickness**.

18.1.2   Ultrasound pulse timing

The ultrasound signal is produced by a high voltage pulse delivered to each element in the transducer array. This produces a **critically damped** ultrasound 'ring' of 2 to 3 wavelengths.   The length of this pulse (spatial pulse length: SPL) and the frequency of pulse production (pulse repetition frequency: PRF) defines certain important image characteristics that have been defined in Chapter 17.

Spatial Pulse Length (SPL)   This is related to wavelength as:

$$SPL = \lambda \times number\ of\ cycles \quad (18.1)$$

Transmission pulses are damped to give 2-3 complete cycles. Three cycles of a higher frequency clearly have a shorter SPL than three cycles of lower frequency (see Chapter 17) but

as the frequency is increased penetration of the ultrasound beam is reduced (absorption increases linearly with increasing frequency). Dimensions are typically between 0.45 and 2.25mm for a diagnostic imaging range.

Pulse duration (PD)   This measures the time period of the pulse. Ultrasound imaging typically uses pulses that are 2-3 wavelengths long.

$$PD = period\ (\mu s) \times number\ of\ cycles$$
$$(18.2)$$

This is typically between 0.5 and 3 μs for current machines.

Pulse Repetition Frequency (PRF)   The transducer element group is excited by an electrical signal which generates the ultrasound **transmission pulse** whose frequency depends on the transducer element dimensions.   A chain of timed transmission pulses is delivered to the transducer while imaging. The timing between the transmission pulses, the **pulse repetition period** PRP, is critical for each transducer type since this determines the rate of image formation or **frame rate** and **imaging depth** D_{max} identified in Fig.18.3(b). If a 1µs transmission pulse is followed by a waiting period of 200µs (receive period) this will give:

$$PRF = 1/(200 \times 10^6) = 5000 Hz \ (5kHz).$$

Typical PRF values range from 2-10kHz for diagnostic imaging. Over 99% of the timing cycle is spent listening for echoes since pulse duration is typically 1µs compared to a pulse repetition period of 200µs. The pulse repetition period (PRP) is matched to the image depth or scan line length (SL) otherwise echo pulses may clash with transmission pulses if the PRP is too short.

Sound attenuation increases with frequency and this is the major determining factor for image depth. The graph in Fig.18.3(b) plots the relationship between PRP and imaging depth for a speed of sound of 1500cm s^{-1}; transducer frequencies used at various PRP values are superimposed on the graph. Various clinical factors decide which frequency is used since higher frequency transducers give improved image resolution and owing to faster PRP are more able to give real time displays and follow pulsatile (cardiac) movement.

Duty factor (DF) This is also the duty cycle and is the percentage or fractional measure of the time that the pulse occupies in the transmit receive cycle. It increases with increasing PRF.

$$DF = \frac{PD}{PRP} \qquad (18.3)$$

Image depth (D_{max}) This can be calculated from the speed of sound in soft tissue (1500m s^{-1}) and allowing for a return path (so halving this distance) then D_{max} = 150000 × 0.5 × PRP or 75000 × PRP cm. For a PRP of 200µs this would give an imaging depth of 15cm.

Alternatively D_{max} can be calculated as 75000/*PRF*. Similarly for soft tissue imaging:

$$PRF = \frac{1500}{2 \cdot D_{max}} \qquad (18.4)$$

Higher frequency transducers have higher PRP values so give shallower image depths as demonstrated in Fig.18.3(b).

Both PD and PRP are measured in µs to give the DF as a unitless fraction. The duty factor is an important measure of ultrasound power used in ultrasound safety.

Bandwidth As improvements are made to transducer materials the characteristic impedance is lowered along with degrees of mismatch. Backing material is used which does not absorb as much sound energy so transducer sensitivity is improved giving increased dynamic range and image depth. Transducer bandwidth is also increased which can be used in one or two ways:

- Operator choice of center frequency in a narrow window moved over the larger bandwidth giving multi-frequency probes and choice of image depth   *or*
- Large bandwidth transmission which gives a wide range of echo information maintaining maximum image depth at all times.

Manufacturers supply variations on these basic properties.

18.1.3 Spatial resolution

Resolution is measured as the minimum distance between objects (in mm) which can be distinguished in the image. Ultrasound transducer resolution is described in terms of:

- Axial
- Lateral
- Section thickness

Axial Resolution (R_x) Axial resolution is measured in the direction parallel to the beam and is illustrated in Figure 18.4(a). It is determined by the **transmission pulse width.** Ideally this should be a single cycle duration of the particular ultrasound frequency. In practice the pulse tends to last for two to three cycles. The backing material is a mechanical damping device for reducing the SPL;

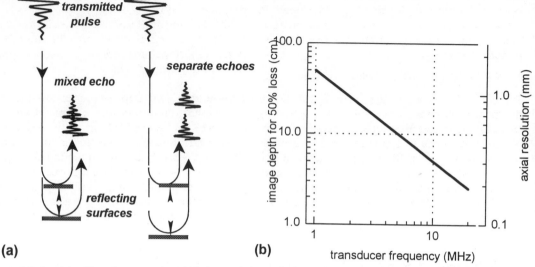

Figure 18.4 (a) Signal separation defining axial resolution. This depends on SPL so the two surfaces could be resolved by using a higher frequency and shorter SPL. (b) PRP and imaging depth for various frequency transducers identified on the slope. Image depth for 50dB attenuation and transducer frequency with approximate axial resolution.

electronic damping is also used to ensure a 2 to 3 cycle SPL.

Axial resolution is measured as the ability to resolve reflecting surfaces along the beam path is determined by the pulse duration (spatial pulse length SPL). Axial resolution R_x is related as:

$$R_x = \frac{spatial\ pulse\ length}{2} \qquad (18.5)$$

Axial resolution can be improved by decreasing the length of the transmission pulse. In practice this can only be achieved by increasing the pulse frequency and thereby decreasing the spatial pulse length (SPL). Figure 18.4(b) indicates that higher frequency transducers have higher axial resolutions but poorer imaging depth. Axial resolutions are on the second y-axis in Fig. 18.4(b) for the range of clinical ultrasound frequencies. Axial resolution varies due to high frequency loss with depth, the center frequency of the pulse decreasing with a consequent broadening of the SPL. **Contrast resolution** is determined by how effective the system is in separating pulse overlap as illustrated in Fig.18.4(a); this is influenced by signal strength and system sensitivity.

Lateral resolution This is governed by the beam width which depends on the number of element groups (the **aperture**) of the transducer during transmission and dynamic focusing during echo reception. Lateral resolution for a linear transducer is identified in Fig.18.5(a); a deeper focal zone would be given by a larger aperture.

Dynamic focusing and dynamic aperture maintains optimum lateral resolution for all depths, which will be described later. Lateral resolution across the beam is determined by the beam width and shape. Beam shape is not a constant dimension and depends on the focal point of the beam. A 3.5MHz transducer has an axial resolution between 0.6 and 0.8mm but lateral resolution is 3 to 5 times larger. Transducer **bandwidth** influences both axial and lateral resolution (Chapter 17).

Slice thickness The slice width or section thickness has already been identified in Fig.18.3(a) and is further defined by the end

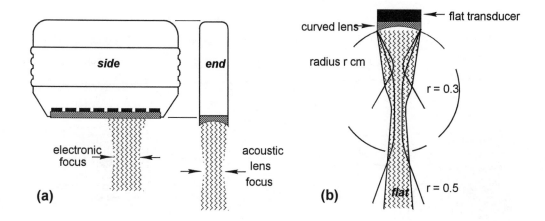

Figure 18.5 **(a)** Lateral resolution is defined by electronic focusing and varies with aperture size. The end view shows the acoustic lens curvature. **(b)** The slice width is determined by the curvature of the acoustic lens

view in Fig.18.5(a). The focal planes which determine slice width are identified in Fig.18.5(b). Beam width in this dimension is achieved by either shaping the transducer crystal or matching layer (see Chapter 17 and refraction). A focused beam is produced by providing a concave crystal and/or a matching layer as a lens system. The concave shape is not ideal for obtaining good contact with the skin. A focused crystal with a convex matching layer will usually provide an adequate amount of focusing and allow good skin contact.

Summary

Lateral resolution
- Is a measure of minimal separation of points across the beam.
- It varies with distance from the transducer (focal region) and aperture.
- It decreases (poorer resolution) with increasing beam width. It increases with frequency.

Axial resolution
- Is the minimal separation of surfaces in line with the beam.

- Governed by SPL as SPL/2 so decreases with increasing SPL (cycles or frequency).
- Imaging depth decreases with frequency.

18.2 IMAGE PROCESSING

The component parts of an ultrasound imaging system is shown in Fig.18.6. The ultrasound signal processing sequences are:

- The **Pulser** consisting of clock and pulse transmitter.
- **Amplification** increases the amplitude of the small echo signals.
- **Time Gain Compensation** where correction is made for tissue attenuation.
- **Signal Compression** reducing the broad range in echo amplitude before displaying the signals as an image.
- **Demodulation** or signal thresholding.
- **Signal Rejection** or filtering prepares the signal for digitization.

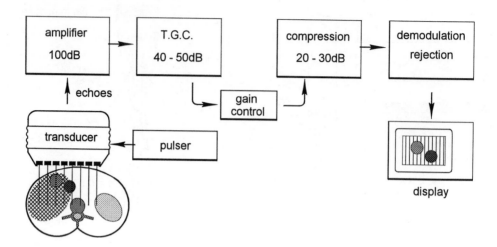

Figure 18.6 A simplified block diagram of the transducer processing circuits. The ultrasound pulse is driven by the pulser and returning echoes received by the amplifier/processing chain. The gain control is operator adjusted for image depth.

The transmitter The heart of the system is the **clock**. This controls all the timing of the transmission pulse, the pulse frequency (PRF), and image data (echo) collection by preparing receiving and digitization circuits. It synchronizes dynamic focusing and the controls the dynamic transducer aperture. The transmitter (combined with the clock as the pulser in the diagram) supplies the electrical pulse to the transducer array at times decided by the clock. Transmitter voltages range from about 5 volts up to a few 100's of volts; this can be operator adjusted. Piezoelectric materials can tolerate field strengths of up to 1kV mm^{-1}.

The receiver The simplest image involves only one reflecting object in the path of the beam but in practice, of course, there are many hundreds. A series of echoes will be received from these objects whose amplitudes will vary in size depending on the size of the echo and the depth at which the echo originates.

18.2.1 Signal pre-processing

Apodization This has been referred to in Chapter 17. The main intensity of an ultrasound beam is directed perpendicular to the transducer face; this is the main lobe. High side lobe and grating lobe level must be kept to a minimum since they will reduce image contrast due to off-axis echo signals which interfere with the main axis signals. Nonlinear signal processing accentuates these off axis signals. Apodization of the acoustic aperture by shaping the electrical pulse applied to the transducer reduces side-lobes in the ultrasound pulse and grating lobes in the multi-element array where the width of each element also influences the magnitude of grating lobe dimensions.

Amplification Small echo signals (μV) undergo linear amplification from a few microvolts to milli-volts so that they can be handled by the signal processing circuits.

Dynamic range This describes the ratio of

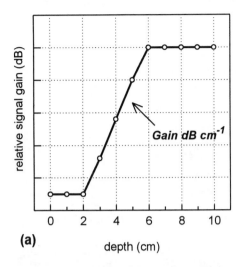

(a)

depth (cm)

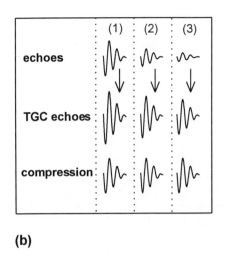

(b)

Figure 18.7 **(a)** TGC curve showing the slope representing dB cm^{-1} gain. **(b)** Time gain compensation altering the signal amplitude where late arriving signals receive more gain than earlier ones, the signals then undergo compression.

the smallest to the largest signals that can be handled by the amplifier. Echoes returning from tissues can have dynamic ranges of between 100 and 150dB giving amplitude differences A of:

$$A = 20 \, log \, \frac{A}{A_O} dB \qquad (18.6)$$

For 100 to 150dB this would represent a signal range of 1µV *to* 316µV. Power differences (intensity) would cover nano-watts to pico-watts. Amplified signals are processed by the signal conditioning circuits before being digitized for computer storage and eventually displayed as gray scale images. Dynamic range is decreased as the signals are processed since small signals carry mainly noise and little information so are rejected so improving the signal to noise ratio. The image depth D of a transducer typically represents a dynamic range limit of 50dB and the depth of penetration based on this figure is plotted in Fig.18.4(b). This is influenced by the at-

tenuation coefficient α in dB cm^{-1} MHz^{-1} and frequency f so that the product α · f · D = 50dB for soft tissue α = 1dB cm^{-1} MHz^{-1} so image depth is related to transducer frequency as:

$$D = \frac{50}{f} \qquad (18.7)$$

A final dynamic range of 50dB is typical of a modern ultrasound systems which would give practical image depths plotted in Fig.18.3(b) and Fig.18.4(b). The displayed dynamic range is operator controlled.

Time Gain Compensation (Swept Gain)
Echoes originating from greater tissue depths will have smaller amplitudes as the sound has undergone attenuation with distance traveled. In order to produce good quality images it is necessary to compensate for echo attenuation and a time varying gain control or time gain compensation **TGC** circuit amplifies the signal depending on time of arrival; later signals undergo greater amplification so cor-

recting signal amplitude loss from tissue attenuation. The process is also known as **swept gain** or **time varied gain**.

TGC techniques amplify the signal proportional to the time delay between the transmission and detection of the ultrasound pulses. In the simplest form of TGC the amplification is linear but modern imaging systems also provide non-linear amplification.   Either analog or digital methods which use look-up tables may be used. This form of signal compensation is illustrated in Fig. 18.7(a) where linear amplification dependent on depth is given to echo-signals originating from 2 to 6cm (in this example); echoes outside this range receive no amplification. The overall effect is illustrated in Fig.18.7(b).

Compression   After TGC the large dynamic range of signal amplitude cannot be displayed effectively so the signal range is compressed using logarithmic amplification represented in Fig.18.8, where smaller input signals (10-20µV) will undergo greater amplification than stronger signals (70-80µV). This increases the amplitude of the smaller signals at the expense of the larger signals and gives the final signal series illustrated by the bottom line of pulses in Fig.18.7(b). Dynamic range is usually reduced to about 20 to 30dB which can be handled more easily by the electronics.

Demodulation and rejection   After compression the signals undergo the equivalent of full-wave rectification which defines their outline or shape (envelope). This is the **demodulated signal**. A threshold is placed on the demodulated signals to reject smaller amplitude pulses which mostly carry acoustic or electronic noise and have very little useful information. The signals above threshold are then digitized.

Phase decoding   The conventional ultrasound image represents changes in signal amplitude, however current developments use information derived from both **phase** and **amplitude** with a consequent improvement in signal to noise ratio (SNR). Both spatial and temporal resolution are improved (faster

frame rates). Dynamic range is also increased to 100dB which improves image depth.

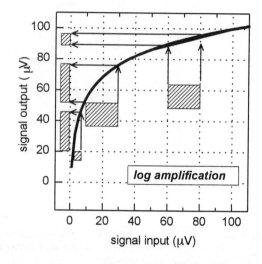

Figure 18.8   Signal compression achieved by logarithmic amplification. Small signal amplitudes are increased, large signals are unaltered.

18.2.2 Signal Digitization

In current ultrasound equipment image formation is controlled by computer and the clinical image is viewed on a video monitor in a continuous or real-time mode. First the echo signals undergo some processing and are then digitized according to echo strength. Figure 18.9(a) indicates how the stored pixel values (*y*-axis) in computer memory relate to echo signal strength (*x*-axis) for three selected dynamic ranges 30, 40 and 60dB. Figure 18.9(b) and (c) show scan line information from each transducer element group is located in an image matrix according to element position (matrix *x*-axis) and echo depth (matrix *y*-axis).   The matrix row (*x*-axis) is **time coded** for echoes arriving at fixed depths. The matrix columns (*y-axis*) are chosen by the transducer **group position**.

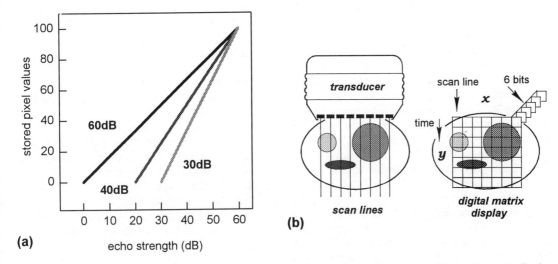

Figure 18.9 **(a)** Echoes are digitized according to time of arrival and strength. Three dynamic display ranges are shown 30, 40 and 60dB. **(b)** Image matrix coding according to scan line position (x-axis) and echo time of arrival (y-axis).

The **echo strength** is stored as a 6, 7 or 8-bit number in each memory location depending on dynamic range. An imaging device which uses a linear probe having 128 parallel beams allocates two columns in computer memory for each beam so the 2-Dimensional image memory has a capacity of 256×256 storage locations.

Locations in the memory array are addressed as columns 1 to 256 and rows 1 to 256. Echoes from *Beam-1* occupy columns 1 and 2, those from *Beam-2* occupy 3 and 4 and so on until beam 128 occupies columns 255 and 256. Each location or address in the 256×256 memory holds a digital number representing echo strength.

Sector scans The production of sector scans (see phased arrays later) follows the same general principle. However in sector scans the relationship between memory location and echo position is by **polar coordinates**. The angle and radius at which the echo occurs defines the memory location. The digital memory (frame) of a modern ultrasound display is typically 512×512 pixels; each pixel is 6,7 or 8 bits deep. Several of

these frames can be acquired each second. If the imaging depth is 15cm then each of the 512 pixels in the y-axis represent 150/512 = 0.3mm; for a 20cm imaging depth each pixel would represent 0.4mm.

18.2.3 Signal post-processing

Many aspects of image presentation are under user control. Echoes emanating from deep structures experience greater signal attenuation than those from superficial structures. Diagnostic imaging equipment allows the user to vary the amplification of echoes from different depths by using variable TGC. (see Fig.18.6 and 7) Usually the amplification increases with depth, however the user may decide not to amplify echoes from a variety of depths depending on whether that information is useful or not.

Sensitivity The simplest image involves only one reflecting surface in the path of the beam but in practice of course there is more than just one. A series of echoes will be received from these surfaces whose amplitudes will vary in size depending on the size of the echo and the depth at which the echo originates.

It may happen that echoes from diffuse structures at depth are so small as to be indistinguishable from the noise level which would also be amplified. The user may vary the depth of field of view by using zoom or expansion controls and, in sector imaging, the **field angle**. In real-time imaging the operator is depth limited, e.g. the depth that can be interrogated while still maintaining real-time or continuous effect. The continuous real-time effect may be sacrificed if extra image depth is required.

Gray scale display Each pixel contains a numerical value representing signal strength; stronger reflections have larger pixel values than weaker reflections. A gray scale display represents echo signal strengths. Pixel depth influences displayed image contrast; more bits per pixel increases this contrast range. Typical pixel depths are:

- 6 bits or 2^6 giving 64 gray scales
- 7 bits or 2^7 giving 128 gray scales
- 8 bits or 2^8 giving 256 gray scales

The binary values in each pixel are converted to analog (voltage) levels for display on a video monitor for visual inspection or film recording. The digital values are fed out from the matrix in sequence into a digital to analog converter (DAC) and the varying analog voltage coded with a video signal to give a video raster display.

18.3 TRANSDUCERS

Mechanical scanning methods previously used in ultrasound imaging have almost entirely been replaced by electronically scanned multi-element array transducers. There are two basic types of electronically scanned transducers:

- Sequenced (switched) transducer arrays (Linear or Curvilinear designs)
- Phased Transducer Arrays (Linear or Annular)

These transducers give different image shapes or scan fields and are shown in Fig.18.10. Each transducer has its own advantages and disadvantages, these are described for each transducer type and typical applications are given.

Sequenced arrays selectively pulse a group of transducer elements. The picture is constructed by moving the group sequence along the transducer. Resolution is determined by the number of scanned lines, field of view and transducer aperture already shown in Fig.18.2(b). The electronic distinction between sequenced and **phased** arrays is decided by the excitation pulse timing.

Annular array transducers differ from these designs since their separate elements form an annulus which is mechanically scanned.

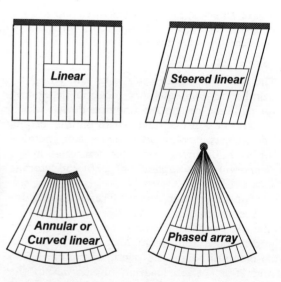

Figure 18.10   Image scan fields delivered by different transducers commonly used in diagnostic ultrasound.

18.3.1 The linear sequence array

The linear array is formed from a large number (up to 128) individual transducer **elements** arranged in groups. During each transmission/receive cycle only one transducer group (from 16 to 32 elements) is ac-

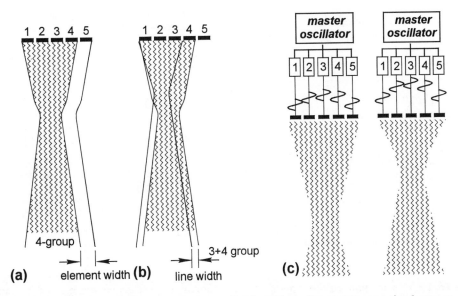

Figure 18.11 **(a)** Linear array beam sequence switching where the aperture varies between 3 and 4 elements which gives **(b)** a scan line separation less than the width of the individual element. **(c)** Varying the delay times applied to each element group influences the depth of focus of the aperture.

tive. The information for each scan line is obtained by switching; a single element is added to the group while the last element is removed.

The transducer group or **aperture** thus advances along the length of the transducer and reconstructs the sectional image line by line defined by the individual element width. The ultrasound field from an individual small element in a multi-element linear array would be a very fine beam. Due to these narrow dimensions the beam would have a very short near field and would diverge very quickly giving poor resolution at depth. This problem can be solved by pulsing groups of transducers in unison; usually 8-32 elements on a 60-120 element array. This produces a wider beam with much improved resolution characteristics at depth. The group size defines the transducer aperture. A scanning motion is obtained by shifting an element one at a time as seen in Fig.18.11(a).

The number of scan lines can be doubled if two groups having different sizes are used. In Fig. 18.11(b), where $n = 3$, if the first group

consists of n elements transmitting and receiving as a unit and the second group has an extra element added, giving $n+1$ elements, then the central axis of this unit only shifts by a ½-element compared with the first group. During each transmission/receive cycle only a single transducer group is active (n or $n+1$).

Although linear arrays can operate in an unfocused mode linear sequential arrays are commonly focused by delaying or phasing the excitation pulses, Fig.18.11(c). This produces either a short or long focal length; the delay pulses have nanosecond timing (10^{-9} s). A focused linear array is sometimes called a **phased linear array**. Pulse delay focuses the beam but the linear array is still operated in a **sequenced** manner.

Linear scanning uses **rectilinear coordinates**; the beam is moved in a rectangular or parallelogram pattern as demonstrated in Fig.18.12(a) giving equal dimensions in the near and far fields seen in the top row of Fig.18.10. The position of the narrow section of the beam at various depths is controlled by

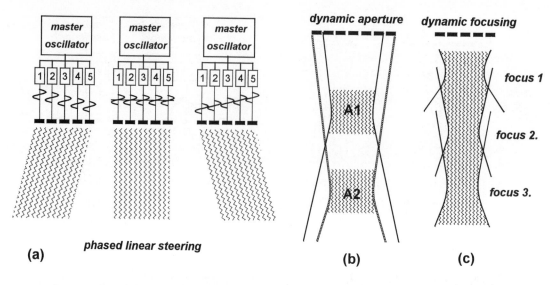

Figure 18.12 (a) Phased steering of the linear array to increase coverage. (b) dynamic aperture achieved during transmission by using different numbers of elements. (c) dynamic focusing achieved by pulse delays.

the **aperture size** (size of element group) therefore the focus at various depths is maintained by dynamically varying the aperture (see Fig.18.12(b)) giving a **dynamic aperture** to the transducer.

Multiple focusing During transmission the focusing can be altered by delaying the pulses in set patterns (focus 1, 2 and 3 in Fig.18.12(c)). The echoes are then received from each focal point before the beam is switched to the next focus. The transducer frame rate is reduced as $1/F_n$ where F_n is the number of foci. **Dynamic focusing** is achieved during echo reception by switching receiver delays so collecting accurately timed echoes from focus points 3, 2 and 1 in Fig.18.12(c).

There is no reduction in frame rate for dynamic focusing during reception. Both dynamic aperture and dynamic focusing maintain optimum image resolution over the entire image depth. The same field dimensions can also be maintained with depth by simultaneously applying **dynamic aperture**.

Frame rate (FR) Several transducer elements provide a scan line (see Fig.18.11(a), (b)) which makes up a sectional image having a typical frame rate of between 25-30 frames per second. Each frame is made up from a complete set of scan lines. The action of the real time transducer moves the scan line prior to the next transmission pulse. The rate of scan-line movement influences the frame rate which is related to the pulse repetition frequency as:

$$\mathrm{FR} = \frac{PRF}{number\ of\ scan\ lines} \qquad (18.8)$$

The frame rate is therefore determined by the PRF and the number of scan lines. The frame time FT is the time taken to acquire the complete image of N scan lines and the frame rate is the inverse of this so:

$$PRP \times N = FT \qquad (18.9)$$

The frame rate should exceed 20fps if image flicker is to be avoided. Frame rate is limited by image depth and number of multiple focuses so that:

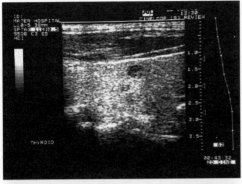
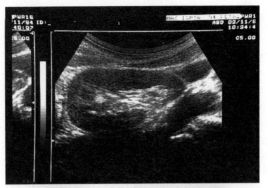
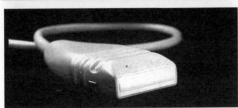
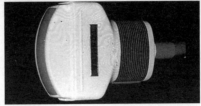

Figure 18.13   Linear array and curved linear array transducers with their respective clinical images.

PRF = *scan lines × number of focuses × frame rate.*   (18.10)

If extra depth is required then the frame rate may be slowed since the PRF must be reduced. Table 18.1 compares frequency, PRF, image depth and frame rate. Each focus during dynamic focusing requires a transmission pulse. If sound velocity is 150000cm s^{-1} for soft tissue and making allowances for the return path then the PRF is determined by the factor: 150000 × 0.5 = 75000 so:

beam penetration × focuses × scan lines × frame rate = 75000   (18.11)

Box 18.1 calculates the frame rate for a 5MHz transducer having 128 elements.

Table 18.1 PRF beam penetration and frame rate.

Frequency (MHz)	PRF (kHz)	Penetration (cm)	FR (100 lines)
3.5	3.8	20	38
5.0	5.0	15	51
7.5	7.7	10	77
10.0	15.4	5	154

Box 18.1

Transducer frame rate.

A 5MHz transducer having 128 elements is required to give a 12cm image depth. What is the frame rate? Sound velocity in soft tissue is 1500m s^{-1}. This is ~13µs cm^{-1} for returning echo so:

$$PRP = 12 × 13 \ = 156µs$$
$$FT = 156×128 = 20ms$$
$$FR = 50Hz$$

Increasing PRP, image depth or scan line density will decrease frame rate.

Linear array specifications   The linear array is commonly used for examining the abdomen. A typical linear transducer would have:

- 60-120 Transducer elements
- 8-32 Group width (aperture)
- 3.5 - 7.5MHz frequency range.
- Element width 1-4l
- Size of footprint from 2×0.6cm to 1.4x10cm

Applications:

- Large body areas such as abdomen
- Gynecology
- Thyroid
- Superficial vessels
- Ultrasound guided biopsy

Advantages are a rectangular field of view which gives good definition to both near and distant anatomy as seen in Fig.18.13 and good image quality across the full image depth and field of view. The disadvantages are a large footprint (surface contact area) and a limited field of view with depth.

Curved Arrays   These are a modification of the linear array design having a convex transducer surface. The scan is produced by sequential element switching as before but a **sector scan** is produced (Fig.18.13) having a curved top. The size of this transducer is smaller than the linear array giving it a smaller footprint (surface contact area). The beam is much wider at depth so gives a larger anatomical image. The size of the sector, which is variable, is determined by the pulse delay variation.

A linear array can give a diverging field of view; this is the **vector array** and the scan lines fan outwards. The image format is similar to the curvilinear array except that the footprint is smaller still and the display format has a flat top.

Specifications   A typical sequenced curved array would have:

- Radius of curvature 40-80mm
- Frequency 3.5-5.0MHz
- Elements >100
- aperture 16 to 32 elements
- frame rate 58 fps

18.3.2 The phased array

The principle of the phased array is shown in Fig.18.14. The transmit pulses are applied to each element via a delay which gives a swiveled (angled) wave-front. The degree of swivel

(±45°) requires very narrow elements of about $\frac{1}{2}\lambda$ dimensions. The effective aperture A' is $A \cdot \cos\varphi$ where A is the total aperture or array length without the swivel. During receive mode the same pulse delays are used.

The phased array can also produce directional and focused beams as used in the sequenced array which moves the focal point to position it shallow or deep giving electronic dynamic focusing in conjunction with beam steering. Unlike the linear sequenced array all the elements are pulsed at the same time during transmission and reception and the phased array image formation is achieved by using polar co-ordinates and not rectilinear.

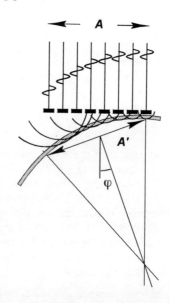

Figure 18.14 Phased array switching giving a planar or focused beam. All the elements usually act in unison.

Phased arrays use a smaller number of elements than a linear array (48 to 128) and consequently their footprint is smaller allowing inspection of more restricted anatomy (between the rib cage). Phased array probes are shown in Fig.18.15(a). A pie-shaped or **sector scan** is obtained which is shown in Fig.18.15(b). The phased array has demanding requirements since separate transmit and

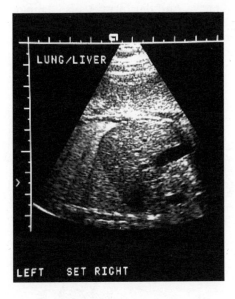
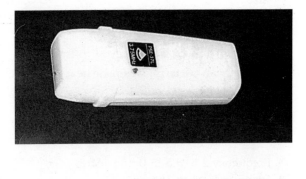
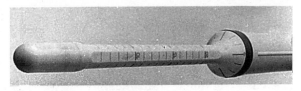

Figure 18.15 (a) Phased array transducers with an example sector display **(b)** Phased array probe geometry. (Courtesy Siemens Inc)

receive delay circuits are present for each element. All elements are pulsed using various delay timings; the pulse rate determines the number of scan lines. The directional characteristic of the elements determines the swivel angle (±45°) which is achieved with very narrow elements ($\sim\frac{1}{2}\lambda$ = 0.22mm for 3.5MHz). In the receive mode delays are introduced into the received signals which enable the transducer to be sensitive to echoes returning from specific directions. These effects produce arrays which are preferentially sensitive to echoes emanating from chosen regions which can be user selected by variation of the delay times. If delay times are changed during the receiving cycle the focal plane can be varied to give **dynamic focusing** but increasing the number of focal planes decreases the frame rate. **Dynamic apertures** are achieved by using a proportion of the total available elements, so in some circumstances not all the elements in a phased array are being used.

Phased array probe The design of the phased array lends itself to miniature probe design for internal examinations (rectum, vagina and esophagus). Tiny catheter sized ultrasound transducers are available for intraluminal inspection of blood vessels.

The geometry of a bi-planar device is shown in Fig.18.15(b). The bi-planar probe allows imaging in transverse (360°) and longitudinal planes (240°); frequency range is typically 5 to 7.5MHz. Acoustic coupling can be obtained either by close application to the epithelial mucous or by inflating an 'on-board' water balloon.

Specifications Small arrays (14mm aperture) are useful for echocardiography. Larger arrays give large field of view pictures of the abdomen and special applications are found in rectal and gynecological probes.

Advantages:

• Large field of view relative to its footprint

size
- Fast frame rate

Disadvantages:

- Sector scan pattern gives poor near field of view

Typical specifications for a phased array would be:

- Frequency 2.5, 3.5, 5.0 and 7MHz
- Frame rate up to 156fps
- Imaging depth 25cm
- Aperture (transducer size) 14-28mm
- Swivel 40-45°

18.3.3   Annular transducer

Instead of individual small linear elements a series of concentric transducers operates as an **annular phased array** (side and plan views given in Fig.18.16(a)). This produces a conical beam section. The concentric rings resemble an optical Fresnel lens. The signals are delayed to each ring in order to give a focused beam Fig.18.16(b) which is mechanically moved in an arc.

Excellent image quality can be obtained from annular arrays since the lateral resolution and resolution at depth can be influenced by signal phasing giving a superior constant focus with depth. The focusing effect is achieved by pulsing the two outermost elements before the two next inner neighbors. The composite wave-front then has a focus along the mid-line. The overall depth of focus is controlled by the delay between pulsing signals.   Annular arrays also provide superior slice thickness uniformity.

Annular arrays cannot be steered electronically as linear phased arrays, so a mechanical 'wobbler' method is employed.   A typical design with the transducer moving within an enclosed bath of transmission oil is shown in Fig.18.16(c). Reduced scan frequency enables increased line density with better resolution. There is a free choice of sector angle and system resolution is optimized by altering scan

frequency. Annular arrays also employ dynamic focusing but due to its mechanical scanning it is difficult to incorporate Doppler scan techniques since the mechanical movement would introduce interfering signals.

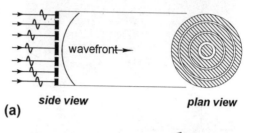

(a)   side view   plan view

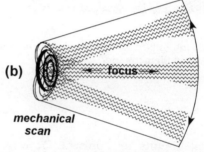

(b)

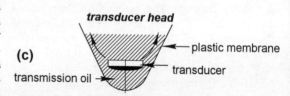

(c)

Figure 18.16   **(a)**   Annular array transducer design and **(b)** the mechanical scan pattern achieved by the mechanical scan head. **(c)** The transducer in its oil bath.

Specifications   Annular arrays are employed whenever fine detail is important such as fetal examinations. They give very good image quality over a long focal length. Their disadvantages are that they require mechanical scanning which restricts their use for Doppler/duplex imaging.   A typical transducer would consist of:

- Annular array 3.5 and 5.0MHz
- Electronic focusing
- Adjustable transmit focus
- Dynamic receive focus
- Imaging depth 25cm (3.5MHz)
- 17cm (5MHz)
- Frame rate 30fps

Examples of clinical images from the transducers described are given at the end of this chapter (see Figure 18.26).

18.4   IMAGE ARTIFACTS

Image artifacts are caused by a variety of technical factors which give false or misleading information in the final image. There are two main sources of artifact in diagnostic ultrasound images due to:

- Propagation
- Attenuation

18.4.1 Propagation errors

Reverberations (multiple echoes) This effect may occur between the face of the transducer and a strongly reflecting surface. The echo signal from this surface returns to the transducer where it is reflected again to the structure surface back to the transducer and so on.   In the image the structure is imaged as expected but it also contains 'structure' at regular intervals (successively reduced in amplitude) due to reverberation of the initial strong reflector.   This occurs because the probe acts as though it has received an echo which has taken twice as long as the first. This is commonly seen in images which include bowel gas or sections of the bladder wall.

Multiple path reflection The incident ultrasound beam may be obliquely reflected onto a second reflector. The echo returns to the transducer via the initial reflecting surface as illustrated in Fig.18.17. There is a miscalculation based on the time taken for the pulse's round trip giving misregistration beyond the oblique reflecting surface causing a ghost or apparent image.

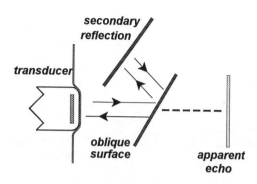

Figure 18.17 The origin of multiple path errors from an off beam reflecting surface giving an apparent echo.

Section thickness /slice width The width of the beam is defined by the acoustic lens as shown in Fig.18.5. Off axis echoes from out side the section thickness appear in regions that should be echo free. This is commonly seen in the lumens of large blood vessels and large cysts.

Refraction This has been described fully in Chapter 17 and is the bending of the ultrasound beam as it passes through tissues having different characteristic velocities. The refracted beam causes echoes to be misregistered. This is commonly seen in tissues having marked differences in acoustic impedance particularly the eye (lens and vitreous humor) and fatty tissues.

Speckle   If the scattering surfaces are spaced at distances less than the axial resolution then echo interference gives constructive and destructive interference patterns which increase image noise seen as speckle on the display.

Beam lobes   The weak echoes from **side** or **grating lobes** are not usually visualized but they become visible from strong reflectors outside the beam section causing misplaced artifacts within the image; commonly seen when imaging the fetal skull.

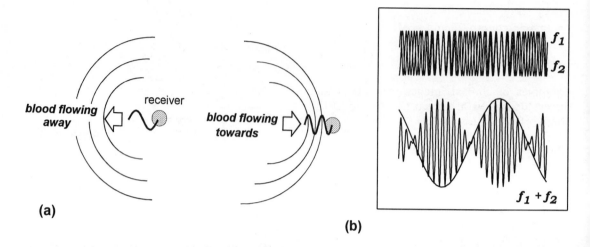

Figure 18.18 **(a)** The Doppler principle showing one sound source traveling away from the receiver and another towards the receiver showing expansion and compression of the wave front. **(b)** Two frequencies f_1 and f_2 mixed to give a beat frequency.

18.4.2 Attenuation errors

Shadowing If several objects of interest are aligned in the path of the beam and the first object in the beam's path is a very strong reflector then almost all of the sound will be reflected at the first object leaving very little to interact with the remaining objects in the path. As a result the area behind the first structure appears uniformly black indicating absence of echogenic structures. These structures are being 'shadowed' by the first strong reflector. An example of this phenomenon is found distally to bone and air structures. One solution is to change the probe's direction or angle of attack.

Enhancement When the beam is intersected by a low attenuation object (traveling between higher attenuation and low attenuation pathways) there is a much lower attenuation for the returning echoes from the

distant wall of this object. These echoes will have abnormally large amplitudes. Commonly seen in fatty cysts and other substances having a high lipid content such as bile.

18.5 BLOOD VELOCITY MEASUREMENT

Blood velocity can be measured very accurately using the **Doppler effect** which is the apparent change in frequency (pitch) when the sound source is moving with respect to the listener (or transducer). This is illustrated in Fig.18.18(a) showing expansion of the wave front (lower frequency of sound sources passing away from the receiver) and compression of the wave front with source moving towards the receiver. A common example of this phenomenon is the change in sound pitch from the siren on a passing ambulance or police car.

18.5.1 The Doppler shift

Figure 18.18(b) shows two waveforms, a transmitted signal and the returning signal, of slightly higher frequency, from a moving object (blood corpuscles). The interference signal has a much lower beat-frequency, its changing frequency giving useful qualitative information to an experienced sonographer when measuring blood velocity.

For a simple case where the transducer is in line with the flowing medium (blood) the apparent frequency f' observed is given by:

$$f' = \left[\frac{v}{v \pm S}\right] \times f_0 \qquad (18.12)$$

Where v is velocity of sound in medium S the blood velocity (+ towards; − away) and f_0 is the transmitted ultrasound frequency. When ultrasound is incident on the moving blood corpuscles there will be a change in the frequency of the returning sound energy. The detected frequency will increase if the blood is moving towards the transducer and decrease if the blood is moving away. For a transducer angle θ the Doppler frequency of the reflected ultrasound is given by:

$$f_D = \frac{2f_0 \cdot v}{c} \times \cos\theta \qquad (18.13)$$

where f_D is the Doppler shift frequency, c is the velocity of sound in the medium and θ is the angle between the direction of the sound beam and the direction of the blood flow. Box 18.2 calculates the frequency change for transducers having different angles to the skin surface using the parameters in Fig. 18.19.

Demodulation   The two signals are mixed electronically in a demodulator to separate the interference or beat signal having a lower frequency, typically in the audible range, which is represented in Fig.18.18(b) as the envelope. The beat frequency changes with the Doppler shift. The source of the echoes for Doppler studies are the blood corpuscles which are very much smaller than the wavelength of the ultrasound. The corpuscles

cause the beam to be scattered and not specularly reflected. The intensity of the scattering increases with frequency f as f^4. Thus higher frequency ultrasound is preferred for Doppler studies. These higher frequencies provide a larger shift in frequency for a given velocity of scatterer. However it should be remembered that the penetration of the Doppler beam would be compromised with increasing frequency.

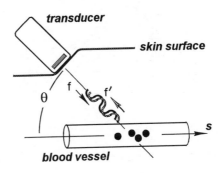

Figure 18.19 The basic Doppler geometry referred to in the text.

18.5.2   Doppler Transducers

Continuous Wave Doppler   The simplest case is where a continuous ultrasound signal is applied to the patient's skin and the change in frequency of the reflected sound is computed; information on any movements in the beam can be determined often as an audible signal such as a fetal monitor. The transducer design is illustrated in Fig.18.20(a). The two signals are mixed electronically in a demodulator to separate the interference or beat signal having a lower frequency in the audible range.

Pulsed Doppler   Using a source of pulsed ultrasound it is possible to select the tissue depth at which echo signals are examined for Doppler shifts. This is achieved by limiting the frequency analysis to echo pulses which

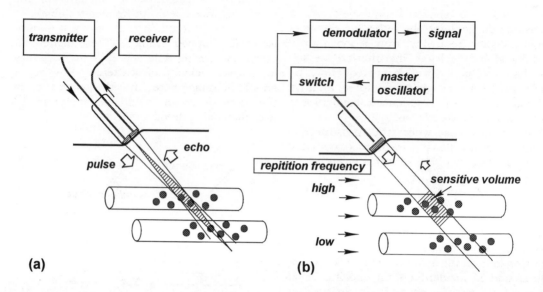

Figure 18.20 (a) Continuous wave Doppler probe showing extended depth of response (b) Pulsed Doppler probe selecting the depth for blood velocity measurements by altering the pulse repetition frequency.

are received at specific time intervals after pulse generation shown in Fig.18.20(b); pulsed wave Doppler probes have a single transmit/receive transducer.

The pulse repetition frequency determines the maximum depth of the sensitive volume.

The time at which the analysis begins and its duration determine the depth and axial length of the volume of tissue which is examined for flow information (the area from which the echoes are received). This is equivalent to opening a signal gate so the procedure is known as 'gating'. It is possible to divide the length of the ultrasound beam into a sequence of gates each having a size of one pixel which provides flow information for color coding.

There are two important limitations on the use of pulsed Doppler ultrasound measurement of blood flow. The maximum depth that can be examined and the maximum frequency shift detected is limited by the pulse repetition frequency. Increasing the repetition

frequency increases the maximum frequency shift that can be detected but decreases the interrogation depth.

Maximum velocity   This depends on the transducer frequency and its PRF. From eqn.18.13 the velocity is:

$$v = \frac{\Delta f \cdot c}{2 f_o} \times \cos \theta \qquad (18.14)$$

For soft tissue c = 150000 cm s^{-1}. So:

$$v = \frac{\Delta f \cdot (7.5 \times 10^4)}{f_o} \times \cos \theta \qquad (18.15)$$

If the Nyquist frequency determines the highest Doppler frequency that can be accurately resolved then this is *PRF*/2; from eqn.18.14 yields:

$$v_{max} = \frac{PRF \cdot c}{4 f_o \cdot \cos \theta} \qquad (18.16)$$

Blood velocity in humans varies between 20

to 200cm s^{-1}. Equation 18.16 indicates that high PRF values are necessary in order to measure fast flow rates, however PRF is also related to image depth, so fast flow rates can only be detected at small distances from the transducer face. The depth of response represented in Fig.18.20(b) can be calculated if the speed of sound in soft tissue is taken to be 1500 ms^{-1} or ~6.5μs in 1cm. Transmission and reception takes about 13μs cm^{-1} so for 6cm tissue depth the **pulse repetition period** must be ≥ 6×13 or 78μs. The PRF is the inverse or 12.8kHz.   Similarly

PRF (kHz)	PRP (μs)	Depth (cm)
5	200	15.4
8	125	9.6
12.5	80	6
15	66	5
20	50	3.8

The maximum Doppler shift that can be detected is half the repetition frequency which is 6.25kHz for a PRF of 12.5kHz so from eqn.18.14 this gives 98cm s^{-1}.

Aliasing   This has been discussed elsewhere (Chapter 14) and concerns signal sampling rate and the Nyquist frequency. Aliasing artifacts in pulsed Doppler give false flow direction signals. The highest Doppler shift that pulsed Doppler can measure is PRF/2 and the maximum repetition frequency is related to maximum image depth (D_{max}). Then maximum recorded velocity and image depth are related as :

$$PRF = \frac{c}{D_{max}} \qquad (18.17)$$

High blood velocities which produce Doppler shifts greater than half the repetition frequency cause an effect known as aliasing, so the frequency shift recorded will incorrectly underestimate the value of the blood velocity.

Box 18.2

Doppler Shift Examples

Basic Equation: $f_D = \dfrac{2f_o \cdot v}{c} \times \cos\theta$

Where
f_D = frequency Change or Doppler Shift
f_o = frequency of ultrasound transmitted beam
c = sound velocity in medium
v = blood velocity
θ = angle between transducer and vessel.

Example:
If the blood velocity is 20cm s^{-1}, the transducer frequency is 5MHz and 60° then 45° angles to the vessel are chosen. What are the Doppler shifts?

$$f_D = \frac{2(5\times10^6)\times20}{15.7\times10^4} \times 0.5 = 637\ Hz\ for\ 60°$$

$$f_D = \frac{2(5\times10^6)\times20}{15.7\times10^4} \times 0.7 = 900\ Hz\ for\ 45°$$

Note:

• Doppler shift increases as transducer is aligned with vessel axis.

• Doppler shift has positive or negative value depending on flow direction + flow toward, − flow away from transducer, these are color coded in Doppler imaging.

• Percentage frequency change is <u>very</u> small:
  637Hz represents **0.0127%**
  900Hz represents **0.018%** of the 5MHz carrier frequency

18.5.3 Duplex and Color Velocity Imaging

Duplex imaging   This combines Doppler information with a real time gray-scale image. A pulsed Doppler transducer is combined in the array (linear or phased) at an angle so that it can be directed into the area of interest as shown in Fig.18.21 The placement of the sensitive area or sample volume is operator controlled so that a particular vessel can be targeted. This technique produces a two dimensional representation of the direction and velocity of blood flow on a gray-scale image. In a typical display blood flowing towards the transducer is coded as red and blood flow away from the transducer is represented as blue.

Various intermediate colors represent the different velocities of the flow. Images of blood flow are produced by examining the change in the echo pattern for each line in the image. The two patterns are examined for differences which would have been produced by movement of blood. Variations in pattern are then color-coded red or blue depending on the direction of the change. The resolution of Doppler flow images is commonly restricted to 128×128 matrices.

Advantages and disadvantages of duplex imaging are given in Tab.18.2

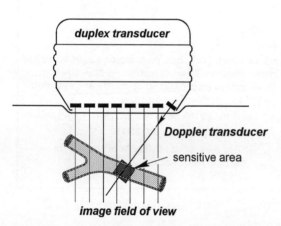

Figure 18.21 Linear array containing a Doppler transducer used for combined color flow in duplex imaging.

Color Velocity Imaging (**CVI**) Other methods are available for measuring blood flow apart from using Doppler techniques. CVI identifies a group of blood cells in a vessel and times their shift. The group, which is identified at time *T1,* has moved to a new position at *T2* and the separation is measured. Figure 18.22 illustrates the basic principle of color velocity imaging. A group of blood cells

gives a unique signal signature which is followed for a fixed time in a 'window'. The blood-velocity is computed from the time taken. The advantages of CVI are:

- Improved spatial resolution of vessels
- A wider color coding in the image
- Low aliasing problems
- Quantitative assessment of blood flow
- Not sensitive to frequency errors

Table 18.2 Duplex imaging

Advantages	Disadvantages
• Visual Display of Blood Flow	• Low spatial resolution
• Rapid localization of Vessel	• Low frame rates
• Flow disturbances visualized	• Aliasing problems
• Small Flow values measured	
• Identification of hypo-echoic plaque	• High power requirements
• Surface features identified	

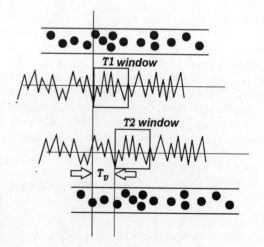

Figure 18.22 CVI principles showing a unique group of blood cells followed for a precise time period.

18.6 SAFETY

The two important mechanisms of potential hazard in diagnostic ultrasound that are considered relevant to present day transducers are **heating** and **cavitation**.

Heating is caused by the conversion of ultrasonic energy to heat in the tissue. The intensity I of ultrasound energy is defined as the energy flux crossing unit area in unit time or the rate of delivery of ultrasound energy per unit area of tissue. Intensity is measured in watts as W cm^{-2} or mW cm^{-2}.

Cavitation or gas bubble growth is related to acoustic pressure p. Intensity and pressure are related as:

$$I = \frac{p^2}{z} \qquad (18.18)$$

where z is the acoustic impedance of the tissue. A typical pulsed beam, as used in diagnostic ultrasound, has an 'on time' or **mark** and an 'off time' or **space**. The mark to space ratio ($m:s$) and **duty factor** $m/m+s \times 100\%$ are important measurements when considering safety factors. Ultrasound **power** is defined as the energy flux per unit time through the whole cross section of the beam.

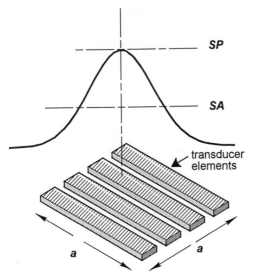

Figure 18.23 Power levels measured in an ultrasound beam

The pulse from a diagnostic ultrasound transducer delivers an acoustic pressure in tissue that alternates between positive and negative values. The major hazards associated with these pressure events is the acoustic output measured in several ways but commonly as the **spatial time averaged intensity** I_{SPTA} in watts m^{-2} and the **time averaged power** measured in milli-watts (mW)

18.6.1 Units of intensity

The beam profile from an ultrasound probe has already been shown in Chapter 17. A modified version in Fig.18.23 is used for defining the basic and derived spatial intensity parameters.

Spatial Peak (SP) This is defined as the peak beam intensity measured on the central axis.

Spatial Average (SA) The mean intensity of the transducer beam.

Ultrasound is delivered in a series of pulses, each giving a peak output. The number of peaks per unit time depends on the pulse repetition frequency (PRF). The pulse train shown in Fig.18.24(a) describes the temporal parameters that are related to the duty factor and **mark : space** ratio which is influenced by the pulse width.

Pulse Average (PA) is the intensity during 'on-time' (mark).

Temporal Peak (TP) is the highest intensity of the pulse. Since the pulse amplitude of Doppler is constant but that of diagnostic ultrasound is varying, the **peak intensity** within each pulse of the diagnostic waveform is the temporal peak *TP* and the average intensity over each pulse is the pulse average *PA*.

Temporal or Time Average Power (TA) This is the intensity of the entire pulse train averaged over time defined as:

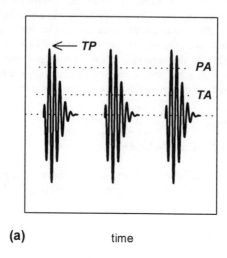 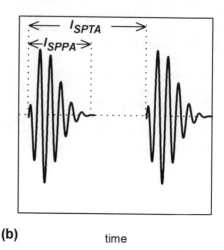

(a)   time   **(b)**   time

Figure 18.24 (a) Peak and average intensities of the ultrasound pressure waveform identified in the text. **(b)** Combination intensity units identified in the text.

$$\frac{total\ power\ per\ frame}{frame\ duration} \qquad (18.19)$$

which gives the average intensity of the pulse train. This gives a guide to the heating effects. It is related to transducer aperture and transducer PRF. As the aperture in linear arrays is increased to access greater depths time averaged power will increase but PRF is reduced with depth so there is a balance. Time averaged power will tend to decrease with depth owing to beam attenuation, however in practice with the use of multiple focal zones (dynamic focusing) which give deeper focus settings, slightly higher time averaged powers will result.

If the *PRF* of the transducer is high then the *TA* will be high; if the *PRF* is decreased then the *TA* will be lower. If the ultrasound is continuous instead of pulsatile (CW Doppler) then the duty cycle is one and *PA = TA*.

18.6.2 Combined intensity units

The Spatial Average *SA* and the Temporal Average *TA* are combined to give a basic overall intensity measurement which is used for deriving other intensity parameters.

Spatial Average Temporal Average Intensity I_{SATA} (mW cm^{-2}):   This is the temporal average divided by the area of the transducer face (referring to Fig. 18.23):

$$I_{SATA} = \frac{TA}{a^2} \qquad (18.20)$$

As a spatially and temporally averaged acoustic intensity it is usually maximum at the surface of the scan head or where the cross-sectional area of the scan profile is smallest. In a linear array I_{SATA} would be greatest at the mechanical focal point given by the acoustic lens previously identified in Fig. 18.3(a). A complete family of other intensity values can be derived from I_{SATA}; some of these are illustrated in Fig. 18.24(b).

Spatial Peak Temporal Average Intensity I_{SPTA} (mW cm^{-2}):   This is derived as:

$$I_{SPTA} = I_{SATA} \times \frac{SP}{SA} \qquad (18.21)$$

This is the time averaged power relating peak power to the pulse width and **duty factor**; a higher PRF will increase the I_{SPTA} value. For a peak power of 1W cm^{-2} and a duty factor of 0.1 the SPTA would be 100mW cm^{-2}, increasing the pulse width or PRF increases this value.

This intensity measurement is a good indicator for heating effects and this together with the time averaged power figures for various investigations is given in Tab.18.3 Absolute maximum values milli-watts per cm^2 that various manufacturers quote are also appended.

Table 18.3 Intensity range in practice

Display mode	TA (mW)	I_{SPTA} (mW cm^{-2})
B-mode	0.5 – 350	1 –1000
M-mode	0.5 – 350	5 – >1000
Duplex/pulsed Doppler	10 – >400	20 – >1000
CW Doppler		
Obstetric	16 – 25	10 – 20
Vascular	2 – 90	20 – 600

Likely manufacturer's limits.

Mode	I_{SPTA} B-mode	I_{SPTA} M-Mode	I_{SPTA} Doppler
Linear Array	3.1	118	
Phased Array	117	243	1266
Annular Array	42	321	

Spatial Peak Pulse Average Intensity (I_{SPPA}) This is a measurement of the maximum mean intensity that occurs within the ultrasound beam at any instant as shown in Fig.18.24(b). It is a good indicator for **cavitation** and other mechanical bio-effects.

Spatial Peak Temporal Peak Intensity I_{SPTP} (W cm^{-2}): Expressed as

$$\frac{I_{SPTA}}{duty\ cycle} \qquad (18.22)$$

This value may be a useful indication for cavitation effects. The **Spatial Peak Temporal Peak Pressure** measured in MPa is similar to I_{SPPA} but refers to the peak pressure.

Spatial Average Pulse Average Intensity I_{SAPA} (mW cm^{-2}): Since $PA = TA/duty\ cycle$ then

$$I_{SAPA} = \frac{I_{SATA}}{duty\ cycle} \qquad (18.23)$$

Intensity magnitudes The magnitude of these intensity values follows the sequence:

$$I_{SPTP} > I_{SPPA} > I_{SPTA} > I_{SAPA} > I_{SATA}$$

The commonly used intensity measures are I_{SPPA} (the maximum transducer pulse intensity) and I_{SPTA}. Both are used in specifying maximum levels by the various national licensing authorities (FDA in USA).

The absolute values will be influenced by focal dimensions. Transducers which have a tight focus in the near field will produce a higher I_{SPTA} value than those which are focused in the far field. Recommended maximum levels quoted by the FDA in America for cardiac, peripheral vascular, ophthalmology and obstetrics are listed in Table 18.4.

Table 18.4 FDA Acoustic output limits

Value	Heart	PV	Op	Abdomen (Fetus)
I_{SPPA} W cm^{-2}	190	190	28	190
I_{SPTP} W cm^{-2}	310	310	50	310
I_{SPTA} mW cm^{-2}	430	720	17	94
I_{SATA} mW cm^{-2}	430	720	17	94

Most machines provide an output control which adjusts the amplitude of the transmitted pulse however at 'switch-on' the power setting is often at maximum.

Scanned mode images (B-mode and color flow imaging) There will be a maximum energy when the axis of the scanning beam passes over a particular point. Beam overlapping will also increase this axial power level. Using linear arrays can increase beam overlap in the proximal image field. For sector scanners the considerable beam-overlap close to the transducer face means the I_{SPTA} value will always be proximal to the focus.

Unscanned modes (pulsed Doppler and CW Doppler) the highest values of I_{SPTA} are seen since tissue points on the beam axis will receive the maximum beam strength repeatedly.

Heating effects   The rate of local heat production is related to the average intensity and the tissue absorption. In the absence of any heat losses the temperature rise depends on the time exposed. There is not a great deal of difference in heat gain for most soft tissues; the important exception is bone.

Thermal effects depend on energy deposited and heat removal (organ blood flow). Both tissue attenuation and transducer frequencies influence heat production; higher frequencies are more attenuated and thus higher energy absorbed. Bone/tissue interface can cause heat build-up. Doppler power outputs can approach hazard levels and also ultrasound probes (rectal, vaginal). A Doppler probe operating in air has given a temperature approaching 80°C. A skin temperature of over 41°C was measured using a 5MHz phased array in pulsed Doppler mode for 30 seconds and a skin temperature elevation of 10°C has been reported at a depth 2mm below the skin surface.

Probe temperature increases are particularly important in intra-vaginal where the probe face may be in close contact to the conceptus. Temperature rise is of most significance during organo-genesis so the embryo is most vulnerable during the first 8 weeks of development. Some proliferating adult tissue (testes, bone marrow) are at risk.

A statement from the American Institute of Ultrasound in Medicine (AIUM) October 1992 states that in the low MHz range there have been no deleterious thermal effects to mammalian tissue due to exposure from:

- *Unfocused beam* intensities < 10mW cm^{-2}
- *Focused beam* intensities < 1W cm^{-2}

Cavitation   At high intensities used in therapy, cavitation (bubble precipitation in liquid) has been demonstrated but it has not been reported at diagnostic intensities. The AUIM and the FDA have introduced a Mechanical Index (MI) derived from peak negative pressure giving an index for cavitation between 0.2 and 1.9 for diagnostic ultrasound.

18.6.3   Bioeffects

Chromosome damage   Single strand DNA breaks have been seen in hymen leukocytes. Various continuous and pulsed frequencies were used but 94W cm^{-2} spatial peak-temporal average (SPTA) at 8MHz continuous wave (CW) yielded consistent breaks associated with cavitation effects. This is much higher power than would be available from diagnostic equipment.

Sister chromatid exchange Most extensive literature deals with sister chromatid exchange in-vitro. The occurrence is small but statistically significant. Because in-vitro and *in-vivo* effects are different, extrapolation should be attempted with caution. The statement from the AIUM is:

"It is difficult to evaluate reports of ultrasonically induced in-vitro biological effects with respect to their clinical significance. The predominant physical and biological interactions and mechanisms involved in an in-vitro effect may not pertain to the in-vivo situation. Nevertheless an in-vitro effect must be regarded as a real biological effect. While it is valid for authors to place their results in context and to suggest further relevant investigations reports of in-vitro studies which claim direct clinical significance should be viewed with caution. "

18.6.4 Safety levels

The boundary of accepted safety levels in the US is given in Fig.18.25. In the low MHz frequency range there have been no confirmed biological effects in mammalian tissue exposed *in-vivo* to unfocused ultrasound with I_{SPTA} below 100mW cm^{-2} for less than 500 seconds or for focused ultrasound with I_{SPTA} below 1W cm^{-2} for less than 50 seconds. Furthermore, for exposure times more than one second and less than 500seconds (unfocused) or 50 seconds focused such effects have not been demonstrated at even higher intensities. The power of current machines however is able to penetrate into the harmful region as indicated by the hatched area on the graph. Biologically sensitive areas would be:

- 1st trimester embryo
- Fetus skeletal heating
- Transcranial Doppler
- Eye
- Intracavitary

Fetal exposure   The calcium channels appear to be the first to develop in the cell membranes of embryos and prolonged ultrasound intensities could have undesirable side-effects not only on embryo-genesis but on late prenatal and postnatal development. There is a growing realization of the potential importance of non-thermal effects and increasing evidence that the temporal peak intensity is potentially related to the production of some effects (cavitation). Doppler flow studies of the fetus are of major concern since this can induce heating in mineralized bone.

A recent safety statement from the Ultrasound Safety Committee states that routine Doppler investigations of the first trimester embryo are inadvisable and that exposure time should be minimized in any pulsed Doppler examination of the fetus particularly if fetal bone is within the Doppler beam. A study of 10,000 pregnancies exposed to ultrasound is currently being carried out in Canada. A preliminary report from this group on 2428 children showed no increase in malformation or other developmental problems. No difference was found between matched pairs of siblings followed up to 6 years of age, one of each pair having been exposed to ultrasound *in utero*.

Summary

There seem to be no limits on acoustic output in most European countries (including Britain and Ireland) but there are limits imposed in the USA and Japan where most ultrasound manufacturers are located.

The USA requires I_{SPTA} and I_{SPPA} levels to be lower than the values in Tab. 18.3 under defined operating procedures (non fetal Doppler) and requires AIUM thermal and mechanical indices to be displayed on-screen. Japan requires an I_{SATA} limit of 10mW cm^{-2} for B-mode and fetal Doppler, 40mW cm^{-2} for M-mode and 100mW cm^{-2} for A mode. A European standard is being prepared which will require an I_{SPTA} <100mW cm^{-2}.

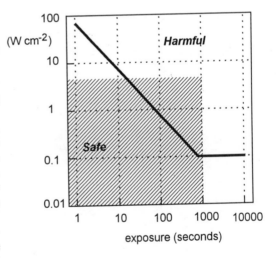

Figure 18.25 The boundary of safe intensity levels for time spent in the examination.

Minimizing risks   Practical general measures to minimize risks in ultrasound scanning would be:

- Do not scan unless there is a clear clinical objective.

- Make sure equipment is regularly checked.
- Discover if the sound output is disabled during freeze frame. If not remove the probe.
- Use the output attenuator to reduce the output to the lowest levels consistent with giving the required quality of image.
- If the output of the equipment exceeds 100mW cm^{-2} calculate the time you can safely dwell at one point before the 50J cm^{-2} limit is exceeded.
- Take special care when scanning sensitive organs (early pregnancy, eye, gonads)
- Keep up to date on scanning techniques to minimize exposure.
- Ensure that trainee radiographers do not spend an undue time on any one patient.
- Keep well informed on experimental findings on the safety of ultrasound.

KEYWORDS

annular array transducers arranged in concentric circles.

aperture (dynamic) change in aperture size during transmission to maintain focus with depth.

aperture the size of the transducer or size of a number of transducer elements

beat frequency a low frequency interference between two waveforms having a different frequent.

cavitation gas bubble production due to rarefaction events in a liquid.

curvilinear array a linear sequence array with a curved outline.

demodulator an electronic circuit which separates a single signal from a mixed signal.

depth of response the point from the transducer face where echoes are -50dB

Doppler (continuous) measuring the Doppler frequency by continuous transmission reception. Separate crystals necessary

Doppler (pulsed) measuring the Doppler frequency by pulsing the ultrasound beam. A single crystal is used.

Doppler effect change of reflected frequency with movement.

duplex imaging combining a gray-scale image with a color Doppler image.

duty cycle (factor) the percentage of time the pulse occupies in the operational cycle.

dynamic range the range of echo intensities. This can be up to 100dB at the input amplifier. 60 to 80dB at the TGC and 50dB after compression.

focus determines the slice thickness by shaping the crystal or matching layer or an electronic focus can influence lateral resolution.

footprint area of transducer in contact with the patient.

frame rate number of complete scanned images per second.

grating lobes side lobes produced by a multielement transducer.

imaging depth visible distance from transducer face determined by the PRP and transducer frequency.

linear array a transducer whose elements are pulsed in a sequence to give a rectilinear shaped image or curvilinear for a curved face.

phased array a transducer where the elements are pulsed together using signal delays to steer the beam in a sector scan.

polar co-ordinates the positional geometry used by a phased array transducer producing a sector scan.

pulse average intensity (PA) average intensity over repetition period.

pulse duration (period) (PD) the time for 2-3 wavelengths typically 0.5 to 3μs

pulse repetition frequency (PRF) 1/PRP typically 2 to 10kHz.

pulse repetition period (PRP) the time between pulses or waiting time for echo collection typically 200μs

rectilinear co-ordinates position geometry used by a linear sequenced array.

scan line produced by a transducer element whose length defines image depth

section thickness the narrowest or focal point of a section or slice.

sector scan produced by a phased or annular array.

spatial average intensity (SA) average intensity over transducer area

spatial peak intensity (SP) highest intensity in beam

spatial pulse length (SPL) the wavelength × number of cycles. Typically 0.45 to 2.25mm.

swept gain (see time gain compensation)

temporal average intensity (TA) time averaged intensity for the time transducer is used.

temporal peak intensity (TP) highest intensity at any time within beam

time-gain compensation (TGC) signal post processing amplification for correcting attenuation loss.

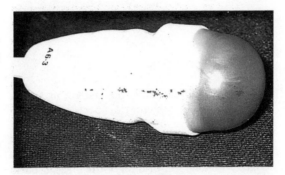

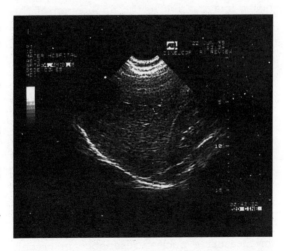

Figure 18.26 Annular probe showing mechanically moved transducer in its hemispherical oil bath and an image from this transducer showing sharp focus with good depth of field.

19
Magnetic Resonance: Basics

19.1 Introduction
19.2 The Proton in a Magnetic Field
19.3 Relaxation time constants

19.4 Pulse sequences
19.5 T1 and T2 signal measurement

19.1 INTRODUCTION

Medical diagnostic imaging uses the upper end of the electromagnetic spectrum almost exclusively for investigating the living body, commanding the shorter wavelengths of x- and gamma radiation. The longer wavelength region embracing the radio-band wavelength 150cm to 150meters (200MHz to 2MHz) has only recently been used by diagnostic imaging due to the application of Nuclear Magnetic Resonance (NMR).

Nuclear Magnetic Resonance does not rely on ionizing radiation (as conventional radiography, CT and nuclear medicine do), nor does it depend on the transmission of energy through tissue like ultrasound. It utilizes an entirely different principle, involving the interaction of atomic nuclei with imposed magnetic fields which cause Radio Frequency NMR Signals. The nuclei studied in NMR all have odd numbers of protons; the most common nucleus is hydrogen: a single proton.

NMR generates very small signals and their strength and frequency give unique information about tissue chemistry. Methods for measuring nuclear resonance in organic materials were simultaneously developed in 1946 by E.M. Purcell and co-workers at Harvard and F. Bloch and his team at Stanford. Both physicists received the Nobel Prize for this work. Since then nuclear magnetic resonance has rapidly become a valuable nondestructive laboratory technique for showing molecular differences in biological materials.

The NMR signal given by a spinning nucleus can be likened to a spinning top, shown in Fig.19.1, which normally spins around its own central axis but when disturbed traces out, or **precesses** at an angle to the vertical axis. This is also shown by a nucleus in a strong magnetic field; when it is disturbed by an opposing magnetic field it will also precess.

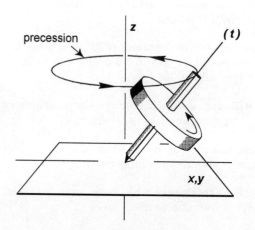

Figure 19.1 Spinning top showing an off center wobble or precession representing a very simple model of the precessing proton.

Image formation Magnetic Resonance Imaging (MRI), introduced commercially in the early 1980s, employs these same NMR signals but in addition provides spatial information that yields tomographic sectional images of the human body in the axial plane (as CT), and also in the coronal and sagittal planes as well as any chosen oblique plane.

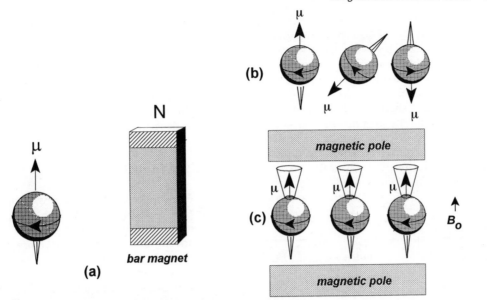

Figure 19.2 (a) The hydrogen proton compared to a bar magnet showing the proton spin creating a magnetic dipole μ analogous to the magnetic pole of the bar magnet. (b) a group of 3 protons showing various orientations of their axis in free space. (c) the proton axis aligned in a strong magnetic field B_O. A smaller proportion take up opposing direction.

The images obtained from MRI convey information that is entirely different from the transmission tomographic images of CT and ultrasound. Magnetic resonance images reflect NMR signal changes that are altered by the chemistry of hydrogen and the configuration of hydrogen atoms within molecules i.e. water, fats, proteins and carbohydrates. Bone, having a relatively poor hydrogen concentration, is poorly displayed and any bony anatomy that is seen is due to fatty marrow or pathological changes that involve invasion by soft tissue.

Before describing magnetic resonance Imaging we must understand the fundamental principles of nuclear magnetic resonance and the basic signals. The principles of nuclear magnetic resonance can be very complex but in order to understand their application to imaging many of the complexities can be stripped away and the basics much simplified. This chapter is therefore an abridged version of the true process. More detailed descriptions are given in books identified at the end of this chapter.

19.2 THE PROTON IN A MAGNETIC FIELD

The phenomenon of nuclear magnetic resonance is not shown by all nuclei; they must contain an odd number of nucleons (protons plus neutrons) and so have a magnetic component or **moment**. The most common is the hydrogen nucleus ^{1}H, which is a single proton. Other physiologically important atoms are ^{13}Carbon and ^{31}Phosphorus.

Since the diagnostic imaging applications of NMR almost exclusively involve the hydrogen proton the following descriptions will use this simple nucleus as a model. The hydrogen proton can be compared to a bar magnet as shown in Fig.19.2(a). It behaves as a dipole having a magnetic dipole moment μ, which is analogous to the bar magnet's pole. Unlike the bar-magnet the proton has spin giving it angular momentum. The proton, in the absence of an external magnetic field, can take up any orientation in free space; three protons are shown in Fig.19.2(b) freely spinning, their axes at different angles.

When the protons are placed in a strong magnetic field B_O, as shown in Fig.19.2(c), the proton axes line up with the magnetic flux lines. In reality protons can adopt two alignment modes: parallel (with the magnetic flux) and anti-parallel (inverted or opposing the flux) however slightly more align with the magnetic field. The proportion that is in alignment varies with the magnetic field strength. In order to simplify the following descriptions only the majority nuclei, parallel to the magnetic field, will be illustrated.

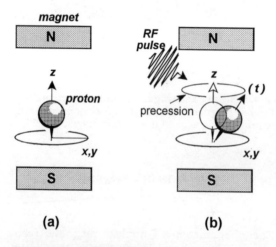

Figure 19.3 (a) The proton in a magnetic field aligned with the longitudinal z-axis, the transverse x, y plane is empty. (b) the RF-pulse displaces the proton axis into the transverse plane.

19.2.1 Precession

The 3-dimensional geometry is represented by three axes, z, x and y in Fig.19.3(a) which shows a proton at equilibrium in a strong magnetic field. The longitudinal z-axis is parallel to the flux lines of the magnetic field and the x and y axes are at right angles to the z-axis in the **transverse plane**. Figure 19.3(b) shows that energy from an RF-pulse has disturbed the equilibrium, displacing the proton axis so that it now occupies part of the transverse plane. The proton loses this excess en-

ergy by precessing (the precession frequency determined by the magnetic field strength) until it regains equilibrium in the longitudinal axis once again. Location (t) denotes position of the proton axis at time t after the RF pulse. There are many protons undergoing this transition in a tissue sample so the sum behavior is best described by using **vectors**.

19.2.2 The NMR Signal

The following descriptions are simplified so that the overall picture can be grasped. The full story involves the complexities of quantum mechanics described in more specialist literature. In order to describe the source of the NMR signal certain parameters must be identified; these are given in Tab.19.1 and identified in the vector diagrams of Fig.19.4.

Table 19.1 Definition of parameters

Symbol	Definition
B_O	static magnetic field.
z	longitudinal plane.
x, y	transverse plane.
M	sum magnetization vector.
M_z	proportion of M in z. longitudinal magnetization
M_{xy}	proportion of M in x, y. transverse magnetization
$M_{(t)}$	M at time t after the RF pulse. Magnitude $\propto$ spin density.

The static magnetic field B_O represents the machine's magnetic field, typically 1 Tesla. The **longitudinal** magnetic plane is z and the **transverse** magnetic plane (at 90°) is x, y.

The simple diagrams in Fig.19.4 use a magnetization vector M to represent the net magnetic moment or the 'sum behavior' of all the protons in the sample. The magnitude of this signal depends on the proton numbers or more correctly the **spin density**. When this aligns with the z axis the **longitudinal magnetization** is 100% (M_z). If this stable configuration is now disturbed by injecting a RF-

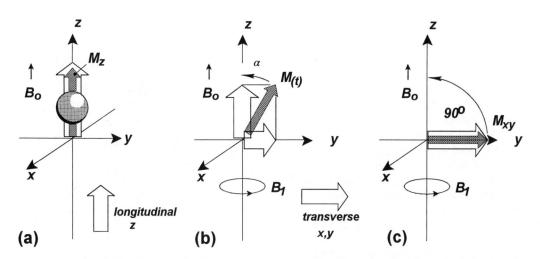

Figure 19.4 (a) The proton in a magnetic field B_0. The total proton contribution is represented by a vector M_z at equilibrium in the z-plane (z-component maximum, x,y component zero) **(b)** An RF-pulse creates the opposed field B_1 displacing M by α degrees; the x,y transverse component has grown. **(c)** A large RF pulse displaces M into x,y (z-component zero, x,y component maximum). Longitudinal recovery now takes place.

pulse M is displaced $M_{(t)}$. The total displacement is proportional to the RF-pulse energy; a 90° RF-pulse will displace M from the z axis into the **transverse** x,y plane ($\alpha = 90°$); the longitudinal magnetization will be 0% and the transverse magnetization will be 100% (M_{xy}).

The intermediate vector position $M_{(t)}$ contains a proportion of longitudinal and transverse magnetization depending on the RF-pulse energy; this decides α the **flip angle**. The speed of relaxation or the time to lose transverse magnetization M_x and regain equilibrium is the **longitudinal relaxation time**. This is an exponential event and is represented by a time constant: *T1*.

The shape and frequency of the RF-pulse is also critical. It is commonly bell-shaped containing a short burst (3 to 4 λ) of a frequency matching the proton's precessional frequency. The various stages of proton interactions within a magnetic field can be described by reference to Fig.19.4.

Stage 1 (Fig.19.4(a))   With the proton axis at **equilibrium** magnetic vector M_z is aligned with B_0. The component of M in the longitudinal plane z is M_z (maximum at this stage), likewise the component of M in the transverse plane x, y is M_{xy} (zero at this stage).

Stage 2 (Fig.19.4(b))   When an external force in the form of an RF pulse imposes a field B_1 on the system perpendicular to B_0 then M acquires energy and moves away from its equilibrium taking up some point $M_{(t)}$. The representative magnitudes of M_z and M_{xy} change as indicated by the white arrows.

Stage 3 (Fig.19.4(c))   If the RF pulse has sufficient energy (90°-RF) then M is projected into the transverse plane x, y and $M_{(t)} = M_{xy}$ having undergone full saturation. A sufficiently powerful RF pulse will invert the proton axis entirely into $-z$ (180°-RF); the magnetic vector will then occupy $-M_z$.

On return of M to its equilibrium value M_z the magnetic vector $M_{(t)}$ undergoes longitudinal relaxation and traces a spiral motion described by the Bloch equations:

$$M_x = e^{-t/T2} \cdot \cos \omega_L t$$
$$M_y = e^{-t/T2} \cdot \sin \omega_L t \qquad (19.1)$$
$$M_z = M_o \cdot (1 - e^{-t/T1})$$

These equations were derived by F. Bloch in 1946 to explain the basic properties of NMR and predicted that the motion of $M_{(t)}$ would be a simple precession (already sketched in Fig.19.3) with a frequency ω dependent on the magnetic field. If proton spins interfere with each other $M_{(t)}$'s precession will lose energy and return to its equilibrium position M_o; this energy loss is the relaxation process.

Two time constants T1 and T2 are introduced to describe this. T1 is the growth in M_z and T2 the decay of the transverse component M_{xy} ; both T1 and T2 follow exponential decay patterns. The Bloch equations have been used to give the tracing in Fig.19.5 showing the spiral pathway during the **free induction decay** (FID), the sum magnetization vector M_{xy} contributing to the transverse relaxation time. From these equations it will be seen that the longitudinal relaxation time T1 represents the time taken for $M_{(t)}$ to reach the position on the curve $1 - e^{-1}$ or 63% of M_o. The **transverse relaxation time** for the FID to decay to e^{-1} or 37% of the M_{xy} value.

The overall signal strength S obtained from $M_{(t)}$ during longitudinal and transverse relaxation depends on three parameters: spin density ρ, T1 and T2 relaxation times, so:

$$S = \rho \times e^{-TE/T2} \times (1 - e^{-TR/T1}) \qquad (19.2)$$

TE and TR are pulse sequence parameters described later.

Flip angles The angle of precession α or the flip-angle, shown in Fig.19.4(b), depends on the RF-pulse energy. If the RF-pulse is less energetic than 90° then intermediate angles of rotation can be induced. If the rotating magnetic field of the RF-pulse is B_1 then the angle of rotation (the flip-angle) is:

$$\alpha = \gamma B_1 t \qquad (19.3)$$

Where t represents the RF-pulse duration.

The flip-angle can therefore be controlled by varying the pulse time or amplitude. After time t the magnetic vector M is orientated at an angle α in the diagram.

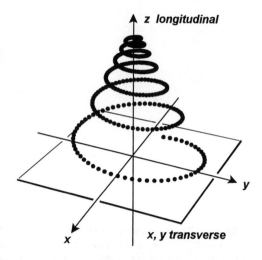

Figure 19.5 The magnetic vector tracing out a spiral path as it regains equilibrium with the z plane

19.2.3 The Larmor frequency

The **precessional frequency f** of the nucleus can be calculated as:

$$f = \frac{\mu B_o}{2\pi L} \qquad (19.4)$$

Where μ is the proton magnetic moment shown in Fig.19.2, L the proton spin angular momentum and B_o the magnetic field strength in Tesla. In order to simplify matters μ and $2\pi L$ can be treated as constants since they are fixed for any particular nucleus (in this case a hydrogen proton). Together they describe the gyro magnetic ratio γ :

$$\gamma = \frac{\mu}{2\pi L} \qquad (19.5)$$

This is a constant specific to the nucleus in question The gyromagnetic ratio for the hydrogen proton is calculated in Box 19.1.

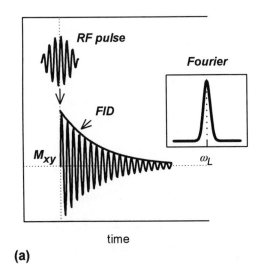

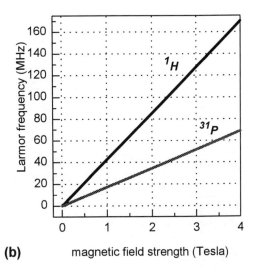

(a)

time

(b)   magnetic field strength (Tesla)

Figure 19.6 (a) Free induction decay. After the RF pulse the proton precession at the Larmor frequency decays yielding the FID. The envelope of this decay measures T2*. The frequency of the FID is measured from its Fourier spectrum (b) Influence of magnetic field strength on Larmor frequency for hydrogen ^{1}H and ^{31}P nuclei.

Simplifying eqn. 19.4 by substituting γ :

$$\omega_L = \gamma B_o \qquad (19.6)$$

This is an important basic equation since it relates the precession frequency to magnetic field strength B_o and is the **Larmor equation**; ω_L is the **Larmor frequency** (J. Larmor 1857-1942, Irish mathematician) where ω represents the angular frequency of precession. In Fig.19.4(b) B_1 will influence M only if it rotates at the Larmor precession frequency ω_L. At 1T ω_L is ~42MHz. When the RF pulse is switched off M regains its equilibrium state M_o by precessing as depicted the figure. Figure 19.6(a) illustrates that after an RF-pulse the NMR precessional signal undergoes **Free Induction Decay** FID and M_{xy} regains equilibrium M_z. This is the **transverse** or **spin-spin relaxation time** where individual protons lose energy to the surrounding tissue. The frequency components of the FID can be identified by Fourier analysis.

Figure 19.6(b) shows the linear relationship between Larmor Frequency (in MHz) and magnetic field strength (in Tesla) for two nuclei : ^{1}H and ^{31}P.

Box 19.1

The gyromagnetic ratio γ for hydrogen.

Proton magnetic moment:
1.41031×10^{-26} J T^{-1}
The proton spin angular momentum is:
0.527×10^{-34}J s^{-1}

$$\gamma = \frac{\mu}{2\pi L} = \frac{1.41\times10^{-26}}{2\pi \times 0.527\times10^{-34}} = 42582252 \text{ Hz}$$

or 42.58... MHz T^{-1}

Clinical magnet strengths

The precession frequency of a ^{1}H (proton) for a

High 1.5 T	f = 42.58 × 1.5	63.87 MHz
Medium 0.3 T	f = 42.58 × 0.3	12.77 MHz
Low 0.064 T	f = 42.58 × 0.064	2.72 MHz

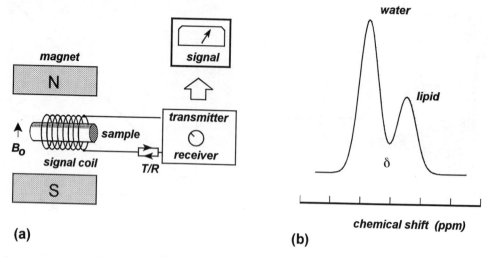

Figure 19.7   **(a)** The basic equipment for generating and detecting the NMR signal from a sample placed in a magnetic field. T/R is the transmit/receive switch. **(b)** Chemical shift between water and lipid measured in parts per million of ω_L.

19.2.4 Signal measurement

Simple equipment for measuring the exact Larmor frequency for any particular substance can be seen in Fig.19.7(a). The sample is positioned in a strong magnetic field B_o surrounded by a signal coil, which acts as a transmitting and receiving antenna. The coil is connected to a variable radio-frequency (RF) oscillator which transmits a series of RF-pulses changing in frequency until resonance is achieved. The weak NMR signals received from the precessing protons are amplified and passed on to a sensitive RF-receiver which measures the strength of the NMR frequency this is highest when the RF pulse frequency is at **resonance** with the Larmor frequency.

The NMR signal strength (amplitude) at resonance depends on hydrogen atom concentration. The Larmor frequency for the same magnetic field strength differs for each nucleus. Table 19.2 lists important physiological elements, their abundance, γ and NMR signal strength relative to hydrogen.

Spin density   The density of the excited spins in a region is one of the major factors influencing MR signal intensity (spin density ρ see eqn.19.2). This influences tissue contrast and depends on the number of hydrogen nuclei and not all the protons as the equation would imply; it is therefore more appropriate to use the term spin density or intermediate scans. The simple equipment illustrated in Fig. 19.7(a) measures the signal from the FID at resonance obtained from a 90° RF pulse. The signal strength is directly proportional to the number of hydrogen protons. Magnetic resonance imaging however does not measure the proton density directly but image characteristics heavily dependent on T1 and T2. This will be described in the next chapter.

This simple equipment contains all the basic components found in larger magnetic resonance imaging machines. They are :

- A strong magnetic field B_o
- Transmitting / receiving signal coil
- An RF transmitter
- A sensitive RF-receiver.
- A display device

Table 19.2 Useful nuclei in NMR

Isotope	Natural Abundance (%)	γ (MHz)	Signal Intensity
^{1}H (Proton)	99.98	42.58	1.0000
^{19}Fluorine	100	40.05	0.8300
^{23}Sodium	100	11.26	0.0930
^{31}Phosphorus	100	17.24	0.0660
^{17}Oxygen	0.037	5.77	0.0290
^{13}Carbon	1.11	10.71	0.0160
^{35}Chlorine	75.5	4.17	0.0084
^{15}Nitrogen	0.37	4.30	0.0010
^{39}Potassium	93.1	1.99	0.0005

19.2.5 Chemical shift (δ)

A typical NMR spectrum is shown in Fig.19.7(b). The precise resonance frequency of a proton is determined by its local magnetic field comprising the static field and its position on the molecule. Therefore all hydrogen protons within a certain tissue do not have exactly the same Larmor frequency. Proton position can be influenced by the magnetic shielding effects of electron orbitals which induce secondary magnetic fields. This effect can either diminish the local field so shielding the proton or enhance the local field so deshielding the proton. The small changes in Larmor frequency or shifts can be represented as a spectrum, the spectrum peak positions proportional to local magnetic field strength differences specified in parts per million (ppm) of the resonance frequency relative to a standard. The chemical shift reference is a compound whose proton Larmor frequency is used as a standard. The reference material is commonly tetramethylsilane $Si(CH_3)_4$ since it exhibits one of the greatest proton shielding, exceeding tissue molecules, so any chemical shift measured would all be moved in the same direction away from this reference peak. By referring to this standard the chemical shift has a constant value independent of machine characteristics (magnetic field strength or radio frequency).

Most molecules of physiological importance have shifts (δ) between 0 and 10 ppm. Water has $\delta = 4.7$ppm so for a 1T magnet with a ω_L of 4.2.58MHz this will give a frequency difference of $(42.58\times10^6)\times(4.7\times10^{-6}) = 200$Hz. Figure 19.7(b) is an NMR spectrum for a mixture of fat and water showing the small separation of about 3.5ppm. For lower magnetic field strengths the frequency difference, and consequently resolution, is less.

Summary

- The proton spin induces a magnetic dipole and the proton axis aligns with the magnetic field.
- Protons align parallel and anti-parallel but more align parallel.
- Proton magnetic vector *M*. At equilibrium this aligns with *z* the longitudinal axis. *x* and *y* axes are at 90° in the transverse axis.
- Protons precess by an RF pulse at resonance with the proton's precessional frequency.
- Resonant frequency is related to magnetic field strength (in Tesla) by the Larmor equation: $\omega_L = \gamma B_0$
- The magnetic vector *M* displaced from *z* into *x, y*.
- Angular displacement of the *M*-vector measured as a tip-angle α
- Gyromagnetic ratio γ is 42.58MHz T^{-1}

19.3 RELAXATION TIME CONSTANTS

Two signals are obtained from the proton's realignment with the static magnetic field. These are measured as time constants:

- The longitudinal time constant **T1**
- The transverse time constant **T2**

T1 and T2 signals are affected by the tissue molecular structure and chemistry. Small changes in tissue chemistry and differences between normal and abnormal tissue can alter the values of T1 and T2.

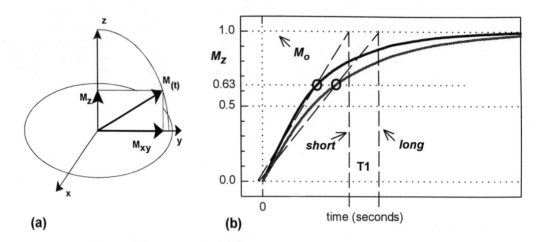

Figure 19.8   **(a)** The vector diagram identifying the proportion of M_z and M_{xy} in the proton magnetic vector M at time t. **(b)** M traces out an exponential decay as it regains equilibrium (M_z = 1). The T1 time is measured at 63% recovery. Both short and long T1 examples are shown.

19.3.1 Longitudinal time constant: T1

The return of longitudinal magnetization M_z to its equilibrium value z-axis requires exchange of energy between the nuclear spins and the material lattice. Following excitation by a 90° RF pulse M_z will return from the transverse plane (M_{xy}) approaching equilibrium with a characteristic time constant. (Fig. 19.8(a)). This spin lattice or longitudinal relaxation time is measured as T1.

The speed of relaxation or the time to lose transverse magnetization M_{xy} and to regain equilibrium is the **longitudinal relaxation time** but since this is an exponential event the time constant itself is measured when the longitudinal magnetization reaches 63% of its original value. Figure 19.8(b) plots this exponential realignment of M with the z-axis and shows that T1 is measured at a point marking 63% of maximum recovery; this is explained in Box 19.2. Both short and long T1 times are shown in the figure.

During longitudinal relaxation the protons lose energy to the surrounding tissue. The rate of proton energy loss depends on the material or tissue composition. Protons lose energy more rapidly to those tissues with greater complexity (T1 time is short). With simple molecular structures (water), the energy loss is slower and T1 is long. The exception to this rule is fat which, in spite of being a simple compound, has chemical bonds at the ends of its fatty acid molecules which have frequencies near the Larmor frequency of hydrogen. These allow fast energy transfer and consequently T1 times are short for fatty tissue. More complex or solid tissue (muscle protein) absorbs proton energy quickly so T1 is shorter for solid tissues. T1 is strongly related to tissue water content; time periods range between 300 to 2000 ms. T1 varies with magnetic field strengths since precessional frequencies increase with B_o (see Larmor Equation) which tends to slow the loss of energy to the surrounding tissues, consequently T1 times increase, approximately as $B_o^{0.1} - B_o^{0.3}$. The broad range of T1 values versus field strength is also plotted in Fig.19.9(a). Table 19.3 gives the values of various tissues for 0.5, 1.0 and 1.5T magnets; the T2 time remains virtually unchanged.

Table 19.3 The variation of T1 with magnet field.

Tissue	T1			T2
	0.5T	1.0T	1.5T	
Fat	210	240	260	80
Liver	350	420	500	40
Kidney	430	590	690	58
Muscle	550	730	870	45
Heart	570	750	880	57
White matter	500	680	780	90
Gray matter	650	810	900	100
CSF	1800	2160	2400	160

Box 19.2

The measurement of T1

After a 90° RF Pulse the M_Z curve = $(1 - e^{-t/T1})$

Calculating $(1 - e^{-t/T1})$

When

		M_Z	
t = T1	$(1 - e^{-1})$	=	**63**
t = 2×T1	$(1 - e^{-2})$	=	86
t = 3×T1	$(1 - e^{-3})$	=	95
t = 4×T1	$(1 - e^{-4})$	=	98
t = 5×T1	$(1 - e^{-5})$	=	99.3

Measurement of T1 time is made when M_Z reaches 63% maximum.

19.3.2 Transverse time constant: T2, T2*

The transverse magnetization M_{xy} is the component of the macroscopic magnetization vector M at right angles to the static magnetic field B_0. During equilibrium recovery precession of the transverse magnetization occurs at the Larmor frequency which is the detected MR signal. After the RF pulse the transverse magnetization M_{xy} will decay to zero with a transverse or spin-spin relaxation time constant T2 or T2* (already indicated by the FID envelope in Fig.19.6(a)).

The overall T2 signal represents the loss of phase coherence among spins orientated at an angle to the static magnetic field. Local deviations in the microscopic magnetic fields generated by interactions between magnetic moments of atoms lead to slight differences in resonance frequencies which cause phase interference or dephasing of the spins. This is demonstrated in Fig.19.9(b) where a single signal in (I) is joined by two others in (II) whose slight differences destructively interfere to yield the sum signal in (III).

The composite signals in (II) **dephase** as the phase diagrams show in Fig.19.9(c) for *t*=0 (FID start), *t*= 0.5 and *t*=1. The FID envelope is again shown in Fig.19.10(a) identifying the T2 time constant measured at 37% of the decay curve. The simple T2 measured here suffers from distortions due to the main magnetic field inhomogeneities and is distinguished by calling it T2* (T2 star, the * denotes a distorted signal influenced by magnetic field inhomogeneities) The additional effect of these inhomogeneities cause M_{xy} to decay far more quickly than the expected T2 so T2*<T2. Image contrast is a function of T2 in spin echo images but T2* determines image contrast in fast sequences or gradient echo images. The pure T2 signal is complex and must be obtained by indirect means, to be described later.

Free Induction Decay From section 19.2.3 equilibrium recovery provides a radio-frequency signal generated by the precessional movement, its decay giving a proton spin-spin relaxation time or T2*.

Figure 19.6(a) illustrates how a 90° RF-Pulse shifts the magnetization vector M into the transverse *x,y* plane M_{xy}. After the RF-pulse the NMR precessional signal undergoes free induction decay FID and M_{xy} regains equilibrium M_Z. This is the transverse or spin-spin relaxation time where individual protons lose energy to the surrounding tissue.

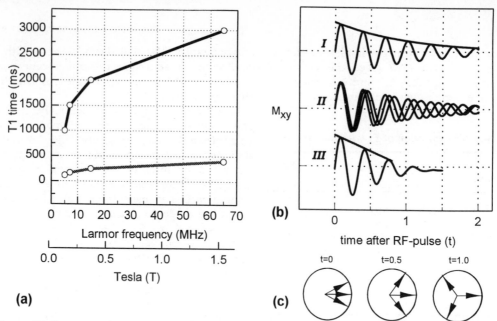

Figure 19.9 **(a)** The variation of T1 time with mag netic field strength for liquid (water, CSF) and soft tissue, other tissues have intermediate values (Table 19.3). **(b)** A single FID (A) and signal interference amongst three FID's (B) having slightly different frequency giving a much shorter time constant (C) **(c)** Phase diagrams for (B) at times 0, 0.5 and 1.0s.

The FID outline or signal envelope of this decay is shown in Fig. 19.10(a) for two tissues with a short and long T2; it follows an exponential slope whose time constant T2* is taken at 37% maximum. Box 19.3 explains why this point is chosen. The Larmor frequency of the FID is sensitive to small magnetic field variations consequently T2 is distorted by small magnetic field inhomogeneities caused both by neighboring protons and the magnet itself. Magnet inhomogeneities obscure the true T2 tissue so the true value of T2 must be separated from magnet inhomogeneities by using a special pulse sequence (described later).

Dephasing The sum effect of frequency and phase differences from neighboring FIDs, demonstrated in Fig.19.9(b), causes mutual interference. Loss of phase coherence occurs exponentially due to spin-spin interference thus the decay time of the composite FID signal is shortened. T2 signal differences in a perfectly homogeneous magnetic field would reflect tissue chemistry.

The FID's undergo less proton **spin-spin in-**

terference in simple compounds (liquids such as CSF) and maintain in-phase conditions for a longer time, so T2 times are longer. T2 for solid material is shorter as protons are in close proximity and the FID's lose phase relationships more rapidly. The loss of transverse magnetization M_{xy} given by T2 occurs relatively quickly whereas longitudinal recovery M_z given by T1 takes a longer time. In order of time-span therefore T1 is longer than T2 which is longer than T2* (T1>T2>T2*). Examples of T1 and T2 times for three main field strengths have been listed in Tab.19.3.

Although the Larmor frequency is very sensitive to changes in magnetic field strength the transverse relaxation time (T2) is not much influenced (unlike T1), indeed spin-spin interactions at higher field strengths may be more efficient and T2 could shorten.

Correlation time τ_c The local magnetic fields produced by various protons are produced by molecular movements or 'tumbling'. Movements at or near the Larmor frequency have the most effect.

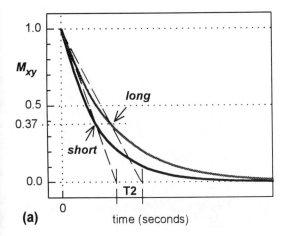

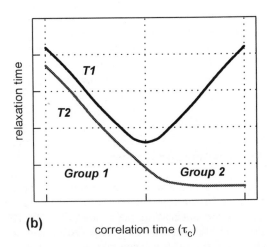

Figure 19.10 (a) The measurement of T2 time from the FID decay envelope (b) Correlation time τc for T1 and T2. *Group 1* are small molecules, *Group 2* more complex molecules including protein and lipids.

Figure 19.10(b) plots the tumbling or correlation time τ_c for a variety of molecular types showing the separation of T1 and T2 times. These can be broadly divided into two groups. Group 1 represents small molecules such as water and CSF with a short τ_c and a long T1 time. As the molecular structure becomes more complex τ_c slows to a rate near the Larmor frequency. Hydrogen protons incorporated into large macromolecules such as proteins and lipids have longer τ_c times (Group 2 in graph) and much shorter T1 times. Molecules with correlation times less than about 500kHz are relatively static in an environment where spins are typically 30 to 60MHz. All molecules in this group (2) give short T2 values. Extremely short T2 values of <10μs are too rapid to be visualized in MRI; these are associated with membrane surfaces and structures having large protein molecules.

Box 19.3

The measurement of T2 from the FID

Figure 19.10(a) FID decays as $e^{-t/T2}$

Calculating $e^{-t/T2}$

$$
\begin{array}{llll}
t = T2 & (e^{-1}) & M_{xy} = \textbf{37} \\
t = 2{\times}T2 & (e^{-2}) & = 13 \\
t = 3{\times}T2 & (e^{-3}) & = 5 \\
t = 4{\times}T2 & (e^{-4}) & = 2 \\
\end{array}
$$

Measurement of T2 time is therefore made when the M_{xy} falls to **37%** maximum

19.4 PULSE SEQUENCES

The subtle differences in tissue chemistry can be thoroughly explored by exposing them to a series of 90° and 180° RF-Pulses of different sequences, altering their strength and time interval. The tissue's response to these pulse sequences, shown by the T1 and T2 signals, can uncover small differences in composition not only between tissue types but within the same tissue perhaps revealing early pathology.

19.4.1 Saturation recovery

Figure19.4(c) shows the movement of the *M*-vector into the *x,y* transverse plane (α = 90°); this is the saturation point and the 90° RF-Pulse is the **saturation pulse**. After the 90° RF Pulse the proton loses energy and recovers equilibrium. The process shown in Fig.19.4(c) is reversed: the *M*-vector regains longitudinal magnetization and undergoes **saturation recovery**. The basic NMR signals given during saturation recovery are:

- The rate of realignment of *M* with *z*. This is **equilibrium recovery**, relaxation time or loss of transverse magnetization and is known as the T1 signal
- During saturation recovery the proton loses energy by emitting an NMR radio-frequency signal. The decay rate of this NMR Signal is known as the T2 signal

Saturation recovery sequence   We have seen that after a 90° RF-Pulse the proton undergoes relaxation, to gain equilibrium, moving from the *x, y* transverse plane towards the *z*-axis. A simple pulse sequence of 90° RF-pulses at fixed TR times in Fig.19.11 (a), (b) show the signal strengths. For long TR times as in (a) protons recover full equilibrium between RF-pulses so each FID is maximum.   For faster TR times as in (b) protons do not recover full equilibrium and the succeeding 90° pulses appear during incomplete recovery ($M_{(t)}$ between transverse

and longitudinal planes); the resultant FID's therefore get successively smaller, shown by the sloping line for each sequence in the diagram.   These are **partial saturation** pulse sequences.

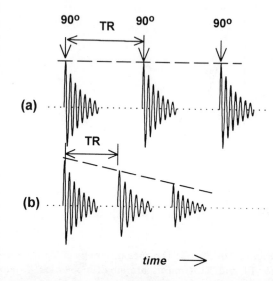

Figure 19.11   Saturation recovery sequence for a sequence of 90° pulses at different repeat times **(a)** long TR **(b)** short TR times

19.4.2 The Spin Echo Sequence

Spin-echo signal   At saturation the protons are precessing in-phase (M_{xy} is maximum) but during saturation recovery ($M_{(t)}$ attaining equilibrium) protons dephase. This is shown again as the phase diagram at the end of the FID in Fig.19.12 (A and B).

Applying a 180° RF-Pulse will achieve proton inversion, shifting the *M*-vector so that it is anti-parallel to the z-axis ($-M_z$).   This has a most valuable property: the phase relationships lost during the saturation recovery process at (B) are regained by reversing the precession, the destructive interference is also reversed. Protons dephased at (B) are inverted by the 180° pulse thus rephasing the signals (C) and so refocusing the protons' precession

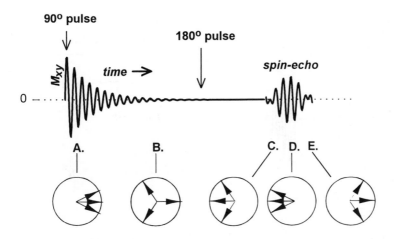

Figure 19.12   The rephasing of the FID by applying a 180° pulse at a predetermined time after the initial saturation 90° RF pulse. The phase diagrams show the phase loss by the FID (A and B) reversed by the 180° pulse (C and D) rephasing in (D) to give the spin-echo signal and again loss of phase (E) as saturation recovery occurs once again.

(D). This gives a strong **spin-echo** signal which again decays due to dephasing (E). Due to the re-phasing of saturation recovery signals after a 180° inversion-pulse, the NMR signals give a spin-echo signal. This echo signal is used in a spin echo pulse sequence (Fig.19.13(a)) which consists of a 90° RF-pulse followed by a 180° RF-pulse; TR time determines the T1 contribution. The time from the 90° pulse to the received echo signal is the **TE** time (time to echo). The larger the TE time the greater the T2 information. The 180° pulse is placed at ½TE, which fixes the time of signal measurement at TE. The spin-echo pulse sequence is a fundamental imaging sequence, TR and TE times determining the proportion of T1 and T2 information (weighting) in the image.

19.4.3 Gradient echo

The spin echo signal can be produced by reversing the direction of the magnetic field, as shown in Fig.19.13(b). This is a much faster technique for obtaining the spin echo signal and is the technique used for fast imaging sequences. The gradient coils are part of the imaging system of a magnetic resonance machine and are described in the next chapter.

19.4.4 Inversion recovery

The inversion recovery process, shown in Fig.19.14(a), resembles saturation recovery but now a 180°-RF pulse places M in the $-z$ axis. During inversion recovery $-M_z$ travels from $-z$, through the transverse x, y plane, reaching equilibrium at the $+z$ axis (M_z). The $-M_z$ realignment is compared in this graph with the 90° RF-pulse saturation recovery. For the 180° recovery the T1 passes through the x, y transverse plane when time t equals $0.693{\times}T1$, completing its recovery when t reaches $4{\times}T1$.

Inversion recovery sequence   Inversion recovery produces a signal that contains more T1 information than the saturation recovery sequence.

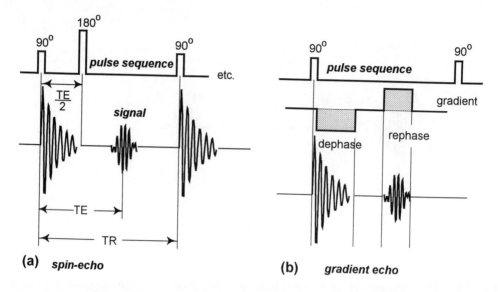

Figure 19.13   **(a)** Spin-echo 90°-180° pulse sequence The spin echo signal is measured at time TE which is operator chosen **(b)** Gradient echo sequence which can replace the spin-echo sequence; the reversed gradient performs the same function as a 180° RF pulse.

The pulse-sequence shown in Fig.19.14(b) consists of a 180° pulse followed by a spin-echo sequence, when the signal strength is measured.   The time period TI between the initial 180° RF-pulse and the 90° pulse is the **inversion time** or τ (tau). Since different tissues will show different T1 times the proton M vector will be at varying intermediate stages of equilibrium depending on the length of TI. The inversion time between the 180° and 90° pulses therefore determines how much T1 information the signal will contain.

19.5   T1 AND T2 SIGNAL MEASUREMENT

For non-imaging chemical analysis exact values of T1 and T2 are routinely obtained. In an imaging system, where short acquisition times are most important, exact measurement is never attempted. A rapid estimate of T1 and T2 are made for image display. A description of the full T1 and T2 measurement is included here for reference.

19.5.1 T1 measurement

The standard indirect technique for measuring T1 uses a series of 90° pulses at specific intervals (TR: time to repeat). If TR is shorter than the T1 recovery time then the resulting peak value of the FID curve will become successively smaller due to incomplete equilibrium recovery. The peak value of the FID signal will follow the T1 saturation recovery curve. Interfering processes will not influence these first peak values. The peak FID values at various TR times provide the signal outline or envelope for accurate T1 measurement. The effect of different TR times is shown in Fig.19.15(a).

   The accuracy of T1 measurement depends on the number of points along the curve; only two readings are taken to obtain an estimated value when imaging. Measurements are repeated a number of times to improve accuracy: this is **signal averaging**.

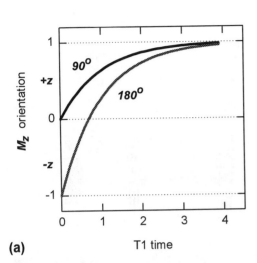

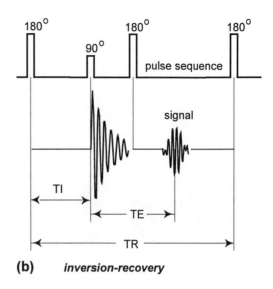

Figure 19.14 **(a)** Comparing 180° and 90° inversion for T1 measurement **(b)** Inversion recovery pulse sequence of 180° followed by 90° after inversion time TI.

19.5.2. Pure T2 measurement

The simple free induction decay (FID) will be influenced by both proton spin-spin interactions (a property of the tissue) and magnetic field inhomogeneities to give the T2* value. Spin-spin interactions cause non-reversible signal dephasing which is retained for some time, consequently repeated 90° RF pulses do not reveal the original signal peak since remnant interference from previous RF-pulses will remain.

If a 180° RF pulse is applied then this remnant dephasing can be reversed and the signals will re-phase to give a full peak signal: this is the spin-echo signal appearing at TE (Figs.19.12 and 19.13). The 90° pulse followed by a series of 180° pulses at time interval TE/2 is the Carr-Purcell sequence. Slight variations in this sequence are sometimes used to overcome inhomogeneities in the signal coils. The envelope of signal decay is now the pure T2 signal, unaffected by remnant phase differences and magnetic field non-uniformities (unlike T2*) reflecting the T2 effects of the tissue itself. Figure 19.15(b) shows this pulse sequence and signal aver-

aging again improves the accuracy of these readings.

Summary

- The 90° RF-Pulse is called the saturation pulse. The precessing proton recovers equilibrium and undergoes saturation recovery.
- A faster 90° pulse sequence will prevent complete recovery and give smaller T1 signals. Partial saturation pulse sequence when 90° pulse timing shorter than T1
- The spin echo sequence is a 90° RF Pulse followed by a 180° Pulse.
- After the 90° RF pulse photons lose phase (are de-phased) and phase differences interfere with individual FID's, shortening T2.
- The 180° Inverting RF-Pulse, re-phases the de-phased protons producing a spin-echo pulse.
- The time between 90° pulses is the Pulse Repetition frequency TR time

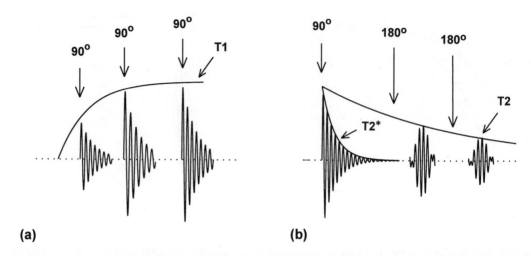

(a)   **(b)**

Figure 19.15 **(a)** Accurate T1 measurement achieved by using different TR times. TR=1 is short, TR=3 is a longer 90° pulse interval. **(b)** Pure T2 measured by a 90°-180°-180° pulse sequence is much longer than T2* measured from the FID.

- After the second 90° the strength of the T1 signal depends on the longitudinal magnetization recovery. Total recovery will be given by tissues with a short T1.
- In a 90°-180° sequence the time from the 90° pulse to reception of the spin echo signal is the TE time
- By increasing the TE times (after the 90° RF pulse) the signals can become increasingly T2 weighted
- T1 weighting is achieved by using short TR time.
- A TR <0.5 second is considered short. A TR >1.5 seconds is long.
- A long TE is about 3 times longer than a short TE (30 milliseconds)

KEYWORDS

angular momentum - A vector quantity given by the vector product of momentum and position. This remains constant until an external force changes the direction of rotation causing precession. Atomic nuclei possess intrinsic angular momentum called spin.

B_0 - the magnetic field measured in Tesla.

B_1 - the radio frequency magnetic induction field opposed to B_0.

bandwidth - a general term describing range of frequencies in a signal.

Bloch equations - describe motion of the magnetization vector. They include precession effects and T1, T2 relaxation times.

chemical shift change in Larmor frequency caused by chemical binding.

Table 19.4 Summary of T1 and T2 properties

T1	T2
• longitudinal relaxation	• transverse relaxation
• spin-lattice	• spin-spin
• water has long T1	• water has long T2
• fat and solids short T1	
• Times between 300-2000ms	• times between 30-150ms
• varies with field strength	• only slight variation with field strength
• related to water content	• variation linked to water lipid and magnet inhomogeneities
• malignant tissue typically has higher T1	
• measured at 63% of maximum	• measured at 37% decay point

diamagnetic - a material with a small negative magnetic susceptibility which will decrease a magnetic field. Water and oxygen rich compounds.

dipole - magnetic dipole.
dipole interaction - interaction between a nuclear spin and its neighbors due to magnetic dipole moments, contributing to relaxation times.

ferromagnetic - a substance that has a large positive magnetic susceptibility e.g. iron.

free induction decay - when transverse magnetization M_{xy} is produced a signal will be produced decaying toward equilibrium M_0 with a characteristic time constant T2 or T2*.

Gauss - G unit of magnetic flux in the CGS system (1 Tesla = 10,000 G).

gyromagnetic ratio γ - the ratio of the magnetic moment to the angular momentum. A constant for a given nucleus.
homogeneity - magnetic field uniformity measured in parts per million of main field

inversion - the magnetization vector orientated opposite to the magnetic field produced by 180° pulse or gradient switching.

inversion recovery - a pulse sequence where the nuclear magnetization is inverted prior to a spin-echo pulse sequence. The time between the 180° pulse and the SE sequence is the inversion time TI.

Larmor equation - this describes the frequency of precession of the nuclear magnetic moment being proportional to the magnetic field: $f = \gamma B_0/2\pi$ Hz.

Larmor frequency - the frequency at which magnetic resonance can be excited; given by the Larmor equation. For H^+ the Larmor frequency is 42.58MHz T^{-1}.

Longitudinal magnetization M_z - the component of the magnetization vector along the static magnetic field. Following the RF pulse M_z will approach the equilibrium value M_0 with time constant T1.

longitudinal relaxation - return of M_z to M_0 after excitation. Requires an exchange of energy between the proton spin and the molecular lattice. Measured by time constant T1.

magnetic moment μ - given by a nucleus (proton) with spin. The associated magnetic dipole moment will interact with an external magnetic field mimicking a tiny bar magnet.

magnetic susceptibility χ - a measure of the ability of a material to become magnetized.

$M_{(t)}$ - M value dependant on flip-angle. Magnitude proportional to spin density.

MR signal - radio frequency electromagnetic signal produced by the precession of the transverse magnetization of the nuclear spins.

M_{xy} - transverse magnetization.
M_z - longitudinal magnetization.

paramagnetic - a material with a small but positive magnetic susceptibility. Paramagnetic substances reduce relaxation times. Gadolinium and manganese are examples.

partial saturation - applying repeated RF pulses at times shorter than T1. Can be used for calculating T1 for the region.

permanent magnet - one whose field originates from a permanently magnetized material.

permeability - tendency of a substance to concentrate a magnetic field. Mu-metal has a high permeability.

precession - the movement of a spinning body which traces out a conical shape. The magnetic moment of a proton with spin will precess at an angle to the magnetic field precessing at the Larmor frequency.

pulse 180° (π pulse) - RF pulse which inverts the magnetization vector as M_z .

pulse 90° ($\pi/2$ pulse) - an RF pulse which rotates M_z into the transverse plane M_{xy} .

pulse length - time duration of an RF pulse. The longer the pulse length the narrower the bandwidth.

pulse sequence - a set of RF pulses, with or without gradient reversal to give an MR signal.

receiver coil - a coil or antenna which picks up the MR signal.

relaxation times - after excitation nuclear spins will return to their equilibrium state where M_{xy} is zero and M_z is maximum. Transverse magnetization returns to zero with a characteristic time constant T2 and longitudinal magnetization returns toward M_o with time constant T2.

resistive magnet - an electromagnet whose magnetic field is due to an electric current which consumes power (unlike superconducting magnet).

saturation - a non-equilibrium state where equal numbers of spins are aligned against and with the main magnetic field; zero net magnetization. Produced by repeated short interval RF pulses compared to T1.

saturation recovery - pulse sequence that achieves partial saturation allowing recovery before next pulse.

sensitive volume - the region from which the MR signal originates. Influenced by shape and bandwidth of RF pulse.

sequence time - or repetition time TR. The period between repeating an identical pulse sequence.

spin - intrinsic angular momentum of a nucleus. Responsible for the magnetic moment.

spin density N - the density of resonating spins in a given volume, determined by the MR signal strength. Measured as moles m^{-3}. For water this is 1.1×10^5 moles H per m^3.

spin echo - reappearance of an MR signal by reversing the dephasing of the spins.

superconducting magnet - a magnet whose magnetic field is obtained from an electromagnet constructed from superconducting materials enclosed in a cryostat (liquid helium bath). No electrical energy is consumed unlike resistive magnet.

T1 - longitudinal relaxation time.
T2 - spin-spin or transverse relaxation time.

T2* - the time constant of the FID which is influenced by a combination of magnetic field inhomogeneities and spin-spin relaxation.

TE - echo time between middle of 90° pulse and middle of spin echo signal.

Tesla - the SI unit of magnetic flux density 1T = 10,000 gauss.

TR - repetition time (see sequence time).

transverse relaxation - loss of transverse magnetization from a non-zero value in the M_{xy} plane.

voxel - volume element, representing matrix resolution and slice depth.

Magnetic Resonance Imaging

20.1 The Main Magnet
20.2 The MRI System
20.3 Imaging Pulse Sequences
20.4 Fast Imaging Techniques

20.5 Image Quality
20.6 Choice of MRI system
20.7 Image Artifacts
20.8 Magnetic Resonance
    Spectroscopy (MRS)

20.1 THE MAIN MAGNET

The phenomenon of nuclear magnetic resonance was developed as an imaging technique in the early 1970's. Its non-ionizing characteristic make it ideal for detailed study of anatomical structures. Present techniques in magnetic resonance imaging (MRI) can display:

- **Chemical Differences** between tissues as changes in a gray scale image (Tumor Pathology).
- **Blood Flow** as a high intensity image of vessels either in thin slices or 3-D images.
- **Axial, Coronal, Saggital** and **Oblique** images from a complete 3-Dimensional voxel data set (Head).
- **Long slices**, particularly in saggital view (spine).

Fast imaging techniques have been developed so that organ movement (cardiac, respiration) can be effectively frozen giving sharp pictures of the heart and abdomen. Fast data collection has enabled clinically routine 3-Dimensional imaging for investigating cranial anatomy and vascular pathways.

MRI does not offer the same clinical information as CT; the latter still provides faster imaging and higher resolution but the non-ionizing properties of MRI are a distinct advantage for imaging sensitive areas (breast). Signal data is related to physiological properties of the tissue unlike x-ray transmission properties shown by CT. Blood flow can be demonstrated by MRI and further refinements to sensitivity enable micro-circulation pathways in the brain to be seen.

MRI System   The complete imaging system consists of:

- A large bore **Magnet** (Resistive, Permanent or Super-conducting)
- Very stable **Power Supplies** for precise magnet control.
- **Transmitter / Receiver** electronics for RF.
- Small Field of View Receiving **Coils** for specific anatomy.
- Imaging **Computer** and **Array Processor** with Fast Fourier Transform (FFT) hard-wired for rapid computation of reconstructed images.

20.1.1   Magnet strength

Magnetic flux density is measured in either Gauss G or **Tesla** T the conversion being: 10000 Gauss equals 1 Tesla so 1 gauss equals 0.1 milliTesla (mT). Tesla is commonly used for describing MRI magnet strengths. Fractions of a Tesla are expressed as milli-Tesla (mT) or micro-Tesla (µT).

MRI magnets have field strengths between 0.2 and 2.0T, the outer interference boundary is 5mT compared to the earth's magnetic field of about 50µT. The choice of magnet strength depends exclusively on the clinical application. This is discussed in a later section.

Low to Medium field have strengths from <0.1 to 0.2T and are mostly *Permanent* or *Resistive magnets* suitable for private clinics or

Medium field have fields of 0.2 - 0.3T and include the largest practical *resistive* and *permanent magnets.* The latter are useful for mobile MRI units where energy consumption is a prime consideration.

Medium to High field The common field strengths are 0.5T, 1.0T, 1.5T, 2.0T and are exclusively **super-conducting magnets** which use liquid helium as a cryogen. Magnet strengths for clinical use can reach 4T.

Magnet field strength has limits depending on the magnet type.

- **Permanent** magnet field strength is restricted to about 0.3T due to weight considerations.
- A **Resistive** magnet is restricted to about 0.3T since power consumption is limited to 100kW which restricts a resistive magnet size and an increased volume can only be achieved by sacrificing field strength.
- **Super-conducting** magnets do not suffer from field strength restrictions or volume size restrictions.

20.1.2   Magnet Types

The largest component of any MRI system is the magnet itself. Three types exist commercially:

- Permanent magnet
- Resistive electromagnet
- Superconducting electromagnet

Permanent Magnet This has considerable advantages in terms of running costs since the generation of its main magnetic field consumes no electricity and Fig. 20.1(a) shows it has a small **fringe field** (external magnetic field) which is a considerable advantage in a small area (mobile installation). There are some major disadvantages however:

- Weight, which can be up to 100 tonnes, needing a strengthened floor.
- Continual loss of magnet field strength throughout its working life.
- Comparatively poor magnetic field uniformity.

In spite of these drawbacks it has become the favorite option for low field machines where the orientation of a permanent magnet MRI machine can be either along the length of the body (Z-axis) or perpendicular to the patient's body (Y-axis) shown in Fig.20.1(b). The latter allows an open aspect which is more convenient for interventional work using a resistive magnet.

Resistive magnet This was a common design in the early MRI machines since it gave good field strengths and had a good power/weight ratio giving medium field strengths. The major disadvantage was its running costs since it can consume in excess of 30kW. The magnet windings offer some electrical resistance so considerable heat is generated which must be removed by water cooling. Some designs use a vertical magnetic field (Fig.20.1(b)) which proves convenient for patient interventional studies. Magnetic field uniformity (homogeneity) is good. Emergency shut down capabilities are important if interventional work is considered within the main magnetic field.

Superconducting Magnet The heat generated by a resistive magnet is caused by the electrical resistance at high field currents. This problem can be eliminated with a superconducting magnet using windings constructed from niobium-tantalum alloy. The winding is divided into several sets in order to create a homogeneous magnetic field and are

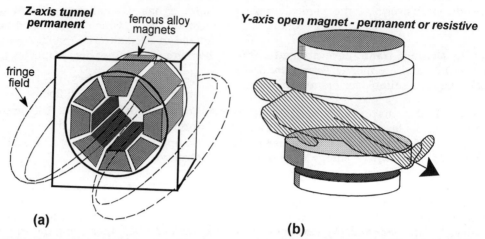

Figure 20.1 **(a)** A permanent magnet design showing the location of the ferrous alloy magnets around the gantry in the Z-axis **(b)** Two separate magnets, top and bottom, giving an open aspect Y-axis design which is used for both permanent and resistive magnets.

immersed in liquid helium which causes the windings to become superconducting (zero electrical resistance). The magnet is now activated by connecting the windings to an electrical supply. The field current (up to 500A) continues to circulate when the supply is removed; electricity costs are therefore minimal. If the magnet temperature rises above the super-conducting limit (~4.2K) then heat is generated and the helium boils off **quenching** the magnetic field (magnetic properties vanish). Helium cryogens used in a superconducting magnet can be recirculated and normally only need topping-up every 6 months or so.

Figure 20.2(a) shows the construction of a typical super-conducting magnet along with its supplementary shielding coils, which significantly reduce the large fringe field. Figure 20.2(b) is a commercial MRI system showing a similar design to a CT machine although the magnet unit is considerably deeper. Table 20.1 lists the basic properties given by the 3 magnet types. The considerable weight (in

tonnes) is a significant consideration when planning a MRI installation.

Table 20.1   Magnet properties

	Permanent	*Resistive*	*Supercon.*
Strength (T)	0.064-0.3	0.1-0.3	0.5-4.0
Fringe Field	small	small	large
Orientation	z or y	z or y	z
Shut down	no	fast	slow
Weight	up to 80t	2t	6t
Energy use	none	large	none
Cooling	none	water	helium

20.1.3   Magnet homogeneity

Uniformity of magnetic field throughout the imaging volume (20-35cm) is essential for good image quality. As the magnet strength increases field homogeneity becomes a major problem. Magnet field inhomogeneities originate from adjacent external influences (high

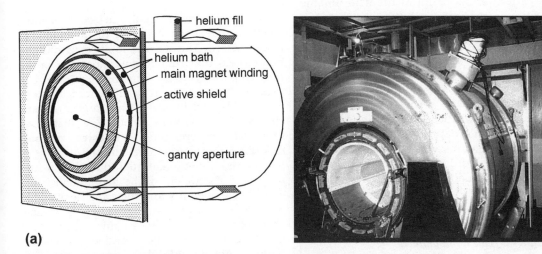

Figure 20.2 **(a)** Superconducting magnet system showing main windings immersed in a helium bath along with active shielding coils. **(b)** A superconducting MRI system.

fields from power lines, elevators and other electric equipment) or ferromagnetic materials (iron pipes or reinforcing rods) within the room. Inhomogeneities can also be caused by small imperfections in magnet construction The resulting main field inhomogeneity requires careful correction by **shimming** to achieve a uniform field.

Magnetic field inhomogeneities are measured in parts per million, a relative measurement independent of field strength, using the reference proton Larmor frequency for water which is 42.58MHz T^{-1}. Worked examples are given in Box 20.1. Magnet inhomogeneities can approach 100ppm even without external influences so shimming the magnet is an essential requirement. It must be very carefully performed since small field inhomogeneities influence nuclei (proton) behavior (T2*). Dislocations in the field homogeneity will influence readout or slice selection gradients. The influence of inherent small non-uniformity after correction can be reduced by increasing the gradient field strengths.

Manufacturers are continuously improving magnet field homogeneity. Methods have been developed for selectively suppressing the fat signal in images and emphasizing water photons. The Larmor frequency difference is 200Hz at 1.5T or 3.5ppm demanding extremely homogeneous magnetic fields and, at the moment, is only possible with small fields of view.

Typical homogeneity values of commercial magnets for MRI is given in Tab.20.2 for two fields of view (FOV) relating to body and head acquisitions. Homogeneity throughout the useful field of view is achieved by the combination of shim coils and iron sheets or foil carefully adjusted within the main winding.

Table 20.2 Magnet homogeneity for 2 field sizes

FOV	Permanent	Resistive	Supercon.
50cm	40ppm	40ppm	15ppm
20cm	10ppm	5ppm	0.25ppm

Shim coils Current carrying coils are arranged cylindrically inside the magnet bore. The pattern or spectrum of the field inhomogeneities is mapped and then corrected by setting the shim-coil currents via a precision power supply. This is **active shimming.**

Iron foil Carefully shaped iron plates can be placed inside or outside the magnet to give **passive shimming.** This method removes major inhomogeneities. Passive shimming is stable and is not dependent on power supply stability. It requires considerable time to fit and adjust; additional coil correction with shim-coils is usually necessary.

Box 20.1

Magnetic field homogeneity

Hydrogen protons have a Larmor frequency of 42.5759MHz T^{-1}. A 200Hz variation would represent a parts per million variation of:

  0.0002/42.5759 = 4.697×10^{-6} = 4.7ppm

Typical magnetic field variations for large fields of view (40cm) are:

Permanent and resistive magnets 40ppm representing a 1.7kHz variation. Over smaller volumes homogeneity is much better.

Superconducting magnets 15ppm representing 600Hz. This reduces to ±3ppm for fat suppression and better than ±1ppm for small volume spectroscopy.

NB
Magnet inhomogeneities are measured in parts per million since this is independent of magnetic field strength.

20.1.4 Shielding

The magnetic field surrounding an MRI installation is hazardous to people and equipment; it will attract ferrous items which can act as missiles endangering staff. External flux lines (fringe field) will interfere with sensitive equipment such as gamma cameras (photo-multipliers) and DSA (image intensifiers). Fringe fields are restricted by means of magnetic shielding, either passively by iron sheets or actively by a supplementary winding.

Figure 20.3 shows the 0.5 mT contour after shielding has been installed on a variety of magnet sizes. The magnet is sited within the building so that this contour does not penetrate important areas. Sensitive equipment is listed in Tab. 20.3 that is influenced by magnetic fields and indicates that nuclear medicine and DSA rooms should be distanced from MRI installations. **Passive or self shielding** requires a considerable number of heavy iron plates mounted directly on the magnet. The weight of the installation is increased significantly and the room floor would require substantial strengthening. A single sheet of iron is sometimes sufficient to shield a particular area i.e. cardiac pacemaker room. **Active shielding** uses an opposing external coil winding included within the cryostat with the main winding. (shown in Fig.20.2). This increases the size and cost of the super-conducting magnet but achieves effective shielding without increasing magnet weight.

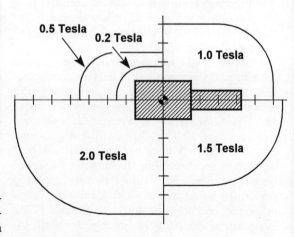

5mT (5G) contours: 2m graduations

Figure 20.3 Magnet shielding. The 0.5mT contour is shown for a variety of magnet field strengths which have had their fringe fields shielded.

Table 20.3   Magnetic field limits

Earth's magnetic field	50µT (0.05mT)
Gamma camera SPECT	50µT
Image intensifier	50µT
X-ray tube	0.2mT
Cardiac pacemaker	0.5mT
Video monitors	1.0mT

Radio frequency shielding   Efficient shielding against Radio Frequency interference (radio, television signals and power switching RF pulses) is essential owing to the high sensitivity of the receiving circuitry for the tiny NMR signals. The shielding factor should be in the order of 100dB for local radio stations.   A copper or aluminum **Faraday cage** is installed which:

- Blocks radio interference from the computer and display units so they do not reach the signal coils.
- Prevents RF pulses from the gradient-fields interfering with other equipment.

A thin (0.5mm) copper foil should completely surround the MRI installation. Gaps in this foil should be carefully filled. Doors should be similarly shielded and cable lengths should also be enclosed so that they do not act as antenna for RF interference. A wire mesh covering the control panel window preserves the integrity of the entire RF cage.

In summary:

- Magnet strength measured in Tesla
- Permanent and resistive magnets have field strengths up to 0.2T
- Superconducting magnets have field strengths from 0.5 to 2.0T
- Superconducting magnet requires liquid helium as a cryogen.
- Superconducting magnet fringe field reduced by active shielding
- Safety contour set at 0.5mT for pacemakers.
- Magnet homogeneity achieved by metal or coil shimming.

- Magnet homogeneity measured in parts per million; independent of field strength.
- RF shielding obtained by using wire-mesh Faraday cage.

20.2   THE MRI SYSTEM

Unlike X-ray computed tomography the image forming signals in MRI are radio-frequencies which convey image information by changes in:

- Frequency
- Amplitude
- Phase

The computations are performed by a dedicated Fast Fourier Transform (FFT) circuit which is part of an **array processor**. This includes a **phase sensitive demodulator** which gives NMR signal frequency and phase information necessary for image formation.

20.2.1   **Magnetic gradients**

NMR signal frequency is directly related to the magnetic field strength (as the Larmor equation explains). A carefully shimmed MRI magnet has an almost perfect homogeneous magnetic field so protons will all have the same Larmor Frequency.

If a magnetic field gradient G is superimposed on the main field B_0 so that there is a small linear increase over the length of the gradient then the Larmor frequency for the proton will vary along this gradient as:

$$\omega = \gamma \, (B_0 + G) \qquad (20.1)$$

where G is the added magnetic field from the gradient. Only those protons in slice location z will resonate at frequency ω as:

$$z = \frac{(\omega - \gamma B_0)}{\gamma G} \qquad (20.2)$$

Protons outside slice position z are unaffected and will give no signal so specific regions can be spatially located.   This was first proposed by P. Lauterbur (USA) in 1973.

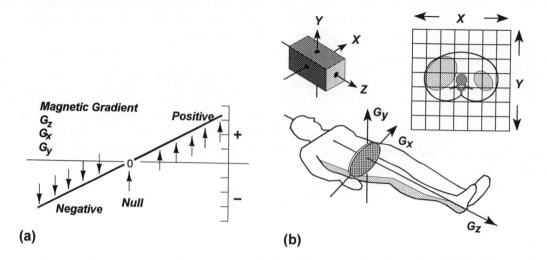

Figure 20.4 **(a)** Superimposing a gradient field on the main magnetic field. The gradient has a central null point; to one side (left) the gradient linearly decreases in strength and to the other (right) it increases. **(b)** *X, Y, Z* image planes used for slice position and decoding the image matrix

Specially constructed **gradient field coils** are placed within the main magnet and superimpose a linear magnetic field gradient on the main magnetic field. This gradient field is very small, typically 5mT to 15mT over the main field of 1T. The main magnetic field must be perfectly uniform otherwise the small variations imposed by the gradient fields will be lost. The gradient magnetic field gives a central null point (Fig.20.4(a)) with a reduced (negative) and increased (positive) magnetic gradient either side of its null point.

Gradient coils serve the three axes making up the patient volume shown in Fig.20.4(b).

- A **frequency encoded** *Z*-axis
- A **phase encoded** *Y*-axis horizontally opposed to the *Z*-axis.
- A **frequency encoded** *X*-axis vertically opposed to the *Z*-axis.

These gradients are termed $\mathbf{G_z}$ $\mathbf{G_y}$ $\mathbf{G_x}$ respectively and enable spatial information to be obtained from the patient. Image data signals

from these axes are produced by switching the gradient field strengths in a controlled sequence.

The gradient coils shown in Fig.20.5(a) are positioned within the main magnet bore and cover the three axes. They are not active all the time (unlike the main magnetic field) but are switched on when required for signal collection. Very large gradient field switching gives the 'machine-gun' staccato sound when an MRI machine is working. When a G_z G_x or G_y gradient is energized the respective linear gradient field is superimposed on the main field.

Gradient field strength must be large enough to overcome magnet inhomogeneities; as the main magnet field strength increases so do the gradient field strengths. Figure 20.5(b) plots this relationship. Gradient strengths are measured in mT per meter (mT m^{-1}); some superconducting magnets have higher gradients in order to achieve thinner sections and better resolution.

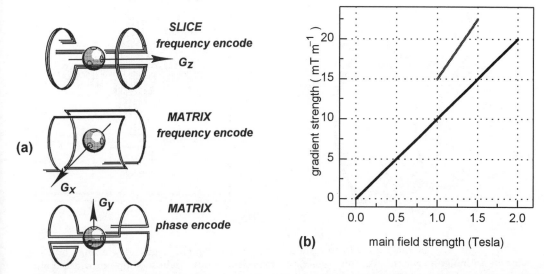

Figure 20.5 **(a)** Gradient coil design. Z axis slice position is frequency encoded x and y gradients encode image pixel position for frequency and phase respectively. **(b)** The main field strength versus gradient strength. The slope can be steeper since large magnets (>1T) can have gradient strengths approaching 25mT m^{-1} (upper gray line).

Complete MRI Inductors (*coils and windings*) The number of windings used in a complete MRI machine are shown in Fig.20.6(a). These are:

- The main **electro-magnet** (resistive or super-conducting coil) which is the largest winding, generating magnetic fields up to 4 Tesla in some large machines but more commonly 0.5 - 1.5T.
- Directly outside the main winding is a smaller winding which acts as the **active shield** in superconducting magnets, constraining the fringe field to within a narrow contour.
- Inside the main winding are various **shim coils** which, together with carefully placed iron sheets, finely adjust the uniformity of the main magnetic field.
- The **gradient coils** then form the complete coil assembly which is fixed within the gantry. The gradient coils are very thick windings since they must carry a current of up to 100 amps.

- The moveable **signal coils** act as transmitter and receiver antenna; these are the body and surface coils respectively.

The receiver coils are placed near the anatomical region of interest in order to improve signal strength.

20.2.2 Eddy currents

These have been described in Chapter 2 as currents induced in a conductor by the varying magnetic field. There is always an electrical field associated with a changing magnetic field; this induces a current to circulate in the volume of adjacent conductive material (patient tissue). These eddy currents interact against the main magnetic field causing interference and inhomogeneities. They are further undesirable because of their energy dissipation. Eddy currents are experienced

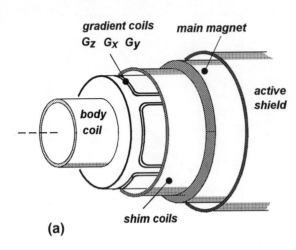

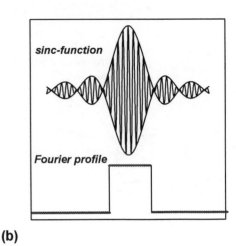

(a)   **(b)**

Figure 20.6   **(a)**   Block diagram MRI System showing the complete family of windings and coils necessary for an imaging system. **(b)** Sinc (*sin x*)/*x* transmission pulse whose shape provides a sharp rectangular frequency distribution for precise slice dimensions (lower trace).

in high field superconducting magnets occurring in only a small way in smaller strength resistive and permanent magnets. They are caused by the switched gradient fields and disturb magnet field homogeneity and require compensation. Eddy currents are a particular problem in fast imaging techniques which use rapid gradient switching. They are also induced by the RF field generating an opposing field which weakens the applied RF; this skin effect causes inhomogeneities in the excitation field.   At high frequencies (above 40MHz) RF field tissue penetration also becomes a problem.

In summary:

- Gradient windings in 3 planes, G_z (slice position and thickness) G_x and G_y (image matrix).
- Gradient has a central null point and imposes a negative and positive magnetic field on the main field either side of the null.

- G_z and G_x encode for frequency. G_y encodes for phase.
- Gradient field strengths are from 10-25mT m^{-1}
- Gradient windings can carry up to 100A.

20.2.3 The radio frequency (RF) pulse

In order to excite a sharp rectangular slice a special pulse shape is used; this is the **sinc-pulse** shown in Fig.20.6(b) and uses the mathematical function (sin *x*)/*x*. The transmitter section of the MRI machine is a computer controlled RF generator whose high frequency can be tuned very accurately for frequency and bandwidth.   The precisely shaped sinc-pulse is amplified to give 90° or 180° power levels or intermediate levels when smaller 'flip-angles' are being used.

The receiver section of the MRI system accepts the high frequency NMR signals which are converted (demodulated) to give low frequency signals before digitization; only frequency and phase differences are important and not the absolute frequency value. Typical specifications for a 1.5T MRI transmitter system is shown in Tab 20.4. The extremely stable frequency is necessary for accurate spatial information.

The **body coil** identified in Fig.20.6(a) is used as the transmission antenna delivering precise frequencies which determine the slice position within the coil (determined by G_z). The NMR signal is picked up by either the same body coil or more commonly by specialized receiver coils designed to cover the anatomy of interest (spine, breast, knee etc.). These surface coils significantly improve signal to noise ratio and hence image quality.

Table 20.4 Specification for RF pulse transmitter

Nominal frequency	63.6MHz
Tunable range	63.4 - 63.8MHz
Bandwidth	400kHz
Stability	4×10^{-9}Hz
Transmit power	10kW

20.2.4   Detector coil design

The detector coil picks up the very small NMR signals from the tissue volume under investigation. For maximum efficiency Q they are tuned to resonate with the selected NMR frequency. The resonant signal is then converted to a lower frequency signal. Most detectors have phase measurement and this information is obtained by using a quadrature demodulator to extract the phase information. A selection of receiver coils is shown in Fig.20.7.

Surface coils   Surface coils are small coils placed immediately adjacent to the body region of interest (spine, neck, knee etc.). They allow the RF signals to be received with excellent signal to noise ratio (SNR) but cover smaller areas than obtained with the standard head or body coils. Most surface coils are used strictly as receivers with the standard body coil as the transmitter. Surface

coils do not surround the body but are placed close to the organ of interest. They have a selectivity for a tissue volume approximately subtended by the coil circumference and one radius deep from the coil center.

A simple arrangement is shown in Fig. 20.8(a). In its simplest arrangement it is a simple ring tuned to resonate at the particular NMR frequency. The sensitivity along the coil axis decreases rapidly with increasing distance from the coil plane. Effective penetration depth is roughly equal to the coil radius. Surface coils are used primarily as detectors; the pulse transmission can be obtained by using the body coil.

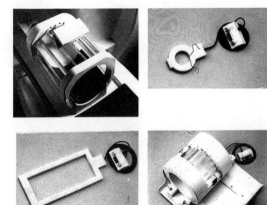

Figure 20.7 Various signal coils available for different organs (Courtesy GE Medical Systems Inc)

Quadrature detectors   By joining a pair of coils at 90° to one another and driving them during the transmit cycle through a power divider and phase shifter a rotating field can be produced that only requires half the RF power (Fig.20.8(b)). In a similar fashion the same principle gives a quadrature detector which is phase sensitive. It is sensitive to the components of the signal which is phase shifted by 90°. Since two separate signals are being obtained from the same tissue volume the SNR is improved by $\sqrt{2}$ or $\simeq 1.4$. Patient motion reduces this value however.

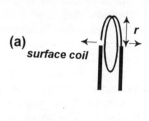

(a) *surface coil*

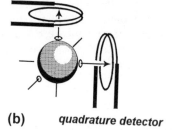

(b)   *quadrature detector*

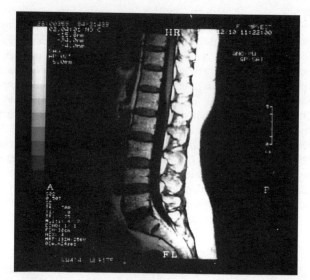

Figure 20.8   Signal coil design showing **(a)** the smaller flat, loop and **(b)** the basic quadrature coil design **(c)** Image examples using surface coils showing much better definition in the locality of the coil. (Courtesy GE Medical Systems Inc)

Surface coils generally improve images of superficial structures.   Figure 20.8(c) gives examples of clinical images taken with anatomically specific coils. Signal reception is increased by proximity of the organ to the receiver antenna and noise and reflections are decreased because signals outside the region of interest are very weak.   Reducing the field of view also improves resolution since there is smaller voxel volume. Signal to noise ratio (SNR) is much improved. Non-uniformity is caused by difference in signal strengths from organs near the coil to ones that are more distant. The surface coil should be chosen for the region of interest; this optimizes the image signal to noise ratio.

Phased array coils These are multiple surface coils, each coil served by a separate detector/receiver.   A typical design consists of six coils that can be combined to give surface or 3D configurations. A large field of view is obtained at high SNR since each coil is an independent detector. Interference between coils is prevented by low impedance receiver matching. They cover a wider anatomical area

reducing imaging time for larger fields of view. Surface coils are available that use a 'ladder' configuration where individual coils are switched through to a common receiver. These are not true phased array coils.

In summary:

- Body coil solenoid coils act as transmitting antennae for the RF pulses
- Specialized surface coils matched to the anatomy act as receiver antennae
- Signal to noise ratio is improved by surface coils
- Phased array coils cover larger areas

20.2.5 Spatial encoding

The three orthogonal axes, which are used for spatially encoding, are shown as a small sketch in Fig.20.4(b).   The three gradient fields G_z, G_x and G_y are switched in a defined sequence firstly to encode slice position and thickness G_z then to encode the x and y positions in the image matrix.   The size of the image matrix has increased with improved accuracy of location from 128 to 256 to 512. The eventual image matrix can be interpolated to a larger size (1024^2) if necessary.

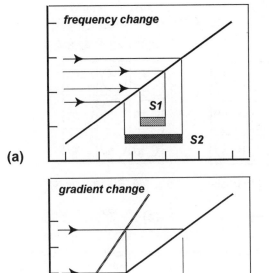

(a)

(b)

Figure 20.9 Slice thickness can be selected by increasing frequency bandwidth or altering the slope of the gradient field

The slice axis G_z (frequency encoded) The protons exposed to the G_z gradient will show differing Larmor frequencies depending on their position along it. The precise frequency of the RF pulse (transmitted via the body coil) will select a specific slice position (see eqn.20.1) described by $\omega = \gamma (B_o + G_z)$. Slice thickness can be altered by:

- Increasing the range of frequencies in the RF pulse; the wider the frequency range the thicker the slice.
- Keeping the bandwidth constant and altering the gradient slope to modify the slice thickness.

These are graphically described in Fig.20.9 and Box 20.2 calculates the frequency difference necessary for defining a 5mm slice. The change is very small and so the magnetic field must be uniform in order to localize the slice position precisely. The transmission pulse should have a narrow frequency range for accurate slice location and thickness and for good SNR. A wide frequency range will excite regions outside the slice of interest causing **cross-talk**. For this reason gaps between slices are maintained, usually between 30-50% of the slice width.

Slice thickness is determined by the gradient strength and the bandwidth of the radio-frequency pulse. The strength of the gradient must be large enough to overcome slight inhomogeneities that are present in the main magnetic field.

Box 20.2

Slice position and thickness

Larmor frequency for a 1T magnet is 42.58MHz T^{-1}. From the slope in Fig.20.5(b) the relative gradient strengths are:

- 0.5T magnet with 5mT m^{-1} (0.05mT cm^{-1})
- 1.0T magnet with 10mT m^{-1} (0.1mT cm^{-1})

What is the frequency range for a 5mm slice thickness using these two magnets?

0.5T magnet (Larmor frequency 21.29MHz)
(0.05/2 mT cm^{-1} for 5mm)
$$21.29 \times 1.000025 = 21.290532MHz$$
$$\Delta f = 532Hz$$
So the central frequency for slice location is chosen with ~ ±250Hz to give the necessary 5mm slice.

1.0T magnet
(0.1/2 mT cm^{-1} for 5mm)
$$42.58 \times 1.00005 = 42.582129MHz$$
$$\Delta f = 2.13kHz$$
So the central frequency for slice location is chosen with ~ ± 1kHz to give a 5mm slice.

Image matrix (G_x G_y phase/frequency encoded) Figure 20.10(a), (b), (c) shows how a combination of G_z G_y and G_x gradients can encode an image matrix. The slice position has already been identified in this example by selecting a hypothetical slice frequency G_z of

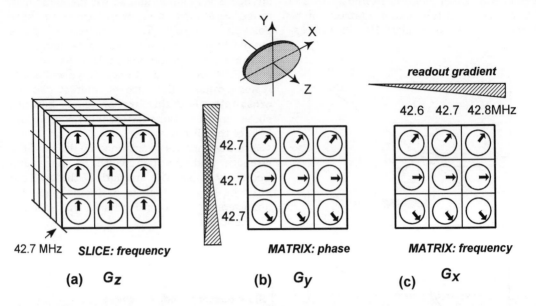

Figure 20.10 Selecting *Z*, *X* and *Y* planes by frequency ω and phase encoding φ. For this example a 42.7MHz frequency selects the slice position in (**a**). The *Y*-gradient (**b**) is switched during acquisition depending on matrix size (3 steps for this simplified example) . (**c**) Larmor frequencies of 42.6-42.8MHz determine the *X*-plane .

42.7MHz The G_y gradient is switched on for a short time which causes another frequency change in the proton signal (after G_z) depending on their position along the vertical *Y*-axis. When G_y is switched off the protons resume their original frequency but they have now lost their phase uniformity; they are now phase shifted according to their position on the *Y*-axis since the momentary change in frequency caused by G_y caused them to be dephased. The phase differences are retained when G_y is switched off and are proportional to the strength of G_y; larger phase differences occur at either end of this gradient. Unlike the other gradients (G_z and G_x), the G_y field is switched in a series of steps in order to decode the full matrix. Step numbers are typically 128, 256 or 512. A 256 matrix having 256 phase encoding steps would mean that each step will cause a phase shift of 360°/256 or 1.4° with respect to its column neighbour. Stepped gradients are represented as a 'ladder' symbol in MRI pulse sequence diagrams.

In the same way that the G_z gradient encodes according to position on the *Z*-axis, the G_x gradient encodes proton frequencies depending on their *X*-axis position, fixing their matrix row position by frequency encoding. The G_x gradient remains switched on while NMR signal frequency measurements are recorded. The frequency changes necessary to separate each pixel are calculated in Box 20.3 and considerable uniformity in the main magnetic field is necessary to achieve good image definition in large matrix sizes. Changes in the phase and frequency of NMR signals are measured by reference to a standard signal. This is usually the pure signal for hydrogen protons at the main magnet field strength (21.29MHz for 0.5T; 42.58MHz for 1T and 63.87 for 1.5T). The calculations are carried out by a Fast Fourier Transform (FFT) in a demodulator circuit.

Gradient sequence The switching sequence of the gradient magnetic fields is controlled and timed by the main system computer. The exact gradient sequence is different from the z, x and y sequence described above. For basic imaging routines a typical sequence could be:

- G_z identifies the slice position. (Fig.20.10(a))
- G_y is now switched on for a short period, causing the protons in the vertical axis to alter frequency momentarily according to their position along the y-gradient.
- The protons resume their pre- G_y Larmor frequency when G_y is switched off but retain a phase difference, depending on their position in the matrix columns. (Fig.20.10(b))
- G_x is switched on causing a frequency difference in the rows, the NMR signal is now measured and the phase/frequency information stored. G_x is therefore the readout gradient. (Fig.20.10(c))

A simplified encoded matrix is shown in Fig.20.11. Each voxel presents a different frequency and phase as encoded by G_x and G_y. This matrix is not the displayed matrix since it carries only frequency and phase information in k-space.

N_x and N_y are often used to signify the number of phase and frequency coded steps; these decide the final dimension of the matrix (256^2, 512^2 etc.).

The two dimensional Fourier Transform (2D.FT) is able to separate the signal into its respective frequency and phase components and using these two components it is possible to identify the two spatial dimensions in the image matrix and so separate the individual voxels in the slice.

After separating the NMR signal according to its frequency and phase characteristics it again undergoes a Fourier Transform which yields signal strength information (amplitude) which is stored as a gray scale value in a pixel display matrix.

Voxel size The matrix dimension m, assuming equal number of phase and frequency en-

coding steps N_x and N_y, and the field of view *FOV* with the slice thickness determine the individual voxel size. For a 50cm *FOV*, which is the typical value, occupying a 512^2 matrix and a 2mm slice thickness, the voxel size would be (*FOV/m*) or approximately 1mm^2 by 2mm deep.

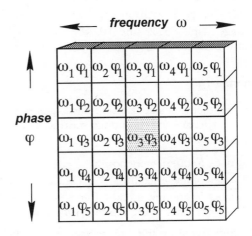

Figure 20.11 The fully encoded matrix where each voxel separates the NMR signal according to phase φ and frequency ω, this matrix is in k-space. A Fast Fourier Transform (FFT) forms the display pixel-matrix.

Box 20.3

Pixel Bandwidth

Pixel selection for 0.5 and 1.0T magnet 15cm field of view (FOV) head coil.

0.5T: (0.1mT cm^{-1})
0.1mT cm^{-1} ×15 = 1.5mT variation over 15cm
　　　21.29 × 1.0015 = 21.3321935
Δf = 32kHz = **120Hz** pixel^{-1} for a 256^2 matrix

1.0T (0.15mT cm^{-1})
0.15mT cm × 15 = 2.25mT variation over 15cm
　　　42.58 × 1.00225 = 42.6758
Δf = 95kHz = **374Hz** pixel^{-1} for a 256^2 matrix
　　　　　 = **190Hz** pixel^{-1} for a 512^2 matrix

The computer system This must be fast

enough for rapid (2 to 4 seconds) image re-construction.   A typical specification would be:

- Central computer using 32 bit or more, architecture
- Data and display memory ~150MBytes
- Reconstruction time for 252^2 approxi-mately 1 sec.
- Disc storage 1.3GByte (magnetic)
- Disc storage 5 - 6GByte (optical)
- Image display 512^2 and 1024^2 (interpolated)

In summary:

Three gradient select z-axis (slice position) and x and y-axes for the image matrix. These are G_z, G_x and G_y.

- G_z uses frequency encoding
- G_y uses phase encoding
- G_x uses frequency encoding and identifies the signal. This is the readout gradient.

Pulse and signal timing can be varied. Gradi-ent fields impose a negative and positive field change with a middle null point where the overall magnetic field is unaltered. Gradient coils switch up to 100amps

20.3 IMAGING PULSE SEQUENCES

The gradient field switching is synchronized with 90° and 180° RF pulses transmitted by the body coil.   These switching and pulse se-quences yield an NMR signal along with its spatial information.

20.3.1 Spin Echo Sequence and 2D.FT

Unlike CT where image reconstruction de-pends on successively rotated projections (polar co-ordinates) MR image reconstruction utilizes Cartesian co-ordinates (x, y and z)

which allows direct reconstruction by means of a 2-dimensional fast Fourier Transform (2D.FFT).

The basic spin echo pulse sequence de-scribed in Chapter 19 is shown again in Fig.20.12(a). This imaging sequence consists of a series of 90° and 180° pulses; the time between the 90° pulses is the time to repeat (TR) time.   After the 90° pulse the proton transverse signal (T2*) will decay at a rate de-cided by tissue characteristics. The 180° pulse rephases the NMR signals so correcting for external magnet inhomogeneities. The NMR signal appears at TE (time-to-echo). The 180° pulse is positioned at half TE: TE/2 time.

Figure 20.12(b) shows the gradient switch-ing G_z, G_x and G_y pulse sequences necessary for image signal collection using a 90°-180° spin echo sequence:

- G_z is applied only when 90° or 180° RF pulses are transmitted. Gradient strength remains constant during data acquisition but changes to select other slices and slice thicknesses.
- G_y is applied after the RF pulses but be-fore the NMR echo is received. It is a stepped gradient, the number of steps depending on matrix size.
- G_x is applied only when receiving signals. This is a constant strength gradient

Since G_y is a varying magnetic field, this is depicted as a stepped pulse in the diagrams. The time of TR and TE in Fig.20.12(a) are termed short and long.   TR is chosen to match the time constant T1 of the tissue of interest. A TR less than 500ms is termed 'short' and >1500ms is termed 'long'. A TE of <30ms is short and >80ms is long. Table 20.5 lists some T1 and T2 times for various tissue types using field strengths of 0.5, 1.0 and 1.5T.

After the protons have been rephased by a 180° inversion pulse an x-gradient G_x is su-perimposed on the main field and the signal echo is collected.   The complete 2D.FT se-quence from Fig.20.12(b) is:

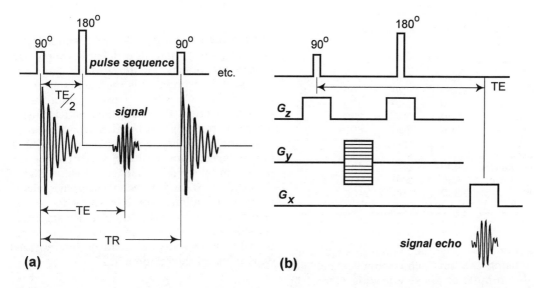

Figure 20.12   (a) The basic spin-echo pulse sequence identifying TR and TE together with τ which is TE/2 (b) The spin echo sequence with gradient switching G_z G_y G_x and echo signal timing which yields the 2D image.

- A 90° RF pulse at a predetermined frequency is transmitted while G_z is switched on.
- The center frequency of this pulse selects the position on the z-axis, its bandwidth determines slice thickness for a given gradient strength.
- G_y is now switched on changing the proton Larmor frequency. When the y-gradient is switched off the protons revert to their original Larmor frequency but they are dephased so giving a phase difference.   A single phase gradient is not sufficient to encode the entire y-axis so it is applied in carefully scaled steps.
- A rephasing 180° signal after time TE/2 re-establishes phase relationships and the photons again have phase coherence.
- Just before TE time the G_x is switched on which distributes the Larmor frequencies depending on proton position along the x-gradient

- Echo signals are received and digitized (fast ADC) and stored in a voxel matrix according to their position determined by their phase and frequency in a k- space (frequency and phase matrix).

This total process is repeated a number of times with further 90°-180° pulse sequences. The following points should be noted about the data stored as phase/frequency information:

- The central voxel represents zero-frequency and zero-phase shift differences.
- The k-space matrix is converted to the conventional display matrix 256^2 or 512^2 which carries gray scale information depending on signal strength.
- A Fourier Transform converts the k-space into and x and y pixel matrix each pixel carrying a gray scale value (8 bits: 256 gray scales).

Table 20.5   T1 in milli-seconds for 3 magnet sizes 0.5, 1.0 and 1.5 Tesla. T2 time does not change.

Tissue type	T1(0.5)	T1(1.0)	T1(1.5)	T2
Body				
Fat	210	240	260	80
Liver	350	420	500	40
Muscle	550	730	870	45
Kidney	440	590	700	58
Heart	560	750	890	57
Brain				
White matter	500	680	780	90
Gray matter	650	810	900	100
CSF	1800	2160	2400	160

Imaging time   The time taken to acquire images using the spin-echo sequence depends on the number of phase encoding steps, signal averaging, and time to repeat. Acquisition time is therefore:

$$M \times N \times TR \qquad (20.3)$$

Where M is the number of phase encode steps which matches the matrix size, N the number of averaging (excitation) times (usually 2 but can be greater), TR the time to repeat. For 256^2 matrix M equals 256 so for a signal averaging of 2 and a TR time of 500ms acquisition time is: $256 \times 2 \times 0.5 = 4.2$ minutes. For longer TR values this can increase to over 12 minutes.

Inversion recovery   This has been described in Chapter 19. The spin echo 90-180° pulse sequence is preceded by a 180° pulse. The proportion of M_Z can only be measured by using the conventional spin echo sequence. The timing of the 180° pulse and tissue type influences the magnitude of M_Z recovery. The negative value of M_Z must pass through zero, continuing until equilibrium M_O is reached. Owing to this increase in recovery time a longer TR period is necessary so the inversion recovery spin echo sequence (IRSE) is a slow imaging process. A modified version is described later called STIR; 'Short T1 Inversion Recovery'.

20.3.2 Multi-image techniques

Multi-slice imaging   During a simple spin-echo sequence there is a delay between successive 90° pulses (TR time) which can be as long as 1.5 seconds. This represents an inefficient duty-cycle which can be improved if data from other slices are collected by using different transmission frequencies; more than one slice can then be decoded from the Z, X and Y image data. Multiple slices can be obtained in a single pulse sequence. Figure 20.13(a) shows a spin-echo multi-slice signal train which allows multiple slices to be collected and the duty cycle efficiency improves considerably. During each TR period other 90-180° pulse sequences can be interspersed depending on the relationship:

$$\frac{TR}{TE \times m} \qquad (20.4)$$

Where m is a constant depending on machine type. For $m = 2$; $TR = 1500$ms and $TE = 30$ms. A theoretical 25 slices can be obtained using a multi-slice sequence.

Crosstalk   It is not possible to obtain ideal rectangular slice profiles since the RF sinc-pulse is foreshortened and not perfect. In MRI the overlap of the slice profiles influences the signals in the adjacent slices. This is slice crosstalk and modifies T1 contrast; it can be minimized by increasing the slice gap.

Multi-echo sequence   A single slice will contain fixed T1 and T2 contributions. Differentiating the T1 and T2 contribution can be achieved by using a 180° pulse train (Fig.20.13(b)). The successive 180° echoes have approximately the same T1 content but will reflect different T2 weighting in the image. Multi-echo techniques can be run with multi-slice routines and will only marginally decrease multiple-slice number.

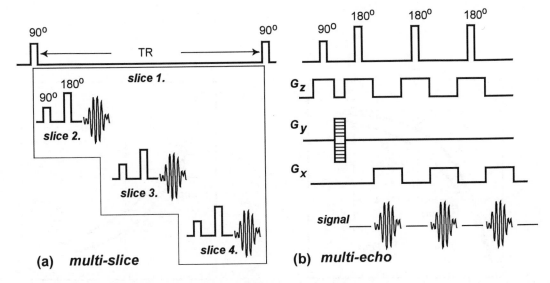

Figure 20.13 (a) Spin echo multi-slice sequence showing 4 separate slices collected during a single TR time (b) Multi-echo sequence giving different T2 weighted images.

In summary:

Select slice with a G_z field super-imposed on main field. Slice thickness can be altered by either:

- Changing the frequency of excitation
- Altering the gradient field slope

The selected slice image matrix uses two other gradient fields:

- X-gradient frequency encoding G_x
- Y- gradient phase encoding G_y

The frequency encoding gradients give different Larmor frequencies. The phase encoding gradient is applied for a specific time by G_y. The gradient is switched off and the protons resume at the original frequency but now have different phase relationships. The fast Fourier transform gives the signal intensities for frequency and phase.

20.3.3 Image contrast

Magnetic resonance signals are influenced by three major parameters:

- The nuclear density (number of protons per unit volume)
- The vertical relaxation time T1
- The transverse relaxation time T2

These 3 qualities are dependent on the tissue type and with a spin-echo sequence the NMR signal S is proportional to:

$$S \propto \rho \times (1 - e^{-\frac{TR}{T1}}) \times e^{-\frac{TE}{T2}} \qquad (20.5)$$

Where TR and TE are the repetition and echo time respectively and ρ is the spin density. The formula indicates that TR and TE settings significantly influence image contrast, controlling the part played by T1 and T2 times and producing **T1 or T2 weighted images**. Optimum image contrast depends on TR and TE timing in order to match the tissue of in-

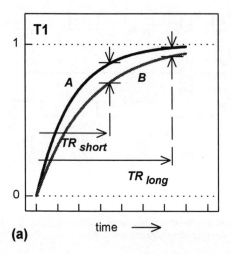

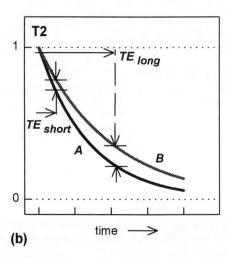

Figure 20.14   (a) Two curves describing longitudinal relaxation with different time constants T1. Tissue A has a **shorter** T1 than tissue B. Their differences are greatest for short TR; the image will be T1 weighted. (b) Two curves describing transverse relaxation with different T2 times; a **longer** TE differentiates between Tissue A and Tissue B; the image will be T2 weighted.

terest and/or pathology. Image contrast is determined by the variation of these parameters to yield T1 or T2 weighted images or a simple proton density image; the relevant time durations are summarized in Tab.20.6. A long TR would be >1500ms whilst a long TE would be >40ms.

Repetition time TR   This is the time interval between consecutive pulse sequences. In the case of the spin-echo sequence it is the time between the 90° pulses as shown in Fig.20.12(a).   T1 contrast is largely influenced by TR. Two T1 curves (A and B) are shown in Fig.20.14(a). A **short** TR time will yield a larger difference between these curves and an image will be T1 weighted for a short TR time although signal intensity will be smaller due to saturation. The minimal TR time depends on the chosen pulse sequence.

Table 20.6 Different combinations of TR and TE

	Short TR	*Long TR*
Short TE	T1 weighted TR 500ms TE 20ms	Proton density TR 2000ms TE 20ms
Long TE	Not valid	T2 weighted TR 2000ms TE 80ms

Echo time TE   This is the time between the center of the excitation pulse and the center of the spin echo or gradient echo. This has also been identified in the spin-echo sequence of Fig.20.12(a).   The T2 contrast is influenced by the length of TE. Two tissue

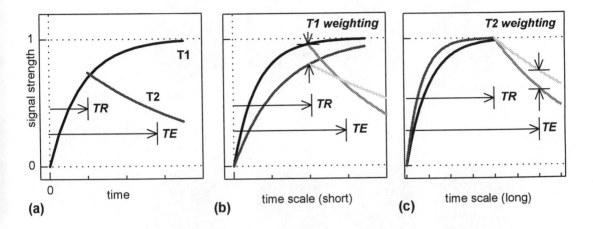

Figure 20.15 **(a)** Combining T1 and T2 curves for a single tissue type, showing TR and TE timing **(b)** Combining two tissue types a short TR time and a short TE time gives a T1 weighted signal **(c)** A long TR time minimizes the T1 differences but a long TE time emphasizes the T2 differences giving a T2 weighted image (the time scale on the *x*-axis is longer).

types (soft tissue and liquid) are shown in Fig.20.14(b). They have different decay times. Differences will be maximum at **longer TE** times. TE times can be chosen by the operator but there is a trade off since T2 signals are rapidly decaying so losing signal strength; there is a practical limit for optimum signal: noise ratio (SNR); a long T2 of 80ms will increase T2 weighting but will also increase image noise. T2 signals are always shorter than the corresponding T1 signals for any given substance. T2 is a measure of how long the substance holds the transverse magnetization and is influenced by the interaction of molecular fields reflecting changes in tissue chemistry. In a liquid the local magnetic fields respond rapidly, their spin-spin interferences are less and dephasing is relatively slow; their T2 times are consequently longer.

Solids have a fixed molecular structure and neighboring protons strongly influence FID phase relationships. After RF excitation protons in solids show spin-spin interference, their FID's rapidly losing phase and producing a shorter T2. Since solids and tissues with low water content have protons that are influenced by their neighbor's small magnetic fields they induce small inhomogeneities in the overall magnetic field so the individual FIDs vary slightly, behaving similarly to out-of-phase signals and giving the same result: shorter T2 times.

T1 and T2 weighted images An idea of signal intensity by altering TR and TE values can be obtained by superimposing the T1 and T2 curves shown in Fig.20.15(a). The TR value determines T1 signal strength as previously seen in Fig.20.14(a) and the superimposed T2 curve seen in Fig.20.15(b) gives the magnitude of the FID signal at this TR time. The TR timing determines the end point of the T1 curve which consequently fixes the start of the T2 signal. The TE period governs the magnitude of the T2 signal (Fig.20.15(c)). Tissue difference (contrast) can therefore be emphasized by using different TR and TE timing. The simulated MR brain images in Fig.20.16(a) and (b) (exaggerated anatomy)

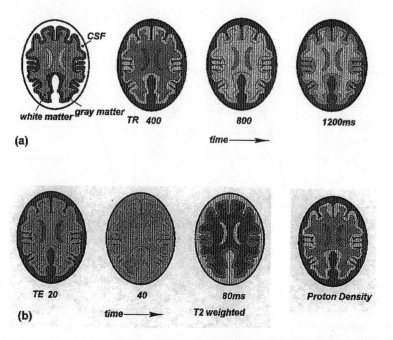

Figure 20.16   Simulated MRI head images (with an exaggerated CSF gap) demonstrating the effect of **(a)** Increasing the TR period which increases T1 information in the image. The gray/white matter contrast alters but CSF remains dark (small signal intensity) **(b)** Short TE where the CSF has a small signal (dark image); for intermediate TE periods overall contrast is poor but at longer TE there is a large signal for the CSF which is now seen as a bright area on the image **(c)** Precise TR/TE timing to give proton density.

show varying TR and TE times altering signal strengths for either T1 or T2 characteristics. Figure 20.16(c) illustrates proton density.

T1 and T2 weighted MR images are shown in Fig.20.17(a) and (b). The T1 weighted image shows dark CSF and the gray matter darker than the white matter. A proton density image would be very similar except contrast between gray and white matter would be reversed since there are more protons (water) in the gray matter, the CSF becomes lighter. Proton density images are not very sensitive to tissue pathology. Figure 20.17(b) is a T2 weighted image where the CSF has a higher signal than the gray or white matter as is ideal for visualizing CSF or edema.

Contrast agents   T1 time can be deliberately altered by using specific paramagnetic contrast agents (gadolinium or manganese compounds). Paramagnetic substances have unpaired electrons causing their magnetic moments to increase by about ×1000; T1 and T2 relaxation times will shorten. Figure 20.14(a) curve 'A' would represent the effect of a contrast agent on T1 timing and T2 timing respectively.

The decrease in T1 and T2 is directly proportional to the concentration of the contrast agent. The effect of contrast agent on T1 times is small for short T1 tissues; their effect on T2 is smaller than T1. At small or intermediate concentrations T1 predominates and

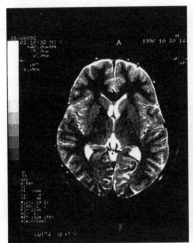 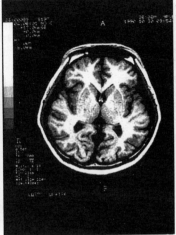 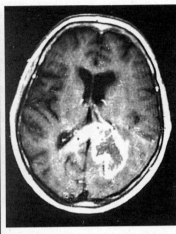

Figure 20.17 **(a)** T1 weighted head image (Courtesy GE Medical Systems Inc) **(b)** T2 weighted head image (Courtesy GE Medical Systems Inc) **(c)** A positive contrast agent (Gd-DTPA) emphasizes this cerebral neoplasm by increasing the T1 effect. (Courtesy Siemens Inc)

faster recovery gives an increased signal strength in T1 weighted images (Fig.20.17(c)). At high concentrations of contrast agent T2 shortening predominates.

Functional MRI (fMRI) This was first attempted by using bolus contrast agents (Gd-DTPA) to study transit through the brain in real time using EPI and mapping blood volume during brain activity (visual cortex) at rest and activity (visual stimulus). This technique bears similarities to PET studies requiring elimination of the agent between acquisitions. PET however operates using agent concentrations many orders of magnitude less than that achievable with *f*MRI.

Current interest concerns the blood oxygen levels. Oxygen is a diamagnetic material (negative susceptibility) so fully oxygenated-blood, oxyhemoglobin, is diamagnetic. Deoxy- or reduced hemoglobin is however paramag-netic due to its unpaired electrons and can be used as an in-vivo positive contrast agent:

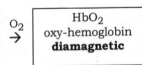

| Hb⁻ deoxy-hemoglobin **paramagnetic** | $\xrightarrow{O_2}$ | HbO₂ oxy-hemoglobin **diamagnetic** |

Its concentration is influenced by variations in oxygenation and tissue metabolism so the acronym BOLD has been given to this technique (Blood Oxygen Level Dependent). As with other paramagnetic substances deoxy-hemoglobin causes a local increase in magnetic susceptibility and consequent T1, T2 shortening. Blood oxygenation reverses this action. Since tissue oxygenation levels depend on changes in perfusion *f*MRI can only show relatively slow events which is an unfortunate limitation.

*f*MRI is restricted to high field strengths. The changes being measured are tiny so it is important to maximize the signal at low noise levels; magnetic susceptibility effects increase with field strength. Most artifacts are due to patient motion since very precise image subtraction is required to reveal the small differences. Shifting the head by a fraction will give false signals.

Both spatial and temporal resolution are critical. Using conventional GRE sequences about 1mm spatial resolution can be obtained but temporal resolution is poor so the study is limited to only a few slices. Faster pulse sequences such as EPI achieve poorer spatial resolution but many more slices can be obtained.

In summary:

- T1 weighted images show fluid (water, CSF, blood) darker than the surrounding tissues.

- T2 weighted images show CSF and liquids as white compared to the surrounding tissues.

20.4 FAST IMAGING TECHNIQUES

Producing a good quality MR image with diagnostic quality resolution and contrast, using conventional T2 weighted spin-echo sequences with long TR (Tab.20.6) takes many minutes. This precludes abdominal imaging which carry respiratory and cardiac movements, particularly those involving 512^2 image matrices. Clinical applications have stimulated the need for fast data acquisition, reducing patient movement in thorax and abdomen images. Time/slice must also be reduced for 3-Dimensional imaging (3D.FFT).

These original imaging pulse sequences suffered from one important drawback: imaging time which is typically between 10 to 20 minutes for a T2 spin echo sequence (SE T2 Tab.20.7). Spin echo contrast is the 'benchmark' by which other image sequence techniques are judged, giving reference quality for T1, proton density and T2 weighted images. T2 weighted images use a long TR and long TE (Tab.20.6) and to give acceptable

contrast TR cannot be made much shorter than 300-400ms giving an image time of 0.4×512×4 or nearly 14minutes. Conventional SE sequences cannot be used for fast imaging.

Fast imaging techniques all have a common disadvantage: reduced signal to noise ratio (SNR) since in approximate terms:

$$SNR \propto \sqrt{Imaging\ Time} \qquad (20.6)$$

Contrast to noise ratio (CNR) is reduced; low contrast detail is therefore poor (see 20.5.2).

Table 20.7 Imaging times for some common fast imaging procedures

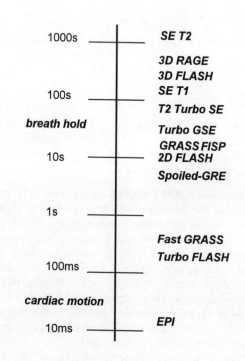

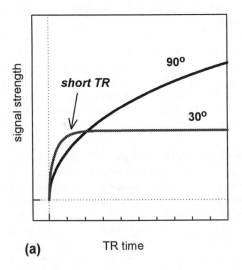
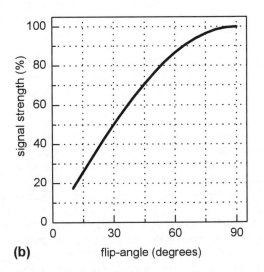

(a) signal strength — 90° — short TR — 30° — TR time

(b) signal strength (%) — flip-angle (degrees)

Figure 20.18 **(a)** Signal strength for short TR is greater for a 30° flip angle than for the conventional 90° saturation pulse. **(b)** Flip angle and signal strength.

20.4.1 Spin echo sequences

Faster spin echo sequences can be obtained by simply using additional 180° pulses following the 90°-180° SE sequence previously shown in Fig.20.13(b); each additional 180° provides an image. An alternative more complex procedure phase encodes these echoes individually; this is RARE (Rapid Acquisition Relaxation Enhancement) and has been marketed as the so called 'Turbo Spin-Echo'.

Scan data can be shortened by acquiring only part of the data and obtaining the remainder by interpolation since data sets are symmetrical. This is the half-Fourier method. Scan time is reduced by nearly half but there is also a concomitant reduction in SNR by 40%.

20.4.2 Gradient echo sequences.

A gradient echo has been described in Chapter 19 where by applying a pair of balanced gradients of opposite sign a gradient or field echo can be obtained. It uses a single RF pulse usually with a flip angle of less than 90°. A major advantage of GRE is the good image quality with very short TR.

Shortening TR below about 0.3s produces problems of rephasing with the 180° pulse and other methods of rephasing must be used. The most common is gradient reversal; echo times are considerably shortened but the disadvantage is that magnetic field inhomogeneities are not compensated. The use of a 180° pulse in the spin-echo sequence corrects for inhomogeneities in the magnet field so a true T2 signal is measured. As the fast pulse sequences do not use a 180° pulse these inhomogeneities are not corrected so the FID loses phase faster; the signal is T2*.

Flip angles When applying a 90° pulse a comparatively long time period must elapse before repeating the pulse train. If a reduced flip angle is used with a GRE sequence then saturation effects are less and the TR can be shortened. Since much shorter flip angles are now used a thick volume of tissue can be interrogated to give a 3-D acquisition. The signal strength depends on TR/T1 timing and also the magnitude of the flip angle. Figure 20.18(a) shows the NMR signal strength for a 90° and a 30° flip-angle. At shorter TR times the shorter flip angle produces the highest signal strength. Figure 20.18(b) indicates the overall loss of signal strength when the flip-angle is reduced below 90°; however the 45° pulse takes half the time of the 90° but returns 70% of the signal strength. There is a practical limit to shortening as the graph illustrates when the returning signal is too weak.

A FLASH (Fast-Low-Angle-Shot) pulse sequence is shown in Fig.20.19(a) where gradient reversal in G_x replaces the 180° rephasing RF-pulse, yielding the signal. G_y behaves the same and spoiler pulses in G_z remove residual transverse magnetization. The faster image acquisition sequences use gradient switching and flip angles less than 90°; these are indicated as α in the diagram. This fast pulse sequence allows breath holding and so makes abdominal studies practical.

Echo Planar Imaging (EPI in Fig.20.19(b)) and Turbo-FLASH increase speed still further to fractions of a second per image but require very fast gradient switching. Image gating (respiration, ECG) improves image quality further at the expense of increased acquisition time.

Spoiled gradient pulses   There is also residual transverse magnetization with short TR intervals so a **spoiler pulse** is introduced into the gradient switching in order to disperse this (Fig.20.19(a)).

The standard 90° flip angle saturation RF pulse power is reduced to give smaller flip angles ($\alpha = 30°$) and the rephasing 180° is replaced with gradient switching since they would not have the previous rephasing effect. This technique removes residual signals which may persist from cycle to cycle in that

Table 20.8 A selection of commonly used fast pulse sequences

Generic	Commercial acronym	Acquisition (seconds)	Flip angle (degrees)	Use
T1 Spin Echo		200	90–180°	T1, proton density,
T2 Spin Echo		1000	90–180°	T2 weighted imaging
Fast spin echo	Turbo-SE RARE	100–300	90–180°	
Gradient echo	PSIF True-FISP T2-FFE	50–60	15–70°	enhanced intensity where T1≈T2 (e.g. CSF)
Spoiled-GRE	FLASH SPGR Spoiled-FAST T1-FFE	10–50	15–70°	T1 weighted contrast, CSF imaging, myelograms, angiography.
Fast-GRE	turbo-FLASH fast-GRASS (FSP-GR)	0.6	6–15°	dynamic perfusion studies of various organs. T1 weighted abdominal images without breath holding.
EPI	Single shot Multi-shot	0.06 8	90–180°	ultra-fast imaging dynamic motion studies
FAT saturation	FATSAT STIR		90–180°	fat suppression
MRS	STEAM ISIS CSI DRESS			spectroscopy

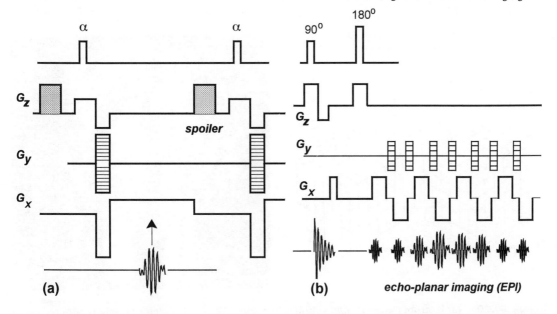

Figure 20.19 **(a)** Fast pulse sequence (FLASH) showing the spoiler pulse which reduces residual transverse magnetization; α is a flip-angle between 15-70°. **(b)** An echo planar (EPI) pulse sequence using 90°-180° flip angles but collecting multiple signal echoes. Very fast gradient switching is essential

before each RF pulse the transverse components of tissue signals have been neutralized ensuring maximum *z* component before excitation.

Spoiling is achieved by randomly changing the phase of the RF pulse which has advantages since it does not produce eddy currents. Reversing the polarity of the phase encoding steps called **rewinding gradients** are applied at the end of each pulse cycle shown in Fig.20.19(a). They ensure the phase stability of the MR signal. Some commonly available pulse sequences and their uses are listed in Tab.20.8.

20.4.3 Fat suppression

The mixed water/lipid spectrum has already been shown in Fig.19.7(b) demonstrating that separation is only 3 to 4ppm. The chemical shift artifact occurs due to the differing reso-

nance of protons depending on their chemical environment. Using the spin echo pulse sequence the 180° pulse causes fat and water to be in phase during each echo signal. Gradient echo pulse sequences which lack this 180° pulse cause fat and water to resonate in and out of phase. This oscillation occurs approximately every 6.6ms for a 1T magnet so this signal cancellation in pixels containing both water and fat is seen as a black border; an example would be the muscle sheath.

Since fat and water spectral peaks can be identified a very narrow bandwidth RF pulse can selectively saturate the fat peak so removing its influence from the image. Careful calibration is necessary in order to select the center frequency of the fat signal. Magnet field homogeneity must be high in order to ensure uniformity of the fat signal and its saturation. For less uniform homogeneity values an inversion recovery procedure is used for nulling the fat signal. Special pre-saturation pulse

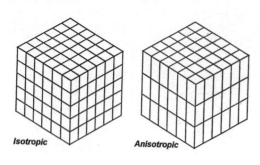

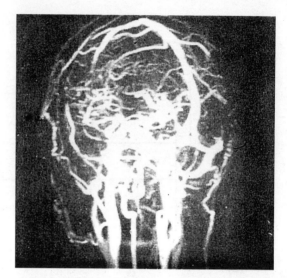

Figure 20.20   **(a)** Isotropic/Anisotropic volume data sets   **(b)**   3D image example produced from a volume data set. (Courtesy GE Medical Systems Inc)

sequences are used to reduce the MR signal from fat. The pulse sequence STIR is a short T1 inversion recovery and is a method for fat suppression using the inversion recovery time previously shown in Fig.19.14(b). Fat has a short TI value of about 250ms and its null point will occur when t = TI or approximately 175ms. An inversion recovery sequence with a TI of this value is the STIR sequence. It has an added property of emphasizing tissues with long T1 times so liquids (blood, CSF) appear as bright areas.

20.4.4 Multi-planar Imaging (3D.FFT)

The 3D data set uses a very broad Z gradient representing the tissue volume to be covered however it differs from the 2D.FFT because both G_y and G_z are now phase encoded. Image data is obtained using gradient echo techniques with TR values of about 50ms. The 3D volume can be acquired in isotropic or anisotropic mode (shown in Fig.20.20(a)). Isotropic volumes have all dimensions identical which gives optimum resolution in all axes

and 2D slices can be extracted without distortion. Anisotropic volumes have one dimension larger than the other. This cuts down the number of phase encode steps which reduces acquisition time significantly but resolution is degraded in this dimension.

It is possible to generate high-resolution 3 dimensional data sets with a voxel size of about 1mm.(Fig.20.20(b)).   From a volume data set any slice orientation can be reconstructed: axial, coronal, saggital or oblique slices.   The complete 3-dimensional volume can also be displayed and rotated.   Three dimensional data sets require a 3D Fast Fourier Transform (3D.FFT) for their reconstruction. Image acquisition is calculated as:

$$TR \times G_z \text{ phase encode steps} \times G_y \text{ phase encode steps} \times \text{signal averaging.} \qquad (20.7)$$

For a 256 volume and a 20ms TR this would require 256 × 256 × 0.02 × 2 = 43 minutes. Smaller volumes (128) reduce this time to 27 minutes using a TR of 50ms.

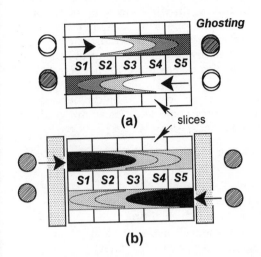

Ghosting

S1 | S2 | S3 | S4 | S5

(a)   slices

S1 | S2 | S3 | S4 | S5

(b)

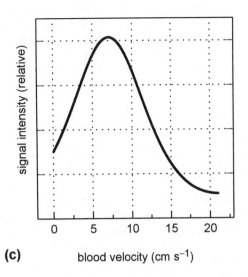

signal intensity (relative)

0   5   10   15   20

(c)   blood velocity (cm s^{-1})

Figure 20.21   (a)   A series of slices containing two blood vessels flowing left to right and right to left, phasing artifacts cause ghosting and vessels are shown as either darker or whiter than the surrounding tissues. **(b)** pre-saturation (shaded slice areas) removes ghosting and gives darker vessels. **(c)** Flow signal strength varying with blood velocity.

20.4.5 Blood flow measurement

The effect of blood moving in and out of slices that are being imaged influences the image in two ways:

- Blood entering the slice brings unsaturated protons
- Blood leaving the slice removes spins in different saturation conditions

Flow influences the NMR signal so that blood movement in vessels can be identified. After a 90° pulse in the spin-echo sequence all the protons within the field are influenced. However the original blood has left the region before the following 180° pulse or gradient reversal. The blood receiving the 180° will not yield a signal so the image will be black in the vessel region; this is the **flow-void** phenomenon. The diagram in Fig.20.21(a) shows blood flowing into a series of slices, both ends having a high signal intensity since spins are fully unsaturated and give the highest signal. Spins within the slice are saturated to various levels and give a lower intensity. The cross sectional diagram illustrates the entrance enhancement along with a ghosting artifact. Because slice selection and frequency encoding gradients are applied for relatively long time periods any motion (blood flow) during G_z and G_x will produce these phase artifacts (in the direction of G_y phase gradient).

If blood enters the excited slice under examination the MR signal is seen to increase at low velocities then decrease rapidly at higher velocities (Fig.20.21(c)). The initial signal increase is called **paradoxical enhancement** and is due to unsaturated nuclear spins flowing into an already excited slice region. At higher velocities excited nuclear spins flow out of the slice so depleting the overall signal strength.

Pre-saturation   (shown in Fig.20.21(b)) suppresses the ghost artifacts by exciting thick slice areas either side of the area of interest. Blood within these regions will be 'pre-saturated' and will give a low signal in the imaged section. The cross section diagrams shows this as a void (low signal). Two techniques are used for vessel imaging: Blood flow direction can be differentiated by pre-saturating either one side or the other of the imaged slice (superior or inferior aspect). Pre-saturation differentiates the blood prior to it entering the imaged slice giving information on flow direction (venous or arterial). Pre-saturation pulses can be applied outside the imaging volume in which case the in-flowing blood will show a signal loss.

Phase shift   Where gradient changes are applied moving spins will show a phase shift while static spins will not. This allows separation of vessels from surrounding tissue giving isolated vessel detail in a 3-D image and also supplying quantitative information about blood velocity depending on the degree of proton saturation.

Magnetic Resonance Angiography (MRA)
Phase Shift imaging using low flip-angles allows thin slices (1-2mm) combined with short echo time imaging. These have been combined to give 3-D angiograms (Fig.20.22). The signal intensity of the stationary tissue remains unchanged so performing a subtraction of two images leaves an isolated image of the blood vessels. MRA is non-invasive and images can be obtained in 6-7 minutes.

In summary:

For fast imaging pulse sequences reducing the TR time has drawbacks. A spin-echo sequence requires a 180° pulse for re-phasing the spins and with very short TR times the time taken to deliver this pulse is a limiting factor (Fig.20.12 revises the spin-echo sequence). With decreasing TR longitudinal magnetization (T1) will have very little recovery so the next pulse will influence it marginally so yielding a poor signal.

These limitations can be overcome if instead of using a 180° pulse a field gradient is superimposed as a pulse giving increased field inhomogeneities in the slice. This causes the

transverse magnetization (T2) to decay faster. The gradient is switched off and then switched on again with opposite polarity and the protons re-phase in a similar way to a 180° pulse: this gives the gradient echo. The poor signal strength can be improved by using flip angles of less than 90° in the range of 10-35°. There is then sufficient remaining T1 signal which can be altered by the next pulse, even after very short TR. These are gradient echo sequences. Also:

- Missing 180° pulse allows much shorter TE but signal depends on T2*
- Shorter flip angles give less T1 weighting
- T2 weighting is not possible; this is replaced by T2* weighting
- Fast pulse techniques enhance blood flow signals (to be described later)
- Fast pulse techniques allow <1second per image.
- Freezes patient movement allowing abdominal and cardiac images.
- Multi-slice techniques are not available

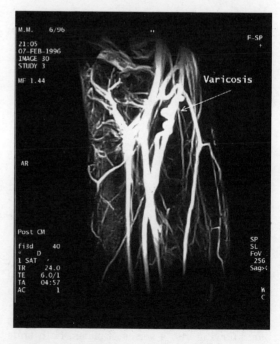

Figure 20.22 Blood vasculature enhanced in a magnetic resonance angiography image. (Courtesy Siemens Inc)

Blood flow imaging can be summarized as:

- Blood brings in unsaturated protons or removes saturated protons from the slice of interest depending on velocity.
- Time of flight uses pre-saturation of blood spins giving it a signal loss. Blood direction can be displayed
- Phase shift differentiates moving and static spins allowing vessel isolation in 3D images.

20.5 IMAGE QUALITY

The x, y and z information during image acquisition must be obtained at the highest signal strength to ensure good signal to noise ratio (SNR), resolution and low contrast differences. In some instances some contrast is sacrificed for fast data acquisition.

Signal to noise is a very complex problem since so many factors play a part so the following assessments and summary are necessarily simplified

20.5.1 Signal to Noise ratio

Signal data is always accompanied by noise. The signal to noise ratio (SNR), which should have a high value, influences both resolution and contrast since any RF noise prevents accurate measurement of small frequency/phase differences. The fundamental limit of SNR is influenced by thermal motion of electrons in the detection coil and Brownian molecular motion of the tissue producing a noise voltage superimposed on the NMR signal. Basic small sample analytical NMR which does not have the added complexity of gradient fields shows an improvement (increase) in SNR with magnet field strength. Many extra factors however are associated with image signal to noise, amongst the most important being: signal frequency (and therefore field strength B_0 and bandwidth), signal coil efficiency, the pulse sequence, tissue characteristics (T1, T2, spin density) and gradient field strength.

Gradient field strength As we have seen by applying a linear gradient each voxel in a slice will have a frequency distribution that depends on the magnitude and steepness of the gradient. When the spin echo is frequency decoded signals from a certain bandwidth can be assigned to each specific voxel. The gradients employed must be large enough to compensate for the main field inhomogeneity and chemical shift artifacts (3.5ppm between fat and water). The inhomogeneity and chemical shift increase with field strength, therefore increased gradient strength (slopes) are necessary to overcome these disadvantages.

RF Pulse bandwidth Pulse bandwidth describes the range of frequencies in the RF pulse. The center frequency selects slice position and the bandwidth determines slice thickness as shown in Fig.20.9. RF pulse bandwidth is dependent on:

$$Bandwidth = \gamma \times G_z \times slice\ thickness \quad (20.8)$$

Increasing gradient strength G_z will therefore increase bandwidth and so decrease SNR.

Field Strengths The graph in Fig.20.23 shows the improvement in SNR, for a selection of tissue types, with increasing main magnet field strength. Larmor frequency (and hence main magnet strength) influences signal to noise as:

$$SNR \propto \sqrt{frequency} \quad (20.9)$$

The square root function causes the curves to flatten with increasing field strength. From Fig.20.23 SNR gains above 1.0 Tesla are slight.

Increasing the magnet field strength increases T1 time and as tissue T1 increases the full SNR cannot be attained without TR increase so patient throughput goes down, however for the same SNR value high field magnets offer a faster patient throughput since signal averaging can be kept to a minimum. Combining the advantage of detection coil efficiency with the disadvantages of signal losses due to greater absorption of higher frequency signals the overall improvement is minimal above 1T.

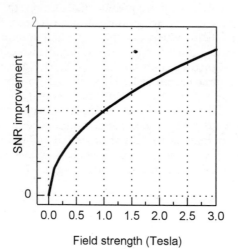

Figure 20.23 The square root function of field strength versus image signal to noise ratio. Above 1T only a small improvement is seen.

Receiver bandwidth The display bandwidth describes the frequency content of the pixel and the pixel bandwidth depends on the number of phase/frequency encoding steps N_{ex} which decides the matrix dimensions and the signal sampling time T_s:

$$Bandwidth = N_{ex}/T_s \qquad (20.10)$$

Image noise approximates to: $\dfrac{1}{\sqrt{T_s}}$

so shorter sampling times increase noise. Signal to noise ratio is dependent on:

$$SNR \propto \frac{1}{\sqrt{bandwidth}} \qquad (20.11)$$

If the receiver circuits are tuned to receive signals having a narrow frequency range (bandwidth) then noise frequencies can be rejected. SNR degrades with increasing pixel bandwidth. Halving the bandwidth (for example from 4 to 2 in eqn.20.11) improves SNR by 1.4 or 40%.

Receiver coil quality For small samples and low Q (efficiency) detector coils the SNR is proportional to (frequency)$^{1.5}$. For high Q coils the SNR figure improves and becomes proportional to frequency. The fixed sample volume seen by the coil influences noise but since this volume is usually large any noise given by the RF coil is dominated by noise from the patient. The receiver Q is improved by choosing a coil to match the anatomy being imaged (matched surface coil).

Signal averaging (n) The SNR can be improved by multiple measurements at the expense of examination time. Signal strength increases with n but the noise increases by $\sqrt{n}$ so SNR improves. Gradient signals are repeated a great number of times and the image signals are collected and the average signal strength used for image formation. The signal noise is decreased but imaging time is increased.

Voxel size SNR is proportional to voxel size. This is determined by field of view *FOV*, matrix size *m*, and slice thickness seen in 20.2.5. The number of measurements performed to obtain a 2DFT slice (M_{2D}) depends on the number of phase/frequency encoding steps in the $x \times y$ matrix which is $N_x \times N_y$. These measurements (excitations or N_{ex}) are repeated in order to reduce noise. The total number of measurements $M_{2D} = N_x \times N_y \times N_{ex}$.

The signal strength is proportional to M_{2D} and the noise proportional to $\sqrt{M_{2D}}$ so:

$$SNR_{2D} = M_{2D}/\sqrt{M_{2D}} = \sqrt{M_{2D}} \qquad (20.12)$$

Three dimensional data sets (3DFT) use a number of slices (N_z) so voxel size $= (FOV/m) \times (FOV/N_z)$. 3DFT imaging is less noisy than 2DFT since the number of slices comprising the 3D volume set N_z decreases the SNR_{2D} in eqn.20.9 so SNR_{3D} is $\sqrt{N_z} \times$ SNR. However the imaging time is increased by N_z which is significant.

Imaging time t The components of image quality are related to the time taken for accumulating 2-dimensional image signals (2D.FFT) by $t = M \times TR \times N_{ex}$ where M is the data matrix size (128^2 or 256^2), *TR* repetition time between pulse sequences. Images having large TR values have better low contrast definition (more sensitive to pathological changes) where N_{ex} is the number of measurements made per voxel. SNR increases with N_{ex} so fewer measurements taken with faster imaging sequences give more noise tending to diminish low contrast detail.

Slice selection By referring to the graph in Fig. 20.9 it can be seen that slice selection can be either:

- Narrow bandwidth/low gradient slope or
- Wide bandwidth using a steeper gradient to give the same slice thickness.

Pixel bandwidth influences noise as eqn.20.8. so choosing a steeper gradient with a narrow bandwidth is preferable. Slice cross-talk has already been mentioned in 20.2.5. Signal strength will be influenced by the slice thickness; thicker slices give stronger signals so less noise.

Overall SNR The overall image SNR is influenced by the above factors as:

$$SNR = \frac{k \cdot voxelsize \cdot \sqrt{Fourier\ terms} \cdot \sqrt{N_{ex}}}{\sqrt{bandwidth}} \quad (20.13)$$

The constant k contains numerous terms related to the physical parameters of the MRI system (magnet strength, pulse sequence etc.) but as a rough guide $k \propto$ magnet strength so SNR tends to improve with increasing magnet field strength. Voxel size determines the volume of tissue from which the signal is derived so larger volumes improve SNR. Fourier terms refer to the complexity of the Fourier reconstruction calculation. Partial Fourier imaging where a restricted data set is used will increase noise. Bandwidth influences SNR adversely. A narrow receiver bandwidth will encompass less noise than a broad-band receiver characteristic. N_{ex} refers to the number of excitations or number of signals averaged for each phase encoding step.

Image reconstruction algorithms These have a significant effect on SNR mainly by controlling the eventual voxel size and whether isotropic or anisotropic image matrices are to be used. Reconstruction filters are designed to reduce SNR.

In summary:

The SNR is reduced if:

- Magnet field strength increased
- Voxel size increased
- Slice thickness increased
- Smaller matrix size
- Increased signal averaging (increase N_{ex})
- Narrow bandwidth
- Increase inter-slice gap

20.5.2 Resolution and contrast quality

This is determined by field homogeneity and steepness of the gradient fields. High resolution MR used for spectroscopy uses steep gradients; SNR decreases so more averaging is needed. The gradient power supply should have a high current (100 amp) and high speed (sub milli-second) for 1mm resolution.

The high frequency signals are converted by **quadrature demodulation** into a low frequency signal before digitization and frequency and phase differences measured prior to image reconstruction. Resolution is dependent on:

- Gradient field strength (slice thickness)
- Receiver coil design
- Signal bandwidth
- Matrix size

The best resolution for general use is 0.5mm to 1.0mm but small FOV and high gradient field strengths can reduce this figure.

Contrast This can be selected by TR and TE timing to influence T1 and T2 differences and blood flow. High field magnets increase T1 time (see Fig.19.9) which tends to decrease image contrast because of increased

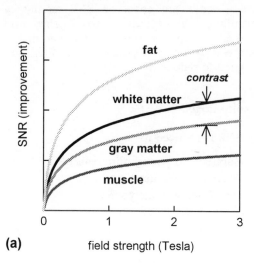

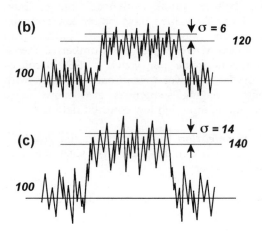

(a)   field strength (Tesla)

Figure 20.24   **(a)** Two profiles showing different SNR values referred to in the text. **(b)** Graph field strength tissue contrast between fat and muscle; **(c)** white matter and gray matter.

saturation of short T1 tissues relative to longer T1 tissues which then reduces the contrast between these tissues. Differences between tissue signals can be treated as a **contrast to noise ratio CNR**; this improves only slightly beyond 1.0T.   Figure 20.24(a) shows the contrast for white/gray matter and muscle/fat versus magnetic strength.

A high SNR on its own does not guarantee good image quality. The differentiation of two tissue types or the contrast between two tissue types depends on the separate SNR shown by the two tissues which gives the CNR. The first tissue may yield a strong signal but the second tissue may give a weaker signal in a poorer noise background. Figure 20.24(b),(c) shows two lesions with different signal to noise values. Their contrasts would be given by C = $(S_1 - S_2)/S_2$ however their contrast to noise value is given as:

$$CNR = SNR_1 - SNR_2 \qquad (20.14)$$

Worked examples in Box 20.4 show that SNR plays a more important role than measured contrast differences in making a lesion visible.

Triggering Data collected from a particular slice at identical points in the lung /heart cycle can be achieved by respiratory and cardiac triggering. Multiple slices combined with triggering causes different slices to hold images of different phases of the cardiac cycle. The R-R interval of the ECG decides the repetition time. Respiratory gating removes organ movement in upper abdomen slices. Fast pulse sequences have reduced the requirement for gating.

In summary:

Noise is influenced by:

- Main magnet field strength. SNR versus field strength Fig.20.23
- Gradient field strength
- Signal coil type and antenna size
- Imaging sequence
- Patient size and composition.
- Spatial resolution
- Scan time
- Slice thickness

Box 20.4

Contrast to Noise ratio (CNR)

From the values given in Fig.20.24

The contrast in (b) is   (120–100)/100 = 20%
The contrast in (c) is (140–100)/100 = 40%

Using eqn. 20.11

Example (b) has a 5% noise figure giving an SNR2 of 20 and SNR1 16.6 so CNR = 3.4

Example (c) has a 10% noise figure giving an SNR2 of 10 and SNR1 of 7.2 so CNR = 2.8

NB
Example (b) has a more visible lesion in spite of its lower contrast.

ments for and against low/high field systems are summarized in Tab.20.9.

Table 20.9

Low Field	High Field
Cheap	Expensive
Short T1	Long T1
Good Contrast	Poorer Contrast (Poor T1 Separation)
T2 Unchanged	T2 Unchanged
No Spectroscopy	Spectroscopy
Low SNR	High SNR
Low Larmor Frequency	High Larmor Freq.
Lower SNR	High SNR (better resolution)

20.6 CHOICE OF MRI SYSTEM

The choice of MRI system will depend on:

- Clinical application (neurological, vascular, pediatric, spectroscopy etc.)
- Image resolution and contrast required (slice thickness)
- Patient throughput/imaging time
- Costs

Other features that would influence choice would be system cooling (water supply), power consumption, degree of field homogeneity and available room size. Some argu-

Since SNR increases with frequency (the gain in SNR is roughly field strength N Fig. 20.23) good thin slice acquisition improves with magnet field strength. To maintain the same contrast behavior at lower field strengths it might be necessary to increase TR at higher field strengths so lengthening examination time but signal averaging is less.

Faster patient throughput and shorter examination times favor higher field strengths. In regions where both water and fat are present the slope of the gradient fields used for encoding X, Y and Z spatial information needs to be doubled to eliminate the chemical shift artifact. Increasing gradient field strength gives:

Table 20.10 Choice of magnet

Property	Superconducting	Resistive	Permanent
Field Strength (T)	0.5–4.0T	0.2T	<0.1– 0.2T
Gradient (mT m^{-1})	10–25	10	<10
Fringe field (0.5mT)	2.5–4m	-	1.5–2m
Power (kW)	28	up to 60	4
Inhomogeneity	<0.5ppm	-	7ppm
Magnet stability	0.1ppm h^{-1}	-	6ppm h^{-1}
Gradient cooling	900m^3 h^{-1}	-	none

- Improved SNR
- Shorter TE time
- More slices per TR time
- Smaller FOV with larger matrix sizes
- Faster 3D FLASH sequences

20.6.1 Low field system (0.1)

Magnet field strengths from 0.1 to 0.2T have certain advantages, perhaps the most important one being capital cost; they also require less room so can be installed safely in a small clinic. These magnets can be designed to have an open aspect y-axis orientation as shown in Fig.20.1 which lends greater accessibility to the patient. The open aspect of this design is popular for interventional work.

Longitudinal relaxation time T1 is proportional to field strength (see Fig.19.9) so low field systems require shorter TR and potentially a shorter imaging time T as:

$$T = M \times TR \times N_{ex} \qquad (20.15)$$

where M is the matrix size which determines the phase encoding steps (e.g. 128, 256 or 512), TR the repetition time and N_{ex} the data averaging or number of excitations. Image SNR however is proportional to field strength so for the same image quality in low field systems more signal averages are necessary so image time must be increased.

Low field magnets require smaller gradient strengths allowing narrower bandwidths with improvement in SNR (eqn.20.8).

Advantages:

- Cheap to run
- Simplified housing (very small fringe field)
- Short T1 time

Disadvantages:

- Long patient imaging time (small patient numbers)
- Poor resolution

20.6.2 A medium field system (0.3-0.5T)

Patient throughput is potentially improved by increasing field sizes up to 0.5T. Permanent magnets are commonly used for some mid-field designs having field strengths of 0.2 to 0.3T. They offer considerable advantages for mobile MRI systems since their power consumption is minimal (gradient coils). Permanent magnets are very heavy however.

Open aspect resistive magnets are also used for interventional work; these have field strengths of about 0.3T. They have high power consumption but resistive magnets have the important ability to be shut down instantly if required. This considerable advantage is not available for permanent or superconducting designs. The gradient field in these systems must be steep enough to compensate for magnet inhomogeneity and chemical shift artifacts, however gradient steepness is proportional to pixel bandwidth so image noise increases as $\sqrt{gradient}$. With an increase in gradient field fast imaging pulse sequences can be more widely used unlike the small field systems.

20.6.3 High field system (above 1-1.5T)

These machines should be considered if spectroscopy is going to be an important application since spectrum resolution improves with increased field strength. Small bore magnets for limb or pediatric investigations are available with field strengths up to 9T.

Their advantages can be summarized briefly as:

- Best image quality
- High gradient field gives thin slices (3D imaging)
- Good magnet homogeneity for fat/water separation.
- Spectroscopy
- Fast imaging
- Fast patient throughput

However they do have disadvantages:

- Superconducting magnet cannot be shut down easily
- Cryogen replacement
- They require a larger room because of their fringe fields

• There are magnet hazards

20.6.4 Harmful effects

The **specific absorption rate** *SAR* is a measure of the energy deposited by a radio-frequency field in a mass of tissue. It is analogous to the radiation absorbed dose the gray used for ionizing radiation. The units for the gray are joules per kilogram, the SAR for radio-frequency is measured in watts per kilogram.

The energy deposited depends on the tissue radius *r*, electrical conductivity σ, the field strength of the magnet B_0 and the flip angle α together with the imaging sequence duty cycle *d* to give:

$$SAR = (r^2\sigma) \cdot (B_0^2\alpha^2) \cdot d \qquad (20.16)$$

The SAR value is markedly increased by:

• Increasing field strength
• Increasing the flip angle: the maximum energy being deposited by 180° RF pulses.
• Increasing the duty cycle

Fast spin echo sequences with multiple 180° pulses are responsible for high SAR values while GRE sequences with low flip angles give small SAR values. Tissues with a high water content have highest conductivity (CSF and blood) and the geometry of the tissue volume may increase SAR non-uniformly and double expected values.

The USA Food and Drug Administration (FDA) guidelines restrict SAR values to 0.4W kg^{-1} for whole body exposure and 3.2W kg^{-1} for brain imaging

RF Pulses These produce warming of tissues and metallic implants since:

$$\text{Heating} \sim \sqrt{Field\ strength}$$
$$\text{Absorbed energy} \sim \sqrt{RF\ frequency}$$

The acceptable limit for energy absorption was set at 0.4W kg^{-1} for whole body imaging and 2W kg^{-1} for smaller organs.

Magnetic field strength The natural magnetic field of the earth is approximately 50mT. and magnetic densities of about 20mT are experienced under high voltage power lines. The highest exposure experienced by humans is given by MRI where patients are exposed to between 0.15 and 2 Tesla. This magnetic field strength has no reported ill effects on the human body. Small bore Field Strengths for whole body imaging (neonates) can reach 6T.

Fast changes of gradient fields These cause Faraday currents in tissues. The most sensitive tissue seems to be the retina which causes flashing sensations. In pacemakers these cause side effects. Large hip prostheses heat up and other smaller metal artifacts (surgical clips) suffer movement, which pose hazards. The maximum rate of change has been limited to 20T s^{-1} (Europe); 3T s^{-1} (USA). Contra-indications for MRI examinations are:

• Pacemaker Patients
• Magnetic Surgical clips.
• Some hip/knee metal prostheses.
• Heart Valve prostheses

Fatalities and injuries have been reported to patients having ferromagnetic implants (aneurysm clips); these have either been displaced in-situ or heated.

20.7   IMAGE ARTIFACTS

These can derive from malfunction of the machine itself or be caused by the patient

20.7.1 Machine Artifacts

Eddy currents cause temporary magnet inhomogeneities and arise from gradient fields and the walls of the cryostat.

20.7.2 Patient Artifacts

Motion Fat layers give high intensity signals and move during acquisition which disturbs frequency and phase encoding especially during long TR routines. This causes 'ghosting' on the images which is reflections of the main signal in the direction of the phase encoding gradient; the reflections are not related to the movement direction. Ghosting can be reduced by using faster image acquisition or physiological gating (respiratory or ECG) but these procedures increase acquisition time.

20.7.3 Chemical Shift

This is visible as light and dark stripes on the image and is caused by the separation of lipid and water components in the frequency encoded read-out gradient (usually G_x). It can cause positional displacement where fat and water are mis-located (commonly seen in head images). The degree of displacement depends on field strength and gradient strength. Box 20.5 gives an example.

20.7.4 Magnetic materials

The magnetic field is distorted by ferrous objects (iron, cobalt, nickel) which are used in the manufacture of surgical wires and clips as well as hip prostheses and stainless steel needles. Eddy currents are also induced in the implanted metal by gradient switching.

Box 20.5

Chemical shift artifact

The chemical shift between water and lipids is between 3 - 3.5ppm; in a 1T field this represents 128 - 150Hz (3 - 3.5ppm of 42.576MHz).

For a read-out gradient of 0.15mT cm^{-1} and 256^2 matrix (see Box 20.3) frequency/pixel is approximately 370Hz so water and fat are displaced by 140/370Hz or a third of a pixel width.

For lower field and gradient strengths displacement is greater and becomes visible. (see Box 20.2).

For 0.5T a 3ppm of 21.287MHz is 63Hz. The frequency per pixel for this matrix is 120Hz so there is a 50% displacement artifact.

20.8 MAGNETIC RESONANCE SPECTROSCOPY (MRS)

For MR imaging the spin echo rather than the free induction decay (FID) is collected. Spectroscopy concerns itself exclusively with the FID which carries the information about the chemical nature of the material. Any NMR sensitive nucleus (H, P, C, F) will give a signal in a strong magnetic field if a RF pulse is applied at the resonant frequency for that nucleus. Tab.20.11 shows the different Larmor frequencies for each of these elements and Fig.20.25 plots these versus field strength.

Table 20.11 Elements important for clinical MRS

Element	MHz T^{-1}
^{1}Hydrogen	42.58
^{19}Fluorine	40.1
^{31}Phosphorus	17.2
^{23}Sodium	11.3
^{13}Carbon	10.7

20.8.1 Signal origin

The local magnetic field varies slightly within the compound molecule due to chemical bonds, size of atoms and position of the atom relative to others. The hydrogen atom in a water molecule will experience a different local magnetic field to a hydrogen atom in fat for example. Since these very small differences in the local magnetic field can affect the Larmor frequency there will be frequency shifts of the NMR signal; this is the chemical shift. A plot of signal intensity versus frequency is the NMR spectrum (Fig.20.25). The area under each peak (integral) is directly proportional to the compound concentration and the position on the frequency axis is its chemical shift measured in ppm.

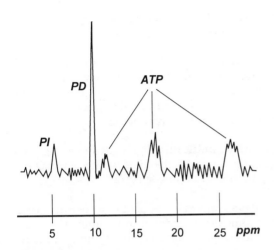

Figure 20.25 Spectrum examples for ^{31}P compounds associated with muscle metabolism displayed using a high field (1 - 2T) magnet.

The degree of shift is characteristic of the chemical bond in which the nucleus is situated. Figure 19.7(b) represents a mixed signal from fat and water which is resolved into its two frequencies by a Fast Fourier Transform (FFT). A chemical shift of about 3ppm separates these signals.

If each separate nucleus precesses at one frequency then the Fourier analysis would yield an NMR spectrum consisting of only one line; no distinction would be observed for different compounds. The local magnetic field varies slightly within a molecule due to chemical bonds and size of various atomic groups; a hydrogen atom attached to an oxygen atom (H–O) will experience a different magnetic field to a H–C bonding. (e.g. water and fat). These small differences in the local magnetic field will influence the individual proton's Larmor frequency; this is the chemical shift.

The range of chemical shifts differs for each type of nucleus and is very small compared to the main frequency (expressed in MHz); chemical shift is given in hertz and this varies with the main magnet field strength so comparison using frequency alone is difficult between two machines having slightly different magnetic field strengths. The concept of parts per million or ppm is introduced. (Box 20.6). Although the term parts per million is not a measure of chemical concentration it is related, since the chemical shift can be changed by chemical dilution. Chemical shift tables give chemical shift ranges for various compounds. Adjacent proton spins interact with each other as well as with the main magnetic field (T1 and T2 times). The extent of this interaction or coupling depends on the chemical bonding. Coupling causes a single line spectrum to be split, producing **multiplets** or groups of lines; a three line spectrum is a **triplet;** four lines a **quartet** etc.

Resolution and sensitivity The resolving power of the spectroscopy system depends on field strength, magnet homogeneity and molecular line width. Large sample volumes decrease resolution since inhomogeneity increases with volume size. Sensitivity (the ability to detect weak signals) depends on SNR which is improved by increasing field strength, concentration of material, volume size and acquisition time. There is therefore a balance between resolution and sensitivity and volume size should be chosen carefully to optimize both resolution and sensitivity.

Volume localization Considerable improvements in acquisition accuracy are required in order to select areas for regional MRS. These include RF Coil design, a very homogeneous magnetic field, stability of magnetic field after gradient switching and elimination of eddy current interference. Special pulse sequences have been developed based on spin-echo (SE) or stimulated echo (STEAM). These are able to give 'volume of interest' spectra of brain or muscle which are better resolved by high field magnets.

In summary, for magnetic resonance spectroscopy:

- The FID signal gives a frequency spectrum representing chemistry.

- The frequency spectra exhibit chemical shifts (ppm)
- The degree of shift depends on the chemical bonding
- Higher field magnets give finer resolution
- Chemical concentration and pH can be measured.

Box 20.6

Signal reference measurement

The frequency difference Δf between water and tetramethylsilane (a reference compound used as a standard frequency) for field strengths of 1.5T and 2.0T :

For 1.5T (where ω_o is 63MHz), $\Delta f = 334$Hz
For 2.0T (where ω_o is 84MHz), $\Delta f = 445$Hz

The Chemical Shift (ppm) is:

For 1.5T: $334/63 \times 10^6 = 5.3 \times 10^{-6} = 5.3$ ppm
For 2.0T: $445/84 \times 10^6 = 5.3$ ppm

Further reading:

Questions and Answers in Magnetic Resonance Imaging.
Allen D. Elster, Mosby (1994)

KEYWORDS

acquisition matrix - the number of independent data samples in each direction.

aliasing: poor sampling increments. Components of the signal are at higher frequency than the Nyquist sampling frequency. In the Fourier transform this gives wrap-around image artifacts.

array processor - dedicated computer for reconstructing the image matrix.

Carr-Purcell (CP) sequence - spin-echo sequence of 90° followed by a 180° pulse.

chemical shift - the change in Larmor frequency of a nucleus due to molecular binding; caused by local alteration in the magnetic field. It is measured in parts per million relative to a reference compound.

chemical shift imaging - an image of a restricted range of chemical shifts corresponding to individual line spectra.

contrast agent - typically a paramagnetic substance (e.g. gadolinium) administered to a patient which shortens both T1 and T2 times.

contrast to noise ratio (CNR) - ratio of the difference between to regions measured by their signal to noise ratios **(SNR)**.

demodulator - a component of the NMR signal receiver that converts it to a lower frequency for analysis. This is also phase sensitive (now called a quadrature demodulator) and will give phase information (detecting phase encoded RF signals).

echo-planar imaging (EPI) - a complete planar image obtained from one excitation pulse. The FID is detected while switching the y-gradient magnet with a constant x-gradient. The Fourier transform of the spin-echo sequence then supplies the image of the selected plane.

eddy currents - electric currents induced in a conductor by a changing magnetic field (e.g. gradient fields).

Faraday shield - metal mesh between an RF transmitter and receiver to block signals such as interfering RF noise from TV, radio and power appliances.

Fast Fourier Transform (FFT) - a modified Fourier transform for computer use.

flip angle - amount of magnetization vector rotation produced by RF pulse. Flip angles of 15 to 30° are used in fast acquisition sequences.

flow - nuclei from liquids moving into an excited slice-region can be distinguished from static tissues.

flow enhancement - the increased intensity that may be seen due to flowing blood due to loss of saturated spins from the imaged slice.

frequency encoding - applying a magnetic gradient causing a consequent gradient in resonance frequency.

gradient coils - coils designed to produce a magnetic field gradient in the Z-axis (slice position) or X and Y-axis (matrix dimensions).

gradient echo (field echo) - spin echo produced by reversing the direction of a magnetic field gradient. A substitute for the 180° pulse in the spin-echo sequence.

G_x G_y G_z - abbreviations used to describe the three magnetic field gradients.

homogeneity - uniformity. Homogeneity of the main magnetic field defines the quality of the main magnet over a large field of view.

inversion-recovery - NMR pulse sequence where nuclear magnetization is inverted before 90° pulse.

multiple slice imaging - sequential plane imaging used with selective excitation techniques that do not affect adjacent slices. Adjacent slices are imaged while waiting for relaxation of the first slice toward equilibrium. Reduces imaging time for a slice set.

partial saturation - excitation applying repeated RF pulses shorter than the T1 time. Causes increased contrast between similar tissue types.

phase encoding - applying a pulsed magnetic field gradient to change frequency for a short time so that after this pulse the nuclei resume their original frequency but now with phase differences.

quadrature detector - a demodulation circuit that detects signal phase by comparing with a reference frequency.

quenching - loss of superconductivity due to temperature rise causing cryogen boil off.

rephasing gradient - magnetic field gradient applied for a brief period after a selective excitation pulse. The gradient reversal rephases the spins forming a gradient echo.

shimming - correction of magnet inhomogeneity; 'active' using shim coils, 'passive' using iron sheets.

signal averaging - combining signals from identical acquisition procedures to reduce signal noise.

spin density - the density of resonating spins which determines the strength of the NMR signal.

spin echo sequence - an RF pulse series having 90° followed by 180° gives the Carr-Purcell Sequence depends strongly on T2.

spoiling pulse - use of a reverse magnetic field gradient to eliminate residual magnetization in the nucleus.

surface coil - a surface coil placed over a region of interest will have a selectivity for a volume approximately subtended by the coil circumference and one radius deep. Improves signal to noise ratio.

Radiation Protection: Radiobiology and risk estimation

21.1 Radiation interaction with tissue
21.2 Biological damage

21.3 Natural and man-made radiation
21.4 Risk estimates

21.1 RADIATION INTERACTION WITH TISSUE

The use of ionizing radiation for diagnostic imaging requires careful thought and handling so that maximum benefit can be obtained for minimum risk. Its use has increased dramatically over the last decade; more and more people are being exposed to medical x- and gamma radiation. Figure 21.1 shows the rapid increase in their use over the past 100 years.

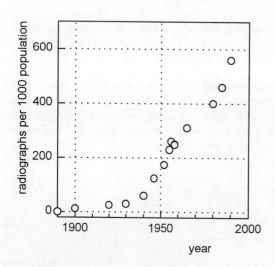

Figure 21.1 The increasing use of x-rays as an imaging medium since their discovery in 1895. (UK data)

Increased machine sensitivity has lowered the dose in diagnostic imaging but exposure even from low levels of radiation is still an unknown risk especially when applied to larger and larger numbers in the population. Although a great deal of knowledge exists about the risks of high radiation levels extrapolation to low doses is fraught with complications.

21.1. 1 Radiation type and interactions.

The degree of radiation damage depends on the density of ionizing events along the radiation pathway in tissue. Figure 21.2 represents these ionization events in tissue; the degree of tissue damage depending on radiation type, which are either particulate or electro-magnetic. Particulate radiation is rarely a feature in diagnostic radiology (Chapter 15: Nuclear Medicine); alpha is almost never encountered and beta radiation only occasionally, either in the form of therapy (^{32}P) or non-ideal imaging nuclide (^{133}Xe).

Alpha particles These are helium nuclei so have a relatively large mass. They are easily stopped by tissue and can scarcely penetrate the dead outer layers of the skin. An α–radionuclide is not hazardous externally but ingestion is of major concern either by swallowing, inhalation or as a result of wound contamination. Alpha particles with their much higher energy cause major radiation damage in tissue over a small range since all their energy is deposited in a very small tissue volume (α in Fig.21.2).

Beta particles These are high energy electrons from radioactive decay. They penetrate only about a centimeter or so of tissue; β–emitters are only hazardous to superficial tissues, unless ingested. The number of ionizing events depends on the β–energy (β in Fig.21.2). Low energy betas (^{3}H, ^{14}C) deposit all their energy in a small tissue volume. High energy β–radiation has a more extensive pathway and produces bremsstrahlung radiation which can be an additional hazard (^{32}P).

In general particulate radiation only has a limited range in tissue so does not constitute an external hazard. They are a major hazard when ingested and feature as therapy agents e.g. ^{32}P, ^{90}Y and ^{131}I.

Electromagnetic radiation This is by far the most familiar ionizing radiation in radiology. Gamma photons are produced by radionuclides and can pass easily through soft tissues only creating a small number of ionizing events (γ in Fig.21.2). X-ray photons are similar but generally have lower energies so are attenuated more easily.

In general both γ– and x-photons leave behind a relatively small number of ionization events but cover a long tissue pathway. It is the density of ionization events that determines tissue damage.

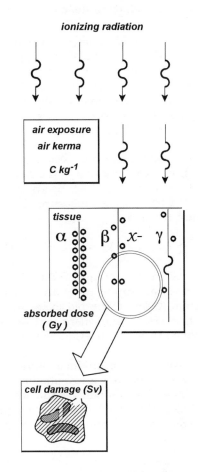

Figure 21.2 Ionizing events in tissue from electromagnetic radiation (γ–, x-radiation) and particulate radiation (β, α)

Table 21.1 Units of radiation exposure

Quantity	Name (Non- SI)	Symbol (Non- SI)	Name (SI)	Symbol (SI)
Exposure	roentgen (R)	1R = 2.58×10^{-4}C kg^{-1} 1R = 8.6mGy	Coulomb kg^{-1} air-kerma (Gy)	1C kg^{-1} = 3876R 1C kg^{-1} = 34Gy
Absorbed Dose	rad	1rad = 0.01J kg^{-1}	gray	1Gy = 1J kg^{-1} 1Gy = 2.9×10^{-2} C kg^{-1} 10mGy = 1rad 1μGy = 115μR
Dose Equivalent	rem	rem = rad × Q	sievert	Sv = Gy × Q

21.1.2 Units of radiation dose

The basic units of measurement for quantities and energies of ionizing radiation are given in Table 21.1. SI and non-SI values are listed since both are in common use. Quantities of radiation may be measured in air (as exposure or air-kerma) or in tissue (as absorbed dose).

Exposure Any ionizing beam passing through air causes ionization of the gas molecules and the formation of an electric charge. This has traditionally been measured in terms of **exposure** E where:

$$E = \frac{Q}{m} \text{ coulombs kg}^{-1} \text{ (C kg}^{-1}) \qquad (21.1)$$

Q is the total electric charge produced and m is the mass of air so the units are coulombs per kilogram (C kg^{-1}). The old exposure unit of 1 roentgen (1R) is equivalent to 2.58×10^{-4} C kg^{-1}. Since 1Gy = 3×10^{-2}C kg^{-1} then 1R $\equiv$ 8.6mGy.

The average energy to produce ionization in air is 34eV so a 100keV x-ray photon would produce about 3000 ion pairs. **Exposure rate** is measured as C kg^{-1} s^{-1}. Since x-ray exposure is represented in mAs a direct conversion exists since:

$$1A = 1C \text{ s}^{-1} \text{ so}$$
$$1C = 1As \text{ then}$$
$$1mAs = 1mC$$

Unit radiation exposure can be given per mAs.

Kerma The amount of energy loss or attenuation in a small air volume is expressed as the kerma (Kinetic Energy Released per unit Mass) which is measured in grays. Kerma is a measure of the **energy released**, including secondary (from photoelectric and Compton events) in a volume of material. The site of the attenuation event (photoelectric/Compton event) may be some distance from the ejected electron when it eventually comes to rest. Kerma takes this into account but it is only relevant for high energy photons. Kerma is an important measure for radiation therapy and is not commonly used in diagnostic radiology. At diagnostic energies the terms are essentially the same since the ranges of secondary electrons and bremsstrahlung are short.

The older term 'exposure' used above only applies to low energy x or γ–photons which are stopped over a short distance in air. The term **air-kerma** does not have these restrictions and can be used for describing all ionizing events and all energies. The output of x-ray tubes is commonly quoted in terms of air-kerma along with skin surface doses. The air-kerma value is measured with a small ionization chamber where the wall of the chamber is an integral part of the device and produces secondary electrons that are important to the measurement.

Box 21.1 uses exposure values to calculate the number of photons of 60keV, 140keV and 1MeV required to give a dose of 10mGy (1rad) to a tissue volume of 1cm^3 (1g). These photon quantities are useful when calculating detector absorption and conversion efficiency of various detector surfaces (image intensifier, intensifying screens etc.) . The output from an x-ray tube is proportional to:

$$\frac{kV^2 \times mAs}{d^2} \qquad (21.2)$$

Where d is distance. This is measured in air-kerma rate. Examples of air-kerma values in practice are:

89kV x-rays at 1m	43 - 52µGy mAs^{-1}
Fluoroscopy	0.5µGy s^{-1} 0.3µGy frame^{-1}
Mammography at 28kV	8.9×10^5 Gy mAs^{-1} or 89µGy mAs^{-1}
Nuclear medicine patient at 1m	15.8µGy h^{-1}

Absorbed dose (gray) (L.H. Gray, British physicist 1905-1965). The definition of exposure given in eqn.21.1 measures the quantity of electric charge (C kg^{-1}) produced by ionizing radiation and is not the same as the energy absorbed, although they are proportional. Absorbed dose is a measure of the **energy absorbed** by a volume of material (air or tissue). The absorbed dose in joules kg^{-1} is the ratio of energy E absorbed by a mass M of tissue: E/M. The SI unit is the gray (Gy) as defined in Box 21.1 and photon flux can be calculated for any particular energy which is useful when estimating dose or detector efficiency.

Box 21.1

Exposure and photon number

Since 1 volt exists if 1J moves 1C of charge, the electronic charge:

$e = 1.6 \times 10^{-19}$C so $1eV = 1.6 \times 10^{-19}$J

Ionization of air requires on average 34eV
Radiation producing 1C kg^{-1} = 34 J kg^{-1} in air.
Since an exposure of 1 gray = 1 J kg^{-1} then an exposure of 1C kg^{-1} = 34 Gy in air

Using practical volumes $1Gy = 1 \times 10^{-3}$J g^{-1}
$10mGy$ (1rad) = 1×10^{-5}J g^{-1}

The number of photons N to produce 10mGy exposure in 1g air where exposure E in air is measured in grays and energy J measured in joules, then:

$$N = E/J$$

Photon energy: 60keV

Since $1ev = 1.6 \times 10^{-19}$J then each x-ray photon of 60keV represents 9.6×10^{-15}J

Incidentally using the basic equation $E = hf$ from Chapter 2 where $f = c/\lambda$ gives λ for 60keV x-ray photons as $1.24/60 = 0.02$nm yielding a frequency of 1.5×10^{19}Hz . Using Planck's constant yields an energy value E of 9.6×10^{-15}J

60keV: Energy is 9.6×10^{-15} J
$N = (1 \times 10^{-5})/ (9.6 \times 10^{-15})$ = **1×10^9photons**

Similarly for 140keV and 1MeV the photon numbers are 4.5×10^8 and 6.3×10^7 respectively

---

Kerma can be treated as identical to absorbed dose for energies <3MeV which would of course apply to diagnostic energies. The average atomic number Z for air is 7.6 which is very close to water and soft tissue: 7.4.

Therefore the mass attenuation and mass absorption coefficients for these materials are very similar and the dose in air can be treated the same as dose in tissue, along with other materials which are tissue equivalent (LiF in dosimeters).

The quantity of energy imparted by ionizing radiation to a unit mass of tissue is the absorbed dose called the gray (Gy) and corresponds to 1 joule kg^{-1} of tissue (Tab.21.1). Since the average energy to produce ionization in air is 34eV the energy absorbed in a unit mass of air during an exposure of 1 C kg^{-1} is 34J kg^{-1}. Therefore 1C kg^{-1} represents 34Gy so 1Gy is equivalent to 0.0294 C kg^{-1}. The non-SI unit, the rad, is equivalent to 100ergs g^{-1} tissue. Equivalent values are therefore 100 rad = 1Gy, 1rad = 10mGy and 1mrad = 10μGy). An unofficial centigray (cGy) is sometimes quoted which allows direct conversion between the rad and the gray (1rad = 0.01Gy or 1 cGy).

Dose measurement The quantity of energy deposited in a tissue by ionizing radiation can be estimated by using tissue equivalent monitoring devices i.e. film dosimeters, thermoluminescent dosimeters, electronic detectors. Figure 21.3 indicates the position in the x-ray beam where relevant dose measurements are made. Both the dose rate and surface dose rate are expressed as air-kerma, tissue dose is expressed in absorbed dose. While Entrance Surface Dose (ESD) is a measure for the individual radiograph the Dose Area Product meter (DAP or Diamentor) gives a reading for the complete study (several radiographs).

When quantities cannot be measured directly, for instance when a radionuclide is deposited in an organ and irradiates that organ with α, β- or γ-radiation, the dose absorbed by that organ is calculated from the known activity of the radionuclide (Chapter 16).

Linear Energy Transfer (LET) This is a measure of the density of ionization events along the ray's path. The LET is correlated with the potential for tissue damage and depends on radiation type e.g. α– β– γ– x– radiation, neutrons, protons and their radiation energy. LET is expressed as the quantity of energy (in keV) deposited per micron (μm) of tissue. Table 21.2 gives the LET for common ionizing radiation and shows approximate tissue penetration. Particulate radiation (α–, neutrons and protons) have a higher LET value since they cause more ionization events over their path than either electromagnetic radiation (γ– and x-rays) or electrons (β–radiation).

Since high LET radiation is more damaging to tissues this radiation is used for radiation therapy. Internal conversion electrons and Auger electrons also have a high LET and this becomes important when considering *in-vivo* radiation dose from various gamma-emitting radionuclides (^{99m}Tc).

Dose equivalent (sievert)   (R. Sievert, Swedish radiologist, 1896-1966)   The lethal dose to humans is about 4J kg^{-1} or 4Gy. This causes an infinitesimal rise in body temperature of about 0.001°C. This tiny heat increase cannot produce biological changes but the method of energy deposition of these ionizing events is significant.

Different types of ionizing radiation (α, β– x- and γ) vary considerably in their tissue damaging properties. The **dose equivalent** allows for this by multiplying the absorbed dose (grays) by a weighting factor which depends on the type of radiation. This is the relative biological effectiveness or **quality factor** (*Q*) and depends on the radiation LET. The product of these two quantities gives the dose equivalent in sieverts:

$$grays \times Q = sieverts \ (Sv) \qquad (21.3)$$

The *Q* values range from 1 for electromagnetic and beta radiation, 10 for neutrons and 20 for α–radiation. The sievert demonstrates that equal absorbed doses do not necessarily have the same biological effect. The *Q* value for α–radiation is 20 so 1Gy of α–radiation represents 20Sv, whereas *Q* is 1 for x-, γ– and β– radiation so 1Gy of x-, γ– or β– radiation ≡ 1Sv. One sievert of α–radiation causes the same biological damage as 1Sv of x or γ–radiation. For practical purposes in radiology the gray and sievert are interchangeable since photons and β–radiation have a *Q* value of 1.

Table 21.2   Average LET for alpha, beta, gamma and x-rays and tissue penetration.

Radiation	Energy (keV)	Average LET (keV μm^{-1})	Tissue Penetration μm or HVL	Example
Alpha particles	5000	95	35	^{241}Am ^{239}Pu ^{238}U
Beta radiation	1	12.3	0.01	Recoil electrons
	10	2.3	1	^{3}H (tritium)
	100	0.42	180	^{14}Carbon
	1000	0.25	5000	^{198}Au ^{131}I
	2000	0.23	10000	85-90$^{}$Sr ^{90}Y ^{32}P
Gamma and	80	1.0	38mm	Diagnostic x-rays
x-rays	120	1.4	43mm	^{57}Co
	140	1.5	46mm	^{99m}Tc
	364	2.8	65mm	^{131}I
	511	3.5	70mm	Positron emitters
	1000	5.2	100mm	^{60}Co

function;   an event that the ICRP calls **deterministic**. Somatic or hereditary effects which may start from a single modified or transformed cell are called **stochastic** effects.

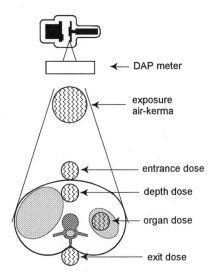

Figure 21.3 The location within the x-ray beam where dose measurements are made. The DAP meter is fixed to the x-ray housing itself.

21.2 BIOLOGICAL DAMAGE

Only a short time elapsed between the discovery of x-rays and reported cases of radiation damage from their use. The workers themselves (clinicians and technicians) who held the film cassettes in the x-ray beam noticed damage to their hands that was slow to heal. Radiation workers were also suffering from general radiation exposure which sometimes lead to cancers and early death. Relatively little radiation biology was done prior to 1940. Fundamental research in this area stemmed from the development of nuclear weapons and the present strict guidelines and controls on the use of radiation originate from that time.

Of the various forms of radiation damage the most important is that to the DNA structure. Damage to the DNA can prevent survival or reproduction of the cell but there is a repair mechanism (see later).   If sufficient cells are killed or damaged there will be loss of organ

21.2.1 Direct and indirect damage

Alpha and beta particles, being charged, lose energy by electrical interactions with the outer electrons of atoms in tissue.   Electromagnetic radiation (γ– and x-rays), being uncharged, can behave differently but both produce ionizing events.   The overall damage may be represented by:

Charged particles (ionization)
$\downarrow$
Electrical interactions
$\downarrow$
Tissue ionization
$\downarrow$
Chemical changes
$\downarrow$
BIOLOGICAL EFFECT

The nuclear protein deoxyribonucleic acid (DNA) is responsible for cell growth and cell-division and is the most important radiosensitive material in the cell. Other radio-sensitive biological molecules are RNA (ribonucleic acid), enzymes and the molecular structure of the cell wall.

DNA may be directly damaged by radiation, causing a break in the chain as shown in Fig.21.4. It can also damage the nuclear cell membrane. Indirect damage is caused by free radicals produced by irradiation of water molecules some distance from the target. Free radicals attack the protein structure of DNA and other important biological complexes by forming unstable and very reactive compounds; these are listed in Box.21.2. Direct damage (stages 1, 2 and 3 in the Box) leads to a chain of destruction involving a peroxy-radical (RO°_2 in stages 2 and 3).

physical reactions are extremely fast, measured in femto-seconds (10^{-15}), these are followed by chemical reactions whose periods are measured in pico-seconds (10^{-12}).

The biomolecular and biological cell damage appear at much slower rates, up to years afterwards, in some cases, which are considered in calculations of population risk.

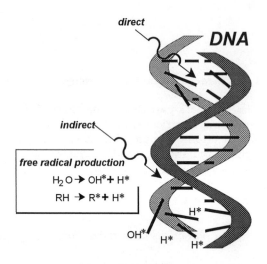

Figure 21.4 Direct damage to the chromosome nuclear material (DNA) from ionizing radiation and indirect damage from free radical production (Box 21.2).

Indirect damage occurs when a charged particle passes through atoms in the tissue transferring some of its energy to atomic electrons in the medium (mostly water) without causing direct effects on radiosensitive targets.

Water molecules, the most common constituent of tissue, enter a state of excitation, forming free radicals (H° and OH°). These are highly reactive and are responsible for indirect protein damage (stages 8 and 9). Simple ionization of the water can also occur ($H_2O \rightarrow H^+ + OH^-$). The main reactions with water are shown in stages 4 - 7. Both indirect and direct reactions can lead to self-perpetuating chain reactions.

Reaction time span Ionizing reactions in tissue can occur almost instantaneously or take place over a longer time. The extreme ranges listed in Tab.21.3 show that the initial

Box 21.2

Direct and indirect damage

Where R represents the target protein (DNA, RNA or enzyme system)

* is a radiation event

Direct Damage:
Where R = protein molecule

1) $RH^* \rightarrow R^\circ + H^\circ$
2) $R^\circ + O_2 \rightarrow RO^\circ_2$
   (Peroxy Radical)
3) $RO^\circ_2 + RH \rightarrow RO_2H + R^\circ$
   (return to start of 2)

Indirect Damage: (the radiolysis of water)

4) $H_2O^* \rightarrow H_2O^+ + e^-$
5) $H_2O + e^- \rightarrow H_2O^-$
6) $H_2O^+ \rightarrow H^+ + OH^\circ$
7) $H_2O^- \rightarrow H^\circ + OH^-$

The ions OH^- and H^+ are removed since they re-combine to form water:
$$H^+ + OH^- \rightarrow H_2O$$
H° and OH° have unpaired electron so are Free Radicals; these extract hydrogen from organic molecules:

8) $RH + OH^\circ \rightarrow R^\circ + H_2O$
9) $RH + H^\circ \rightarrow R^\circ + H_2$
(joins chain reaction in 1 above)

Level of damage The radiation harm to a living cell depends on the level of differentiation (complexity); whether a single cell, a group of cells or the whole organism. Frequency of cell division is also important. Radiation damage at the molecular and cellular levels can eventually become evident within the population. This progression is shown in Tab.21.4.

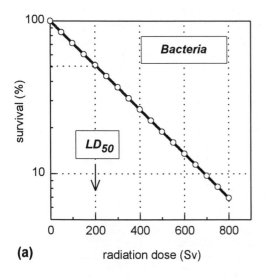

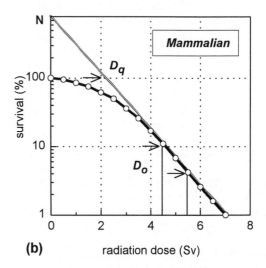

Figure 21.5   **(a)**   A simple exponential dose survival curve for haploid cells (bacteria). **(b)** Dose survival curves for diploid cells (mammalian) showing a repair 'shoulder'. D_q at point 100% and D_o, the dose reducing survival by 37%

Table 21.3   Time Span of radiation damage

Damage	Time Span	Effect
Initial	10^{-17} to 10^{-15}s	• Ionization • Excitation
Chemical	10^{-14} to 10^{-3} s	• Free radicals • Excited molecules
Biomolecular	Seconds to hours	• Protein damage • Nucleic acid split
Biological	Hours to decades	• Cell death • Malignancy • Animal death

21.2.2 Cellular response to radiation

The radiation sensitivity of a cell depends on whether it is haploid (unpaired chromosomes, e.g. bacteria) or diploid (paired chromosomes, e.g. mammalian cells).

Bacteria   The response of simple bacterial cells to radiation damage shows a single exponential relationship. (Fig.21.5(a)). This is the **dose-response or survival curve**, the survival axis is plotted on a logarithmic scale and the radiation dose on a linear scale.

The overall effect of cellular damage is measured at the point where radiation dose causes a 50% cell loss. This is the **lethal dose** for 50% death or the LD_{50} point. Bacterial cells can survive high radiation doses (hundreds of sieverts). The LD_{50} for bacteria is typically 200Sv; for viruses it is much more.

Mammalian cells   These show a more complex dose-survival response to radiation than the simple single event exponential curve shown by bacteria. It is a multi-event response (Fig.21.5(b)), where cellular repair at low radiation doses gives a shoulder to the start of the curve; this is characteristic of mammalian cells. The LD_{50} for mammalian cells show they are more radiosensitive than bacteria (less resistant to radiation damage); the LD_{50} is between 3 and 5Sv depending on the animal and cell type. From the curve certain important parameters can be identified: N, D_q and D_o.

The shape of the graph is described by reference to the two parameters N and D_O. The dimension D_O is the slope of the exponential function (a straight line on this log-linear plot) and represents the dose necessary to reduce the surviving cell fraction by $1/e$ or 0.37 (37%); D_O represents the mean lethal dose. If the exponential part of the curve is extrapolated toward the y-axis it will cross this axis at some point which is called N. This is a measure of the shoulder size of the curve. Where this line crosses the 100% survival point (arrow in Fig.21.5(b)) is the threshold dose D_q, which approximates to the sublethal radiation dose.

The radio-sensitivity of a cell or tissue affects the shoulder dimension and is proportional to its mitotic activity and inversely proportional to its state of differentiation. Rapidly dividing cell populations within an organ are most radiosensitive (bone marrow, GI mucosa); tissues with little mitotic activity (brain, muscle) are more resistant. Following a radiation exposure the radio-sensitive tissues will contain more target points and so suffer more damage than radio-resistant tissues. Table 21.5 gives radiation exposure levels and their observed effects on humans

Table 21.4 Effects on biological materials

Level of complexity	Radiation effects and damage
Molecular	Macromolecules (enzymes RNA DNA)
Sub-Cellular	Cell membrane, nucleus, chromosomes, mitochondria, lysosomes
Cellular	inhibits cell division, cell death, transformation, mutation
Tissue and Organ	Nervous system , bone marrow , intestinal tract, cancer induction
Whole individual	death, life shortening
Populations	genetic change, mutations

Table 21.5 Damage to human tissues (conversion factor Gy = R × 0.0088)

Exposure R	C kg^{-1}	Human exposure
0-25	0 - 0.0065	No effect detected
25-50	0.0065 - 0.013	Some blood changes
50-100	0.013 - 0.026	Blood changes and nausea
100-200	0.026 - 0.05	Nausea, diarrhea, life shortening
400	0.1	Death in 50% of the population in 30 days
600	0.15	100% death in 30 days
1000	0.25	Death in 2 weeks
3000	0.8	Death in 2 days

21.2.3 Organ response to radiation

A cell modified by radiation damage may transmit flawed genetic information via its DNA to other cell generations. This can cause both somatic and hereditary effects which may start from a single modified cell; this is the **stochastic** effect where radiation causes potential harm even at low doses. If enough cells in an organ or tissue are killed or prevented from functioning normally there will be a loss of organ function; this is the **determi-**

Target theory The mammalian cell survival-dose curve(s) suggest a multi-target model and the shoulder represents a repair process which becomes ineffective at higher doses. A simple multi-target model can be represented by incorporating the parameters N and D_o into an equation describing the surviving fraction s after a dose D:

$$s = 1-(1-e^{D/Do})^N \qquad (21.4)$$

nistic effect where there is a threshold dose (Fig.21.6(a)) below which these effects are not seen (e.g. cataracts and erythemas); a linear response region may still exist. These two radiation effects are illustrated in Fig.21.6(a) where stochastic describes a linear relationship showing no lower limit or threshold to radiation damage; breast cancer and leukemia would be examples.

These effects are a valuable guide to personnel radiation protection recommendations indicating maximum permissible radiation doses. Radiation protection measures aim to prevent deterministic (non-stochastic) effects and reduce the probability of stochastic effects to acceptable levels. Deterministic effects are shown where a loss of tissue function is seen at doses of a few hundred mSv (100mSv = 10rem). These are characterized by a dose-frequency relationship for which a dose threshold exists.

Table 21.6   Deterministic thresholds Sv for acute tissue (H_T) and chronic whole body (E) exposure.

Tissue and effect	Brief exposure H_T	Long exposure $E\,y^{-1}$
Gonads		
Testes:		
Temporary	0.15	0.4
Permanent		
sterility	3.5-6.0	2.0
Ovaries:		
Sterility	>2.5	>0.2
Lens		
opacities	2–10	>0.1
cataract	>2.0	>0.15
Bone marrow		
hematopoesis	>0.5	>0.4

In order to produce a scheme for radiation protection it is necessary to know the probability of stochastic effects for a certain radiation dose (**risk estimates**). For healthy workers the probability for deterministic effects will be zero for doses up to hundreds of milli-sieverts but will increase steeply above this threshold. Table 21.6 lists some estimated dose levels for deterministic effects taken from ICRP60.

21.2.4   Population response to radiation

The response by human beings to low doses of radiation has been the subject of much study. Most hard evidence about radiation damage to human populations comes from high exposure rates (Japanese bomb survivors, therapy data, etc.) and estimated damage from low exposure rates is obtained by extrapolation from these high-dose data points. This provides much controversy and several theories exist which attempt to predict radiation damage to populations exposed to lower dose levels. The three possible curve shapes that can represent population dose responses are shown in Fig.21.6(b).

Linear   This is the simplest response. Radiation induced breast cancer is an example of a disease showing a linear dose relationship. Radiation protection standards take a linear response as their reference so that low dose responses can be simply calculated from high dose data. i.e.

- 1000 people exposed to 1Sv (100 rem) show an increased cancer incidence of 20 cases.
- 10,000 people exposed to 100mSv or 100,000 exposed to 10mSv would show the same incidence.

Quadratic   this is proposed for describing the reduced damage shown by certain tissues (skin) to low radiation levels.

Linear quadratic is an combined linear and quadratic model which takes into consideration the repair mechanism shown by diploid cells (Fig.21.6(b)). which would not be included in a purely linear model. Leukemia induction is an example of a disease showing a linear-quadratic dose response.

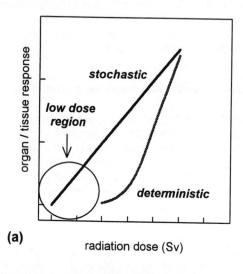
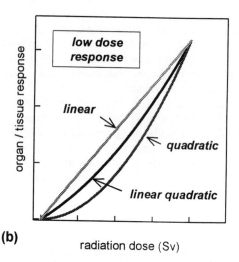

Figure 21.6   **(a)**   A stochastic effect with organ or tissue response at all dose levels. A deterministic response is seen when the dose reaches a certain threshold. **(b)** Three probable types of low-dose stochastic response. Linear and two non-linear models: quadratic and linear-quadratic.

21.2.5 Somatic and genetic effects

Radiation can damage both body tissues causing somatic effects seen mainly as carcinogenesis in individuals or populations, or affect his/her offspring causing genetic effects which are hereditary defects seen in populations.

Somatic cell damage This is the damage that is apparent during the life-time of the organism, exclusive of effects on the reproductive system. Somatic cells include all cells except gametes. A great variety of changes can be seen, some temporary and others permanent, the latter often leading to cell death.

Somatic cells most commonly survive low radiation dose rates since the damage at molecular and sub-cellular levels is mostly repaired.   Somatic damage could result in leukemia, breast cancer and other adult carcinomas in individuals and populations. Non-carcinoma damage, for instance cataract or pulmonary fibrosis, is seen in people exposed to local high radiation levels. Somatic effects occur mainly as a result of acute (short time-span) doses from atomic weapons or therapy. Chronic radiation exposure data from large populations in USA and China have failed to show any unequivocal evidence that high natural background radiation levels increase the incidence of somatic or genetic effects.

Radiologists prior to 1921, exposed continuously to quite high levels of soft (low-energy) radiation, were seen to have an increased cancer mortality.   This is not seen in present day radiologists owing to safer equipment and decreased radiation exposures; indeed they may illustrate a 'healthy worker syndrome' as they have a lower incidence of cancer than the general population.

Somatic changes are seen in radiation sensitive adult tissues having high proliferation rates, for instance bone marrow, breast and

GI mucosa. Less damage is done to slowly proliferating cells as in the adult central nervous system. Somatic damage is most dangerous at the embryo and fetus stages where cells have multiple descendants.

Inhibition of cell division by radiation mostly leads to cell death but some radiation damage causes cell transformation where normal cell functions are altered and carcinogenesis initiated. Soft radiation (UV, electrons), or soft (low energy) x-rays give a high surface dose and these would promote skin cancer.

The small incidence of **radiogenic** cancer that may be present in a population is indistinguishable from naturally occurring cancers (leukemia, breast, sarcoma, lung) and since the natural cancer rate is about 16% per 100,000 (16000 deaths) the effect of low level radiation on the population (cancer incidence) is almost impossible to detect with statistical confidence.

Germ cell damage The influence of radiation on the gonads (testes or ovaries) can lead to inherited malfunction. Damage to reproductive cells (gametes) may be heritable, and could cause an abnormally functioning genotype, i.e. genetic effects. Most concern was initially focused on genetic damage to populations from radiation. Careful observation over a long period of time however has not established any trend in populations exposed to high levels of radiation (atomic bomb survivors and areas of high natural radiation) so inherited damage has been down-rated as a serious threat.

Genetically significant dose GSD This is a measure of genetic hazard to the population from radiation exposure, particularly medical radiation, and assumes a linear dose-effect relationship.

If the mean gonad dose to patients undergoing radiological examinations (between 0.5mGy and 20mGy) is received by every member of the population it would be expected to produce the same total genetic effect on the general population. So if 10% of the population received ×10 the mean gonad dose the effect would be the same as the total population receiving just the mean dose. If, for instance, the average gonad radiation dose to a relatively small exposed patient population is about 10mGy then the GSD adjusts this to give the same relative hazard to the entire population. The genetically significant dose (GSD) also takes into consideration the child bearing potential of the patient population. It is derived as:

$$SD = \frac{\sum\left[N_{xy}P_{xy}D_{xy}\right]_m + \sum\left[N_{xy}P_{xy}D_{xy}\right]_f}{\sum N_x P_x} \quad (21.5)$$

Where

N_{xy} : The number of patients in age groups x undergoing patient examination y

P_{xy} : The child expectancy for persons in age group x undergoing examination y

D_{xy} : The average gonad dose for patients in age group x undergoing examination y

N_x : The number of persons of age group x in the population.

P_x : The child expectancy for age group x.

The subscripts m and f denote male and female groups.

The GSD value has steadily declined over the years. However there are differences between countries depending on the frequency of radiological examinations and techniques used in the different age groups:

Sweden	0.46mGy
Germany	0.41mGy
USA	0.20mGy
Japan	0.17mGy
UK	0.12mGy.

The genetic effects of low dose rates are exceedingly rare compared to the natural mutation rate. The current incidence of genetic linked disease is 10% of the population.

21.3 NATURAL AND MAN-MADE RADIATION

Background radiation both natural and man-made is a consistent source of low exposure to all members of the population. Some areas of very high natural background levels (up to 100mSv per year in Kerala, India and some regions of Brazil) have served as benchmarks for studying population low dose exposure. The general population is exposed to a variety of natural and man-made radiation sources. These are listed in Table.21.7 for a typical location and represented as a pie chart in Fig.21.7.   The US values tend to be higher for radon (up to 55%) with proportionally less internal, external and cosmic; the medical percentage is about the same but is seen to be increasing generally in the western world.

sign. A radon concentration of 200Bq m^{-3} is currently considered a suitable limit.

A large variation in population dose arises from radon exposure and in some instances (hard rock areas i.e. granite) this can be responsible for an individual annual dose of up to 100mSv. Data on population exposure from all sources of radiation in most countries give an overall whole body dose of   2.5-4mSv. About 85% comes from natural sources, half of this from radon exposure in the home.

Table 21.7   Typical proportions of natural and man-made radiation in Europe (whole body dose)

Source	Dose (μSv)	%
Natural radiation		
Cosmic radiation (solar activity)	310	13
Terrestrial gamma radiation (Soils, rock, water)	380	16
Radon decay products (houses and work area)	800	33
Internal radiation (^{40}K, ^{14}C, etc.)	370	15
Total natural exposure	1860	78%
Man made radiation		
Medical procedures	500	21
Weapons fall out	10	0.4
Nuclear power	3	0.15
Occupational	9	0.36
Air-travel	8	0.34
Total man-made	530	22%
Natural and man-made	2390	100%

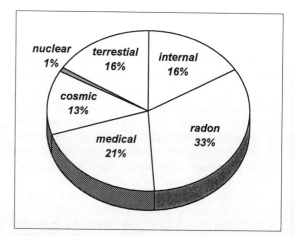

Figure 21.7   Components of natural and man-made population exposure in the UK. The total dose range is between 3-10mSv. The small sector represents exposure from nuclear products which is <1%.

21.3.1 Natural radiation

The largest contributing factor to population exposure from natural radiation comes from radon gas (^{222}Rn), a decay product of uranium, a natural component of most soils and rocks. The exposure to other natural radiation sources normally cannot be altered but radon exposure is influenced by building de-

21.3.2 Man-made radiation

Background radiation acts as a reasonable benchmark for judging staff and patient radiation doses from medical exposures. Medical exposure accounts for a population dose of typically 20% of the total man-made radiation; nuclear discharges (in spite of popular misconception) add only a further 1%. Doses from individual medical exposures can range from 0.2mSv for a chest radiograph to 10 or 20mSv for extensive fluoroscopy.

21.4 RISK ESTIMATES

The slight increase in the incidence of cancer following irradiation can only be detected by studying large populations. It is from these studies that risk estimates are made. The largest set of data comes from the health records of atomic bomb survivors who lived in Hiroshima and Nagasaki and radiation risks for medical workers are estimated from this comprehensive information. Box 21.3 gives a worked example of risk estimation showing that cancer induced from low radiation levels is almost impossible to detect within the high natural cancer incidence.

The two reports from the International Commission on Radiological Protection **ICRP** which have most influenced radiation dosimetry are ICRP26 (1977) and ICRP60 (1990). ICRP26 is based on the early risk estimates from the original atomic bomb survivor data (T65DR 'old' dosimetry). These data were reassessed during the 1980's, in the light of fresh information concerning the type and mixture of radiation given by the two nuclear explosions (DS86 'new' dosimetry). Based on the findings of DS86 the cancer risk associated with radiation was increased by about ×2 and recommendations to this effect were published in ICRP60. The new calculations were necessary because the contribution from neutron radiation to the total population exposure was far less than originally thought. This increased the emphasis on gamma exposure and consequently the risk associated with gamma radiation were scaled upwards. There is still controversy over the neutron : gamma mix so ideas and recommendations may undergo more change. Although the new evidence has increased somatic risk the radiation risk associated with gonad exposure and hereditary defects has been derated.

21.4.1 Risk comparisons

The population is exposed to many risks. Some carry a beneficial component (car or air-travel), others do not (e.g. aging). Table 21.8

compares a variety of radiation and non-radiation risks to the population. The risks are expressed as a 'risk-ratio' : 1.0×10^{-2} or 1 in 100 (1:100).

Table 21.8 A comparison of fatal risks

Event	Risk	Risk ratio
Anesthetic Death	40×10^{-6}	1 : 25000
Car Driver (10000 miles)	200×10^{-6}	1 : 5000
Age 55 years	10000×10^{-6}	1 : 100
1 mSv exposure	10×10^{-6}	1 : 100000
50mSv exposure	1.5×10^{-3}	1 : 700

Radiation risks are usually standardized for a 1 Sievert exposure. Risks for exposure levels less than this are derated linearly, demonstrated and calculated in Box 21.3.

Box 21.3

Radiation induced cancer risk

The risk for radiation induced cancer in 100,000 people exposed to 1Sv would be 1250

$$(1.25 \times 10^{-2} \text{ Sv}^{-1} \text{ or } 1:80)$$

For a lower dose of 1mSv this would be 1.25 for 100,000 people exposed

$$(\sim 1 \times 10^{-5} \text{ mSv}^{-1} \text{ or } 1:100,000)$$

This has been revised by ICRP60 and the risk for a 1mSv exposure is now:

$$3.0 \times 10^{-5} \text{ mSv}^{-1} \text{ (1:33000)}$$

21.4.2   Calculation of risks

If an irradiated group of people are studied (radiotherapy patients, atomic bomb survivors etc.) and the radiation doses that they have received are known with a fair precision then if the number of cancers exceeds the number that would be expected (calculated from an identical unexposed population) then the excess number of cancers may be attributable to radiation effects and the risk of cancer per unit dose can be estimated. This is the risk factor and these form the basis of all radiation protection directives. There is a great deal of uncertainty in these calculations since the radiation dose to the population is not known accurately and the unexposed control is hardly ever identical to the exposed group. Box 21.4 calculates cancer induction from low dose levels and illustrates how difficult it would be to detect this cancer increase in a population.

Box 21.4

Risk assessment

500,000 people are irradiated and receive 15mSv whole body irradiation. They show 4 more cancers than normal:

$$\text{Risk Factor} = \frac{\text{increased cancer incidence}}{\text{population} \times \text{dose}}$$

$$= \frac{4}{500000 \times 0.015} = 5.3 \times 10^{-4}$$

$$\sim 1 \text{ in } 2000$$

Since there is a spontaneous cancer incidence of about 1600 per 10,000 of the population there would be an expected cancer rate of 80,000 in 500,000 people. A population dose of 15mSv would add 250 to this total and would be well hidden by the statistical fluctuation.

Estimation of acceptable risk   For the purpose of dosimetry a risk can be:

- Unacceptable: which would unreasonably increase harm to a population.
- Not-unacceptable: where the small level of increased harm is balanced by a great deal of benefit.

An increase in perceived somatic risks has placed more restrictive limits on worker and public exposure levels; these recent risk estimates are listed in Table 21.9.

Table 21.9   Risk Estimates (ICRP60)

Risk	Risk estimate	
Exposure at 50mSv	1.5×10^{-3}	(1 in 700)
Workers annual risk		
Unacceptable	10^{-2}	(1 in 100)
Not unacceptable	10^{-3}	(1 in 1000)
Exposure at 15mSv	5.0×10^{-4}	(1 in 2000)
Public risk		
Unacceptable	10^{-4}	(1 in 10,000)
Probably acceptable	10^{-5}	(1 in 100,000)
Exposure 1mSv	3.0×10^{-5}	(1 in 33,000)
Exposure 0.5mSv	1.4×10^{-5}	(1 in 70,000)

The re-evaluation of the Japanese data suggests a fatal risk of ~ 3 in 100,000 mSv^{-1} or $\sim 1: 33,000 \text{ mSv}^{-1}$ (previously 1 in 100,000)

The new data suggested that members of the public exposed to 1mSv had a new risk estimate of 1 in 33,000 which was thought to be unacceptable, so the recommended maximum public exposure was lowered to 0.5mSv, decreasing the perceived risk to 1 in 70,000.

Nominal risk coefficients   Since there is still uncertainty in the risk estimates given in ICRP60 the probability of a fatal cancer was renamed the nominal risk coefficient (nominal: not real or actual). The nominal life-time cancer risk coefficient for an adult is:

$$4 \times 10^{-2} \text{ Sv}^{-1} \ (1{:}25) \ (1{:}25000 \text{ mSv}^{-1})$$

and for the whole population:

$$5\times10^{-2} \text{ Sv}^{-1} \text{ (1:20) (1:20000 mSv}^{-1})$$

The nominal hereditary coefficient is much smaller:

$$1\times10^{-2} \text{ Sv}^{-1} \text{ (1:100) (1:100,000 mSv}^{-1})$$

Risk limit This is now analogous to the dose limit. The recommended long term dose limit for occupational exposure is:

$$\sim 8\times10^{-4} \text{ (1:1300 } \approx 25\text{mSv per year)}$$

and for the public:

$$\sim 3\times10^{-5} \text{ (1:33,000 } \approx 1\text{mSv per year).}$$

These are maximum values. By practicing the ALARA principle, a typical diagnostic department can achieve 1.5×10^{-4} (1:7000 $\approx$ 5mSv) for workers (technicians and radiologists) and 1.5×10^{-5} (1:70000 $\approx$ 0.5mSv) for the public (non-radiation workers). Table 21.10 summarizes the risk estimates associated with radiation dose limits.

Table 21.10 Summary of risks for various doses

Acceptable risk	Annual exposure (mSv)	Risk
Worker		
1:1000		
	50	1.5×10^{-3} (1:700)
	25	7.5×10^{-4} (1:1333)
	20	6.0×10^{-4} (1:1666)
	15	5.0×10^{-4} (1:2000)
Public		
1:100000		
	5	1.6×10^{-4} (1:6000)
	1	3.0×10^{-5} (1:33333)
	0.5	1.4×10^{-5} (1:70000)

Risks to the fetus Current information indicates that radiation risks to the developing fetus are small from diagnostic radiology. The probabilities, given in Table 21.11, are for developing cancer or an organ malfunction in later childhood. The natural incidence of these abnormalities in the western world is 4.07% or approximately 1 in 25 live births. This incidence is hardly influenced even with an exposure of 10mSv which would represent a fairly extensive abdominal x-ray investigation.

The risk of cancer induction in children from high level exposure *in-utero* is $\sim6\times10^{-2}$ Sv^{-1} (1:17); half these cases are expected to be fatal. There is also a risk of adult cancers originating from fetal exposure. There is a deterministic (non-stochastic) threshold of between 200-400mGy for severe mental retardation resulting from fetal exposure.

Table 21.11 Added risk to fetus from radiation

mSv	No Abnormality	Increased Risk
0.0	95.930%	0.0
0.5	95.928%	0.002
1.0	95.922%	0.008
2.5	95.910%	0.02
5.0	95.880%	0.05
10.0	95.830%	0.10

Cumulative Risk The risk of damage to the gonads or fetus during diagnostic investigations are cumulative and patients who are undergoing successive investigations during diagnosis and follow-up will increase their risk of radiation damage to $\sim1\times10^{-2}$ (1:100). This is obviously more serious in young patients under going repeat investigations and the level of risk must be justified by clinical benefit. The reduction of patient radiation exposure in diagnostic radiology is the prime responsibility of radiology staff since there are real risks to young patients and the population as a whole.

Dose rate effectiveness factor (DREF) This has been introduced so that high-dose tissue responses, obtained from measurements, can be used to estimate low-dose effects which cannot be easily measured. The DREF allows for the enhanced effect seen at high dose rates (Japanese bomb survivors) so that risks for lower dose exposure can be derived.

A DREF value between 2 and 4 is commonly

used as a divisor. A cancer mortality of: 2.5×10^{-2} Sv^{-1}(1:40) seen in bomb survivors, is reduced to 1.25×10^{-2} Sv^{-1}(1:80) (DREF value of 2). There is considerable debate concerning the proper choice of DREF for human risk calculations.

The latent period The **reaction time span** (21.3) already describes the delay between radiation exposure and its effect (cancer or tissue damage). The time delay is the latent period. The latent period for leukemia is shorter than for other cancers; a minimum time of 2 years and a peak incidence at 8 years following high radiation doses. For other cancers 10 years and 15 years are typical minimal latent periods. Cancer risk can persist for a further 40 or more years.

KEYWORDS

absorbed dose - the ratio of energy absorbed by a volume of tissue. The unit is the gray (Gy).

air-kerma - the energy released from all ionizing events in a volume of air. The unit is C kg^{-1} or Gy.

air-kerma rate - measured as μGy mAs^{-1}.

ALI - annual limits on intake for internal exposure based on committed effective dose of 20mSv.

deterministic - loss of organ function due to many cell damage. Deterministic effects have a threshold below which no effect is seen.

diploid - relates to cells having a double set of chromosomes, usually relates to all mammalian cells except gametes.
D$_o$ - the dose that gives (on average) one lethal event per cell reducing survival to 37% of its previous value.

dose equivalent (H$_T$) - the product of the absorbed dose in tissue and quality factor.

Measured in rem (non-SI) and sievert (SI).

DREF - dose rate effectiveness factor corrects for extrapolation from high to low dose effects.

exposure - measured in roentgen (R) or air-kerma.

free radical - a chemical compound containing an unpaired electron.

germ cell - pertaining to the gametes: sperm, ovum or a cell from which they originate.

gray (Gy) - a measure of absorbed dose 1J kg^{-1}

haploid - relates to single stranded DNA cells: bacteria and gametes.

hereditary - affecting future generations.

LD$_{50}$ - the lethal dose for 50% cell or population death

linear energy transfer LET - a measure of the density of ionizing events along a radiation path as keV μm^{-1}

quality factor Q or w_R - a dimensionless value used for weighting absorbed dose according to the radiation's biological effect. Now called the radiation weighting factor w_R.

radiation weighting factor (w_R) - as listed in Tab. 22.1 from ICRP60. (see quality factor above)

röntgen (R) - 2.58×10^{-4} coulombs kg^{-1} of air.

sievert (Sv) - A measure of dose equivalent. gray × Q or w_R.

somatic - pertaining to all cells except reproductive cells
stochastic - somatic or hereditary effects which may start from a single cell. There is no threshold.

tissue weighting factor - (w_T) as listed in Tab. 22.3 from ICRP60.

Radiation protection : Clinical practice

22.1 Dosimetric quantities

22.2 Staff radiation exposure

22.3 Patient radiation exposure

22.4 Hospital radiation protection

22.5 The x-ray room

22.1 DOSIMETRIC QUANTITIES

X-radiation, and to some extent gamma radiation, undergo three interactions which are important to diagnostic radiology:

1. **Transmission** through tissue, the fluence variations carrying information that forms the image.
2. **Absorption** by the tissue, influencing image contrast but also causing radiation damage to the patient.
3. **Scatter** within the tissue, spoiling image contrast, increasing patient radiation exposure and contributing to staff radiation exposure.

All three can be optimized by employing the most efficient imaging equipment (fast film-screens or digital imaging) and scatter minimized by careful preparation.

The aims of radiation protection is to provide an adequate standard of safety for workers without unduly limiting its beneficial use as a clinical tool, both diagnostic and therapeutic. The dose restrictions currently applied to the workplace are sufficient to avoid deterministic effects and ensure that ionizing radiation remains a minor risk in the hospital.

22.1.1 Organ and tissue dose

There are two dose quantities for describing energy deposited in a tissue and distinguishing the effects of different radiation on tissue:

- the absorbed dose, measured in grays
- the equivalent dose, measured in sieverts

Both describe radiation damage to individual organs or tissues

Absorbed dose The definition of exposure given in eqn.21.1 measuring the quantity of electric charge (C kg^{-1}) produced by ionizing radiation is not the same as the energy absorbed by tissue although they are proportional. Absorbed dose is the ratio of energy absorbed by a unit mass measured as J kg^{-1}. This is a fundamental quantity in radiation protection and is called the gray (Gy) normally describing average dose to an organ or tissue.

Radiation weighting factors w_R The basic units for air-kerma, LET and absorbed dose do not allow for factors which differentiate the type of radiation. The probability of tissue radiation damage depends not only on the absorbed dose (Gy) but also on the type and energy of the radiation. The effect of radiation type (α–, β–, γ or x-radiation) is introduced as a radiation weighting factor w_R formally called quality factor. The absorbed dose must be weighted to take account of the nature of the radiation. The factor is selected for the type and energy of the radiation incident on the body, or emitted by a source within the body.

The value of the radiation weighting factor has been selected by the ICRP to be representative of the relative biological effectiveness for inducing stochastic effects at low doses. The values of w_R are broadly compatible with the quality factor Q which are related to the LET.

Table 22.1 Radiation weighting factors w_R

Type and energy range	w_R
X- and gamma-rays	1
Electrons and betas	1
Neutrons	5-20
Alphas and fission fragments	20

Equivalent dose (H_T) This is the absorbed dose averaged over a tissue or organ and weighted according to the radiation type (w_R in Tab.22.1). In previous ICRP publications the weighting factor referred to as the quality factor (Q) has been applied to the absorbed dose at a point and not over the organ as a whole; this was the dose equivalent (restating eqn.21.3) as $Gy \times w_R$ measured in sieverts (Sv). It has now been replaced by the average dose for the organ or tissue: the **equivalent dose** H_T which is the equivalent dose in tissue T for an absorbed dose D_T from a radiation having a weighting factor w_R:

$$H_T = \sum D_T \cdot w_R \quad \text{(Sv)} \quad (22.1)$$

The equivalent dose is measured in sieverts (Sv) and forms the foundation unit for other parameters in radiation protection.

Some variations on the basic equivalent dose term are defined in Tab.22.2 taking account of **deep** and **shallow** doses. ICRP60 considers these other quantities describing them as individual dose equivalent (penetrating or deep dose) and individual dose equivalent (superficial or shallow dose). A further quantity expressed as an eye dose equivalent is sometimes used.

The equivalent dose measurement does not consider the different radio-sensitivities of each tissue or organ so a further tissue weighting factor w_T is used which allows for the different radio-sensitivities of the various organs and tissues.

Table 22.2 Equivalent dose variants

Variant	Definition
Shallow dose equivalent H_s	Skin or extremity; 0.07mm tissue depth ($7mg\ cm^{-2}$)
Deep dose equivalent H_d	Whole body; 10mm tissue depth ($1000\ mg\ cm^{-2}$)
Eye dose equivalent	Dose equivalent to eye lens; 3mm tissue depth ($300mg\ cm^{-2}$)

21.1.2 The whole body dose

Equivalent dose H_T enables individual organ or tissue radiation exposure to be described independent of radiation type using weighting factors w_R. However each tissue has a different radio-sensitivity and in order to recognize these different sensitivities (e.g. for breast, lung, bone etc.) a tissue weighting factor w_T is used, which represents the risk of stochastic effects resulting from irradiation of that organ or tissue as a total risk figure for stochastic effects if the whole body had been irradiated uniformly.

Table 22.3 lists the radio-sensitivity of organs defined by tissue weighting factors w_T. The radiation referred to is that incident on the body or emitted by a source within the body. The values of w_T are used for calculating the **effective dose E or effective dose equivalent (EDE)**.

Tissue weighting factors (w_T) Values for w_T listed in Tab.22.3 have been obtained from a representative population (wide age range and both sexes). The values which range from 0.01 for the skin up to 0.2 for the gonads. The weighting factors listed have been estimated for important tissues. For purposes of calculation the remainder consists of adrenals, brain, intestine, uterus and other separate organs. The dose equivalent in the remainder is the estimated mean dose equivalent over the whole body excluding the specified tissues.

The values have changed from their introduction in ICRP26 (1977) to revised values in ICRP60 (1989). The list includes those organs that are likely to be selectively irradiated and some of these organs are known to be susceptible to cancer induction. As more investigations are made and other tissues more closely investigated, and their radiosensitivity identified, they may also be included in later lists for w_T. Both w_R and w_T may change from time to time as new evidence is obtained, so derived quantities that rely on these parameters may also change. This is the case for previous values of w_T published in ICRP26 (1977) which were reviewed giving the revised figures published in ICRP60 (1990).

Table 22.3 Weighting factors w_T (ICRP60)

Tissue or organ	w_T
Gonads	0.20
Bone marrow (red)	0.12
Colon	0.12
Lung	0.12
Stomach	0.12
Bladder	0.05
Breast	0.05
Liver	0.05
Esophagus	0.05
Thyroid	0.05
Skin	0.01
Bone surface	0.01
Remainder	0.05
Whole body	1.0

Effective dose (E) or effective dose equivalent (EDE) This is a quantity which describes the dose to the whole body and is derived from the equivalent dose. This quantity expresses the overall measure of health detriment associated with each irradiated tissue or organ as a whole body dose and considers the radio-sensitivity of each irradiated organ or tissue. Both equivalent dose (for a single tissue or organ) and effective dose (for the whole body) are quantities intended for radiological protection use, providing a method for estimating the probability of stochastic effects at low doses.

If the risks per equivalent dose for the various exposed tissues of the body ($H_T \times w_T$) are summed, a value is obtained for the overall risk per Sv of irradiating the whole body (defined in Tab.22.4). This sum is the effective dose E, and represents the summed organ or tissue doses as an overall whole body dose:

$$E = \sum H_T \cdot w_T \qquad (22.2)$$

Using the figure obtained from effective dose a radiation burden to the individual can be compared between various patient investigations, for instance a whole body dose from a nuclear medicine bone scan and a chest radiograph. In both cases the patient dose can be compared as the same effective whole body dose E using eqn.22.2.

As a simple example, a chest radiograph having a measured organ dose of 0.2mSv and a w_T of 0.12 (from Tab.22.3) would represent a whole body dose equivalent of 0.2×0.12 or 0.024mSv. Box 22.1 calculates E from eqn. 22.2 for a nuclear medicine study and a chest radiograph involving multiple organs. The weighted sensitivities listed in Tab.22.3 relate to a reference population of equal numbers of both sexes and a wide range of ages.

22.1.3 Accumulated dose

If a person is subjected to a radiation burden over a period of time then **committed** dose quantities are used. The time integral for the equivalent dose is the **committed equivalent dose** $H_{T(\tau)}$. If τ is not specified then it is assumed the dose is received over a 50 year period (70 years for children). Similarly the **committed effective dose** E_τ is accumulated over a defined time period τ. This would describe long-term x-ray exposures in a radiology department to a member of staff where the time period is defined.

The U.S. Nuclear Regulatory Commission (NRC) defines very similar quantities to ICRP. The committed dose equivalent ($H_{T.50}$) is the dose equivalent to organs or tissues during a 50 year period. Similarly committed effective dose equivalent ($H_{E.50}$) is $\sum H_{T.50} \cdot w_T$. The NRC also defines the **total effective dose equivalent** (TEDE) as the sum of the **deep dose** H_d for external radiation (Tab. 22.2) and **committed effective dose equivalent** $H_{E.50}$ for internal radiation exposure (Table 22.4).

22.1.4 Population dose

For the purposes of assessing the overall effect of radiation dose on a large group of people or entire populations the individual equivalent or effective doses described in the previous section are multiplied by the population number exposed. This gives a collective dose figure. Overall increases or reductions in dose to the population can then be assessed and, in some instances, a financial costing given to attempts at exposure reduction.

Collective effective dose (S) This is the whole body exposure to a **population group** exposed to radioactive materials in the environment and can cover successive generations of the population being studied. An example of collective effective dose using this measurement would be a community of 40,000 people receiving 2mSv and another 20,000 who receive 4mSv. The collective dose in each case is 80 man-sieverts (population × dose) which on present estimates would result in one radiation induced cancer. Incidentally the expected natural cancer incidence in a normal population of 40,000 would be 6,400. so the effects of this low radiation dose could not be distinguished.

The UK population of 60 million people who receive approximately 2mSv background radiation have a collective dose of 120,000 man-Sv. On the above estimate this would result in 1500 radiation induced cancers over a period

Table 22.4 Individual dosimetric terms

Measure	Unit	Derivation	Application
1. Absorbed dose D	gray	Energy/mass $J\,kg^{-1}$	Average dose to organ
2. Equivalent dose H_T	sievert (rem)	$H_T = \sum D_T \cdot w_R$	Radiation dose independent of radiation type
3. Effective dose E (Effective dose equivalent: EDE)	sievert	$E = \sum H_T \cdot w_T$	Whole body dose (see Box 22.1)
4. Committed equivalent dose $H_{T(\tau)}$	sievert	$H_{T(\tau)} = H_T \times \tau$	Equivalent dose H_T to single organ over stated time τ
5. Committed effective dose $E_{(\tau)}$	sievert	$E_{(\tau)} = E \times \tau$	Effective dose to whole body over stated time τ
6. Collective effective dose S	man-sievert	Population × E $S = E_{(\tau)} \times N$	Dose to the whole body for a population

of time (road deaths 6000 per year).

The United States population of 240 million people exposed to a similar background would have a collective dose of 480,000 man-sieverts giving 6000 radiation induced cancers (44,500 road deaths in 1990).

Box 22.1

Effective dose equivalents E

Nuclear Medicine
Nuclear Medicine Bone investigation where 700MBq (20mCi) ^{99m}Tc-MDP is estimated to give the following dose equivalents:

Organ	Dose	w_T
Bone Marrow	11mSv	0.12
Bone Surface	16mSv	0.01
Bladder	68mSv	0.05
Gonads	4mSv	0.2

The effective dose $E = \sum H_T \times w_T$
$= (11 \times 0.12) + (16 \times 0.01) + (68 \times 0.05) + (4 \times 0.2)$
$= 5.68mSv.$

Radiology
A high voltage chest x-ray gives the following doses:

Organ	dose	w_T
Breast	0.05mSv	0.05
Lung	0.15mSv	0.12
Bone Marrow	0.01mSv	0.12
Stomach	0.05mSv	0.12

$E = \sum H_T \times w_T = 0.0217mSv$

22.2 STAFF RADIATION EXPOSURE

The simple reduction of intensity from an isotropic source obeys the inverse square law, which was derived in Chapter 1, which is:

$$I_d \propto \frac{1}{d^2} \quad \text{or} \quad I_d = \frac{I_0}{d^2} \qquad (22.3)$$

where I_0 is the intensity of the source and I_d the intensity at distance d. However a more common problem in radiology is for an intensity to be given at a reference distance d and the intensity to be calculated for another new distance d_n. If the new intensity is I_{dn} then

eqn.22.3 can be restated as:

$$I_{dn} = \frac{I_0}{d_n^{\,2}} \qquad (22.4)$$

Rearranging eqns 22.3 and 22.4 yields intensities $I_0 = I_d \times d^2$ and $I_0 = I_{dn} \times d_n^2$ which together give:

$$I_{dn} = \frac{I_d \times d^2}{d_n^{\,2}} \qquad (22.5)$$

Examples using this formula for problems commonly encountered in radiological protection are given in Box.22.2

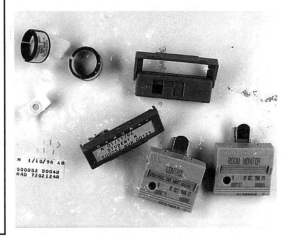

Figure 22.1   A selection of film and TLD radiation monitoring badges.

22.2.1 Radiation monitoring

Radiation doses to designated workers are monitored on a regular basis by means of dosimeter badges which integrate the worker's radiation dose over a fixed period of time, usually one month, but could be over a shorter period (2 weeks for pregnant staff as mentioned) or longer (2 months for occasional exposure i.e. ancillary staff). There are three methods available for monitoring radiation:

1. Film (film badge dosimeters).
2. Thermoluminescent dosimeters
3. (TLD badges).
4. Direct readout electronic monitors.

Personal dosimeter Film was the earliest form of radiation dosimeter. Commercially available film dosimeter badges have a sensitivity of 0.1mSv over 1 month. Thermolunescent dosimeters are also commonly used based on lithium fluoride; they have a similar sensitivity. The design of these two dosimeters is itemized in Tab.22.5 and a selection shown in Fig.22.1.

TLDs are more versatile than film dosimeters since they can be manufactured in smaller dimensions, providing extremity readings (finger doses) as well as the usual whole body dose. They are however more expensive than film and need an expensive reading device. The fluorescent material lithium fluoride (LiF) used in badges has a sensitivity slightly higher than film at 0.08mSv. It also has a radiation absorption close to tissue; it is **tissue equivalent**.

Box 22.2

Radiation exposure and distance

Example 1

The dose at 60cm from an x-ray tube is 250µGy, the dose rate at 75cm using eqn.22.5:

$$I_{dn} = \frac{I_d \times d^2}{d_n^{\,2}} = \frac{250 \times 60^2}{75^2} = 160\mu Gy$$

Example 2

The measured dose at 60cm for a mammogram tube is 250µGy. What is the dose during a magnification view at 50cm? $I_{dn} = 360\mu Gy$

Example 3 (rearranging eqn. 22.5)

The distance limit can be found which reduces a dose rate of 1000µSv h^{-1} at 30cm from a radioactive source to 7.5µSv h^{-1} . This is:

$$d_n^{\,2} = \frac{I_d \times d^2}{I_{dn}} = \frac{1000 \times 30^2}{7.5} = 346cm$$

Electronic monitors Electronic pocket dosimeters are expensive but give immediate readout of radiation doses being received. Their accuracy is low being typically ±20% up to 500mSv h^{-1}. The detector used in older models was a small calibrated Geiger tube but more recently PIN semiconductor diodes have been used complete with energy filters. They are able to measure deep and shallow dose and can store their readings in an on-board memory for subsequent readout. An example of a particular model is shown in Fig.22.2. Dose range displayed is typically 1µSv to 1000mSv and their response is from 20keV to 1.5MeV. Overall accuracy ranges from ±10 to ±20%.

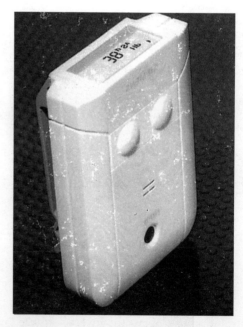

Figure 22.2 An electronic dosimeter capable of storing dose information (courtesy Siemens Inc.)

A staff-dose record from a personal dosimeter system should be kept for archive purposes (data-base) extending many years so a radiation exposure history is available. Staff who change jobs are required to carry a record of their radiation exposure with them so continuity of exposure record is maintained.

Table 22.5 Dosimeter properties

Film	Attenuation	Measures
Window	None	All radiation
Thin Plastic	Low β	High energy β
Thick Plastic	β–, low γ–	Low energy x-rays
Dural	β–, x-rays	High energy x-rays and low γ
Cd-Pb	β–, x- rays some γ	Slow neutrons
Sn-Pb	β–, x-ray	Uniform response to γ

TLD	Filtration	Estimation
Open window	none	skin dose
Thick plastic	700mg cm^{-2}	whole body dose.

In summary film dosimeters have the following points:

Advantages	Disadvantages
• Cheap	• Not tissue equivalent
• Wide range of intensities	• Long delay before result (~1 month)
• Mixed doses identifiable	• Interpretation difficult
• Robust detector	• Can be used once only
• Permanent record	• Film varies in sensitivity.

22.2.2 Classification of radiation workers

A radiation worker is normally defined as an individual engaged in work under license issued by a national agency. The occupational dose is the dose received in the course of employment and does not include dose received from background radiation.

Dose limits There is a legal requirement for classifying radiation workers in both Europe and America. Estimated risks for radiation induced cancer increased by a factor of 3 to 4 since ICRP26 making it necessary to reconsider the annual dose limits for workers which is now presented in ICRP60 (Tab.22.6). The restrictions on effective dose for workers are sufficient to ensure that deterministic effects will be avoided in all tissues and organs except the lens of the eye (which makes no contribution to the effective dose) and skin which may be subjected to localized high exposures such as radionuclide dispensing and angiography; separate equivalent dose limits are imposed on these tissues. Previous reports (ICRP26) divided workers into:

- Category A worker, who is likely to receive a major proportion of the dose limit.
- Category B worker, who is likely to receive a minor proportion of the radiation dose

This clear division does not appear in ICRP60 but it probably could continue in a modified form in order to distinguish those workers who are liable to receive higher radiation doses (fluoroscopy).

Category A These workers would receive three-tenths of any maximum. They are not normally seen in diagnostic radiology but high radiation levels can be approached in nuclear medicine (hands of radio-pharmacist) and in biplanar cine-angiography (cardiologists' eyes). They would receive up to a maximum of 15mSv whole body according to ICRP60. High exposure to the extremities can also place a worker in this category.

Category B This is the general category commonly found in diagnostic radiology. Previous definitions (ICRP26) imposed dose limits for this category as above one-tenth but below three tenths of any maximum. Most recent definitions redefine this category for a worker who does not exceed 5mSv per year. The bar chart in Fig.22.3 shows the overall reduction in yearly radiation dose to workers in hospitals as monitored by film dosimeters in the 1970s and 80s. Since 1986 the greatest proportion of radiology workers return readings less than 1mSv per year.

Table 22.6 Worker Limits (ICRP60)

Application	Occupational	Public
Whole body	100mSv in 5y	1
Eye lens	150	15
Skin (100cm^2)	500	50
Hands	500	50
Mean fetal dose		5

Accumulated evidence from film badge reports are now a more significant driving force for staff exposure reduction than recommendations from national and international radiation commissions and have encouraged constraint levels to be maintained in radiology departments.

Dose limits imposed by some authorities (USA) still retain the recommendations given by ICRP26 (Tab.22.7) although modifications have been made and the two sets of worker dose limits are now very similar except for the whole body dose figure. An **agreement state** in the US complies with or exceeds federal standards which are basically ICRP26.

Table 22.7 Alternative dose limits

Category	Dose (mSv)
Dose equivalent to eye	150
Effective dose equivalent EDE	50
Dose equivalent to any organ except eye (deep dose)	500
Dose equivalent to skin (shallow dose)	500
Minor (<18y) respectively	5, 50, 15, 50
Embryo or fetus	5mSv/9m
Public	1mSv y^{-1}
Unrestricted area	20μSv y^{-1}

Constraint   The new recommendations introduce the term constraint which indicates a restriction to be applied to individual doses. A constraint on the upper limits of dose is seen as a regulatory requirement and should be set by regulatory agencies based on experience of the level of exposure likely to be met in the day to day operations. This is **ALARA** (as-low-as-reasonably-achievable)   principle in operation and can be viewed as a type of risk estimate.

The ICRP26 report used dose limits, the use of constraint should give more control where dose limits are unnecessarily high. The trend shown by the readings plotted in Fig.22.3 indicates that low values can be implied and Tab.22.8 suggests practical constraints which may be applied to clinical radiology. These are annual maximum dose limits that should not be exceeded routinely.

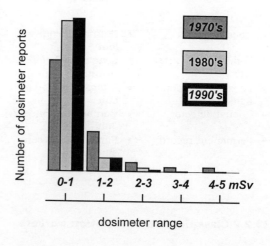

Figure 22.3   Yearly film records collected from radiology sources for 1970's, 80's and 90's showing a sharp decline in high dose rates over these decades.

Table 22.8 Recommended constraint levels

Radiotherapy staff	10mSv
Diagnostic radiologists	5mSv
Diagnostic radiographers	1mSv
Nuclear medicine staff	5mSv
Other hospital staff	1mSv

Public The public are here defined as other hospital staff members (secretarial, portering and nursing) who visit the radiology department from time to time and may become exposed. It also includes accompanying persons with the patient who either wait in the department or assist with the investigation (mothers of pediatric patients). Radiation exposure limits for the public are needed since maximum worker limits will not necessarily protect against deterministic effects. An arbitrary reduction to 10% of the lens and extremity doses has been imposed; this would apply to nursing staff who assist from time to time in radiology procedures. The whole body limit has been reduced from 5 to 1mSv per year with a recommendation that this limit be reduced still further to 0.5mSv y^{-1}. Other variations include a short term dose rate of 20μSv h^{-1} which defines an unrestricted area.

22.2.3 Staff pregnancy

In the radiology workplace the ICRP recommends no particular restriction on women of child bearing age who are not pregnant. Radiology staff consistently show very low levels of radiation exposure therefore the previous controls for occupational exposure of women of child bearing age working in diagnostic radiology is no longer thought necessary at present. The consequence, however, of ICRP60 and future legislation may affect future working practices for pregnant staff. The European current maximum for pregnant staff is 10mSv however since the fetus is to be treated as a member of the public its limit should be 1mSv. ICRP60 requires that once pregnancy has been declared the conceptus is protected by applying an equivalent dose limit to the surface of the abdomen of 2mSv for the remainder of the pregnancy. The personal dosimeter record therefore should not exceed 0.14mSv per month if the declared term exposure (7months) is not to exceed 1mSv.

The principle criterion is that employment should be of a type that does not carry a significant probability of high accidental staff doses (e.g. fluoroscopy and perhaps nuclear medicine). Personal dosimeter records should be reported at 2 week intervals for this individual instead of each month.

Table 21.11 gives the expected natural incidence of abnormality for the fetus as 95.93% or 1:24.6. An exposure of 10mSv increases this risk to only 1:23.9, however it has been estimated that a **risk of malignancy** before the 15th birthday from a 6mSv exposure during the 3rd trimester increases the nominal life time cancer risk to about 1:3000; of which half will be fatal.

22.2.4 Working environment

Exposure levels vary in radiology departments depending on equipment type and usage. There are also rooms within any department (offices and public waiting areas) that should not receive any radiation exposure.

Specified areas where radiation exposure will be experienced fall into categories of high and low exposure rates. These have been designated **controlled** and **supervised** areas respectively. This has been abandoned in ICRP60 however and it is now recommended that design features or local (hospital) authorities should decide operational limits. These limits should be based on ambient exposure to radiation and intake of radionuclides. A controlled area could be defined as one where routine environmental monitoring is not sufficient to predict doses to individual workers. A supervised area could be one where doses can be predicted with confidence but may exceed the dose limit for members of the public.

Established definitions for a controlled area required workers to observe safety procedures in order to reduce their radiation exposure. These would be classified persons or patients undergoing investigation. Previous radiation thresholds required that these areas would have an exposure rate exceeding 0.3 of any maximum dose. Since the established maximum for ICRP26 was 50mSv one third is 15mSv which gives an hourly exposure figure of 7.5µSv h^{-1}. The following were commonly designated as controlled areas:

- ^{99m}Tc Generator Room
- Immediate vicinity of any x-ray machine (including mobiles)
- Nuclear medicine waste store

Lower radiation levels established definitions for a supervised area where the dose level is liable to exceed 0.1 of the maximum dose; usually between 1 and 2.5µSv h^{-1}. The area surrounding the control panel of x-ray equipment, would be typically 1µSv h^{-1}. Supervised areas would include:

- X-ray rooms
- Radio pharmacy
- Nuclear medicine waiting rooms

Definitions commonly applied to radiation work areas are listed in Tab. 22.9.

Table 22.10 Alternative classification of radiation areas.

Area	Exposure
1) Radiation area	50µSv h^{-1} at 30cm
2) High radiation area	1mSv h^{-1} at 30cm
3) Very high radiation area	5Gy h^{-1} at 1m

1) Controlled area	Likely to exceed 0.3 of any limit
2) Supervised area	Likely to exceed 0.1 of any limit
3) Restricted area	Access limited by licensee
4) Unrestricted area	Uncontrolled access <20µSv y^{-1} (2mrem y^{-1})

ICRP60 recommends these measures are kept under review but special procedures are not warranted. Controlled and supervised areas can be used as normal rooms when the x-ray units are switched off. This, of course, does not apply to nuclear medicine laboratories. Other radiation areas are distinguished in some US regulations: a **radiation area** would be where a dose rate is measured of 50µSv h^{-1} at 30cm from the source (or barrier), a **high radiation area** where this is 1mSv h^{-1} at 30cm and a **very high radiation area** where 5Gy h^{-1} at 1m can occur.

Room monitoring equipment Specification of radiation areas is given by the hospital radiation protection committee and decisions are made usually after long-term monitoring (typically a month).

An easy method for deciding whether a room should have restricted access and be designated a controlled or supervised area is to position TLD badges on the walls. Immediate measurements can be obtained by a sensitive survey meter which has a large volume ionization chamber (350cm^3 minimum). Large volume chambers have an almost flat response with energy levels from 12 to 300keV so are ideal for low level monitoring surveys. They have typical sensitivities from 3µSv to 30mSv min^{-1}

The exposure rates which define three important threshold levels are given in Box 22.3

22.2.5 Protective shielding

Machine shielding Local shielding around equipment (under and overcouch fluoroscopy or cantilevered C-arm) can significantly reduce radiation dose to staff. The undercouch design usually comes equipped with a flexible lead-screen surrounding the image intensifier. The overcouch unit can have a short flexible lead-curtain fitted to the tube housing. Ceiling mounted lead-glass shields, in the close vicinity of the x-ray housing can be used for cine-angiography.

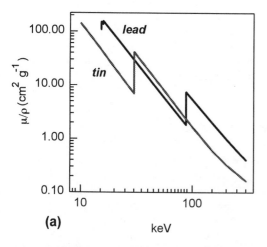

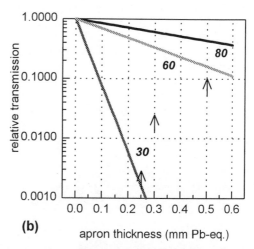

Figure 22.4   (a) The mass attenuation curve for lead and tin showing position of the K-edges. (b) The reduction in transmission for 0.25, 0.3 and 0.5mm Pb equivalent protective aprons (arrows) at 30, 60 and 80keV$_{eff}$.

Protective clothing   Staff working in controlled areas must wear protective clothing in the form of lead-aprons. Several designs are available from complete wrap-around aprons to those that only cover the front of the body. The lead-equivalent thicknesses are normally 0.25, 0.33 and 0.5mm Pb-equivalent. Lead as an attenuating medium has an inconvenient K-edge position as indicated in Fig.22.4(a). Energies above 88kV are better attenuated than the lower energy scatter radiation. Composite aprons have been introduced manufactured from a lead/tin mixture. Tin has a lower K-edge of 29keV (Fig. 22.4(a)) which compensates for the higher K-edge of lead. Over the range of 30-80keV tin has a better attenuation than lead for a greatly reduced weight. Composite aprons therefore give improved protection over a fixed energy range than pure lead aprons, however they are inferior to 0.5mm Pb equivalent aprons which should always be used for high dose procedures (e.g. fluoroscopy). The approximate weights for the different aprons are:

- 0.5mm Pb eq. 5.4kg m^{-2}
- Composite (0.4mm Pb eq.) 3.6-4.5kg m^{-2}
- 0.3mm Pb 3.24kg m^{-2}

Personal dosimeter position   When measuring staff exposure radiation dose the position of the dosimeter on the clothing is important. Figure 22.4(b) shows the relative transmission for 30, 60 and 80kVeff x-rays. The arrows indicate the common apron equivalent Pb thickness of 0.25, 0.3 and 0.5mm. An apron having a Pb-equivalent of 0.3mm reduces transmission at these energies to 0.0002, 0.3 and 0.58 so a dosimeter badge placed under the apron would underestimate radiation exposure to the extremities.

The ICRP 35 report of 1982 recommended that more than one dosimeter may be required. When wearing protective lead aprons a single dosimeter should be worn outside high on the trunk (collar level) to give an eye and skin unshielded dose. A dosimeter placed outside the lead apron at collar level will also

554 *Physics of Diagnostic Imaging*

give a better idea of ambient exposure since most of the scattered radiation is low energy and will be stopped by the apron itself, however this dosimeter will overestimate the effective dose by about ×5 so a second 'under apron badge' may be required. The reading from this will be the true whole body dose for record keeping.

- Wear a protective lead-apron (0.5mm Pb equivalent)
- Make use of image storage systems for review monitoring
- Exposure timing devices should have an audible warning
- Display elapsed fluoroscopic time on monitor screen

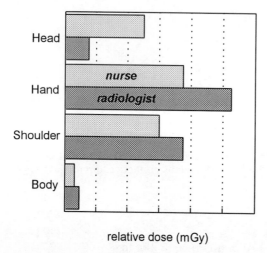

Figure 22.5 Relative doses to radiologist and nurse during fluoroscopy/angiography examination showing considerable greater radiation exposure to the extremities.

An 'above apron' badge is a very good indicator of efficient use of fluoroscopy equipment when used in parallel with a dose area product area meter for the patient dose record. In some cases it is good practice to use an electronic dosimeter for recording individual doses since these can give an immediate idea of radiation exposure. The histogram in Fig.22.5 shows relative radiation exposure for the body, shoulder, hand and head for a radiologist and nurse during a fluoroscopy study. A reading from the body region would give a false idea of radiation exposure to the extremities; a shoulder badge position gives a better idea of radiation doses to the upper third of the body.

A summary of staff dose reduction for fluoroscopy examinations would be:

Box 22.3

Exposure rates

1.0 μSv h⁻¹
General public

Time	Total Dose
8 hour day	8μSv d⁻¹
5 day week	40μSv w⁻¹
1 month	160μSv m⁻¹
50 week year	2mSv y⁻¹

2.5 μSv h⁻¹
(maximum for diagnostic staff)

Time	Total Dose
8 hour day	20μSv d⁻¹
5 day week	0.1mSv w⁻¹
1 month	0.4mSv m⁻¹
50 week year	5.0mSv y⁻¹

7.5 μSv h⁻¹
(Category A worker)

Time,	Total Dose
8 hour day	60μSv d⁻¹
5 day week	300μSv w⁻¹
1 month	1200μSv (1.2mSv m⁻¹)
50 week,	15mSv y⁻¹

22.3 PATIENT RADIATION EXPOSURE

Diagnostic Radiology is the largest man-made source of radiation exposure to the population. It contributes approximately 20% to background radiation, world-wide. In western countries this can be nearer 50%. A serious attempt should always be made to reduce patient radiation exposure whenever possible providing it does not compromise image quality.

RADIOGRAPHY

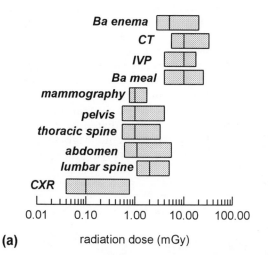

NUCLEAR MEDICINE

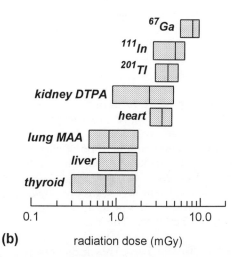

Figure 22.6 **(a)** The range of radiation doses found in some typical diagnostic investigations. **(b)** the patient radiation dose (mGy) in nuclear medicine for recommended activities of ^{99m}Tc. Other isotopes are also given ^{201}Tl, ^{111}In and ^{67}Ga.

Table 22.10 Procedures for reducing patient dose

Method	% dose reduction
1. Eliminate unjustified examinations	100
2. Minimize films per examination	20
3. Minimize fluoroscopy time	30
4. Reduce repeat rates	5
5. Availability of previous films	100
6. Collimate beam effectively	20
7. Shield sensitive organs	25
8. Patient compression	50
9. QC program	influences No. 2 and 3

Unnecessary investigations It has been estimated that at least 20% of X-ray exami-nations currently carried out in some western countries are clinically unnecessary. Further unnecessary exposure results from repeat films due to film loss or poor image quality Box 22.4 uses the man-sievert to estimate dose savings in radiology and Tab 22.10 lists procedures for reducing patient dose. Table 22.11 suggests some equipment modifications which have a significant effect on overall pa-tient dose reduction. Costs in this area can be justified from ALARA principles.

Table 22.11 Patient dose reduction (equipment)

Method	Potential reduction (mSv)
Carbon fiber components	4000
Rare earth screens	3000
Film processor temperature	2000

22.3.1 Range of doses from diagnostic examinations

Examples of radiological investigations and their typical doses reported in the literature are shown graphically in Fig.22.6(a). The highest doses are for fluoroscopy and CT investigations; the lowest for chest radiography (CXR). Lowest patient dose levels are given by high voltage CXR techniques and successive increases in kVp give substantial saving in radiation dose; high voltage chest radiographs should always be the method of choice.

Nuclear medicine studies, shown for comparison in Fig.22.6(b), give much lower whole body doses than investigations involving x-rays, equivalent doses to target organs may be higher however. The percentage collective dose of various radiological examinations is given in Tab.22.12. This indicates the relative contributions made by various diagnostic x-ray investigations to the total patient collective dose and identifies those investigations which need careful planning in order to give a significant reduction in patient radiation exposure. Radiological investigations involving computed tomography (CT) have become major additions to this collective dose figure.

Suggestions for collective dose reduction by modifying techniques have already been given in Box 22.4. Equipment modifications also achieve significant reductions but at some cost. A list is given in Tab.22.11 (UK figures). Carbon fiber materials for x-ray table tops and cassette construction have a major effect. Rare earth screens and maintaining film processor temperatures at their recommended levels also play an important role.

Suggested dose levels for various investigations (NRPB (UK)) are listed in Table 22.13, which should be easily maintained in a radiology department employing dose reduction methods.

Table 22.12 Collective dose per examination

Examination	Frequency	% Collective dose
CT	2.0	20
Lumbar spine	3.3	15
Barium enema	0.9	14
Barium meal	1.6	12
IV urography	1.3	11
Abdomen	2.9	8
Pelvis	2.9	6
Chest	24.0	2
Extremities	25.0	1.5
Skull	5.6	1.5
Thorax	0.9	1
Dental	25.0	1
Nuclear medicine	2.0	1

Box 22.4

The man-sievert

The annual collective dose for radiological examinations in the UK is 16000 man-Sv of which 70% is film radiography, 30% fluoroscopy. Smaller contributions are made by nuclear medicine (1000 man-Sv) and dental studies (200 man-Sv).

Dose Reduction	Collective dose saving
Unnecessary Investigations:	3200
Maintain number of films to national mean value (NMV):	2500
Reduce fluoroscopy time to NMV:	1500
Reduce dose per exam to NMV:	1300
Reduce repeat rate from 10 to 5%:	600

Conclusion:
For no financial outlay the collective dose to the patient population could be reduced by between 7000 to 8000 man-Sv (~40%) with a concurrent reduction in staff dose.

For the US population (230 million):

Radiology	92000 man-Sv
Nuclear medicine	32000 man-Sv

Table 22.13 Suggested reference doses (NRPB)

View		Standard dose (mSv)
Lumbar spine	AP	10
	Lat	30
Abdomen		10
Pelvis		10
Chest	PA	0.3
	Lat	1.5
Skull	AP	5.0
	PA	5.0
	Lat	3.0

22.3.2 The pregnant patient

The stages of pregnancy for the first trimester are given in Fig.22.7. The period of organogenesis are identified between days 13 and 50. The effects of high levels of radiation exposure to the developing fetus, obtained mostly from A-bomb data, are listed in Tab.22.14. Patients are routinely asked if there is any chance that they might be pregnant. If the answer is 'no' the radiological examination can proceed. If there is uncertainty the radiographer is asked to check the date of the last menstrual period. If this is overdue consideration should be given to delaying the examination and make a future appointment (if the clinical conditions allow). This is the so-called '28-day rule' and a suggested questionnaire is given in Fig.22.8. There is accumulating evidence that the incidence of childhood cancer may be increased following *in-utero* irradiation before a period has been missed.

There may therefore be a case for restricting high dose examinations such as CT, which can give *in-utero* radiation doses between 20-50mGy. A '10-day rule' could be employed in such cases which restricts high dose investigations to the first part of the menstrual cycle. If the patient is comatose (trauma patient) or clinical conditions demand a radiological investigation then the lowest possible radiation doses should be employed.

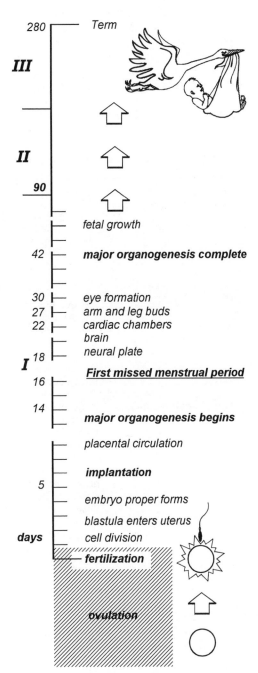

Figure 22.7 The timing for ovulation and embryo/ fetus development in days after fertilization, and stages important to radiation protection protocols. Trimester divisions I, II and III are not to scale

Skeletal surveys can be achieved by employing the 'scout-view' or 'Toposcan' longitudinal scan given by a CT machine. This is a very low dose technique giving typical dose levels of 40μGy (4mrad). Other investigations in the abdominal region should use the fastest screen/film combinations that give a diagnostic image. Chest and extremity investigations are not restricted since the dose to the conceptus or fetus is negligible.

Table 22.14 Effects of irradiation on the human embryo

Days after fertilization	Period of development	Effects
1 to 9	pre-implantation	Most probable effects: death with little chance of malformation
10 to 12	implantation	Reduced lethal effects; malformation unlikely; intra-uterine growth retardation predominant effect
13 to 50	organo-genesis	Production of congenital malformation; retarded growth
51 to 280	fetal	Effects on CNS; growth retardation at high doses
All	fetal/neonate	Increased incidence of cancer and leukemia

The '10 Day Rule'   An early recommendation from the ICRP for examinations involving the lower abdomen of women:

.... is least likely to pose any hazard to a developing embryo if carried out during the 10-day interval following the onset of menstruation....

This recommendation was adopted by certain national regulatory organizations but was subsequently questioned since it was found that the developing ovum prior to fertilization was equally radio-sensitive.   The shaded portion in Fig.22.7 represents the stage of follicle production and ovulation prior to fertilization which can be threatened by radiation exposure.

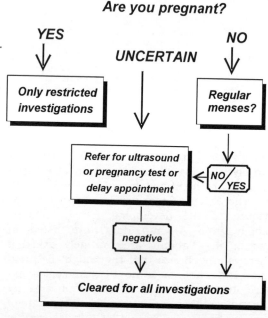

Figure 22.8   A series of questions for the female patient who may be pregnant; the so called '28-day rule' identifying the first missed period.

Patient dose reduction techniques   Fluoroscopy is a particularly high dose rate procedure. Dose reduction could be obtained by:

- Short periods of screening exposure.
- Digital image store.
- Temporary removal of anti-scatter grid (less radiation needed for film exposure but poorer image quality).
- Automatic brightness control influencing x-ray exposure for different anatomy (varying absorption).
- 90kV at 0.5mA should be the exposure level delivering 10mGy min^{-1} surface dose.

Collimating the beam to the smallest field with mA and kV as low as possible is also a very effective dose reduction technique using automatic collimation where possible.

Image storage devices added to fluoroscopy equipment can give major dose reduction for patient and staff (Chapter 10). If a non-storage system needs a 5 second screening exposure, a 'last image hold' would only require a 2 second exposure recognizing image content and then storing: this reduces the dose to 40%. Digital storage only requires 1 second exposure reducing the dose still further to 20% of continuous non-storage fluoroscopy.

Dose-area product meters (DAP/Diamentor)

The dose-area product is measured with a special ionization chamber fixed to the x-ray tube housing shown in Chapter 21. It enables the total surface dose to be recorded for each examination; it can also display the total elapsed fluoroscopy time. With regular use the dose-area product meter can compare exposures for different patients and different techniques; particularly useful for training.

The detector consists of a large parallel-plate ionization chamber feeding a high input impedance amplifier. The chamber is fixed close to the x-ray tube where the x-ray dose is high and back-scattered radiation from the patient is minimal. The factors that alter the dose area product are

- Tube kilovoltage   (kVp)
- Tube current   (mA)
- Filtration   (mm Al)
- Time   (minutes)

The dose measurement is independent of distance from the x-ray source (Fig.22.9) since for an isosceles triangle $d \propto a$. Since the chamber is transparent it does not interfere with any light beam positioning device. Under-couch (under-table or UT) fluoroscopy units are not ideal for dose-area product meters since the table acts as an additional filter in front of the patient. A selection of common examinations with their typical dose-area values in Gray cm^2 are given in Tab.22.15.

Table 22.15 Reference values for dose-area-product per examination

Examination	DAP value (Gy cm^2)
Lumbar spine	15
Barium enema	60
Barium meal	25
Intravenous urography	40
Abdomen	8
Pelvis	5

22.3.3 The nuclear medicine department

Staff doses   These can be higher than conventional radiography staff doses if high activity patients (e.g. 600MBq ^{99m}Tc bone or cardiac) are present in large numbers at any one time. Table 22.16 gives an indication of air-kerma rates from such patients and if a radiographer/technologist/nurse is in close proximity, as a routine, then doses could exceed the annual radiation constraint value. For example a department handling 25 such patients and the average proximity being 0.5m, then over a working year this could contribute over 6mSv to the staff member. The recommended limit for classified workers (as a result of ICRP60) is likely to be 6mSv.

Finger doses from syringes during dispensing and injection is reduced significantly by using syringe shields. Locating a 'butterfly needle' in the chosen vein prior to the injection also reduces the handling time of the loaded syringe and this practice can contribute quite a large dose savings. The annual dose limit for skin (the hand) is 500mSv and this can be exceeded if an individual carries out most of the elution and dispensing. A finger dosimeter should be regularly worn in order to monitor these doses.

Waiting rooms   Radiation dose transfer from injected patient to adjacent patient is usually small provided the seating is separate and the waiting times short. Total doses range between <5µSv to 35µSv for the duration.

Outpatients   The major clinical advantage of nuclear medicine is its availability as an out patient service. Non-hospitalized referrals are injected with a radionuclide preparation, undergo an imaging procedure and are then free to leave. The short T½ of ^{99m}Tc ensures minimum radiation exposure to other members of the public but family members should be aware of contamination hazards from incontinent patients and proper precautions issued. Outpatients undergoing ^{131}Iodine therapy are a very real hazard to the general populus and clear instructions should be made available before sending them away.

Table 22.16 Staff exposure from ^{99m}Tc patient 600MBq

Distance	$C\,kg^{-1}\,h^{-1}$	Air-kerma $\mu Gy\,h^{-1}$ (mR)
0.25	1.70×10^{-6}	58 (6.6)
0.5	0.92×10^{-6}	31 (3.6)
1.0	0.46×10^{-6}	15.8 (1.8)
2.0	0.13×10^{-6}	4.5 (0.5)

22.4 HOSPITAL RADIATION PROTECTION

The proper implementation of safety measures throughout a hospital, including radiology, nuclear medicine and laboratories using radiation equipment is the responsibility of a committee or informed group appointed by the hospital board.

22.4.1 The radiation safety committee

Every hospital that uses radiation equipment or substances must establish a hospital radiation protection committee comprising radiologist, hospital administrator, physicist and radiation safety officers from each department using radiation. There should be definite pathways to this committee for any member of the hospital staff who wishes to clarify problems or events concerning radiation exposure to either staff or patients.

Radiation safety officers are sometimes termed 'authorized' users, either a licensed physician certified in radiology, radiation oncology or who has been trained and certified in the use of radiation or radioactive materials and listed in the hospital's license. Hospital doctors, other than radiologists, who are responsible for using or directing medical exposures (e.g. orthopedic surgeons) should undergo a recognized training course.

Hospital and local regulations   A set of simple instructions to staff members must be published in-house for reference. Controlled and supervised areas can be defined in this document along with procedures for the safe use of radiation.   Brief 'local-rules' for each laboratory or section of radiology should be displayed along with the name(s) of the safety officers. Suggested outlines for radiographic local rules would be:

- Close the room door before making an exposure
- Staff not taking part in a procedure to be behind control panel shielding
- Gonad shields to be used on patients whenever appropriate
- Beam field size to be collimated consistent with investigation. Fluoroscopy procedures should operate under limited tube current (1mA at 100kV)
- Staff who are needed to support patients during an exposure must wear a lead-fabric apron (0.3mm Pb equivalent). Lead-fabric gloves may also be necessary.
- A record of the dose should be made.

22.5 THE X-RAY ROOM

The design and construction of an x-ray room decides not only the safe working conditions for the radiology personnel working in that room but also for non-radiological staff (secretarial, porters and nurses) outside the immediate vicinity. Visitors and general public are also afforded optimum protection.

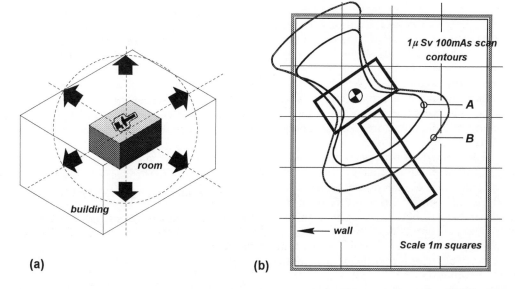

Figure 22.9 **(a)** Room position within the building. Radiation from the x-ray machine will penetrate walls, floor, ceiling into adjacent areas (offices etc.) **(b)** The radiation air-kerma figures for two types of CT machines A and B, showing wall penetration by the contour for machine B; the CT gantry would need repositioning in this case.

Over specification is unnecessary since lead-sheet and barium plaster are very heavy and require substantial and very expensive foundation support. Lead-lined doors should only be specified if essential since these too are very expensive and because of their inertia when closing can constitute a hazard in themselves.

22.5.1 Room Layout

The position of the x-ray room within the building identifies adjacent areas which may need particular attention (offices, kitchens etc.); radiation will penetrate walls, ceilings and floors into these localities (Fig.22.9(a)).

The principles associated with room design and equipment layout generally cover the following points:

- Construction of barriers to attenuate both primary (direct beam) and secondary (scatter) radiation.

- Restriction of x-ray beam dimensions (collimation).
- Observing the inverse square law during planning stages and equipment positioning.
- Using the minimum radiation for the diagnostic information required.
- Warning signs and indicator lights in operation.

When designing radiation protection for a room the following points should also be known:

- The Workload expected in the room in mA min per week (mA min w^{-1}; Tab.22.17).
- The Direction of the primary beam.
- The Occupancy factor of the x-ray room and any adjoining non-x-ray rooms (Tab.22.18).

The use factor is given to the exposed surfaces (floor, walls, ceiling) so that the amount of shielding can be calculated. The expected workload in mA min per week can be estimated from the x-ray examination and the number of patients examined. It is categorized in terms of usage: low, moderate and high. The limits are given in Tab.22.17 and examples given in Box 22.5.

The general design of a room housing an x-ray unit should consider easy access for the staff behind the shielded area of the control console. The primary beam of the x-ray unit should be restricted so that occupants in adjoining rooms are not exposed. Ideally the room should be of adequate size 36m^2 (350ft^2) ceiling height 3.6m (12ft) and any external windows 2 meters (7ft) above ground level. The walls should be concrete block or brick; particular attention should be made to the corridor wall. There should be a shielded cubicle surrounding the control panel with a clear lead-glass observation window of adequate lead-equivalent thickness (typically 1.5 −2mm Pb-equivalent).

The primary beam should be directed away from doors and the control cubicle. Wall areas that may be exposed to the primary beam should be adequately shielded depending on the activity in the next room. The doors leading into the room should be lead-lined but this is not necessary for the staff access door since this should already be protected by the shielding of the control area.

Box 22.5

Workload estimation from Tab.22.17

Low use: 100 patients x-rayed in ICU per week. Average exposure 15mAs. = 1500mAs or **25mA min w^{-1}.**

Moderate use: 15 patients undergo fluoroscopy per week. Each patient exposed to 3-5 minutes screening at 3mA giving 15mA min. per patient maximum giving **225mA min w^{-1}**.

High use: 10 patients per week undergo cineangiography. Five cine runs per patient, 5s at 1200mA or **5000mA min w^{-1}.**

Table 22.17 Fluoroscopy workload

Usage	Remarks
Low 30mA min w^{-1}	• Theaters and Intensive Care Units need no special construction requirements. • Staff and patient protection guidance from local rules. • Adequate clearance between beds.
Moderate 30 - 300mA min w^{-1}	• Theaters should have walls, ceilings and floors 1mmPb eq. • Restricted access. • Screen protection for adjacent patients.
High >300mA min w^{-1}	• Walls, ceilings and floors 2mmPb eq. • Warning lights on outside doors.

Site of x-ray equipment Special cases exist for equipment that is operated outside the radiology department (wards, clinical rooms, operating theaters etc.) and also radiology rooms housing equipment that has a high radiation output (CT and some fluoroscopy equipment). Table 22.17 defines the necessary shielding and precautions for workload.

CT rooms The 'bow-tie' shaped contour surrounding the gantry center is usually shown for 'dose/1000mAs'. A typical figure for medium sized machines would be 10μSv for 1000mAs. In order to calculate the weekly dose rate at this contour the following parameters are used:

• Exposure per slice typically 210mAs
• Number of slices per patient ~ 20
• Exposure per study: 210×20 = 4200mAs

For a weekly workload of 20-25 patients this

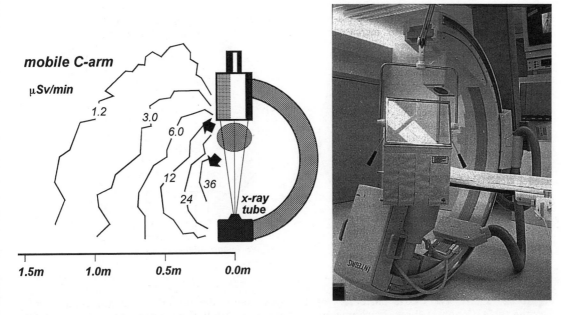

Figure 22.10 **(a)** Mobile C-arm radiation contours, showing the low dose rates at 1.5m from the machine **(b)** An example of moveable shielding around a cantilevered C-arm machine.

would represent ~100,000mAs, giving a dose rate at the contour of 1mSv per week. The German DIN6812 tables use shielding calculations based on a higher value of 300,000mAs per week. For this higher mAs figure an office wall, 2m from the gantry, will require 1.5mmPb equivalent shielding. Figure 22.4(a) shows the increased absorption after the K-edge at 88keV so less thickness is needed in rooms using higher kV techniques (chest units).

22.5.2 Machine safety

Mobile x-ray machines The use of small mobile x-ray machines outside the radiology department need pose no radiation exposure problems since these machines are deliberately designed to have a decreased primary beam intensity. Portable machines can be found in intensive care units (ICU's) which

use mobile x-ray units operating at 60 to 80kVp with a low tube current. Rare earth screens should always be used with these units. Unprotected members of staff should be 2 meters from the tube housing; at this distance scatter radiation is negligible. An example of local rules for the use of portable equipment in wards would be:

- The primary beam should only be directed at the patient
- Ward staff should stand at least 2 meters from the machine unless contrary to the patient's well being. Aprons and gloves should be available in this case.
- The radiographer or technician must wear a protective apron (0.25mm Pb).
- Small mobile screens should be available if adjacent patients need to be protected.

Surgical units Mobile C-arm fluoroscopy units are used for orthopedic and cardiac pacemaker work.

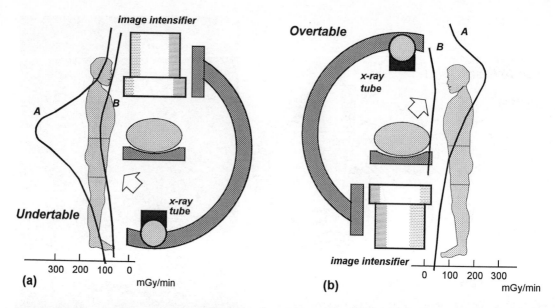

Figure 22.11   Two C-arm positions **(a)** the x-ray tube under the table and **(b)** the x-ray tube over the table. Contours show the change in radiation exposure to the operator with (B) and without (A) shielding. (Courtesy GE Medical Systems Inc)

The exposure from these machines shows that at 2m the scattered radiation is negligible (Fig.22.10(a)). Three categories define C-arm use, depending on workload in mA-minutes shown in Tab.22.17.

Large cantilevered C-arm machines which are tending to replace fixed under or over-table units present their own problems for staff radiation protection. Figure 22.11 shows a typical unit being used with the x-ray tube both under-table (a) and over-table (b). The contour A in both cases shows significant radiation dose rates to the operator without local machine shielding. Contour B shows the marked reduction in dose rate when a 1.5 - 2mm Pb-equivalent acrylic shield is used. This type of shield is shown in Fig.22.10(b).

22.5.3 Protective radiation shielding

Although the ALARA principle should always be applied when designing rooms for x-ray use it must be borne in mind that this princi-

ple contains the phrase :

'..social and economic factors taken into account....'

Lead (Pb) is the usual shielding material being high density and easily worked. Sheet lead is fixed inside a plywood sandwich (plymax) forming ideal material for partitions. Thicknesses range from 1 to 2mm for diagnostic radiology. Other materials used as effective shielding are concrete and brick. Their shielding efficiency is expressed as '**lead-equivalent**' in mm-Pb ranging from 0.5mm to several millimeters.

Primary barrier   protection from the primary beam must be incorporated into any part of the ceiling, floor and walls that the primary beam can be directed toward. The equipment itself will be supplied with shielding for the tube housing, image intensifier and table covers. In order to limit the radiation dose to an acceptable level shielding must be provided to walls, floors, ceilings and room doors:

- **Walls**: Shielding should take into ac count the distance between the x-ray tube and the type of adjoining room.
- **Floors and Ceilings**: These are commonly made from concrete and usually need no additional material. The level of extra shielding depends on the occupancy in areas below and above the x-ray room. If concrete construction has not been applied then local lead shielding may be necessary above and below the x-ray unit.
- **Doors**: Both single and double width patient access doors should be lead lined; this can be 1mm in most cases since distance from the equipment would have reduced scattered radiation reaching doors.

Lead-lined doors are very expensive and should be planned with care. Warning lights outside doors are essential. The doors should be lockable on the inside. The upright cassette holder/chest stand should have a primary shield (2mm lead) on the wall behind.

Primary barrier calculation The information that is necessary in order to calculate the primary barrier requirements is:

- Weekly staff dose limit (P)
- Workload in mA-minutes per week (W)
- Maximum kilovoltage likely to be used
- Occupancy factors for adjoining rooms (T)
- Use factor (U)

The workload is measured in mA-minutes. A 5 minute screening at 5mA is 25mA-minutes per patient. For 20 patients a week this would be 500 mA-minutes per week.

The maximum kilovoltage is usually taken as 100kV for routine diagnostic work but 50 and 75kV are considered. The allowable transmission B for maintaining radiation levels is calculated within the set limits from factors listed in Table 22.18:

$$B = \frac{Pd^2}{WUT} \qquad (22.6)$$

Where *d* is the distance from the x-ray tube housing. The *B* factor is translated into lead-thickness by reference to Fig.22.12. The shielding for a primary barrier specification is

calculated in Box. 22.6 using the graph in Fig.22.12.

Secondary barrier This protects personnel from scattered radiation and applies to any part of the room receiving scatter. Barrier requirements are far less than for primary barrier since scattered radiation one meter from the x-ray source has an intensity about 0.1% of the primary beam. Secondary shielding is typically half the shielding thickness of primary barriers and is normally satisfied if the walls are brick or concrete.

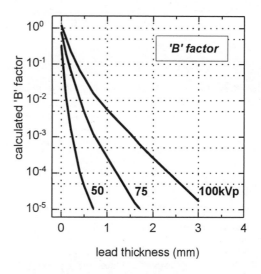

Figure 22.12 Factor 'B' calculated in Box 22.6 related to shielding thickness (mm-Pb) for energies 50, 75 and 100kVp. A constant current supply is assumed.

Scatter levels have steadily become lower due to the introduction of faster film screens, modern machine design and more effective collimation of the beam but although calculated barrier requirements have decreased, the patient safety levels have become more stringent requiring greater safety levels for staff and public areas. Safety measures that influence patient dose reduction have a direct effect on radiation exposure to staff.

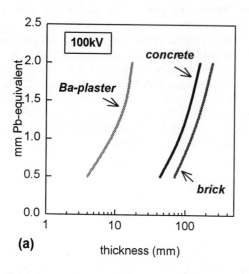 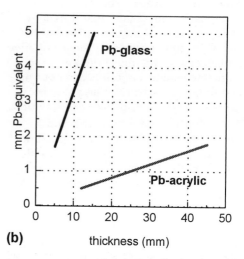

Figure 22.13   **(a)** Brick, concrete and baryta-plaster compared to lead in mm-Pb equivalence. Barium Plaster density 3200kg m³; concrete 2300kg m³ and brick density 1600kg m³ **(b)** Lead-glass and Lead-acrylic (plastic), and their various thicknesses compared to their Pb-equivalent. (mm-Pb).

Table 22.18 Parameters used in eqn.22.6

P : weekly dose (mSv)

1.0	areas for Category A personnel
0.3	areas for Category B personnel
0.1	control areas in x-ray room
0.03	public areas in radiology dept.

T : Occupancy

1.0	control areas and offices
0.25	corridors and wards
0.0625	toilets and outside areas

U: Use factor

1	surfaces exposed to the primary beam
0.25	areas not exposed to the primary beam
0.625	occasional exposure (ceilings)

22.5.4   Shielding materials

Lead   Sheet lead between 1.5 and 2.5mm conveniently sandwiched between plywood is the simplest installation for shielded room partitions. This ease of installation may offset its expense but although other materials are cheaper they are more labor intensive.

Building materials The effectiveness of baryta-plaster, concrete and brick as shielding materials and their lead-equivalence (mm-Pb) are compared in Fig.22.13(a). It is worth noting that with adequate room sizes and modern machines, concrete block or brick construction offers a very effective barrier against scattered radiation. The added expense of baryta-plaster (materials and fixing-time) seldom warrants the added protection and should be cautiously specified. Mobile lead-screens or strategically placed lead-sheet plywood (plymax) can usefully be installed in sensitive areas or as room partitions for temporary room designs. Sensible and informed planning can save a great deal of unnecessary cost.

Lead-glass and lead-acrylic windows
Shielded observation windows as secondary barriers can be provided by both lead-glass and lead-plastic. Glass impregnated with lead and barium oxides or acrylic-plastic impregnated with an organo-lead compound can be used. Plastic has the advantage of less cost, so larger areas are possible allowing large open plan room designs. It is shatter proof, unlike glass, and can be machined. Lead equivalence for these materials is given in Fig.22.13(b).

FURTHER READING:

An Introduction to Radiobiology
AHW Nias   John Wiley 1990

Low Level Radiation Effects
AB.Brill Society of Nuclear Medicine

ICRP Report number 26   1977
ICRP Report number 60   1989
Pergamon Press

A Rational approach to Radiodiagnosic Investigations
Technical Report 689 WHO Geneva

Patient dose reduction in diagnostic Radiology:
Documents of the NRPB 1:3 1990

NCRP Report 93 September 1987

BEIR V 1989

Biological Risks of Medical Irradiations
AAPM Monograph 5.

Box 22.6

> ***Primary barrier thickness***
>
> Calculating the radiation shielding necessary for screening a control area using eqn.22.6
> A fluoroscopy clinic sees 20 patients per week and gives 5 minute screening at 5mA. Maximum workload (W) is then 500 mA-min per week at 100kVp. The distance to the control room window is ~ 4m. It is not exposed to the primary beam so U = 0.25; the occupancy T is 1 and it is a controlled area so P is 0.1.
>
> $$B = \frac{P \times d^2}{WUT}$$
>
> $$= \frac{0.1 \times 4^2}{500 \times 0.25 \times 1} = 0.0128$$
>
> Point 0.0128 on the y-axis of the graph in Fig.22.12 corresponds to a thickness of 0.75mmPb or equivalent material. In practice this would be 1mm Pb-eq. glass or acrylic

KEYWORDS

ALARA - As-Low-As-Reasonably-Achievable. Making every reasonable effort to reduce radiation levels below the stated dose limits.

ALARP - As Low As Reasonably Practical. The limiting factor being existing facilities due for update or replacement. (unofficial term)

ALI - Annual Limit on Intake. The derived limit for amount of radioactive material taken in by the body (ingestion or inhalation) per year.

becquerel (Bq) - a measure of radioactivity: one disintegration per second, 1 dps.

BEIR - Biological Effects of Ionizing Radiation

collective dose - Sum of individual doses received by a population in a given time from a specified radioactive source.

committed dose equivalent (H_{T50}) - The dose equivalent to organs or reference tissues that will be received by an individual over a 50 year period from the initial intake.

committed effective dose equivalent (H_{E50}) - The sum of the products of the weighting factors w_T to each organ or tissue and the H_{T50} to these organs or tissues so:

$$H_{E50} = \sum w_T \cdot H_{T50}$$

controlled area - An area with limited access within a department.

curie (Ci) - (non-SI unit): 3.7×10^{10} becquerels

deep dose equivalent (H_d) - External whole body dose-equivalent at 1cm depth.

diploid - Relates to cells having a double set of chromosomes, usually relates to all mammalian cells except gametes.

D_O - The dose that gives (on average) one lethal event per cell reducing survival to 37% of its previous value.

dose equivalent (H_T) - The product of the absorbed dose in tissue and quality factor. Measured in Rem (non-SI) and Sievert (SI).

DREF - Dose rate effectiveness factor corrects for extrapolation from high to low dose effects.

effective dose equivalent (H_E) - The sum of the products of the dose equivalents and the weighting factor (w_t) for each organ or tissue

so: $\qquad H_E = \sum w_T \cdot H_T$

eye dose equivalent - External exposure of the lens of the eye. The dose equivalent at 0.3cm depth.

free radical - A chemical compound containing an unpaired electron.

gray (Gy) - a measure of absorbed dose 1J kg^{-1}

haploid - Relates to single stranded DNA cells: bacteria and gametes.

ICRP - International Commission on Radiological Protection.

NCRP (US) - National Council on Radiological Protection and Measurements

NRPB (UK) - National Radiological Protection Board

radiation area - an area within the department where individuals could receive 0.05mSv h^{-1} at 30cm (50µSv or 5mrem) from the radiation source.

radiation weighting factor (w_R) as listed in Tab. 22.1 from ICRP60.

restricted area - a limited access area where exposure to individuals may occur.

röntgen (R) - 2.58×10^{-4} coulombs kg^{-1} of air.

shallow dose equivalent (H_s) - the external exposure to the skin is the dose equivalent at a tissue depth of 0.007cm averaged over an area of $1cm^2$

sievert (Sv) - A measure of dose equivalent. Gray × relative biological effectiveness of the radiation.

Total effective dose equivalent (TEDE) - The sum of the deep dose equivalent (external exposures) and committed effective dose equivalent (internal exposures).

tissue weighting factor (w_T) as listed in Tab. 22.3 from ICRP60.

23

Basic quality control procedures

23.1   The quality assurance program
23.2   Quality control equipment
23.3   Conventional radiology
23.4   Film image
23.5   Mammography

23.6   Fluoroscopy
23.7   Computed tomography
23.8   Nuclear medicine
23.9   Ultrasound
23.10 Magnetic resonance imaging

23.1 THE QUALITY ASSURANCE PROGRAM

A quality assurance program (QA) combines the many aspects of equipment monitoring to ensure consistent performance from equipment purchase to its eventual scrapping. The program is organized by a small group within the department. A full QA program should cover:

- Acceptance testing
- Equipment commissioning
- Routine quality control including after repair.
- Decommissioning or scrapping equipment

23.1.1   Organization

Acceptance where specifications at purchase are checked and all extras (additional items above the basic system) have been installed and are operating. When this has been satisfied the machine enters its commissioning period.

Commissioning The equipment is accepted for routine clinical use and then must prove reliable over a certain period (usually 1 month). The machine then enters its warranty period during which the manufacturer is liable for the cost of repair.

Routine QC   A quality control program is started for each machine and a log-book kept.

Post-repair QC When a machine malfunction has been reported the engineer should be notified and the machine repaired. Before accepting the repair, test programs should be performed which will confirm safe operation of the equipment.

Decommissioning   Old machines that have passed their useful life span should have a written report itemizing the reason for scrapping. The regulatory authority usually requires to be informed.

23.1.2   QC Program

Quality control can be a basic service or more complex depending on the size of department and available budget.   Basic QC programs that should be set up for routine monitoring by the QA group insure safe equipment operation. More detailed tests are described in publications listed at the end of this chapter.

Quality control sheets (as foundation examples) are given at the end of this chapter. Tests can be divided into primary and secondary tests depending on the frequency of use and specificity. Simple primary tests are usually adopted as routine for confirming malfunction before more complex secondary tests are used to pin-point the fault.

Primary tests These will identify equipment operating outside tolerance limits established either at purchase or with older machines immediately after a full service. They are mostly non-specific that do not directly identify the source of malfunction. These primary tests can be carried out rapidly by the radiologist, radiographer or technologist to check the day-to-day or weekly running of the equipment and identify those aspects of system performance which are most likely to deteriorate. It is also a good idea to run these tests after a service/maintenance visit. Primary tests for **x-ray equipment** would be:

- Inspection of a reference test object or phantom for resolution and contrast
- Linearity between x-ray exposure (mAs) and measured radiation output (mR or micro-grays)
- Linearity between kVp and the factor mR per mAs (mR/mAs)
- Automatic exposure control linearity

These tests require the minimum of equipment and time. Primary tests for **film image/ processor** would be:

- Developer temperature
- Optical density for test exposure (sensitometry)
- Film screen contact

Fluoroscopy equipment is complex and the primary tests rely mainly on subjective display observation so would include:

- A reference test object video display noting resolution, contrast and field distortion
- An entrance radiation dose measurement

The routine testing of **CT** and **MRI** would measure field of view uniformity using the QC equipment supplied with the machine. These tests are usually standard for the machine and involve automatic QC program protocols. **Nuclear medicine** gamma cameras should be tested each day for field uniformity and **ultrasound** should have beam registration accuracy (position) measured on a routine basis together with gray scale.

Secondary tests If machine deterioration has been detected by the relevant primary test then an appropriate secondary test should be performed by a technologist, physicist or hospital engineer. They mainly concern x-ray equipment since CT, MRI, nuclear medicine and ultrasound would commonly require specialist knowledge only available to the manufacturer. Secondary tests are designed to identify the machine fault. Some of them are rather complex and publications at the end of this chapter should be consulted. Simple tests are described (i.e. kVp measurement) which use straightforward digital meters. Some common secondary tests for x-ray equipment would be:

- X-ray beam quality (half-value layer)
- kVp measurement
- detailed exposure rate measurements
- X-ray beam alignment
- Radiation leakage
- Film processor refreshment rate
- Mammography image quality and dose
- Fluoroscopy dose and video performance

23.1.3 Reporting format

A record of the measurements should be kept on an easy to understand form. The hospital and equipment should be identified along with room details and personnel involved.

The report forms can be generated either as a set, representing the department as a whole, or as individual QC log books kept with each separate machine so that trends and comparisons can be made more readily for different dates.

A suggested sample report is given at the end of each section where the readings obtained are placed alongside acceptable limits for each measurement. Computerized QC packages are available that will accept measurements from the monitoring equipment and present these in tabulated format with various comments. These can mostly be customized for any particular quality assurance program using available database software. Table 23.1 shows a basic header for a QC sheet which will be kept in a central location. It serves to identify hospital, relevant staff, room and equipment type as well as keeping a record of previous visits.

Table 23.1 Sample report header block

Hospital:.....	Date:.....
Address:.....	Department:.....
Technician/radiographer:	Phone/Fax:.....
Radiologist/clinician:......	Phone/Fax:.....
Room:	
Machine make (x-ray unit):......	Model: ......
Serial #:......	
Machine make (generator):.......	Model: ....
Serial #:.......	
Previous visits: / / / /	

23.2 QUALITY CONTROL EQUIPMENT

The equipment used for quality control can be divided into general and specialized. The general equipment is simply operated without a great deal of careful setting up and tests can be quickly performed. This equipment should be top of the purchasing list:

- Digital radiation monitor with additional remote ion chamber.
- Aluminum filters 3×3″ (8×8cm) having 0.1, 0.5, 1.0 and 2.0mm thickness for HVL measurement.
- Digital kVp meter covering the range 60-125kVp.
- Aluminum step wedge
- Large wire mesh ⅛″ (3mm) pitch for screen film contact tests.
- Lead sheets for masking cassettes
- Fluoroscopy test pattern
- Sensitometer for film processor checking

- Tissue equivalent plastic blocks for testing linearity of automatic exposure control (AEC)

Radiation exposure levels and exposure rate are still given in a mixture of non-SI (roentgen as R or mR) and SI units (gray as μGy and nGy); the conversion factors in Tab.23.2 can be used for standardizing.

Table 23.2 Conversion non-SI to SI units.

Non SI	SI
1R = 0.87rad	8.7mGy
	$\sim 2.6 \times 10^{-4}$C kg^{-1} or 0.26mC kg^{-1}
1mR	8.7×10^{-6}Gy (8.7μGy)
1μR	8.7×10^{-9}Gy (8.7nGy)

Specific tests may be required for identifying the precise fault (timing, focal spot, automatic exposure device etc.). The necessary equipment would be:

- Electronic or mechanical x-ray exposure timer
- Focal spot test tool
- Light beam diaphragm and beam alignment template
- Digital thermometer
- Stopwatch
- Storage oscilloscope

This equipment is usually acquired when necessary particularly by a large radiology department. It will quickly pay for itself by identifying faults quickly or plotting trends (degrading focal spot sizes) so that remedial action can be taken before breakdown. The equipment also serves a very useful purpose: checking that engineers have repaired a machine as quoted and left it clinically safe (i.e. filters replaced).

23.2.1 X-ray generator performance

These are only outline descriptions, the instruction manual should of course be studied for each piece of equipment.

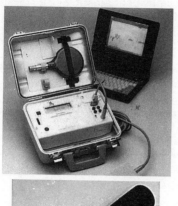
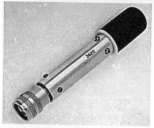
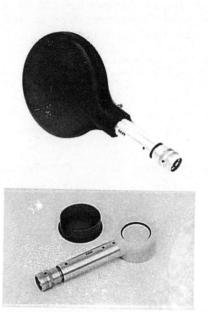

Figure 23.1 **(a)** Digital radiation meter Dose (mR or µGy) and dose rate (mR or µGy min^{-1}) can be measured. **(b)** Selection of ion chambers for different sensitivities for (from the top) in-beam, leakage and mammography work (courtesy Radcal Corporation).

Radiation monitors (Figure 23.1(a)) These are digital meters, some of them with a built-in detectors which make them convenient for primary test in-beam measurements. Certain applications (mammography) require a thin walled remote ion chamber (shown in Fig.23.1(b)) and specifications for some common ion chambers for QC measurements are given in Table 23.3.

Table 23.3 Specifications for separate ion-chambers.

Chamber	Energy range and sensitivity	Use
Pancake (400cm^3)	0.02–1.3 MeV 0.1mR h^{-1}	Beam leakage and fluoroscopy
Thimble (6cm^3)	0.02–1.3 MeV 1mR min^{-1}	Tissue dose and general use
Low energy (6cm^3)	10–40keV 1mR min^{-1}	Mammography

Very precise radiation measurements are re-quired to record equipment radiation leakage or patient/staff dose. The greater sensitivity given by the large volume detector listed in Tab.23.3 is necessary. This equipment would only be suitable for trained staff and would form a secondary testing schedule.

Kilovoltage measurement Early methods for measuring kVp relied on a kVp test cassette with specially calibrated copper filters; this was the Adrian-Crookes penetrometer. It requires very careful exposure to give acceptable accuracy so is very time consuming. Its accuracy is ±3kVp over the range 50-150kVp. A mammography version covered the lower range of 24 to 40kVp with similar accuracy. These have been superseded by digital meters offering greater accuracy, particularly important when measuring mammography x-ray units.

Figure 23.2 shows two types of kVp meter and specification for a conventional meter is given in Tab.23.4 (50-160kVp) along with a mammography meter (22-45kVp).

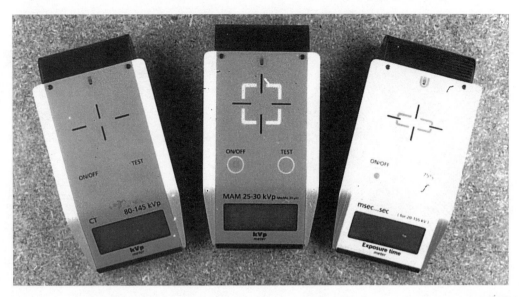

Figure 23.2   A selection of digital meters suitable for (from the left) conventional kVp (60 to 125kVp) and mammography kVp measurement and exposure time.

Combination meters for measuring a variety of machine outputs are also available from various manufacturers. The output can be interfaced to a personal computer and report sheets generated with acceptance limits built into the test.

Table 23.4 kVp meter basic requirements

Conventional
Range	50 – 160kVp
Accuracy	±2kV or 2%
Reproducibility	0.5kV
Resolution	0.1kV

Mammography kVp meters
Range	22 – 45kVp
Accuracy	±1kV

Exposure timers   Earlier versions of exposure timers used a spinning top driven by a synchronous motor to give a moving circular slit whose image was captured on film. The angle of the slit gives a fairly accurate measure of the exposure time. It can give a

best accuracy between 7ms-8ms. As they require careful film exposure to obtain a good test image they have become less popular.

A digital timer (essentially a stopwatch) is activated by the x-ray beam and is the simplest method for measuring exposure time being ideal for checking very fast timing from high-kV chest units (~20mS). Timer ranges are typically 0 to 2000mS and 0 to 20 seconds and have an accuracy of 0.1mS or 1mS depending on the scale used (Figure 23.2).

23.2.2 X-ray tube

Focal spot size   The simplest test for indirectly assessing focal spot size uses either a line pair or a star-pattern grating to give a film image (Fig.23.3(a)).

A variation of this uses a series of bar patterns etched in tungsten, held in a 15cm (6″) plastic tower which is placed on a film cassette. The bar patterns vary from 0.6Lp mm^{-1} to 3.35Lp mm^{-1} in eleven groups. A chart relates the visible bars to focal spot size. Correct film exposure is essential for all these tests.

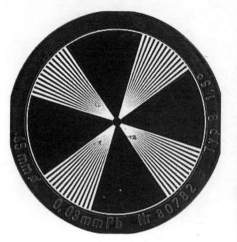
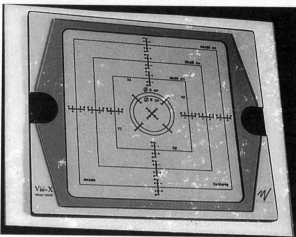

Figure 23.3   **(a)** A line pair grating extending to 10LP mm^{-1} for measuring the resolution limits of an imaging system. The star pattern grating allows estimation of the focal spot size from the formula described in the text (eqn.23.1). **(b)**   X-ray beam alignment with light beam diaphragms is quickly checked using a calibrated fluorescent screen (courtesy VISI-X, RTE Electronics)

A pinhole camera can be used to give a direct image of the focal spot; this allows more accurate measurement but the set-up is far more complex and the procedure can damage the x-ray target in inexperienced hands.

X-ray beam alignment and collimation
Both can be measured together and so require just one film exposure. The beam alignment device is two ball bearings one exactly over the other separated by about 15cm and held in a plastic tower. A perpendicular beam will give superimposed dots on the film; any misalignment will reveal two dots. This device is located on a plastic template with printed metal lines for measuring any light beam/collimator misalignment. Exact coincidence between illuminated area on the template and blackened area on the film image should be obtained. A more recent version uses a luminous plate which doesn't require a film image; this is represented in Fig.23.4(b).

23.2.3 Film image quality

Diagnostic sensitivity in radiology depends on the final image. If this is a film image then a great number of variables effecting photographic quality can go wrong. Maintaining a routine quality control program for judging the formation and processing of the film image should be the first priority for any radiology department. The film processor particularly should be subjected to a daily QC check and results recorded so that trends can be detected and avoiding action taken.

Film sensitometer   This is a stable calibrated light source that places a gray scale wedge on film (Fig.23.4(a)). The film is then developed in a day-light developing system and the gray scale read with a densitometer.

The film is exposed in a darkroom (no safe lights) and several sheets can be exposed together and kept as stock test film.

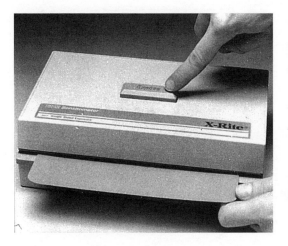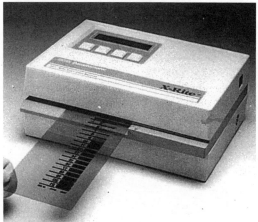

Figure 23.4 **(a)** A film sensitometer able to expose a graduated scale on either blue or green sensitive film. **(b)** A spot densitometer with a constant light source used for reading a gray scale in terms of optical density (courtesy X-Rite Inc.)

Both blue or green light is provided by most sensitometers (blue at ~455nm and green at ~520nm) so blue sensitive (mono-chromatic) and green sensitive (ortho-chromatic) film can be tested. A precise gray-scale of 21 or 24 steps is usually produced.

Film densitometer There are various designs. Spot densitometers have their own reference light source and allow precise small areas to be measured (Fig.23.4(b)). Hand held densitometers are used in conjunction with an external light source (viewing box). Densitometers with automatic motor drive can read the film gray scale as a strip and plot the characteristic curve. Top specifications are essential for meaningful results; a recommended list is given in Tab.23.5.

Digital thermometer Complete film processor assessment requires knowledge of the developer temperature (fixer and wash temperature are not so critical). Developer temperature variation by 1°C can significantly

alter film density particularly in mammography. The digital thermometer should have a robust probe, ordinary glass thermometers must not be used. Temperature reading should be a regular part of film processor quality control.

Table 23.5 Specifications for sensitometer and densitometer

Sensitometer	
Gray scale	21 step 0.15 OD per step
Blue peak	460nm
Green peak	510nm
Repeatability	±0.02 log E
Densitometer	
Range	0 to 4 OD
Accuracy	±0.02 OD
Repeatability	±0.01 OD
Zero stability	±0.02 OD

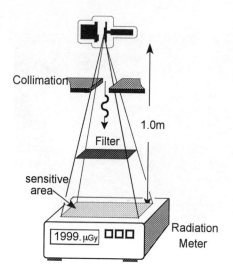

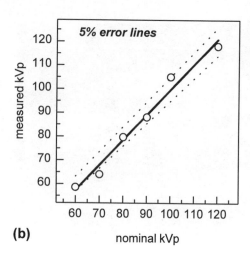

Figure 23.5 **(a)** General equipment set-up for measurements. A narrow beam geometry (carefully collimated) should always be used for measurements to reduce interfering scatter radiation. **(b)** Nominal versus measured kVp and the ±5% limits. In this example the 70 kVp measurement would be outside the limit.

23.3 CONVENTIONAL RADIOLOGY

QC equipment layout The general arrangement used for assessing equipment performance is shown in Fig.23.5(a) using a digital radiation meter with built-in ion chamber. A 1 meter focus to meter distance ensures reproducibility for follow-up studies. The x-ray beam should be closely collimated to the area of the detector. The 1m distance does not apply to kVp measurements since the meter should be much closer to the tube housing for successful operation.

The generator output for an x-ray tube must deliver stable voltage and current for a precise time period. Exposure times range from 0.01 s (10ms) to many seconds (2-5s) depending on image requirements and generator power. The timing precision is controlled by the automatic exposure control (AEC), separate timing devices in the generator have now been superseded. Any timing errors would therefore indicate AEC malfunction.

X-ray output; quantity and quality The consistency and quality of the x-ray beam must also be within tight specification; this is determined by measuring the quality and quantity of the x-ray beam. The following non-specific tests will measure consistency of radiation output (quantity):

- mR and mAs linearity
- mR/mAs versus kilovoltage linearity

If non-linearity exists in these measurements then (assuming the kV is reliable) the following specific quantities should be measured to identify the fault:

- exposure control from the AEC
- tube current

X-ray beam **quality** is assessed from the half-value layer (HVL) which indirectly measures beam filtration. HVL has an important influence on patient radiation dose and image contrast.

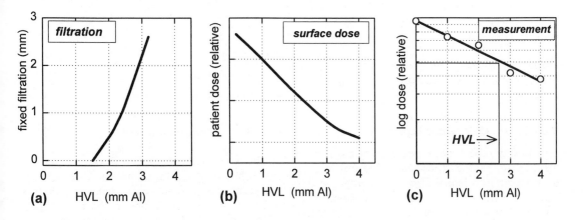

Figure 23.6 **(a)** The relationship between the half-value layer, as measured, and the tube fixed filtration. **(b)** The sharp reduction in patient entrance dose and increasing HVL. **(c)** HVL measurements from Table 23.6 plotted. The half-value-layer is 2.7mmAl which is acceptable for 80kVp.

Other important tests which investigate the mechanical and safety characteristic are:

- focal-spot-size
- X-ray beam alignment
- radiation leakage

Focal spot size and alignment will strongly influence image resolution. Radiation leakage from the tube housing influencing safe machine operation

23.3.1 QC tests: Conventional equipment

There is an example QC report sheet at the end of this chapter (QC 1.) which can form the basis of a routine inspection program. For more complex tests the relevant specialist publications should be consulted. QC report sheets should be simple to follow and contain concise directions about setting up the test equipment so that a standard approach is adopted.

Test 1: ***Kilovoltage***

This test relates the nominal (control setting) kilovoltage value against an accurately measured value. An example result is plotted in Fig.23.5(b).

Equipment:

- Digital kVp meter

It is important that the kVp meter has been calibrated since additional beam filtration (aluminum plate) may be necessary to improve the meter accuracy to within a ±5% variation.

Method: Place the meter in the primary beam close to the tube housing, open the light diaphragms until the top is completely illuminated. Choose dial kVp values of 60, 70, 80, 90, 100 and 125kVp. The mAs values are quite large at 60kVp (~100mAs) and much lower for the higher kVp's (~20mAs) depending on meter sensitivity.

Limiting value: Each reading should be within ±5kV of the indicated voltage and ±5 to10kV is acceptable; greater than 10kV is poor. Some regulatory bodies are more strict and require ±3kV below 100kVp and ±6kV above. The should be easily achieved by current HF generators.

Frequency of test: Yearly for current equipment having electronically controlled HF generators.

Test 2:   *Half value layer*

The quality of the x-ray beam is measured by placing increasing thickness of aluminum (1 to 4mm) in the beam and measuring the decreasing intensity with a digital dosimeter. The thickness of aluminum that reduces the intensity by half is the half-value layer (HVL). It can be used to estimate the total beam filtration (Fig.23.6(a)) The HVL also indicates the relative quantity of soft radiation that increases patient dose without playing any part in image formation; it is wholly absorbed by superficial tissue Fig.23.6(b).

Equipment:

• Digital radiation dosimeter.
• Aluminum absorbers consisting of 0.5 and 1mm sheets cut to fit the detector area

Method :   With reference to Fig.23.5(a) the tube is raised until the focal point is 1 meter above the detector. The beam is collimated so that only the area of the aluminum filter is covered. It is important that no stray radiation by-passes the aluminum filter. Results are plotted on log/linear paper to give the HVL (Fig.23.6(c) gives an HVL of 2.7mm Al).

Limiting value: The mean value of multiple readings will improve accuracy but precision is usually acceptable from single values. The suggested tolerance for conventional equipment is ±10%. Table 23.6 gives the minimum values for selected kV.

Frequency of test: Every six months or after equipment maintenance.

Table 23.6 Minimum values of HVL versus kV

kVp	Minimum HVL
30	0.3
50	1.2
70	1.5
80	2.5
100	2.8
120	3.2

Test 3:   *Focal spot size*

As the x-ray tube ages the anode target becomes pitted which broadens the focal spot so degrading image resolution. Focal spot measurement should be performed on a regular basis in order to detect this degradation.

Equipment:

• **Line pair grating**: A line pair grating gives a direct reading of image resolution so a high definition 'detail' cassette should be used (Fig.23.7(a)).
• **Bar-pattern test tool**: The bar-pattern indirectly indicates the focal spot range by reference to the manufacturer's conversion table (Fig.23.7(b)).
• **Star pattern**: The effective focal spot size *f* is estimated from the blurring diameter as:

$$f = \frac{2\pi D}{180} \times \frac{1}{(M-1)} \qquad (23.1)$$

Where *D* is the blurring diameter and *M* the geometric magnification of the image

Method: The **line-pair grating** can be used for assessing conventional and mammography focal spot sizes (Fig.23.7(a)). It should be centered on the cassette (or surface plate of the mammography unit) and a low exposure made (2-3mAs). The plastic tower containing the **bar-pattern** tool is carefully centralized in the field of view and leveled. The focal spot marking on the tube-housing must be 1 meter from the pattern surface. A low exposure level is chosen (60kVp at 2-3mAs).

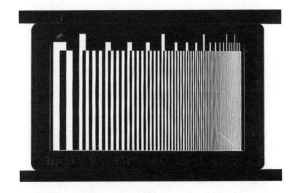 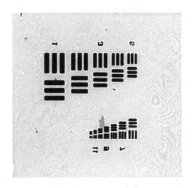

Figure 23.7   **(a)** Line pair grating showing difference between a mammography and conventional x-ray tube **(b)** Bar set example from two x-ray tubes showing: a tube having good resolution and unacceptable degraded focal spot size

The **star pattern** test grating (Fig.23.3) is supported 30 to 50 cm from the focus and a magnified film image produced from a detail screen cassette. The film cassette should be 1m from the tube focus.

Limiting value: The line pair grating should show at least 5Lp mm^{-1} on the film image; for the bar-pattern the manufacturer's conversion table or nomogram should be consulted.

The International Electro-technical Commission (IEC) specification gives the following limits outside the nominal value:

- measured size ×1.5 nominal is acceptable
- ×1.5-×2.0 more than nominal is poor
- greater than ×2.0 would be unacceptable and the tube needs replacing.

Frequency: This test should be performed at least twice a year.

Test 4: Automatic exposure control (AEC)

This test can be applied to most designs of exposure control systems met in conventional radiography. AEC complete breakdown of the AEC device can result in prolonged patient exposure if the design is not 'fail-safe'. Routine testing can reveal unreliable and inconsistent operation.

Equipment

- Two blocks of tissue equivalent material (PMMA) 2.5 or 3.0cm thick.
- Radiation dosimeter

Method: Film holders (Bucky's) normally carry three exposure control devices (see Chapter 4). Before carrying out the following tests ensure that a particular detector is active as an AEC. Filter the x-ray beam with a 1mm copper foil and shield those AEC ion chambers that are not being tested with a 2mm lead sheet. Make an exposure at 80kVp/200mA with the entire Bucky in the beam. If the exposure time is less than 0.5s then the AEC is working. Repeat this for the remaining ion chambers.

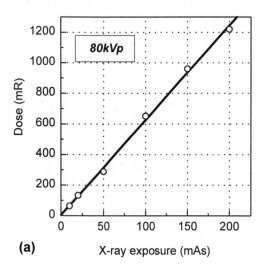
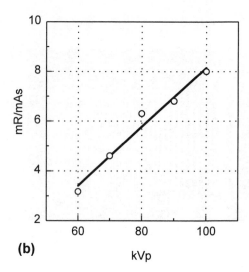

(a)   **(b)**

Figure 23.8 **(a)** mR plotted against mAs from the results calculated in Box.23.1. The overall linear relationship is just within ±5%. **(b)** The results for mR/mAs versus kVp showing a good linear relationship.

The most straightforward method of quantifying AEC response is to note the mAs reading on the machine.

Limiting value The variation in exposure levels should be no more than ±10%.

Frequency of test: Twice a year or after maintenance.

Test 5:   *Output linearity (mR/mAs)*

Linearity of exposure (mAs) with radiation output (mR/μGy) and kilovoltage. Radiation output varies with kVp, mA and exposure time; for a fixed kVp the radiation dose output (mR/μGy) should vary linearly with exposure (mAs). The test should be performed approximately once a month as part of the routine QC monitor program.

mR/mAs: This is measured in air and should show a linear relationship across the full range of exposure settings; an example is shown in Fig. 23.8(a).   A non-linear mR/mAs reading but acceptable timer test would indicate tube current inconsistencies.

mR/mAs versus kVp: This more comprehensive test requires that the kVp is changed for a fixed mAs reading. It is a rigorous test for generator consistency showing up any changes in tube current for change in kVp setting which should be controlled by the kV compensation circuit. The plot of mR/mAs versus kVp should show a linear relationship. The example in Fig 23.8(b) is obtained from data in Box 23.1.   Non-linearity here would indicate variable kVp with tube current. Although both of these are non-specific tests they give a good general indication of generator performance (mA, timing and kVp). A one meter FFD is used for both these readings so follow-up comparisons can be made.

Equipment:

• Digital radiation meter
• Steel tape measure

Method: Repeated measurements using a dosimeter at constant exposure (80kVp 200mA at 0.2s) Place the meter in the primary beam 1m from the focus. Open the light diaphragms until only the detector area is illuminated.

- *mR versus mAs:* For a constant kV and exposure time (80kV and 0.2s) a linear variation in output with changing tube current (mA) should be noted. For machines which only have a single mAs control this should be varied over a wide range (5- 200mAs). The plot of output (µGy or mR) versus mAs should be linear.

- *mR/mAs versus kV:* For a constant mAs (between 20 and 50mAs) the kVp is varied over 60 to 120kVp and the output measured at each 10kV step.

Box 23.1

Calculation of mR/mAs for kVp

The following mR values were obtained for a standard 20mAs (with different tube currents and times) at 60, 70, 80, 90 and 100kVp :

mA	sec	60	70	80	90	100
100	0.2	65	91	125	135	162
200	0.1	64	92	126	137	158
400	0.05	63	92	127	134	160
800	0.025	62	92	126	136	161
	Mean	63.5	92	126	136	160

The mR per mAs for each kV setting is calculated as mR/20, which yields:

	60	70	80	90	100
mR/mAs	3.17	4.6	6.3	6.8	8.0

These values are plotted in Fig.23.8(b).

Limiting value: A 10% change in mR/mAs value would be visible on the film image. Linearity should be within ±5% for modern equipment. The percentage variation in the readings (reproducibility) is :

$$\frac{maximum - minimum}{maximum + minimum} \times 100\% \qquad (23.2)$$

The results from the calculated mR/mAs versus kVp plotted in Fig.23.8(b) show an acceptable linear relationship.

Frequency of test: Twice a year or after machine maintenance.

Test 6: Exposure time

Calibration of generator timer over the range 0.025 to 1 or more seconds in dial setting intervals. This test is necessary if the mR versus mAs test proves non-linear. If the timing is shown to be accurate then the tube current should be suspect. The frequency of testing is dictated by non-specific tests or after servicing. Most exposure times are controlled by an automatic exposure control (AEC).

Equipment:
- Digital timer (the simplest method requiring no film exposure)

Method: The digital stopwatch is placed centrally within the x-ray beam and a succession of exposure times selected for testing. If the mAs setting can only be altered then several values should be selected to cover a wide range.

Limiting value: The time periods should be within ±5% of the nominal value for current equipment. Any variation from this would indicate a faulty timing circuit or AEC.

Frequency of test: Yearly

Test 7: Beam alignment and collimation

The alignment of the x-ray beam perpendicular to the table surface is essential for optimum image resolution. Registration of the illuminated area with the x-ray beam is necessary for accurate positioning and protection of patient anatomy outside the beam ('coning-down'). Both tests can be performed at the same time.

Equipment:
- Beam alignment test tool (Fig.23.9).
- Calibrated template (Fig.23.3 or similar)
- Detail screen cassette

Method: The template is placed on the film cassette and the plastic tower containing the alignment tool is located carefully over the central target area on the template. The light diaphragms are opened until the inner square is exactly covered. A small spirit level ensures that the top of the plastic tower is exactly level. The tube focal spot is positioned 1m above the tower

Limiting value: The light beam diaphragm should be within 1cm of the setting at 1m and the x-ray beam should be misaligned by less than 4%. (example Fig.23.9).

Frequency of test: Once a year or after machine servicing.

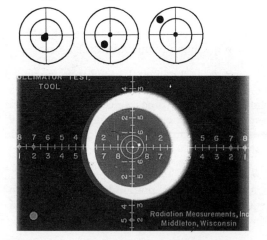

Figure 23.9   Radiograph of x-ray beam alignment using a ball-bearing alignment tool. Borderline acceptance would be 2%. Outside this is the etched boundary for light beam collimation measurement.

Test 8:   *Radiation leakage*

Leakage radiation around an x-ray tube housing increases the radiation exposure to the staff particularly at head-height where personal dosimeters may not register. It is good practice to locate 2-3 TLD badges on the inside walls at locations near the machine. These will give a continuous assessment of scatter radiation in fluoroscopy and cine-angiography rooms.

Equipment:

- Loaded film cassette
- Radiation monitor with large volume pancake detector

The existence of leakage can be established by positioning 3 to 4 cassettes around the tube housing and making a 60kVp at 20mAs exposure. The film image will show the extent and position of the leakage.

Method: The general set up is shown in Fig.23.10. In order to ascertain whether leakage radiation exists around an x-ray housing four film/screen cassettes can be used to 'box-in' the housing and an exposure made with the collimators closed. If leakage radiation is present the film image will show dark lines of varying thicknesses. The radiation dose rate should then be measured with a large volume 'pancake' ion chamber at a fixed distance (30cm) and the reading converted into μGy h^{-1} at 1m.

Limiting value: A maximum limit of 1mGy h^{-1} averaged over a 3 minute period at 1m is generally accepted but equipment is usually better than 0.25mGy h^{-1} at 1m. Certain legislation requires a much lower level of 1μGy h^{-1} at 1m so the relevant national legislation should be consulted.

Frequency of test: Usually once a year or when any maintenance work has been carried out.

Test 9: *Room safety: ambient radiation*

New equipment or room design alteration require comprehensive monitoring both immediate and long term. Badge dosimeters should be a permanent feature for fluoroscopy and nuclear medicine departments in order to monitor safe practice.

Equipment::

- TLD or film badge for long term monitoring
- Large ion chamber (100 – 350cm^3) for immediate measurements.

Method: The dosimeter badge is fixed to the wall and its exact position noted. For extra sensitivity the badge should be kept in place for between 2 to 3 months. For these low radiation doses it is important that matching control badges are kept in a non-radiation area so that normal background during monitoring and during transport between department can be allowed for; particularly relevant in a nuclear medicine facility.

Limiting value: Behind control panels in diagnostic x-ray rooms $1\mu Gy\ h^{-1}$ is attainable. Outside corridors and windows should register below $0.5\mu Gy\ h^{-1}$ averaged over one minute if using the ion chamber monitoring equipment. Special aluminum oxide low noise TLD's should be employed in these low radiation areas otherwise LiF TLD's or even film dosimeters can be employed to measure higher radiation levels.

Frequency of test: Continuous program.

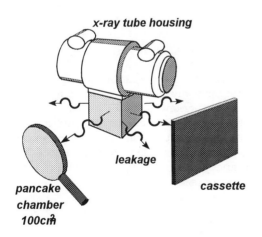

Figure 23.10 Radiation leakage can be detected generally by using a film cassette and accurately measured using a $100cm^3$ ionization detector placed 1 meter away.

23.3.2   Portable x-ray units

The tests already described for mR/mAs linearity, kVp, HVL and light beam registration apply to portable x-rays sets. Capacitor discharge generators will register lower kVp than the nominal value. The standard 80kVp would measure as ~72-75kVp. Most recent high frequency portables should give kVp readings within ±5kVp and give QC values as good as conventional x-ray units.

Electrical safety should be carefully checked on portable machines. Loose cables can become dangerously frayed and broken.

23.4   FILM IMAGE

The image quality: resolution, contrast and noise, must be maintained at an optimum level for reliable and consistent diagnostic sensitivity. Quality control sheets are given at the end of this chapter (QC 2.) which can be used for entering daily measurements. Film and film processing performance will be shown as changes in contrast and speed, film storage problems will be shown as changes in base-fog and inconsistent exposure for standard conditions shown as changes in AEC mAs values.

23.4.1   Film sensitometry

The film image quality is crucial to the diagnostic radiology department. Even the best imaging equipment (conventional, DSA or CT) will give mediocre results if film processing is sub-standard. The majority of departments operate daylight-loading film processors where routine cleaning and chemical replenishment should be established.

Current high frequency x-ray equipment gives very constant output with very little variation so x-ray sensitometry can safely be carried out using a 21 step aluminum wedge. This will give density increments of 0.15 (a variation of $log\sqrt{2} = 0.15$) which will embrace the entire characteristic curve of the film as shown in Fig.23.11(a).

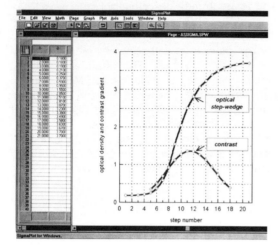
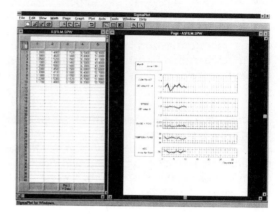

Figure 23.11 **(a)** Computer QC program showing film characteristic curve with computed contrast gradient curve measured by sensitometric step-wedge. **(b)** The same QC program displaying the daily chart of film processor performance and AEC constancy.

This curve gives a speed index of 2.2 (allowing for base + fog), where the curve coincides with the mid-step 11. A base-fog reading of 0.22 at the zero exposure level (step 1) indicates both film quality (age) and developer performance; if either of these deteriorates the base-fog index will increase. The film D_{max} is 3.6 and the contrast gradient is calculated from the exposure levels between steps 4 and 10 or the peak value of the contrast curve which is part of the computer control sheet example in Fig 23.11(a).

Test 1. Film characteristic curve

Variation in processing influences film image quality. Test films are supplied by manufacturer's or film can be exposed directly with a sensitometer wedge.

Equipment:
- Sensitometer
- Box of x-ray film   or
- Box of test films

Method: The sensitometer is used to expose two gray scale wedges on a sheet of film. This test film, or the commercially prepared test film, is then located in a cassette and fed into the daylight processor. The gray-scale step is accurately measured using a densitometer and the results plotted on the appropriate QC graph paper or entered into the computer data-base (QC.2).

Limiting value: A variation within ±0.1OD for a step midway up the gray scale is acceptable. An experienced observer can visually detect this change by comparing with a reference exposure but densitometry is necessary if the results are plotted on a QC sheet. The acceptance limits are then marked on the graph paper (see example sheet).

Frequency of test: Film processor performance should be recorded as a daily routine. The results from the QC measurements: film contrast, speed, base-fog, developer temperature and AEC stability are plotted on a QC graph as shown in Fig.23.11(b).

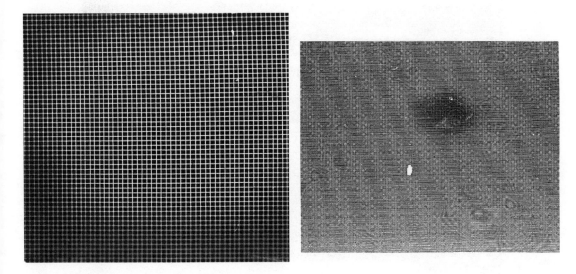

Figure 23.12   Film and screen contact tool showing bad contact in **(a)** conventional and **(b)** mammography cassettes.

This routine lends itself to computer data entry so that performance trends can be identified.

Test 2. Film-screen contact

The film cassettes should be inspected regularly since they receive a great deal of abuse and the intensifying screen should be cleaned on a regular basis with an appropriate screen cleaner in order to remove dirt specks which give image artifacts.

A fine mesh is used to test contact between screen and film; particularly important in automatic chest x-ray equipment where the screens can become dislodged (Fig.23.12).

Equipment:

- Fine copper mesh 3mm pitch for conventional cassettes and 1mm pitch for mammography cassettes.

Method: Place the cassette outside the Bucky holder on the table surface. The mesh is then positioned directly on the cassette. Use a low exposure level of 60kVp at 5mAs (27kVp in the case of mammography units).

Limiting value: The developed film should show a uniform sharp image of the mesh. Any screen-film contact problems will show up as dark areas.

Frequency: All the cassettes should be inspected on a yearly cycle or when damage is suspected.

23.4.2   The Film Processor

Two critical components of film processor operation is the developer freshness (replenishment rate) and working temperature. The replenishment rate depends on film throughput measured in square meters (Tab.23.7) and alters depending on film sizes being used.

Fixing and washing cycles determine the keeping quality of the film image and test films from the processor should be observed over a long period in order to judge archival quality. If fog levels increase then fixing and washing are below acceptable levels.

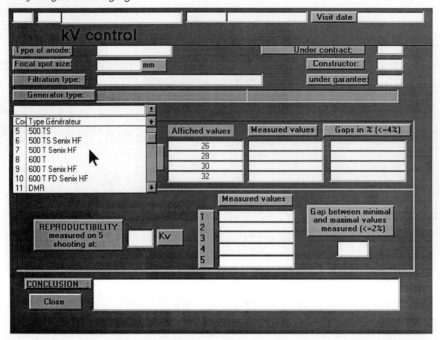

Figure 23.13 Data input handling by a computer data-base QC program designed for mammography (courtesy Hoptaux de la Timone Group, Marseille, France).

Table 23.7 Films processed for 400ml replenishment per m² film.

Film size	No. films
35 × 43cm (14″×17″)	7
18 × 24cm (8″×10″)	25

Test 3,   Developer temperature

Film processors can be fitted with temperature indicators, in which case a separate digital thermometer is not necessary.

Equipment:

- Digital thermometer having ±0.1°C accuracy. The temperature sensor should be at least 10cm long for easy location in the developer bath.

Method: The temperature probe should be placed in the volume of developer actually in contact with the rollers. Make a note of the steady reading and enter this on the QC daily log. (sheet QC 2. example).

Limiting value: The film manufacturer's recommendations should be followed. A typical value would be 35°C for most film types and developer chemistry.

Frequency: Daily

Test 4. Refreshment rate

The developer and fixer refreshment rate is fixed in agreement with the engineer but should be increased for certain developers. It can be measured by carefully running a volume of developer or fixer into a measuring cylinder when the pump is operating during film processing. The manufacturer's specifications will change for different 'chemistry'.

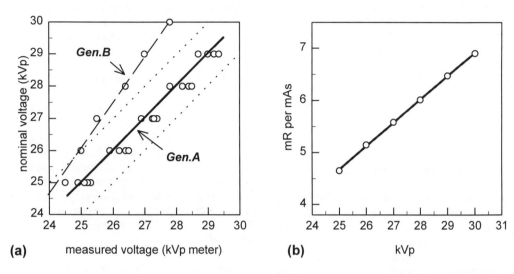

Figure 23.14 **(a)** The kV accuracy of an HF mammography generator (Gen.A) compared to an old model 3-phase machine (Gen.B) which exceeds acceptable limits. **(b)** expected mR per mAs linearity for mammographic range.

23.5 MAMMOGRAPHY

It is accepted that strict quality control objectives are essential if premium image quality is to be achieved in mammography. Since image formation depends almost exclusively on photoelectric reactions within soft tissue in order to get optimum contrast for lowest radiation dose all aspects of the equipment whether it be the x-ray machine or film processor must be working at their peak performance. Several computer packages are available designed for accepting QC data into a data-base. Separate machines can be accommodated and so comparisons between machine types, their performance history, trends and other relevant data can be readily displayed. An example of computer input format is shown in Fig. 23.13 and QC 3. suggests some basic tests that should be routinely performed.

23.5.1 The x-ray machine

The following tests should be carried out on a regular basis throughout the year. Daily checks would involve a mammography phantom with a gray-scale insert so that film contrast, speed and fog can be measured.

Test 1. Kilovoltage accuracy

When monitoring older machines a kilovoltage calibration check should be performed with a meter capable of at least ±1kVp accuracy. Electronic controlled high frequency generators are very stable and routine kVp tests are somewhat redundant since the internal monitoring carried out by the machine is more precise than an external kVp meter reading.

Equipment:

• Digital kVp meter with kilovolt range from 20 to 40kV with a quoted accuracy of ⩽±1kV and a reproducibility of ±0.3kV

Method: Select a fixed high mAs value in order to operate the meter. Lower mAs may not be sufficient. Greater sensitivity is obtained if the meter is supported just under the x-ray tube housing

Limiting value: Each reading should be within ±1kVp of the indicated voltage. K-edge filters that are automatically moved into the beam complicate this otherwise simple measurement. Figure 23.14(a) compares the results from a machine with precise specification with a machine giving unacceptable performance tolerances

Frequency of test A kVp check should be carried out after any maintenance.

Test 2. mR/mAs output versus kVp

The procedure outlined in Section 23.3.1 for output linearity (Test 5.) should be followed for a restricted range of kVp values; say from 24 to 30kVp. The plot of mR per mAs versus kVp should be linear to within ±5%; most current machines can better this figure. Inaccuracies are mostly due to measuring equipment drift, so only radiation monitoring equipment with good specifications should be used. Figure 23.14(b) shows the linearity that should be obtained.

Test 3. Exposure times

The time taken for a routine exposure is important since if the generator is under powered the necessary mAs product for thick breasts is achieved by increasing the time of exposure; movement artifact would be a serious problem.
Equipment:

• Radiation timer
• 4 and 6cm plastic absorber blocks

Method: Measure exposure times using the two plastic blocks using AEC at the clinical settings (27-28kVp).

Limiting value: Exposure times for current x-ray units vary between 0.15 and 1.17s for a 4cm absorber and between 0.6 and 6.0s using a 6cm absorber. There is a lack of guidance on acceptable exposure times but reasonable values would be 0.3 to 0.5s for the 4cm ab-

sorber and 1.5 to 2.5s for the 6cm block.

Frequency of test: This is an acceptance test and should be used for assessing the suitability of x-ray units for clinical use.

Test 4. Half Value Layer (HVL)

In order to reduce low energy radiation in the incident x-ray beam and so reduce breast surface dose the total beam filtration should be 0.5mm aluminum or 0.03mm molybdenum. This level of beam filtration would give an HVL for aluminum greater than 0.3mm at 30kVp. Higher values of HVL will indicate that lower photon energies are being removed and image contrast will be affected.
Equipment:

• Thin walled ion chamber (see Fig.23.1(b))
• Pure aluminum foil 2×0.1mm and 1×0.5mm

Method: This is measured using a setting of 28kVp and the compression paddle in place. The equipment is set up as described previously in Section 23.3.1 for HVL measurement. Three radiation readings are taken:

• No filter in place (Y_0 mR)
• Filter X_1 mm yielding Y_1 mR (0.1mm for mammography)
• Filter X_2 mm yielding Y_2 mR (0.5mm for mammography)

These are used for computing accurate HVL measurement in the formula:

$$\text{HVL} = \frac{X_1 \times \ln\left[\frac{2 \times Y_2}{Y_0}\right] - X_2 \times \ln\left[\frac{2 \times Y_2}{Y_0}\right]}{\ln\left[\frac{Y_2}{Y_1}\right]} \quad (23.3)$$

This formula is used in a program for precise computation of HVL for mammography given at the end of the chapter.

Limiting value: New anode materials and filtration are from time to time introduced which will influence the HVL reading. K-edge filters are automatically moved into the beam which complicates this otherwise simple measurement. The IEC has produced a list of the common combinations:

Anode and filter	HVL (mm Al) at 28kVp
Mo + 30μm Mo	0.32
Mo + 25μm Rh	0.40
W + 60μm Mo	0.37
W + 50μm Rh	0.51
W + 40μm Pd	0.48
Rh + 25μm Rh	0.39

Frequency of test: Generally twice a year is sufficient or after machine maintenance.

Test 5. Focal spot size

The 'gold standard' for measuring focal spot size is the slit camera, however this requires considerable expertise. In the wrong hands this can damage the x-ray tube due to heavy tube currents. A simpler technique uses a magnified line pair image.

Equipment:
- Line pair grating having 15Lp mm^{-1}
- Routine film screen cassette
- 40mm absorber block
- magnifying lens

Method :   The cassette is placed on top of the support above the grid and the line pair grating placed on the cassette face. A low mAs (4–6) is chosen at 28kV to give a clear image. The procedure is repeated using a 40mm absorber block.

Limiting value: The full line pair grating should be clearly visible up to 15Lp mm^{-1}. Scatter performance using the absorber block should give at least 10Lp mm^{-1}.

Frequency of test: Depending on equipment use. Units used for screening should check resolution on a monthly basis.

23.5.2 Film processor and image quality

Since the mammogram is most sensitive to machine variability both x-ray machine and film processor should be tested on a daily basis using a QC program that is simple and comprehensive. The major variables affecting image quality in current film mammography are:

- Film and intensifying screen type
- Processor chemistry
- Developer temperature and refreshment rate
- Automatic Exposure Control

Current x-ray systems using microprocessor controlled high frequency generators are extremely accurate and do not drift with time so an x-ray reference image could be used for checking film processor performance as a daily routine.

Test 6.   Image quality; high and low contrast resolution

A comprehensive and well designed mammography phantom having tissue characteristics similar to breast (5cm tissue equivalent) can show low contrast and resolution performance of both the x-ray machine and the film/screen combination. The breast phantom should contain small details that push the imaging system to the limit of its capability and beyond so that improved performance can be observed when updating equipment.

Equipment:
- Mammographic phantom (Fig.23.15) representing 5cm tissue equivalent thickness (50% adipose) having aluminum step wedge, line-pair grating, micro-inclusions and low contrast detail.
- Densitometer

Method: The test object is placed on a 40mm absorber block and exposed at 28kVp under AEC control. The mAs reading should be noted and plotted on the daily QC chart (Fig.23.11(b) and sheet QC 2.). Densitometric measurements are made on the contrast items and step wedge. High contrast detail is examined parallel to and perpendicular to the tube axis.

Limiting value: The majority of the phantom

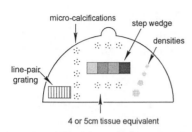

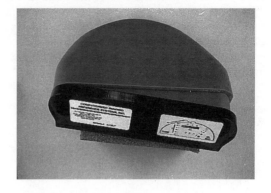

Figure 23.15   A tissue equivalent breast phantom with the diagram showing position of inserts, gray scale wedge and line pair grating

detail should be visible and the AEC exposure reading should not have varied by more than ±10%.

Frequency of test: Daily

Test 7. Film density

In order to encompass the full dynamic range of mammographic image a median density of about 1.5OD should be maintained.

Equipment:
- Routine screen film cassette
- 4cm plastic absorber or step wedge
- Film densitometer

Method: Expose the absorber or step wedge (which can be part of the breast phantom in Test 6.) using routine settings for AEC and processing the film under normal conditions. A gray-scale step should be chosen representing a middle value.

Limiting value: The optical density should be 1.5±0.05.

Frequency of test: This should be performed at the start of each week in order to check reliability of film processor chemistry. The film processor QC described in Section 23.4.2 is a most important daily routine for mammogra-

phy and results should be carefully plotted as the film speed (see QC chart).

Test 8. AEC compensation

Patient radiation dose is kept to optimum levels by the automatic exposure device situated underneath the film cassette (see Chapter 9: Mammography). It is essential to monitor its performance as any malfunction usually gives a large radiation exposure since signal feedback from the device would stop. This test should be a routine daily check.
Equipment:

- Routine mammography cassette and film
- 40mm and 6cm plastic absorber
- Densitometer

Method: Film densities obtained by using a 40mm plastic absorber under AEC clinical settings are measured at fixed locations on the film. Exposure settings are adjusted one step above and below the routine setting. The procedure is repeated using the 6cm block.

Limiting value: Film density maintained within 10% of the optical density values

Frequency of test: This should be performed on a daily basis.

23.5.3 Radiation dose

Test 9. Radiation output

A high radiation output is desirable for short exposure times and reduction in patient movement artifacts.

Equipment:

- Radiation dosimeter with mammography ion chamber.

Method: Measured at 28kV and 40mAs using a dosimeter with a mammographic quality chamber (Fig.23.1(b)). The distance from the focal spot to the center of the chamber is used in the calculation for µGy mAs^{-1} at 1m.

Limiting value: Greater than 45µGy mAs^{-1}. Current machine outputs vary from 20 to 70µGy mAs^{-1}. Table 23.8 lists acceptable values for machine specifications.

Frequency of test: This should form part of the acceptance testing.

Test 10. Entrance and Mean Glandular Dose

The entrance and mean glandular dose for a fixed optical density (usually 1.5OD) is influenced by a number of parameters amongst them being kV setting, film/screen type and film processor chemistry, temperature and process time. Although the mean glandular dose is the relevant measurement for a standard 5cm thick absorber the entrance dose is a quick method for giving indications of change.

Equipment:

- 5cm thick breast phantom
- mammography ion chamber with dosimeter
- routine film/screen cassette

Method: The breast phantom is placed in position on the support platform and the ion chamber placed on top. For a standard AEC setting an exposure is made at 27-28kVp. The air-kerma dose is noted and the film processed in the normal way. The background optical density of the phantom is measured and the mean glandular dose calculated from published tables using the HVL figure as measured above.

Limiting value: The acceptable entrance surface dose for current machines is between 4 - 6mGy for an optical density of between 1.3 and 1.4OD; the mean glandular dose would be 1.2 - 1.8mGy. When this is corrected for an optical density of 1.5OD the values are between 1.33-1.9mGy. It should not exceed 3mGy with the grid in place.

Frequency of test: This should be performed approximately every month or when film processing or film/screen details are changed.

Table 23.8 Some desirable values for mammography from European Guidelines.

Parameter	Desirable value
X-ray source	
misalignment of x-ray field	<5mm
radiation leakage	<1mGy/h
output	>40µGy/mAs
output rate	>10mGy/s
Tube voltage	
reproducibility	<+0.5kV
accuracy (26-30kV)	<+1.0kV
AEC	
reproducibility (on film)	<+0.15OD

23.6 FLUOROSCOPY

Although modern fluoroscopic equipment delivers a very low radiation output, its continuous operation (several minutes in some examinations) can give a high total dose to the patient when compared to film/screen or 100mm spot film studies. Three basic fluoroscopic models exist that have been described in Chapter 10:

- An under-couch (table) design where the

x-ray tube fires upwards through the table top.

- An over-couch design with the x-ray tube in a conventional downward pointing position.
- A C-arm design either used for cine-cardiology or as a smaller mobile version.

The under-couch design poses problems when performing QC measurements since the test gear needs to be inverted.

23.6.1 Image intensifier parameters and controls.

Conversion factor   This is a complex measurement which is not practical for general QC program.

Automatic exposure control. There are three main types:

- Automatic Brightness Control (ABC)
- Automatic Dose Control (ADC)
- Automatic Gain Control (AGC)

The ABC and ADC are automatic exposure controls and adjust kV and or mA to maintain sufficient radiation for image quality. The AGC controls the video camera which affects the brightness of the video monitor. The image intensity is kept constant regardless of dose which sometimes gives noisy images in low dose examinations. It has a much faster response than the automatic exposure controls and will keep the image intensity constant while they are adjusting.

Test 1.   Resolution/contrast, frame distortion and field size

A simple test for fluoroscopy resolution can be performed by using a graduated wire mesh (Fig.23.16). The mesh sizes are usually given in inches; the approximate equivalent to millimeter values are given in Tab.23.9.

General fluoroscopic performance is best assessed by using a phantom containing test patterns having low contrast objects and a line pair grating. A common phantom design is shown in Fig.23.17 (Faxil TOR—TVF Leeds'

phantom). These circular phantoms come complete with a 1mm copper filter, to simulate patient absorption.

Equipment:

- Suitable circular phantom containing contrast and resolution information

Method: Using adhesive tape stick the phantom to the image intensifier face. Place the 1mm copper filter as near to the x-ray tube as possible. Collimate the edges of the phantom and select 70kVp. Operate the screening control and note that the ABC is operating. Record the mA and kV. Store the image to allow inspection. Record the smallest mesh size or the limit of resolvable lines together with the number of contrast discs visible. The line pair grating may need a lower kV setting. Note the distortion to the phantom outline.

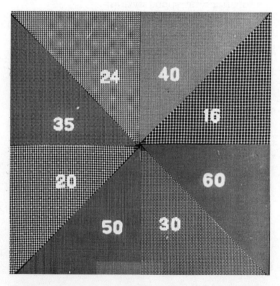

Figure 23.16 Resolution mesh showing sectors having pitch sizes 16 to 60 lines to the inch. Equivalent metric conversion given in Tab.23.9.

Limiting values: There should be no geometric distortion to the phantom outline. All the contrast discs should be visible. The resolution depends on the display line standard. For 1024 lines this should be at least 2Lp mm^{-1} with up to 5Lp mm^{-1} visible with higher resolution displays.

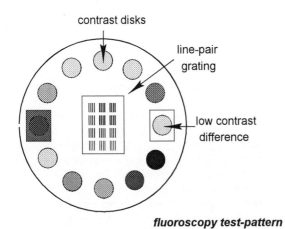

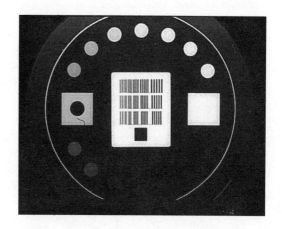

fluoroscopy test-pattern

Figure 23.17 Diagram of a fluorography test object and a radiograph of the test object from a digital fluorography machine showing the low contrast discs.

Table 23.9 Mesh size conversion

Lines per inch	Lines per mm
16	0.6
20	0.8
25	1.0
30	1.2
35	1.4
40	1.6
50	2.0
60	2.4

The visible mesh sizes should be:

- Under/overhead fluoroscopy: 35-40
- Cine and Mobile C-arm: 40-50

Frequency: Twice a year.

23.6.2 Automatic exposure (brightness) control

The AEC ensures that a given output signal from the image intensifier or the video camera is maintained regardless of absorber (patient) thickness. This is achieved by varying tube kV and/or mA (see Chapter 10). The level of control is measured as air-kerma rate $\mu Gy\ s^{-1}$ at the surface of the image intensifier. The method measures minimum and maximum dose rates and working dose rates with equivalent absorber in place.

Test 2. Image intensifier entrance dose

An ion chamber for these measurements should not have large metal connectors or cable which would produce significant x-ray attenuation. Changing (zooming) the image intensifier field requires an increase in entrance dose rate. A change from 18 to 13cm requires a dose increase of $18^2/13^2$ or approximately ×2. The general set up is shown in Fig.23.18(a).

Equipment:

- Large area pancake detector capable of recording very low dose rates ($10\mu R\ s^{-1}$ or ~90nGy).
- Copper discs 0.5mm thickness

Method: Move the image intensifier at least 70cm from the tube focus. If possible the grid should be removed from the x-ray beam. Place the copper sheet on the x-ray tube. Place the ion chamber as near to the image intensifier face as possible and collect dose rate while depressing the screening button.

Since the air-kerma rate is very low for selected frame rates it is necessary to sum over several frames and calculate an average dose per frame exposed.

Limiting value: Within the range 430 to 1740nGy per frame for single film and serial fluorography (screening) and 87 to 348nGy per frame for cine-fluorography. The dose rate will increase with decreasing field size (zoom setting) unless an automatic iris is operating.

Frequency of test: Twice yearly

Test 3. *Maximum output dose rate*

To ensure that the x-ray output is sufficient for the largest patient. If the maximum value is low then image quality will be poor and the image intensifier, or video chain, wrongly suspected.

Equipment:

- Radiation meter with fluoroscopy ion chamber
- 2mm lead-sheet
- plastic or wooden support blocks

Method: Figure 23.18(b) sketches the general set up. Place the chamber in the center of the field (confirm this by screening and placing in center of display). Set to automatic exposure. Set kVp and mA to maximum (i.e. 100kV at 6.5mA). Support the lead-sheet above the ion chamber using blocks. This protects the image intensifier. Expose for several seconds so that AEC stabilizes and record dose rate as mR (μGy) min^{-1}.

Limiting value   The maximum exposure level should not exceed 50mGy (5R) min^{-1} with modern equipment.   If the field size can be changed then the patient dose rate increases as the inverse ratio of the square of the areas in order to maintain the same brightness.

Modern digital fluorography equipment is extremely sensitive and typically gives values between 1.5 and 2mR (15-20μGy) min^{-1} at a setting of 73kVp and 1-2mA

Frequency of test: Yearly

Test 4. *Patient entrance dose*

Improved radiation protection is achieved by reducing the total radiation output from the fluoroscopy machine. Unlike conventional film radiography where a single exposure is made the patient undergoes continuous radiation exposure (often several minutes) the image being viewed on a video monitor.   Owing to the sensitivity of the fluoroscopy system the dose level is kept low (70-100kVp at 4mA).

It is desirable to measure the total dose received by the patient during a complete examination.   This can be achieved by fitting a large area (15×15cm) transmission ionization chamber to the aperture of the x-ray housing and connecting it to a continuously recording radiation dosimeter (dose-area-product or Diamentor™).   The read-out is given as total radiation received as a dose area product in Gy cm^{-2}. Continuous monitoring will reveal excessively long procedures that perhaps can be fore-shortened.

The lowest possible working level should be known and kept as a reference to monitor future performance of the machine. This test should be carried out twice yearly or after maintenance. Table 23.2 gives the conversion factors that can be used when working with non-SI units.

Equipment
- Radiation meter
- Body/tissue equivalent material 20cm thick plastic.
- support stand

Method   Support the chamber in the center of the field (confirm this by screening and place in center of display) as close to the image intensifier face as possible (Fig.23.18(c)). Place the absorber over the x-ray tube. Set to automatic exposure and set the kVp and mA

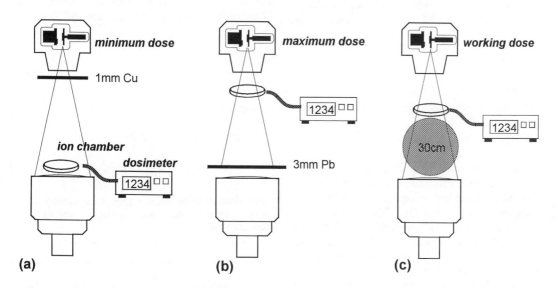

Figure 23.18   Fluoroscopy equipment QC set-up for measuring **(a)** image intensifier entrance exposure rate, **(b)** maximum and **(c)** working exposure rates. The ion chamber is not the same but should be chosen for its suitability.

to routine setting. Expose for several seconds so that AEC stabilizes. Record dose min^{-1}.

Limiting value: The suggested working level for image intensifier input exposure rate, achieving optimum video image quality, is usually quoted by manufacturers to be:

- 12-24µGy (1.2 to 2.4mR) min^{-1} or
- 0.2-0.4µGy (20µR-40µR) s^{-1}

The level of the automatic control should be set to no more than 1µGy s^{-1} (100µR) for a 23cm image intensifier field size.

  Table 23.10 lists absolute maximum radiation levels for patient entrance dose rates, that have been acceptable, but current machines can operate at much lower dose rates as mentioned above.

Frequency of test: This should be performed on a yearly basis or when the machine has received any servicing.

Table 23.10 Entrance exposure to the patient.

Parameter	Dose mGy (R) min^{-1}
Maximum output	100 (~10R)
High Level Control	
Can exceed	440 (~50R)
Suggested upper level	200 (~24R)
Recommended	100 (~12R)
Routine exposure	
20cm phantom	10-20 (~1-2R)
Maximum	44 (~5R)
Image intensifier input	0.2µGy s^{-1}
Unacceptable	>1µGy s^{-1}

Test 5. Flare or veiling glare

The image contrast deteriorates with aging of the electronics, particularly the image intensifier – video chain.

Equipment:

- 4cm lead square 2mm thick
- Storage oscilloscope capable of recording video bandwidths
- BNC T-piece

Method: The lead strip is placed in contact with the image intensifier face. The oscilloscope shares the video signal line at the back of the display (using the BNC T-piece). A screening program is selected (70-100kVp at 4mA) and measurements made of V_{min} and V_{max}. (Fig.23.19). The contrast can be calculated from the formula:

$$Contrast = 1 - \frac{V_{min}}{V_{max}} \times 100\% \qquad (23.4)$$

Where V_{min} is the video voltage behind the lead-strip and V_{max} the maximum white signal as identified in the diagram.

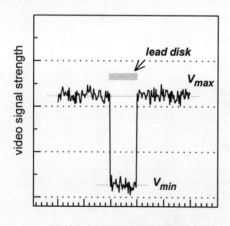

X axis on intensifier face

Figure 23.19 Video waveform showing the maximum signal: V_{max} and the signal peak behind the lead-strip: V_{min}.

Limiting value: The contrast is measured as detailed in the boxed example (Box 23.2). Current machines should achieve >80%.

Box 23.2

Contrast calculation

Example $\quad V_{max} = 0.7$volts
$\qquad\qquad V_{min} = 0.3$ volts

Contrast $= 1 - \dfrac{0.3}{0.7} = $ **57%**

A modern system should give a 70 to 80% contrast figure so this result would be unacceptable

---

23.7 COMPUTED TOMOGRAPHY (CT).

The CT machine should come complete with phantom test objects for measuring machine performance. A computer program handles the data and displays the results (Box 23.3). A full program test takes some time, should only be performed by a skilled engineer and is only necessary when the machine is giving trouble or during scheduled maintenance. Field uniformity over a 30cm diameter is a good general indication of machine performance.

Test 1. Field of view uniformity

The uniformity of CT number values throughout the entire field is a comprehensive check of the CT machine performance. Figure 23.20 shows the placement of regions of interest as recommended by the manufacturer. Detector or mechanical faults are immediately visible as irregularities.

Equipment:

- 30cm water filled phantom as supplied by the manufacturer

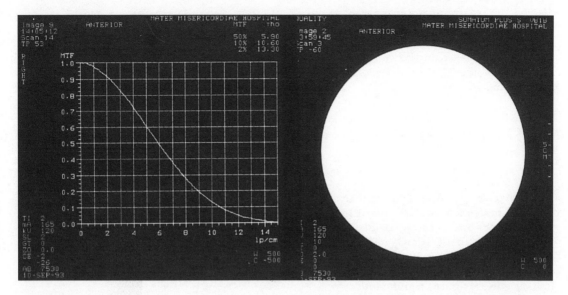

Figure 23.20   Quality control for uniformity and modulation transfer function taken from the manufacturer's test kit.

Method :   Locate water phantom exactly in the center of the gantry aperture. Choose 2mm slice thickness and a standard scan time (2-5 seconds). The procedure is usually governed by the quality control program supplied with the machine. Cross field uniformity is obtained by selecting five regions of interest; each ROI is approximately 5% of the total 20cm area of the phantom.

Limiting value: Variation between the 5 regions of interest over the phantom field should not be more than 2HU (CT numbers) and is typically <1HU. Increasing standard deviation values or variation between ROI's is apparent as an x-ray tube becomes older. A replacement is usually necessary after 60 to 80,000 slices when the coefficient of variation figure becomes large.

Beam hardening problems will show up as vignetting (variation in image density). Detector malfunction will show visible ring artifact formation. Pixel noise is also measured with a large area ROI on the 20cm phantom and the standard deviation should be within 10HU. The noise is influenced by slice dose D and slice thickness n as:

$$pixel\ noise \propto \sqrt{\frac{1}{D \times n}} \qquad (23.5)$$

so either a higher slice dose or thickness will improve the noise figure.

Test 2. Integrated CT dose index. (CTDI)

Surface dose to the patient can be measured by fixing small TLD badges to the area in question. A depth dose can be obtained by integrating the radiation exposure of a series of slices (e.g. spiral acquisition). The line of integrated dose must be of sufficient length to include primary and scattered radiation.

Equipment:
- A long ion chamber probe at least 10cm with a volume of 3.2cm³
- A CT dose phantom (PMMA or acrylic) diameter 16 and 32cm containing a central hole and several at the periphery 1cm from the edge.

Method: The manufacturer's instructions usually describe the FDA procedure conforming to their regulation (21 CFR 120.33). The probe is placed in the central or peripheral hole and the CT Dose Index calculated for 14 slices as:

$$CTDI = \frac{1}{T} \int_{-7T}^{+7T} D_z \, dz \qquad (23.6)$$

Limiting value: The expected dose from current machines would be 12mGy per 100mAs for 8mm slices using the 16cm phantom and about 10mGy per 100mAs for 1mm slices using the 32mm phantom. Scan protocols, trading dose for image quality, will influence these figures significantly.

Frequency: Yearly or when a new scanning procedure is required. A complete dossier of slice doses should be kept for the most common scan procedures, particularly pediatric protocols.

Box 23.3

Monthly quality check sheet

Slice thickness

Desired	10.00	5.00	3.00	2.00	1.00
Actual	9.85	4.99	3.05	2.05	1.23

Water value

	1	2	3
Water	0.18	0.20	-0.34
SD	11.32	10.80	19.51
kV	124.60	135.80	80.00

Homogeneity (differences ΔD from central ROI)

Location	3	6	9	12
ΔD1	-0.40	-0.37	-0.39	-0.51
DD2	-0.27	-0.32	-0.28	-0.35
DD3	-0.29	-0.34	-0.38	-0.36

MTF

Lp/cm at	50%	10%	2%
	5.90	10.60	13.30

23.7.1   Secondary tests

Resolution   The manufacturer's MTF phantom should be used and should show ~1Lp mm^{-1} at 2% MTF using standard filters. Values at 10 and 50% are often quoted (Fig.23.20).

Low contrast   A modern machine will show 0.4% contrast on a 3mm object (10mm slice, 2 second scan time).

Slice thickness   This is the FWHM measured with an aluminum plate at 30° in the center of the field of view. The slice profile should be ±2% of the stated value.

23.8 NUCLEAR MEDICINE

Planar imaging: Basic imaging systems should have regular measurements made of:

- Intrinsic uniformity
- Intrinsic resolution
- Intrinsic spatial linearity

Acceptance testing would involve measurement of:

- collimator resolution
- collimator sensitivity
- dead time

Tomographic (SPECT) systems require additional regular measurements:

- tomographic resolution
- tomographic uniformity
- center of rotation

Acceptance testing for SPECT machines would require checking of attenuation correction software

23.8.1   Routine QC: Planar

Test 1. Intrinsic uniformity

The sensitivity of the gamma camera should be uniform over the entire field.   Intrinsic uniformity is measured without the collimator.

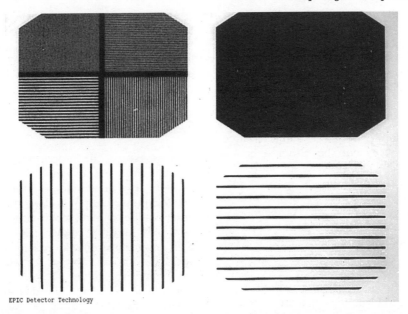

EPIC Detector Technology

Figure 23.21 (a) Gamma camera uniformity measured with the manufacturer's program (b) resolution image using a bar phantom

Equipment
- Point source ^{99m}Tc or ^{57}Cobalt 200kBq (5μCi)

Method: Remove collimator and carefully position the camera head horizontally. Place the point source 2-3 meters from the center of the camera. Collect 5 million counts using a 64×64 word matrix for planar imaging (Fig.23.21(a)). Use the QC program that is usually incorporated into a nuclear medicine system to estimate non-uniformity. If the camera has more than one head then the time taken to collect the set count should be noted for each head.

Limiting value: With the correction circuits intrinsic uniformity should be <±2%. Sensitivity between heads measured as counts per unit time should be ≤±5%

Test 2. Intrinsic resolution

This method describes a visual appraisal of resolution. If a NEMA specified line source is available then an MTF measurement can be performed which will give a quantitative measure of resolution.

Equipment:

- Source of ^{99m}Tc in an elution vial 20MBq in 1ml.
- Resolution bar or pie-sector (Anger) phantom.

Method: The collimator is removed and the detector head placed facing upwards. The resolution phantom is placed carefully on the surface of the crystal. The ^{99m}Tc source is suspended about 2m centrally above the camera. Between 1 and 2 million counts are collected and a film image taken for reference.

Limiting value: The 3 or 4mm holes or bars should be distinguishable. The linearity of the bars should also be noted (Fig.23.21(b)).

Frequency of test: This should be performed about once every 2 months in order to detect any degradation.

23.8.2 Acceptance test: Planar

The following collimator tests need only be carried out when new equipment is purchased. These tests should be performed for each collimator type.

Test 3. Extrinsic (collimator) uniformity.

System uniformity requires a disc source of radioactivity. This can be either a commercially available solid uniform source (^{57}Co) or made up as a liquid source in a flat plastic container. The latter has problems with uniform mixing; both have problems with radiation safety since surface dose rates can be as high as 900μSv h^{-1}.

Equipment:

- Suitable disc source (^{57}Co or ^{99m}Tc) having a uniform activity distribution better than 1%.
- Collimator of choice

Method: The manufacturer's computer software should contain a QC program which will give integral and differential uniformity measurements for both the useful and central field of view (UFOV and CFOV).

Limiting value: The system uniformity should comply with the manufacturer's specification. This is usually better than ±5% for the useful field of view measurements.

Test 4. Extrinsic (collimator) resolution.

The procedure described for the intrinsic resolution can be adopted using a bar phantom. The pie-sector hole phantom will give moiré interference patterns with the collimator holes and should only be used for intrinsic resolution assessment.

Spatial resolution (MTF): Using a carefully collimated line source and collecting LSF image data on a 256×256 matrix the MTF program listed at the end of this Chapter can be used for giving a comprehensive measure of intrinsic and extrinsic resolution. The precise FWHM can also be obtained from the LSF.

Limiting value: The manufacturer's collimator specifications should be consulted. A typical figure for a general purpose collimator is currently 10mm FWHM without scatter material.

Test 5. System sensitivity.

This measures the proportion of gamma radiation captured by the collimated gamma camera. It is measured as counts per second per MBq (cps MBq^{-1}) and will depend on collimator type; a high sensitivity collimator will obviously have a higher sensitivity than a high resolution collimator. The gamma energy spectrum and window width will also significantly alter the value.

A plastic container of sides 100mm or diameter 150mm should be used for good collimator coverage, overcoming any collimator non-uniformity. The source activity should be carefully measured in a dose calibrator. If a solid flood source is accurately calibrated, used in the system uniformity, then this could be used.

Equipment:

- A known activity giving a count rate of about 10,000 cps. A suitable activity would be about 50 to 200MBq.
- Collimator of choice.

Method: Note the recorded count rate for several measurements. The sensitivity can be measured as a relative value M/A where M is the measured count rate and A is the total activity (allowing for 2π geometry losses) or the activity can be represented in absolute terms of cps MBq^{-1}.

Limiting value: Most ^{99m}Tc collimators fall into the following sensitivity ranges:

- High resolution: 50 to 145 cps MBq^{-1}
- General purpose: 100 to 200 cps MBq^{-1}
- High sensitivity: 180 to 300 cps MBq^{-1}

For non-SI measurements the conversion factor is cpm per μCi ×0.45 = cps per MBq.

Test 6. Temporal resolution (dead time)

Gamma camera count rates respond linearly with activity until an activity is reached that produces 'pulse pile-up' and so individual events are missed. Current cameras have a very high counting capability for high activity clinical studies such as dynamic blood pool imaging and cardiac studies. The response shown in Fig.23.22 shows the reference linear response bordered by lines marking 10% and 20% losses.

Equipment
A series of 5 elution vials containing exactly equal activities of ^{99m}Tc so that all 5 vials will exceed the camera count rate.

Method: Place the sources in sequence about 2m from the uncollimated camera face; first one then two then three etc. noting the count rate each time. The first vial should be treated as the reference true count rate. Repeat the exercise with the camera in high count mode.

Limiting value: Standard settings should give at least 100,000 cps for a 20% loss. High count mode increases this to ~ 200,000 cps.

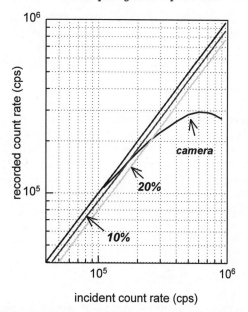

Figure 23.22   The count rate response of a gamma camera showing the 10% and 20% thresholds for count loss. This camera can capture 200,000 cps for a 20% loss. Its maximum count rate is 300,000 cps.

Energy resolution   during uniformity measurements the photo-peak should be measured

Table 23.11   Summary of nuclear medicine gamma camera parameters

	Parameter	Central field of view	Useful field of view
Intrinsic			
Uniformity			
	(integral)	±2.5%	+4.5%
	(differential)	±2.0%	+3.0%
Resolution	(spatial)		
	FWHM	4.0mm	4.1mm
	FWTM	7.6mm	7.8mm
Resolution	(energy)		10.6%
Spatial linearity			
	(absolute)	≤0.35mm	≤0.7mm
	(differential)	≤0.15mm	≤0.2mm
Count rate			
	(20% loss)		85kcps
	(maximum)		135kcps
Extrinsic			
System sensitivity (GP collimator)			286 cpm µCi^{-1} (128cps MBq^{-1})

from the camera display and a FWHM figure obtained. An acceptable value would be about 12% or less.

A list of standard requirements for a current gamma camera specification is given in Tab.23.11.

Dose calibrator accuracy The ion chamber used for measuring the activity of labeled radiopharmaceuticals should be checked for accuracy (twice yearly). A 10MBq (250µCi) calibrated ^{137}Cs source is used as a reference. Adjustments are made as described in the manufacturer's handbook.

23.8.3 Routine QC: SPECT

Gamma camera testing basically measure the intrinsic and extrinsic performance of the system.

Intrinsic tests are carried out with the collimator removed. It is essential to take great care with these tests since the exposed scintillation crystal is only protected by a thin aluminum cover; it is very easily damaged. Extrinsic tests include the camera collimator and should be repeated for all collimators that are used with the camera. Measuring the camera's uniformity of response gives a good general appraisal of camera sensitivity over the field of view and between heads, if more than one camera head is fitted for SPECT work.

Test 7. SPECT uniformity

A non-uniformity value of 5% may go undetected in planar imaging but this degree of non-uniformity will cause significant distortion in a tomographic slice. The commercially available sources (^{57}Co disc or rectangular sources) must have an overall non uniformity of ⩽1% for checking camera uniformity for SPECT work.

Equipment:
- 400kBq (10mCi) ^{57}Co or ^{99m}Tc point source
- 20mCi uniform disc source or the SPECT phantom (<1% non-uniformity)

Method: A point source at >2m will serve as a uniform source of activity for intrinsic measurements. A high count density is required, at least 30 million counts collected on a 64×64 word matrix. This will give 7324 counts per pixel yielding a noise figure of $\sqrt{7324} = 85$ or 1%. The source should have an activity of at least 400-800MBq (10 to 20mCi) so that a system uniformity matrix (with collimator) can be collected in a reasonable time.

Limiting value: The manufacturer's literature should be consulted but no visible non-uniformity should be present

Frequency: This is not likely to change for the same camera collimator combination but should be checked on a monthly basis.

Test 8. SPECT Resolution and contrast

A special SPECT phantom containing different diameter objects (Jaszczak Phantom, Nuclear Associates) should be used for assessing overall image quality including uniformity, resolution, contrast and ring artifact presence (Fig.23.23(a)).

Equipment:
- Jaszczak phantom filled with recommended activity concentration of ^{99m}Tc eluate.

Method: The same radius of view should be used (15 or 20cm) each time and reference images kept for comparative purposes.

Limiting value: Most of the resolution objects should be visible but these will vary with collimator type. A representative sample series of images should be collected

Frequency: A SPECT phantom lends itself to a weekly routine check of SPECT performance.

Test 9. SPECT: Center of Rotation COR

The calibration needs to be performed for each collimator. COR errors lead to degraded

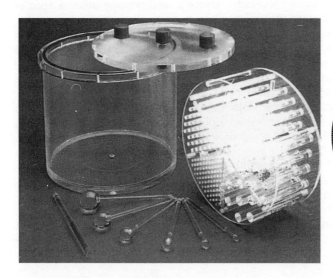
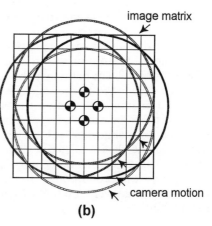

Figure 23.23 **(a)** Jaszczak phantom commonly used for SPECT quality control measurements for uniformity and resolution showing simplified internal construction. **(b)** The consequences of a center of rotation misalignment with reference to the image matrix.

spatial resolution and reconstruction artifacts (Fig.23.23(b)).

Method: Each manufacturer has their own method for performing this most important calibration and their instructions should be followed carefully. Some require multiple point sources placed in a plastic frame, others require just a single source, either a point or line source.

Equipment: See manufacturer's instructions.

Limiting value: The minimum error should be <0.5 pixel if image artifacts are to be avoided.

Frequency: Each week.

23.8.4 Radiopharmaceutical QC

Although licensed manufacturers of radio-pharmaceuticals take every measure to produce the highest quality of chemical and biological product for use in nuclear medicine

there are still very valid reasons for the purchaser to carry out routine tests to ensure that labeling these compounds is as near 100% effective as possible.

When reconstituted, radiopharmaceuticals have a limited useful life of only a few hours before breakdown products are produced. These products have no organ specificity and so increase background activity adding to image noise and producing indistinct organ/tissue scintigrams (e.g. bone, liver, lung images) or poorly resolved time/activity curves in dynamic studies (e.g. renograms).

The principle of radiopharmaceutical quality control using chromatography was introduced in Chapter 16, Section 16.1.4. Chromatography separates components of a mixture (labeled radio-pharmaceutical in this case) on an adsorbent surface exploiting differences in affinities for the absorbent material (stationary phase) and a developing solvent (mobile phase). A sample of the reconstituted compound (radiopharmaceutical) is placed at the bottom (origin) of a strip of adsorbent material (Gelman silica gel paper or Whatman No.1 filter paper).

The dried preparation is then placed in a small tank of solvent (saline, acetone or methyl ethyl ketone: MEK). The substance's retardation factor (*Rf* value) determines separation of its constituent parts. The *Rf* value is the ratio of distance moved by substance to distance moved by solvent so if the substance moves with the solvent boundary the ratio will be 1:1, the substance having an *Rf* = 1. If the substance remains at the origin the ratio will be 0:1 and the substance *Rf* = 0. Table 23.12 shows that by using different solvents components can be distinguished. This can be used for estimating the percentage labeling efficiency and the proportion of free pertechnetate and breakdown products (hydrolysed pertechnetate).

Table 23.12 The *Rf* values of some radiopharmaceuticals and breakdown products.

Solvent	Substance	Rf value
Normal saline (0.9%)		
	DTPA	1.0
	MDP/HDP	1.0
	$^{99m}TcO_4$ (free)	1.0
	colloids	0.0
	MAA	0.0
	$^{99m}TcO_4$ (hydrolysed)	0.0
Acetone or MEK		
	$^{99m}TcO_4$ (free)	1.0
	DTPA	0.0
	DMSA	0.0
	MDP/HDP	0.0

Test 1. Chromatography (qualitative)

Equipment:

- 10cm strip of Gelman silica gel paper marked in soft pencil at source (1cm from end) and marker pen 1cm from end of strip.
- acetone or MEK solvent

Method: Using a 2ml syringe place a spot of the radiopharmaceutical on 1cm pencil line. Place in capped cylinder holding 0.5cm solvent. When the solvent marks its presence by smudging the marker pen remove and dry the strip. Fix a high resolution collimator on the camera and protect with a plastic sheet. Place the Gelman strip across the center of the field of view. Collect 100,000 count image and draw profile through the center of the source.

Limiting value: Visually inspect the profile for activity at the finish.

Frequency: This is a quick method for confirming breakdown of radiopharmaceutical and the presence of activity away from the source

Test 2. Chromatography (quantitative)

Equipment:

- a series of small (5cm) Gelman strips marked with a pencil 1cm at one end. The halfway point is similarly marked. Commercially available as Tec-Control™ (Atomic Products Corp.)
- saline solution
- acetone or MEK
- small universal capped plastic containers

Method: Using the same procedure as in Test 1 spot the radiopharmaceutical at the start on two of the small strips. Place one in a universal container containing acetone and the other containing saline. At the end of the run remove strips, cut in half. The acetone halves are designated 1(source) and 2 (finish). The saline halves are designated 3 (source) and 4 (finish). They are placed in separate small tubes and the activity measured using a well counter. Figure 23.24(a) and (b) outlines the procedure. From the counts the following calculations can be made:

$$free\ ^{99m}TcO_4 = \frac{counts\ from\ 2}{counts\ from\ 1 + counts\ from\ 2}$$

$$hydrolysed\ ^{99m}Tc = \frac{counts\ from\ 3}{counts\ from\ 3 + counts\ from\ 4}$$

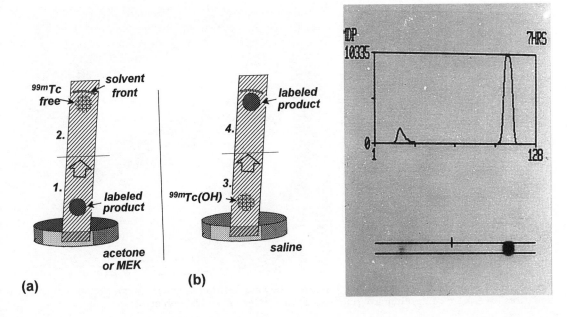

Figure 23.24 **(a)** Radiochromatogram obtained from a gamma camera image profile **(b)** Quantitative estimation of free and hydrolysed pertechnetate.

labeling efficiency = 100 − *(free + hydrolysed)*

Limiting value: Impurity levels should be less than 5% and the labeling efficiency should be better than 90%.

Frequency: The quantitative procedure should be routinely applied to all reconstituted radiopharmaceuticals.

23.9   ULTRASOUND

There are several quick methods for testing the integrity of transducer arrays. Individual transducer operation can be quickly checked by running a thick wire (metal paper clip or thin screwdriver) along the transducer face, watching the individual spikes that should be visible. However more involved image quality tests should be performed for linear arrays,

sector and annular arrays which give a measure of:

- Image resolution
- Beam registration
- Dead zone
- Dynamic range
- Swept gain (time gain compensation)

It is also possible to measure geometric distortion and caliper accuracy. Damage to the transducer and poor performance by both receiver and transmitter can affect sensitivity and dynamic range. Registration is compromised in multi-element probes by changes in the amplifier and transmitter electronics.

Resolution, likewise, can be degraded by faults in the focusing circuits. Caliper calibration alters if velocity/distance computation circuits develop faults. Many of these parameters can be measured with a good ultrasound phantom.

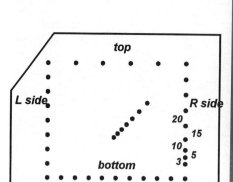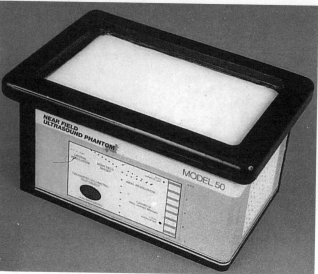

Figure 23.25 **(a)** The AUIM ultrasound phantom showing position of beam registration and resolution wires **(b)** A more comprehensive phantom having differing contrast objects.

23.9.1 The ultrasound phantom

The American Institute of Ultrasound in Medicine (AIUM) has designed a basic phantom consisting of metal wires regularly placed around a plastic container. This can be used for checking registration and resolution. Figure 23.25(a) shows the general design. There are
five sets of wires:

1. Surface wires for dead zone measurement.
2. Side wires for vertical caliper accuracy
3. Bottom wires for horizontal caliper accuracy
4. Axial resolution is measured using the middle diagonal wires.
5. Lateral resolution can be judged from the side wire width.

A typical ultrasound phantom is filled with tissue equivalent material having an attenuation of between 0.5–0.7dB cm^{-1} MHz^{-1}. Speed of sound is approximately 1540m s^{-1}. It holds various test objects. Some phantom models contain calibrated reflectors of various dB values for gray scale calibration (Fig.23.25(b)). The top of the phantom should be a soft membrane so all shapes of transducer can be tested.

23.9.2 Power output

Ultrasound transducers show a wide range of output power levels. This range is indicated in Fig.23.26(a). In some instances the levels shown by Doppler devices exceed the maximum power limits indicated by the dotted line in the graph of Fig.23.26(b). The recommended maximum intensities from the Food and Drug Administration (FDA) are given in Tab.23.13. Power outputs from a transducer can be measured by:

- calorimetry
- radiation balance
- hydrophone

None of these are suited to routine quality control tests. An estimate of power output is displayed on the ultrasound image.

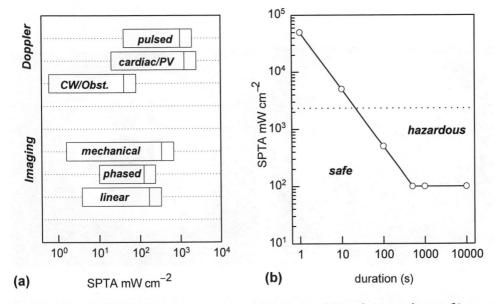

Figure 23.26 **(a)** Power output from current imaging and Doppler transducers **(b)** power output limits that should not be exceeded. The dotted line indicates the maximum output from Doppler transducers.

Table 23.13 FDA recommended limits.

Application	I_{SPTA} in water (mW cm^{-2})
Cardiac	730
Peripheral vascular	1500
Ophthalmic	68
Other imaging *	180

* including fetal, breast, abdomen and pediatric investigations.

23.10 MAGNETIC RESONANCE IMAGING

The MRI machine requires periodic checking in order to ensure optimum image quality. The parameters that are recommended for a quality assurance program are:

- Resonance frequency,
- SNR,
- Field uniformity,
- RF pulse shape,
- Environmental RF noise,
- Gradient pulse shape,

There are basic tests that should include detail and contrast resolution, image and field uniformity, spatial distortion and slice thickness. Commercial phantoms exist for subjective measurement of image quality. These are cylindrical plastic blocks (Fig.23.27) with various inserts that register different T1/T2 times when imaged. The simulation solutions mimic adipose tissue, liver and white/gray matter for normal and abnormal brain. This enables an estimation of machine stability, evaluation of different imaging pulse sequences, T1/T2 weighting as well as comparison of machine to machine differences.

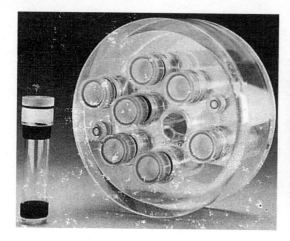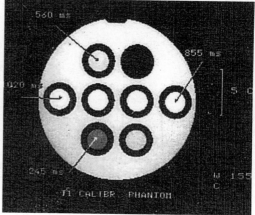

Figure 23.27 An MRI phantom with inserts giving different T1 and T2 times with resulting image (courtesy Computerized Imaging Reference Systems Inc. CIRS).

FURTHER READING:

Quality Control in Diagnostic Imaging. Joel Gray et al.   University Park Press.

The Institute of Physical Sciences in Medicine (UK). Various reports on quality control in radiology, nuclear medicine and ultrasound.

American Association of Physicists in Medicine: Performance specifications and equipment requirements for mammography. AAPM 1991

A Categorical Course in Physics. Technical Aspects of Breast Imaging. Radiological Society of North America Syllabus 1993.

A Review of Mammographic Equipment and its Performance. National Health Service Breast Screening Programme (UK). Publication 24 1992. Also Publications 33 and 35 (1995)

European Guidelines for Quality Assurance in Mammography Screening. Office for official publications of the European Communities. 2nd Edition 1996.

Performance measurements of scintillation cameras. National Electrical manufacturers Association (NEMA) NU-1-1994

KEYWORDS

accuracy - The close of a measured value m of a quantity to the true value t. Measured as the percentage of the difference $(m-t)\times100/t$.

baseline value - the value that is used for comparison when no absolute limiting value is present.

deviation -   the percentage difference between measured value and prescribed value.
entrance surface air kerma (ESAK) - air

kerma value measured in free air, without back-scatter, at a point in a plane corresponding to the entrance surface of a specified object e.g. patient skin or phantom.

entrance surface dose - absorbed dose in air including back-scatter, measured at a point on the entrance surface of the patient or phantom.

net optical density - optical density excluding base and fog.

optical density (OD) - the logarithm of the ratio of the intensity of the incident light on a film to the light intensity transmitted by the film. OD differences are measured in a line perpendicular to the tube axis to avoid influences from the heel effect.

PMMA - the plastic material used for manufacturing tissue equivalent absorbers. Also known as Lucite, Perspex or Plexiglas.

precision - the variation in observed values.

reproducibility - the reliability measured as the precision.

typical value - the common or expected value found in most facilities.

DERIVED UNITS

	Quantity	Units	Dimensions
1.	Area	square metre	m^2
2.	Volume	cubic metre	m^3
3.	Force	newton (N)	$kg\ m\ s^{-2}$
4.	Pressure	pascal (P)	$N\ m^{-2}$
5.	Weight	mass × gravity	kg
6.	Density	mass / volume	$kg\ m^{-3}$
7.	Work/Energy	joule (J)	$J = kg\ m^2\ s^{-2}$
8.	Speed	metre second	$m\ s^{-1}$
9.	Linear Velocity	metre second	$m\ s^{-1}$
10.	Angular Velocity	radian second	$rad\ s^{-1}$
11.	Acceleration	metre/ second/second	$m\ s^{-2}$
12.	Momentum	mass / velocity	$kg\ m\ s^{-1}$
13.	Electric Charge	coulomb (C)	$A\ s$
14.	Power	watt (W)	$J\ s^{-1}$
15.	Voltage	volt (V)	$J\ C^{-1}$
16.	Resistance	ohm (W)	$V\ A^{-1}$
17.	Thermal Conductivity	watt/m/kelvin	$W\ m^{-1}\ K^{-1}$
18.	Frequency	herz (Hz)	s^{-1}
19.	Radioactivity	becquerel (Bq)	s^{-1}
20.	Luminous Flux	lumen (lm)	$cd\ sr$
21.	Illuminance	lux (lux)	$lm\ m^{-2}$
22.	Magnetic Flux	weber (Wb)	$V\ s$
23.	Magnetic Flux Density	tesla (T)	$Wb\ m^{-2}$
24.	Radiation Dose	gray (Gy)	$J\ kg^{-1}$

Supplementary Units (dimensionless)

Plane Angle	Radian	rad
Solid Angle	Steradian	sr

ELEMENTS IMPORTANT IN RADIOLOGY

Atomic Number	Element	Symbol	Atomic Mass	Density kg m-3	Mt. Pnt. K	K-Edge keV
1	Hydrogen	H	1.0	0.089	14.0	
2	Helium	He	4.0	0.166	0.95	
4	Berylium	Be	9.0	1800	1550	
6	Carbon	C	12.0	2300	>3800	
7	Nitrogen	N	14.0	1.165	63	
8	Oxygen	O	16.0	1.33	55	
13	Aluminium	Al	26.9	2700	933	1.6
22	Titanium	Ti	47.9	4500	1948	5.0
28	Nickel	Ni	58.7	8900	1726	8.3
29	Copper	Cu	63.5	8950	1356	9.0
39	Yttrium	Y	88.9	4600	1768	17.0
40	Zirconium	Zr	91	6500	2125	18.0
42	Molybdenum	Mo	95.9	10200	2880	20.0
45	Rhodium	Rh	102.9	12500	2230	23.2
46	Palladium	Pd	106.7	11900	1825	24.3
47	Silver	Ag	107.8	10500	1234	25.5
50	Tin	Sn	118.7	7310	505	29.1
53	Iodine	I	126.9	4950	387	33.2
56	Barium	Ba	137.3	3500	1000	37.4
57	Lanthanum	La	138.9	6200	1190	39.0
64	Gadolinium	Gd	157.2	8000	1585	50.2
68	Erbium	Er	167.2	9000	1770	57.4
69	Thulium	Tm	168.9	9300	1818	59.3
73	Tantalum	Ta	180.9	16600	3269	67.5
74	Tungsten	W	183.8	19300	3650	69.5
75	Rhenium	Re	186.2	20800	3450	71.6
78	Platinum	Pt	195.0	21450	2042	78.4
79	Gold	Au	197.0	19400	1336	80.7
82	Lead	Pb	207.2	11340	600	88.0
92	Uranium	U	238.0	19000	1405	115.6

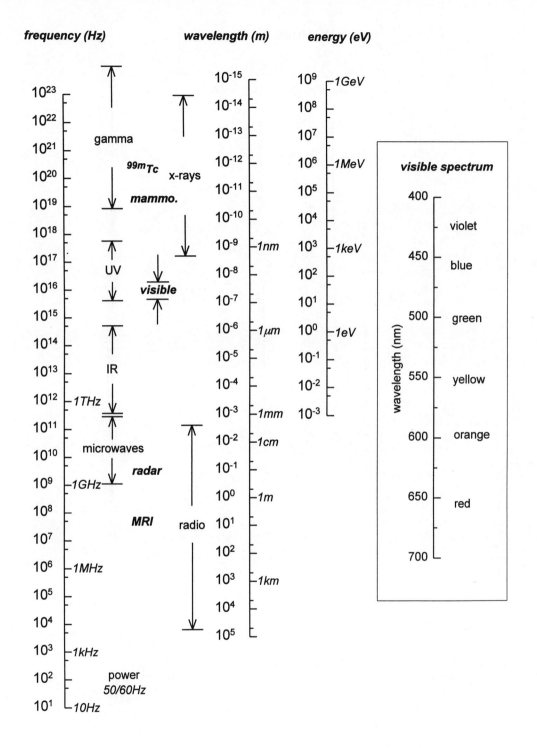

scales for dB

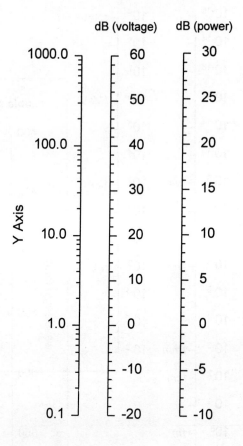

Program for Computing the Modulation Transfer Function from a set of Line Source values obtained as a digital profile

Program Introduction:

- The resolution of each channel in the profile should be known (line 13).
- The basic frequency unit (lines mm^{-1} or lines cm^{-1}) is requested (line 14).
- The values for a set number of profile channels is then fed in (line 12 and 20).

The program is written in easily understood BASIC which can be translated into other formats.

Design explanation:

D(J) increments the basic frequency unit Δx = Q. The following equations have been introduced in Chapters 1 and 8.
The fundamental MTF equation :

$$\text{MTF} = \frac{\sum_{j=1}^{m} L(x_j, z) * (\cos 2\pi\, vx_j - i\, \sin 2\pi vx_j)}{\sum_{j=1}^{m} L(x_j, z)}$$

Where $L(x_j, z)$ are m individual line spread function values (B(K)) at a sampling interval Δx and v is the cycles/cm computed (A).

In the program this breaks down as:

$$\sum_{R}^{1} \cos(2\pi * D * A) = C \qquad \text{(line 28)}$$

$$\sum_{R}^{1} \sin(2\pi * D * A) = E \qquad \text{(line 29)}$$

$$I = \frac{C}{\sum(B(K))} \qquad \text{(line 34)}$$

$$M = \frac{E}{\sum(B(K))} \qquad \text{(line 34)}$$

$$L = \sqrt{I^2 * M^2} = \text{MTF} \qquad \text{(line 36)}$$

```
10.  REM ## DATA INPUT ##
11.  DIM   Y(50), D(50), B(50)
12.  INPUT "Number of LSF Values"; R
13.  INPUT "Resolution as Measured"; A
14.  INPUT "Frequency Unit"; Q
15.  REM ## CALCULATION OF MTF ##
16.     FOR J=0 TO R
17.     D(J)=Q*J
18.     NEXT J
19.     FOR K=1 TO R
20.     INPUT "LSF value"; B(K)
21.     NEXT K
22.  REM ## Initialization for sine and cosine
        summation ##
23.  P2=2*3.14159265
24.     FOR J = 0 TO R
25.     C = 0: E = 0: H = 0
26.  REM ## K loop is the MTF calculation ##
27.     FOR K=1 TO R
28.     C = C+B(K)*COS(P2*D(J)*A*(K-1))
29.     E = E+B(K)*SIN(P2*D(J)*A*(K-1))
30.  REM ## Sine and cosine summation ##
31.     H = H+B(K)
32.     NEXT K
33.  REM ## Sigma cosine and sine divided by
        Sigma (L(X) ##
34.     I = C/H:   M=E/H
35.  REM ## Calculate modulus of real and
        imaginary parts ##
36.     L = SQR(I*I+M*M)
37.     Y(J) = L
38.  REM ## Print out      J, B(J), D(J), L
39.     NEXT J
40.  END
```

Example input from gamma camera line source:

No. (J)	Data (B(J))	Frequency (D(J))	MTF value (L)
0	0	0.00	1
1	64	0.15	0.985
2	576	0.30	0.942
3	2704	0.45	0.874
4	6344	0.60	0.786
5	12768	0.75	0.686
6	17112	0.90	0.579
7	17880	1.05	0.473
8	13808	1.20	0.372
9	8336	1.35	0.282
10	3376	1.50	0.206
11	912	1.65	0.144
12	152	1.80	0.0963

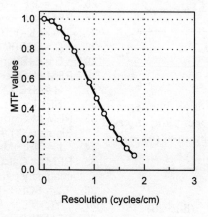

Precise measurement of Half Value Layer by computation

Introduction
Narrow beam geometry must be used in order to reduce scatter interference
Two absorber thicknesses are required and three measurements:

1. The incident radiation dose without absorber (Y_0 mR)
2. The radiation dose after X_1mm filtration (Y_1 mR)
3. The radiation dose after X_2mm filtration (Y_2 mR)

The formula uses natural logarithms to compute the half-value-layer:

$$HVL = \frac{X_1 \times Ln\left[\dfrac{2 \times Y_2}{Y_o}\right] - X_2 \times Ln\left[\dfrac{2 \times Y_1}{Y_o}\right]}{Ln\left[\dfrac{Y_2}{Y_1}\right]}$$

BASIC PROGRAM.

```
5      REM**** HALF VALUE LAYER COMPUTATION ********
10     INPUT " Maximum Dose reading without absorber:";Y0
20     INPUT " First Absorber thickness (mm):";X1
30     INPUT " Dose obtained for first thickness:";Y1
40     INPUT " Second Absorber thickness (mm):";X2
50     INPUT " Dose obtained for second thickness:";Y2
60     TOP = X1*LOG(2*Y2/Y0)-X2*LOG(2*Y1/Y0)
70     BOT = LOG(Y2/Y1)
100    PRINT USING " Half Value Layer : #.### mm.";TOP/BOT
200    STOP:END
```

EXAMPLE: (from Mammography Unit)

Maximum Dose reading without absorber:	718
First Absorber thickness (mm):	0.1
Dose obtained for first thickness:	583
Second Absorber thickness (mm):	0.5
Dose obtained for second thickness:	275
Half Value Layer:	0.358 mm

QC 1. - X-RAY

kVp with Digital Meter (*Meter make and model if more than one* **)**
Recommended limits: ±5kV from nominal value

Date:						
60 kVp 200mAs						

Date:						
70 kVp 100mAs						

Date:						
80 kVp 40mAs						

Date:						
90 kVp 20mAs						

Date:						
100 kVp 20mAs						

Date:						
120 kVp 10mAs						

Half Value Layer: (at 80kVp measured). *Recommended value 2.6 - 3.0mm Al*

Date:						
0mm						
1mm						
2mm						
4mm						
HVL:						

Focal Spot Size (RMI Model #112)   *Recommended value: 0.6 - 0.8mm*

46cm (18") FFD, 60kVp at 2mAs 4/3 magnification (4cm between markers)

Date:						
Smallest Group						
Focal Spot						

Beam Alignment (RMI Model #162)   *Recommended limit: <4%*

FFD 1metre (40") 60kVp at 2mAs

Date					
Inner Circle 1%					
Inner Circle Edge 2%					
Outer Circle 4%					
Comments					

Light Diaphragm (combined with above tool)   *Recommended limit: <1cm*

60kVp 2mAs Align with copper edge in X and Y axes

Date:						
±1cm (1%)	X Y	X Y	X Y	X Y	X Y	X Y
±≥2cm (>2%)	X Y	X Y	X Y	X Y	X Y	X Y
Comments						

Tube current and timer

mR/mAs Linearity at 20mAs   DATE:

20mAs mA seconds	60kVp	70kVp	80kVp	100kVp
100 0.2				
200 0.1				
400 0.05				
800 0.025				
Mean mR÷mAs				
Linearity				

(Repeat this Section for different dates)

QC 2. - FILM PROCESSOR

Month: *June 199-*

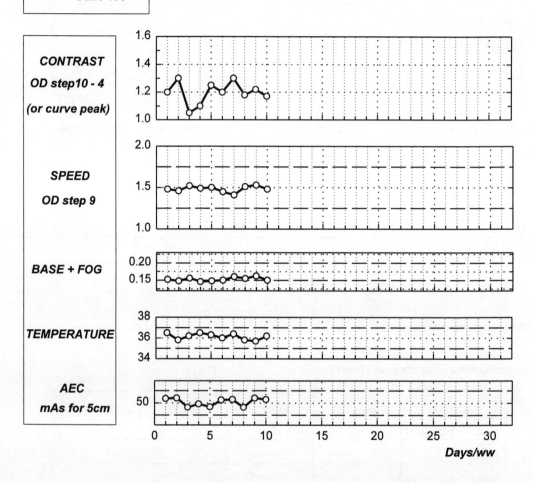

CONTRAST
OD step10 - 4
(or curve peak)

SPEED
OD step 9

BASE + FOG

TEMPERATURE

AEC
mAs for 5cm

Days/ww

QC 3. - MAMMOGRAPHY (Basic)

<table>
<tr><td>HEADER BLOCK HERE</td></tr>
</table>

kVp WITH MAMMOGRAPHY DIGITAL METER (Model ....)

Date:						
30kVp 100mAs						

RESOLUTION LOW CONTRAST (Model of breast phantom...   )

Low Contrast Discs Visible (27KvP)

Date:						
Discs visible						

Resolution (Line pairs visible 27KvP)

Date:						
lp/mm just visible						

Entrance dose, AEC consistency and Mean Glanular Dose

Date:						
Air kerma for 1.0 OD						
mAs for 5cm phantom						
MGD (TLD group)						

HALF VALUE LAYER (ALUMINIUM):   AT 30KVP (MEASURED)

Date:						
0mm						
0.1mm						
0.2mm						
0.5mm						
HVL:						

QC 4. - FLUOROSCOPY

```
┌─────────────────────────────────┐
│     BASIC TEST FOR SIX VISITS    │
│       HEADER BLOCK HERE          │
└─────────────────────────────────┘
```

RADIATION DOSE RATE (Meter make and model if more than one)

Maximum Dose-Rate

(2mm lead-plate protecting image intensifier)

Date:						
80kVp at.................mA						

Working Dose-Rate

(20 cm tissue equivalent material over image intensifier)

Date:						
80kVp at.................mA						

Entrance Dose-Rate

(1mm copper plate on x-ray tube)

Date:						
80kVp at.................mA						

(Repeated for film and cine output)

RESOLUTION LOW CONTRAST PHANTOM
(identify test object type here with photograph or diagram if possible)

Contrast Discs Visible (70kVp + 1mm Cu disc)   Field Size:

Date:						
Discs Visible						

Resolution (Line pairs visible @ 50kVp)   Field Size:

Date:						
lp/mm just visible						

Image Distortion (test object circular outline)   Field Size:

Date:						
XY						

Index

Absorbed dose (Gy) 124, 526, 528
- energy 124
absorption 107
- coefficient 116, 147
- edge 116
- image formation 123
- photoelectric 113
- tissue 212
absorber 108
- thickness 109, 165
acoustic (also see sound)
- impedance 419
- lens 438, 441
- limits 461
- modulus of elasticity 418
- pressure 417
active shielding 529
activity
- concentration 354
- residual 355
- specific 354
ADC (analog to digital converter)
afterglow
ALARA 567
ALARP 567
algebraic reconstruction, xx
ALI 567
aliasing 275, 337, 457
alpha detection
- decay 347
- particle 346, 347, 526
alternating current 56
- power 58
aluminum 108
- absorption 112
- filters 77
ampere 53
amplifier 51, 139, 441, 442

amplitude resolution 443
angiography 105
angstrom units 29
angular momentum 482
annular array 452
anode 70
- angle 70, 321
- bearing 102
- compound 101
- construction 70, 211
- cooling 86, 87
- current 82, 83
- design 101, 103
- heat capacity 87
- rotating 70
- rotor 71
- size 70
- stationary 70
- stress relieved 71
- track 70, 73
antenna 472
aperture 437, 440, 448
apodization 431
array 436
- curved linear 450
- focusing 451
- linear sequence 446, 449
- phased 450
- phased linear 447
- processor 270, 276, 491
- sector scan 450
artifact
- cupping 322
- image 338, 453
- misregistration 307
ASCII 256
atomic number 49
- structure 47
- weight 49

attenuation 8
- coefficient 107, 109
- correction 403
- errors 454
Auger electron 114, 115
automatic
- brightness control 246
- dose control 99
- exposure control 220, 225, 246
- gain control 244
auto-transformer 90

Background
- counts 27
- radiation 537
- scatter 190, 404
back
- projection 330
- scatter 123, 141
band
- conduction 49
- forbidden 49
- valence 49
bandwidth 10/13
- pixel (MRI) 499
- receiver 516
- RF 515
- ultrasound 430
barium
- contrast material 113, 115, 118
- plaster 566
barrier 561
- materials 566
- primary 564
- secondary 565
base-fog 155, 584
Bateman equation 360
baud 265
beam
- collimation 75
- energy 76
- filtration 77
- hardening 322, 339
- homogeneity 79
- lobes 453
- quality 78
- quantity 80
beat frequency 454
becquerel 29, 128
beryllium filter 211

beta 346, 349
- decay 348
- dose 349, 527
- particles 348, 527
- penetration 353
biased 61
biological
- damage 531
- half-life 345
biplane system 249
bit 255
Bloch equation 470, 482
blood
- flow 513
- flow void 513
- velocity 454, 456
blurring (see unsharpness)
bone 121
- dose 126
bremsstrahlung 65, 351
Bucky factor (see grid factor)
byte 255

C-arm fluoroscopy 248, 249
cabling 55
- high tension 96
calculus 11
- differential 11
- integral 13
calcium tungstate 162
carbon- fiber 216, 555
cardiac imaging 398
carrier free 358, 359
cassette
- design 166
- mammography 216, 167
- spot film 242
cathode 69
- assembly 68
cavitation 459
$CaWO_4$ (see calcium tungstate)
Celsius 34
center of rotation 401
cesium iodide detector 118
- iodide (image intensifier) 230, 233
characteristic
- curve 155
- modulation
- radiation 76, 115
charge coupled device (CCD) 239

chemical shift 473, 522
chest radiography 184, 222, 223
chromatography (QC) 604
cine-fluorography 242, 249
coherent scattering 117
coefficient of variation 26
coils 486
 - detector 495
 - gradient 492
 - phased array 496
 - shim 490
 - surface 495
collimator
 - CT 319, 320
 - gamma camera 377, 378, 379
 - x-ray 74
color velocity imaging 458
Compton
 - scatter 117, 122
 - scatter image formation 223, 225
computed tomography 317
 - CT number 327
 - CTDI 340
 - dose 340
 - dose index 657
 - fan beam 317, 320
 - field of view 656
 - image 336
 - room plan 562
 - sampling 319
 - slice 658
 - slip ring 326
 - spiral 324
 - system 335
 - x-ray tube 320
computer 254
 - bulk storage 256
 - code 265
 - communication 265
 - CPU 256
 - languages 265
 - memory 259
 - operating systems 265
 - processor 257
 - radiology 270
 - word 255
conductor 55
conservation of momentum 30
constraint 550
continuous spectrum 54, 55, 66
contrast 186, 517

 - agents (MRI) 506
 - agents (x-ray) 123
 - detail diagram 201, 338
 - gradient 157
 - improvement 195
 - objective 188
 - resolution 440
 - radiographic 188
 - ratio 237
 - subject 122, 187, 222, 225, 217
 - subjective 188
 - to noise ratio 518
 - visual 176
control
 - high voltage 96
 - feedback 244
 - filament 97
 - starter 97
conversion efficiency 46
conversion factor 233
 - units 234
convolution 331
 - kernel 331
correlation 28
 - time 476
cosine 18
 - law 364
coulomb 51
 - field 52
counting
 - loss134, 373
 - statistics 24
coupling gel 427
cryogen (cryostat) 488
curie 345
current
 - alternating 56
 - eddy 493
 - tube (see x-ray tube)
CW Doppler 455
cyclotron 356, 408

DAC (digital to analog converter) 279
data
 - analysis 25
 - compression 289
 - retrieval 262
 - sampling 274, 338
 - spread 22
 - storage 327

- transfer 257
dead time 134, 146
decibel 7, 420
decimal place 2
demodulation 444
densitometer 160
density 32
    - optical 156, 186, 188
    - material 109, 165
derivative 13
detective quantum efficiency (DQE) 202, 234
detector 142, 323
    - $2\pi/\ 4\pi$ 16, 144
    - efficiency 16, 143, 145, 146
    - gas 129, 131
    - Geiger 130, 133
    - image 177
    - ionization 130
    - luminescent 134, 138
    - non uniformity 339
    - probe 366
    - proportional 130, 132
    - scintillation 139
    - semiconductor 142
    - sensitivity 142, 147
    - surface 177
    - xenon 131
deterministic response 535
developer 151, 159, 586
diaphragm 74
DICOM 271
digital image 274
    - compression 289
    - contrast 280, 281
    - filtering 282, 284
    - matrix 276, 302
    - noise 279
    - processing 281, 302
    - resolution 280, 292, 301
    - storage systems 288
    - storage 278, 279, 301
digital fluorography 299
    - specifications 300
digital subtraction angiography (DSA)
    - cardiac 311
    - data processing 302
    - dose 312
    - dual energy 309
    - filter 303
    - imaging chain 296

    - motion correction 303, 307
    - programs 308
    - road mapping 309
    - specifications 297
    - system 304
digital to analog converter (see DAC)
diode 61
dipole moment 467
direct
    - current 53
    - direct current generator 55
disk 261
    - floppy 261
    - hard (Winchester) 261
    - optical 263
dispersion 434
display 264
    - analog 370
    - digital
    - stations 291
    - video 180
distortion
    - image intensifier 239, 592
distribution 22
    - binomial 10
    - normal (Gaussian) 22
    - Poisson 21
    - sample 19
divergence (ultrasound) 432
DNA 532
dominant region 245
doping 135
Doppler 451
    - continuous wave (CW) 455
    - effect
    - pulsed 455
    - shift 455
    - signal 455
    - transducer 455
dose 124, 388
    - absorbed 124, 526, 528
    - accumulated 545
    - area product 100, 559
    - deep 545
    - diagnostic 556
    - effective (EDE) 527
    - entrance 218, 226, 529, 531, 577, 593, 594
    - exit 531
    - genetic 536

- genetically significant 537
- limit 550
- maximum 594
- mean glandular 219, 591
- monitor 132, 367, 552, 547
- nuclear medicine 559
- patient 217, 226, 391
- permissible 550, 551
- population 535, 546
- rates 130, 563
- shallow 545
- somatic 536
- whole body 544
dose calibrator 131, 365
dosimeter
- electronic 548
- film 548
- personal 141, 548
- thermoluminescent 141
DREF 541
duplex imaging 457
dynamic
- aperture 451
- focusing 451
- range 189, 328, 443, 450

ECG triggering 399, 518
echo
- time 415
- planar imaging (EPI) 524
eddy current 493
efficiency
- conversion 136, 146
- detector 143
- extrinsic 143, 146
- geometric 143, 144
- intrinsic 143, 145
elastic scattering 117
electric
- charge 51
- current 53
- field 52
electromagnetic
- induction 50
- radiation 46, 49
- spectrum 43
- units 44
electrostatics 51
electron 47
- beam 65

- binding energy 47
- bound 113
- capture 351
- density 118
- emission 60
- focusing 68, 69
- free 113
- momentum 47
- orbit 47
- recoil 117, 118
- source 68, 356
- spin 47
- traps 134-7
- volt 53
elution 350
emission 60
- temperature 70
empirical 10
emulsion (film) 149
energy 31
- effective 76
- equivalent 79
- fluence 80
- flux density 80
- kinetic 31
- potential 31
- radiation 43
- resolution 147
- spectrum 139
- transformation 31
- wavelength 43
enhancement 454
environment (radiation) 551
equilibrium
- transient /secular 361
equivalent
- committed dose 530
- dose 544
- energy 79
error
- quantization 275
escape peak 141
excitation 48
expansion 37
exponent 4
exponential 7
- attenuation 108
- decay 9, 13
- e 6
- growth 14
- law 9

- log(n) 6
exposure 124
    - control 99
    - film (see film)
    - pediatric 391
    - rate 528
    - time 98
extrapolation 10

Falling load 85
fan beam 320
Faraday shield 491, 524
fast Fourier Transform (FFT) 333
fat suppression 511
f-factor 125
fiber optic 45
field
    - central 374
    - gradient 491
    - of view (FOV) 374
    - strength 487
    - useful 374
filament 68
    - circuit 97
    - current 81
    - heating 69
    - supply 68
    - transformer 97
file server 268
film
    - changer 242
    - characteristic 154, 155, 584
    - contrast 158, 178
    - density 7
    - detector 129
    - dynamic range 157
    - emulsion 149
    - gamma 157
    - image 178
    - latitude 156, 157
    - monochromatic (blue) 153
    - orthochromatic 153
    - panchromatic 154
    - processor 585
    - resolution 151
    - response 151, 159
    - sensitivity 158
    - sensitometry 154, 159, 161
    - speed 158, 178
    - storage 153
    - structure 152
    - type 153
film screens 138, 152, 154, 164, 585
film processor 159, 168
    - developer temperature 586
    - refreshment rate 596
filter
    - Butterworth 283, 405
    - CT 322
    - fixed 75
    - Hamming 405
    - Hanning 405
    - high pass 282, 283
    - inherent 75, 77
    - K-edge 78
    - low pass 282
    - mammography 213
    - ramp 405
    - reconstruction 405
    - spatial 282, 303
    - temporal 284, 303, 304
    - total 578
FISP 510
fission 359
fixer 137
FLASH 511
flicker 181, 182
flip angle 469, 509
floating point 3
flow
    - rephasing 514
fluence (x-ray) 80
    - energy 80
    - photon 80
fluorescence 134, 136, 161
fluoroscopy
    - AEC 592
    - cine 242, 249
    - contrast 592
    - controls 244
    - conversion factor 233
    - entrance dose 593
    - exposure level 245
    - image chain 243
    - maximum dose 594
    - over table (couch) 247
    - patient dose 252, 594
    - resolution 592
    - staff dose 250
    - system 237
    - under table (couch) 248

- veiling glare 596
- x-ray tube 238
flux (x-ray) 80
- density 80
- energy 81
- photon 80
focal spot 72, 211
- dual 73
- effective 72
- geometry 72-3
- image resolution 302
- real 72
- size 224, 321
focusing
- coils 239-240
- dynamic 448
- electrode 230
- multiple 448
- transducer 441
focused
- cathode 69
- collimator 379
- grid 191-2
force 40
footprint 437
Fourier transform 18, 333
fraction 3
- error 4
frame 249, 278
- rate 448
Fraunhofer zone 431
free induction decay (FID) 470, 475
frequency
- and wavelength 40, 44, 418
- beat 42
- Larmor 470
- precessional 470
- range 43, 415
- relaxation 424
- sound 415
Fresnel zone 431
friction 31
fringe field 488
full-wave rectification 91
full-width
- at-half-maximum (FWHM) 140
- at tenth-maximum (FWTM) 372

Gadolinium
- contrast agent 506

- intensifying screen 163
gain
- minification
- flux 232
gamma camera 368
- dead time 373
- detector 368
- electronics 369
- energy resolution 372
- field of view 374
- resolution 371, 375
- uniformity 374
gamma radiation 352
- spectrum 139
gas laws 33
generator
- constant potential 90
- control 96
- high frequency 93, 214, 326
- performance 94
- power 94, 95
- single phase 91
- switching 96
- three phase 92
Geiger-Müller counter 133
gradient
- coil 492
- echo 479, 509
- field 515
- magnetic 494
- sequence 499
- spoiled 510
grain
- size 149, 151
graphs 9
- linear 9
- logarithmic 10
- non linear 9
- semi log (log/linear) 11
GRASS 508, 510
grating lobes 453
gray (Gy) 124, 528, 543
gray
- scale 207, 415, 448
grid 82, 190
- contrast improvement 195
- design 191
- factor 208
- focused 192
- high kV 224
- lines 193, 208

- mammography 216
- misalignment 196
- moving 193
- ratio 194
- selectivity 196
- septa 192
- specifications 194
grid-controlled x-ray tube 69
GSD 537
gyromagnetic ratio 471

Half
- amplitude 420
- power distance 420
- value-layer (HVL) 8, 79, 110
- wave rectification 91
half-life
- biological 345
- physical 345

hard copy 206, 241
heat 34
- absorption 37
- conduction 34, 35
- convection 36
- latent 35
- loss 88, 101
- radiation 36
- storage capacity 86
- transfer 35
- unit (HU) 4
heel effect 73, 217
histogram equalization 286
homogeneity
- magnetic field 488
Hounsfield Units 327
hybrid subtraction 309

Illuminance 150
image
- analysis 312
- archiving 288
- artifacts 453, 521
- compression 289
- contrast 186, 280, 338, 503
- density 77
- depth 415, 430, 431, 439
- diagnostic 178, 204
- distortion 239, 592
- duplex 457

- filtering 334
- fluoroscopic 228
- formation 123
- lag 244
- magnification 184, 215
- matrix 329, 394
- transmission 290
- noise 188, 234, 279
- planar 394
- processing 281, 332, 441
- quality 182, 197, 225
- reconstruction 330
- resolution 183, 198, 280, 301
- storage 278, 293, 301
- transmission 290
image intensifier 228, 296
- contrast 235
- dose response 235
- field size 238
- input 229
- output 230
- performance 238
- resolution 236
image plate 141, 169
- selenium 172
- x-ray absorption 170
impedance
- acoustic 152
- electrical 57
integer 2
integral (integration)
- definite 14
- infinite 14
integration time 177
intensification factor 164
intensifying screens 138, 154, 161, 164, 165, 179
interface 264
interference
- constructive/destructive 41
- RF 491
interlace 208
internal conversion 353
internet 270
interpolation 16, 281, 287
inverse square law 5, 9, 354
inversion recovery 479, 502
iodine
- K-edge 115
- contrast agent 117
ionization 48

- chamber 131, 133
- current 132
- gas 129
- detectors 130
iris diaphragm 298
I$_{SAPA}$ 461
I$_{SATA}$ 460
isomeric transition 352
isotope 344
- generator352, 362, 363
isotropic 15, 364
I$_{SPPA}$ 461
I$_{SPTA}$ 460
I$_{SPTP}$ 461
iterative reconstruction 330

Joule 30

K- edge 116
- absorption 48, 162
- filters 78, 213
K-electron
- binding energy 48
- capture 351
kelvin 34
kerma 528
kernel 331
kilovoltage (kV)
- effective (kVeff) 76
- equivalent (kVeq) 79
- high 222
- low 210
- maximum 75, 82
- minimum 75
- peak (kVp)
kilowatt
- rating 83
kinetic
- blurring
(see movement unsharpness)
- energy 31, 65

Lanthanum
- intensifying screen 163
Larmor
- equation 471
- frequency 470
- precession 471
laser
-imager 207

- disk 263
last image hold 250
latent
- heat 35
- image 151
latitude (film) 156
layer thickness (tomography) 315-6
lead (Pb)
- absorption 116
- aprons 553
- content (of grid) 192
- density 118
- equivalent 564
- filtration 595
- glass 566
- K-edge 116, 118
- plastic 566
- shielding 564
leakage radiation 583
least significant figure 2
light
- exposure 150
- diaphragm 581
- optics 44
- reflective layer 164
line
- focus principle 72
- pair 177, 281
- spread function (LSF) 199
linear
- absorption coefficient 166
- array 446
- attenuation coefficient 107
- energy transfer 126, 127, 536
- graph 9
- tomography 314
lithium fluoride 137, 548-9
loadability
- batch 104
- long term 84, 86, 104
- short term 83, 104
logarithm 5
- base$_{10}$ 5
- natural 6
logarithmic subtraction 306
longitudinal
- magnetization 478
- relaxation time 469, 474
look-up table (LUT) 284
low frequency drop 236
luminance 175

luminescence 134
- photo-stimulated 170

Magnet 486
- homogeneity 488
- permanent 487
- quenching 488
- resistive 487
- shimming 489
- strength 50, 486, 520
- super-conducting 487
magnetic
- field 515
- flux density 486
- gradients 491
- induction 50
- materials 522
- moment 467
- permeability 484
- plane 468
- shielding 490
- tape 262
magnetic resonance imaging (MRI) 486
- angiography (MRA) 513, 514
- detector coil 495
- fast imaging 508
- functional (fMRI) 507
- image quality 517
- image time 516
- pulse sequence 500
- QC 548
- signal origin 522
- signal to noise 515
- slice selection 517
- spatial encoding 496
- spectroscopy (MRS) 522
- system 486, 519
mains (supply) 56
- cable resistance 55-6, 96
- voltage 59
mammography 167, 210, 211
- AEC 220, 590
- anode 211
- dose 217, 218, 219, 590
- exposure time 588
- film density 589
- focal spot 589
- grids 216
- HVL 588

- image quality 215, 589
- machine design 222
- kVp 587
- output 587
- spectrum 212
- system 221
Marinelli 389
mAs 580
masking
- unsharp 284, 304
- DSA 304, 306
mass 30
- absorption coefficient 119, 127, 147
- attenuation coefficient 111
- scattering coefficient 120
mantissa 2
matrix 276
- size 277
mean 24
median 24
memory 259
- cache 259
- read only 260
- virtual 260
MIRD 389
mode 25
modem 265, 270
modulation transfer function (MTF) 199
modulus of elasticity 418
mole 29
moment of inertia 30
momentum 30
monitoring
- contamination 367
monochromatic light 153
mottle 153
multi
- echo sequence 502
- format camera 206
- image techniques 502
- planar imaging 512
- pulse generator 92, 93
- slice imaging 502
- tasking 266

Near field 431
netware 266
network 267
neutrino 348

neutron 47, 358, 363
newton (N) 30
NMR (see nuclear magnetic resonance)
noise
- quantum 189
- spectrum 201
normalized 5
notation
- conventional 2
- scientific 2
nuclear
- decay 345
- reactor 358
- structure 344
nuclear magnetic resonance (NMR) 467
- signal 468
nuclear medicine imaging
- center of rotation 603
- extrinsic resolution 600
- extrinsic uniformity 600
- intrinsic resolution 599
- intrinsic uniformity 598
- PET 407
- planar imaging 394
- QC 598
- sensitivity 600
- SPECT 399, 602
nucleus 46, 49
number
- complex 4
- irrational 2
- negative 4
- rational 2
Nyquist frequency 275

Ohm 54
oil cooling 74, 86
operating systems 265
optical
- density 7, 154, 156
- disk 263
orthochromic film 151
orbit
- center of rotation 400
- non circular 400
outlier 28
output screen 230

PACS (picture archiving
and communication systems) 287
pair formation 120
paradoxical enhancement 513
parallel hole collimator 378
parametric 27
partial volume 339
particle acceleration 356
pascal 29, 33
patient
- dose reduction 558
- pregnancy 557
- radiation exposure 545
penetration depth (ultrasound) 415, 431,
439
penumbra 184
percentage 4
- change 4
permissible dose 550-51
personal monitor 141, 548
phantom
- fluoroscopy 592
- mammography 589
- SPECT 602
phase
- decoding 444
- diagram 19
- single (supply) 91
- three (supply) 91, 92
phased array 450
phosphor 162, 179
- crystal size 165
- input 230
- pigments 165
- thickness 165
phosphorus (NMR signal) 523
phosphorescence 134, 135, 161
photocathode
- image intensifier 230
- photomultiplier 139
photochemical process 150
photoelectric
- absorption 113
- effect 113
photoelectron 127
- recoil 117, 119
photomultiplier 100, 139

photon 42
- absorption 107
- density 529
- energy 118
- fluence 80
- flux 80
- scattered 107, 127, 165
- transmitted 211
photon interactions
- nuclear 113
- general 107, 121
- atomic 112
- electron 112
- probability 122
photopeak 140
piezoelectricity 426
pipeline principle 327
pixel 276
Planck's constant 44
planar 333
- imaging 394
plaster (barium) 566
plumbicon 239
plutonium 348
p-n junction 61
point spread function (PSF) 197
population response 535
positron 120, 349
- camera 408
- emission tomography (PET) 349, 407
- nuclides 410
- range 408
potassium-40 538
potential energy 31
power 31, 32
- a.c. 58
- loss 55-6
- law 12
- real/apparent 58
- transmission 55-6
precession 466, 468
pregnancy
- patient 557
- staff 551
presaturation 513
pressure 33
primary
- radiation 190
- barrier 560
program

- computer *11.5*
- QC 569
propagation velocity 416
proton
- bombardment 359
- charge 47
- mass 47
pulse
- bandwidth 429, 440
- duration 438
- duty factor 439, 459
- height analyzer 370
- length 429
- pile up 146
- power 460
- repetition frequency 438
- repetition period 439
- RF 494
- sequence 500, 509, 510
- shape (ultrasound) (MRI) 428, 494
- six/twelve 92
- timing 438
- width 140
pulsed Doppler 455

Quadrature detector 495
quality control 570
- AEC 579
- beam 574, 581
- conventional 577
- equipment 576
- exposure time 573, 580
- film 574
- focal spot 574, 578
- HVL 578
- kilovoltage 572, 577
- output 580
- radiation 582
quality factor 530
quantiles 23
quantitative analysis 594
quantum
- noise 189, 234
- sink 232
quartiles 23
quench 488

Rad (radiation absorbed dose) 124-5
radian 17

radiation 528
- (machine) 563
- area 551, 552
- cellular response 534
- characteristic 66, 76, 114, 115
- detector 128
- energy 43, 64, 125, 346
- gamma 64
- leakage 582
- man made 537, 538
- monitoring 547
- monitors 572
- natural 537, 538
- organ response 534
- quality 79, 110
- quantity 80
- room plan 561
- safety committee 560
- scattering 117
- weighting factor 543
- workers 549
- x-ray 64
radio nuclide
- clinical 362
- dosimetry 387, 389
- impurities 361
- production 356
- transport 393
- waste 392
radio-pharmacy 392
radio-pharmaceuticals 383, 386
- QC 387, 603
rating 83, 224
- curve 84-5
- electrical 83
- thermal 85
ratio 5
rayl 419
Rayleigh scattering 117
ray sum 318
readout gradient
real time (ultrasound) 448
receiver 416
- coil 516
- gain 442-3
- bandwidth 516
reciprocals 5
reciprocity loss 214
recoil electron 117-18
reconstruction 329

rectification 59
rectifier 91
reflection 421
- multiple path 453
- non specular 421
- specular 421
refraction 38, 423
refractive
- angle 39
- index 39
regions of interest (ROI) 396
regression 28
relative biological effectiveness (RBE) 530
relaxation time 473
- longitudinal 469, 474
- transverse 470, 475
- spin/spin 471
rem (radiation equivalent man) 546
repetition time
resistance
- electrical 54
- sound 419
resolution
- axial 432, 439
- energy 140, 147, 372
- lateral 432, 440
- spatial 179
- temporal
- visual 177
resolving power
resonant frequency 430
RF
- pulse 494, 515
- shield 4911, 524
ripple 92, 93, 96
risk
- comparison 539
- radiation 539
- calculation 539
- coefficient 540
- cumulative 541
roentgen (R) 528
ROC (receiver operating characteristic) 202, 205
ROI (see region of interest)
root-mean-square (RMS) 58
rule
- 10 or 28 day 558
run-length encoding 290

saturation
- current 82
- recovery 478

scan
- time (frame) 448
- lines 436, 437

scattered radiation 117

scatter 178
- absorption 123
- angle 120
- coefficient
- Compton 117
- elastic (coherent) 117
- image formation 123
- mammography 216
- SPECT 404
- to primary ratio 190

screen-film
- efficiency 162
- thickness 165
- unsharpness 183, 186

section (see slice)

sector scan 445

secular equilibrium 361

semiconductor 61

semi-log plot 11

sensitivity
- detector 147
- and specificity 203
- visual 175

sensitometer 159

Shannon sampling theorem 275

shaped filters (CT)

shielding
- cyclotron 358
- generator 388
- machine 552
- materials 560
- protective 552, 564
- room 560
- syringe 388, 559
- tube 74

SI symbols 29

sievert 530
- man 556

signal
- averaging 516
- coils 493

- compression 423, 444
- demodulation 444
- digitization 444
- dynamic range 442
- NMR 468
- post-processing 332
- preprocessing 332, 442
- to-noise ratio (SNR) 188, 515

silver
- halide 149
- recovery 169

sinc pulse 494

sine 17

single tank generator 94

slice thickness 440
- CT 598
- linear tomography 315
- MRI 517
- SPECT 402

Snell's law 39

sound 38
- absorption 424
- amplitude 39, 418
- diffraction 423
- frequency 415, 417, 424
- intensity 39, 418, 419
- power 418, 419
- propagation 416
- reflection 38, 421
- refraction 38, 423
- transmission 423, 427
- velocity 38, 427
- wavelength 426

space charge 69, 212

spatial
- average (SA) 459
- encoding (MRI) 496
- peak (SP) 459
- pulse length (SPL) 429
- resolution 179

specific
- gamma ray constant 125, 366
- heat 34

speckle 422, 453

specifications
- ion chambers 572
- kVp meters 573
- nuclear medicine 601

- sensitometry 575
spectrum
        - continuous 65
        - electromagnetic 43
        - gamma 140
        - x-ray
spin
        - density 472
        - echo 478, 509
standard
        - deviation 23
        - error 25
steradian 15
stochastic response 534
STP 34
swept gain 422

T1 480, 503, 505
T2 480, 481, 505
TR 504
TE 504
tangent 17
technetium
        - generator 383, 393
        - oxidation states 385
teleradiology 291
temperature 34
temporal
        - filter 284
        - peak (TP) 459
tesla 486
thermal
        - capacity 34, 35
        - conductivity 35
        - noise 515
        - transfer 35
thermionic emission 60
thermoluminescence 134, 137
three dimensional reconstruction 512
three-phase supply 56-7, 93
threshold dose 535
time
        - access 261-2
        - activity curve 398
        - average power (TA) 459
        - gain compensation 443
        - of flight 8
        - seek 262
        - transfer 261, 279, 301

tissue
        - equivalent 137
        - weighting factor 544
tomographic plane 315
tomography 411
        - CT 317
        - linear 314
        - PET 407
        - ray sum 318
        - SPECT
total reflection (fiber optic) 45
transducer (also see array)
        - annular 452
        - focusing 448
        - crystal thickness 426
        - Doppler 455
        - real time 437
        - ultrasound 446
transformer 56, 90
        - filament 97
        - high tension 94
        - high frequency 57, 93
transient equilibrium 361
translation-rotation system 317
translation table 285
transmission 423
        - coefficient
        - layer 426
        - pulse 494
transmitter 416, 486
transport (radioactivity) 394
transverse
        - magnetization 468
        - relaxation time 470

Ultrasound
        - bandwidth 430, 439-40
        - bioeffects 462
        - Doppler shift 455
        - duty factor 439
        - echo 445
        - field 432
        - frame rate 436
        - image 441, 453
        - image depth 431, 439
        - phantom 606
        - power output 606
        - pulse 429, 431, 438
        - pulse timing 438

- resolution 429, 432, 439
- resonance 430
- safety levels 463, 607
- transducer (see also array and transducer) 425, 426, 437, 446
umbra 184
- penumbra 44
Unix 266
unsharpness 215
- geometric 183, 184
- movement 183, 186
- radiographic 183, 186
uranium series 346

valency 47
veiling glare 231, 237
velocity
- angular 19
- blood 454
- maximum 456
vidicon 239
video
- bandwidth 181, 240
- camera 296
- disc 241
- film formatter 206
- image 180, 239
- recording 241
- resolution 240
- standards 181, 298
- waveform 180
volume 14
- 2π and 4π 15, 16
- element (VOXEL) 499, 516
- sample 366
volt (voltage) 52
- high 60
- low 61

water
- absorption curve
- equivalent material
- electron density
watt
wave 2.7
- damping and resonance 40
- front 437
- harmonic motion 40

- interference 41
- length 119
- longitudinal
- periodic 18
- radio 46
- transverse
waveform
- analysis 18
Weber-Fechner law
Wehnelt electrode
well counter 365
Wiener spectrum
window 286, 303
- CT 333
- x-ray 75

X-ray
- beam
- detector
- energy
- equipment 102
- exposure
- generator 571
- intensity 66, 223
- quality 576
- quantity 576
- sensitometry 155
- spectrum 66, 75
- transmission 110
x-ray tube 67, 101
- current 77, 82, 83
- enclosure 74, 101
- filter 75, 77
- lifetime 69
- load 71, 103
- power 83
- rating 83
- specifications 105
- starter 97
- voltage 81, 223
- window 75
- workload 103

zonography 316